Skills for
Midwifery Practice

Skills for
Midwifery Practice

Fourth Edition

Ruth Johnson BA (Hons) RGN RM

Clinical Midwife
Formerly Senior Lecturer Midwifery,
University of Hertfordshire and Supervisor of Midwives

Wendy Taylor BSc (Hons) MSc RN RM

Formerly Senior Lecturer Midwifery,
University of Hertfordshire,
now clinical midwifery educator in Whangarei, New Zealand

ELSEVIER   Edinburgh   London   New York   Oxford   Philadelphia   St Louis   Sydney   Toronto   2016

ELSEVIER

First edition 2000
Second edition 2005
Third edition 2011

ISBN 978-0-7020-6187-5

British Library Cataloguing in Publication Data
A catalogue record for this book is available from the British Library

Library of Congress Cataloging in Publication Data
A catalog record for this book is available from the Library of Congress

Notices
Knowledge and best practice in this field are constantly changing. As new research and experience broaden our understanding, changes in research methods, professional practices, or medical treatment may become necessary.

Practitioners and researchers must always rely on their own experience and knowledge in evaluating and using any information, methods, compounds, or experiments described herein. In using such information or methods they should be mindful of their own safety and the safety of others, including parties for whom they have a professional responsibility.

With respect to any drug or pharmaceutical products identified, readers are advised to check the most current information provided (i) on procedures featured or (ii) by the manufacturer of each product to be administered, to verify the recommended dose or formula, the method and duration of administration, and contraindications. It is the responsibility of practitioners, relying on their own experience and knowledge of their patients, to make diagnoses, to determine dosages and the best treatment for each individual patient, and to take all appropriate safety precautions.

To the fullest extent of the law, neither the Publisher nor the authors, contributors, or editors, assume any liability for any injury and/or damage to persons or property as a matter of products liability, negligence or otherwise, or from any use or operation of any methods, products, instructions, or ideas contained in the material herein.

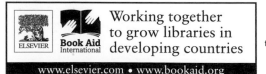
Printed in China

Contents

Contents

Preface

Welcome to the fourth edition of this text, we hope that you enjoy it and find it informative for your practice as a midwife. On each occasion when we rewrite this book, we are surprised at just how much has changed and how much new material has been published. This is encouraging, as we all strive to achieve the best possible care for women, babies and their families. And keep reading, some parts of this text will be superseded in the years to come, new findings will advance midwifery practice yet further and, we trust, will see mothers world-wide healthy and happy in their roles with healthy babies.

As in previous editions, we acknowledge the contribution of all midwives, whatever their gender. However, purely for the purposes of clarity this text considers midwives to be female and babies to be male. We are also aware that there are many more skills that midwives utilise than are featured here. Some of them are implied, e.g. communication, rather than featured. There are frequent encouragements to 'gain informed consent'; this is a standardised way of noting the significance of good communication that allows the woman/parents to make decisions following a full, open and honest conveying of the facts for their consideration.

Student midwives will be able to undertake many of the skills detailed in this text, but with the overseeing and guidance of qualified midwives. This is particularly the case for the countersigning of records and for actions such as 'Document the findings and act accordingly'. In taking action with regard to a particular response, it is the midwife who carries the responsibility and so acts according to knowledge, experience and local and national protocols.

Best wishes to you in your practice,

Ruth Bowen & Wendy Taylor

Acknowledgements

The authors gratefully acknowledge the unstinting support of family and friends, namely (for Ruth Bowen): Robbie, Hannah, Daniel, Jean & Harold, Wendy Taylor; (for Wendy Taylor): Ian, Helen, Ann & John, Ruth Bowen. We are also sincerely grateful for the professional expertise and kind assistance from: Dr Stephen Rowley, Clinical Director, ANTT; Colette Palin, Infant Feeding Lead, Mid Cheshire Hospitals NHS Foundation Trust; Liz Hemmingway B.Pharm, MRPharmS, Women & Children's Divisional Pharmacist, Mid Cheshire Hospitals NHS Foundation Trust, Melinda Jordan, Resuscitation Officer, Whangarei Hospital; and Library staff at the JET Library, Mid Cheshire Hospitals NHS Foundation Trust. This edition is dedicated to mothers, who make our personal and professional lives so special.

Chapter | 1 |

Principles of abdominal examination: during pregnancy and labour

LEARNING OUTCOMES

Having read this chapter, the reader should be able to:

- discuss the indications for abdominal examination in pregnancy and labour
- discuss the different components of an abdominal examination, indicating the nature of the information sought and the rationale for it
- describe the ways in which the fetal heart can be auscultated
- explain the indications for using a CTG, how it is applied and how to interpret the tracing
- describe the criteria used to identify normal, non-reassuring and abnormal CTG tracings
- describe how uterine contractions are palpated in labour, why this is undertaken and the significance of the findings
- explain the midwife's role and responsibilities in relation to each of these aspects of care.

Abdominal examination is a skill that is used to assess fetal growth during pregnancy, to determine the presentation, position and lie as the pregnancy progresses towards term and at the onset of labour, and to auscultate the fetal heart sounds. Palpation of contractions during labour also involves abdominal palpation. This chapter considers the skills of abdominal examination during pregnancy and labour, focusing on how and why this is undertaken and the significance of the information obtained. The different ways of assessing the fetal heart rate will be discussed and related to the significance of cardiotocograph (CTG) interpretation.

ANTENATAL ABDOMINAL EXAMINATION

Traditionally midwives undertook an abdominal examination at every antenatal visit to assess fetal growth, the presentation, lie, and position of the fetus and to auscultate the fetal heart; however, this is no longer current practice within the UK. NICE (2008) recommend fetal growth is assessed by measuring the symphysis–fundal height at each antenatal appointment from 24 weeks' gestation but advise the presentation does not need to be assessed until 36 weeks' gestation or later. This is the point where the presentation may affect the birth plan; e.g. a breech presentation at 28 weeks is not significant, but at 36 weeks enables the woman to consider whether she would like to have an external cephalic version attempted at 37 weeks' gestation.

NICE (2008) further suggest assessment of presentation should not be offered routinely before 36 weeks' gestation because it can be inaccurate and uncomfortable. Some women may want to know more about which way round the baby is and the midwife can undertake this earlier but needs to discuss the significance of doing so at an earlier gestation than recommended and the possibility of the information changing as the pregnancy moves towards term. Certainly when the woman presents in labour, the lie, position, and presentation should be determined as they can affect the course of labour.

Auscultation of the fetal heart at each antenatal visit is no longer recommended by NICE (2008) as they advise it has no predictive value. A discussion on fetal movements may provide more information on fetal wellbeing than listening to the fetal heart rate for 1 minute. Many women, though, will want to hear the heart rate as they find this reassuring and if requested by the woman, the midwife should auscultate the fetal heart with a device that enables the woman to hear the sounds. Regular auscultation of the fetal heart rate is required during labour.

To summarize, the recommended components for abdominal examination during pregnancy (NICE 2008) are:

- measuring and recording of symphysis–fundal height from 24 weeks' gestation (RCOG 2013)
- assessment of fetal presentation at and after 36 weeks.

It is recognized that the skill of abdominal examination will improve with both knowledge and experience and while the current recommendations for undertaking this in pregnancy are limited, the authors recognize the need to maintain the skill (for the times when it is much needed) or risk losing it!

Indications for abdominal examination

- At each antenatal assessment from 24 weeks of pregnancy, adapted according to gestation.
- Prior to auscultation of the fetal heart and use of CTG equipment.
- Before a vaginal examination.
- Throughout labour.

Contraindications

As the uterus can be stimulated when this examination is performed, it should be undertaken cautiously when there is:

- placental abruption
- preterm labour.

ABDOMINAL EXAMINATION: PRINCIPLES

This examination is not undertaken in isolation but involves consideration of the woman and how she is looking and feeling, and what is revealed through discussion. For example if the woman describes experiencing indigestion, breathlessness, and the baby pushing under her ribs, the midwife may wonder if the fetus is in a breech presentation.

The procedure should be explained to the woman, particularly that there may be some discomfort associated with it and the rationale for undertaking the procedure, so that her informed consent is obtained. The examination should begin with an exploration of the woman's perception of the growth and movement of her baby as this is a two-way sharing of information (Blee & Dietsch 2012). The discussion should be continued throughout so the woman is aware of what will be happening and what has been identified, and the woman given the opportunity to feel where the head or buttocks are, and what position the baby is in. Nishikawa & Sakakibara (2013) found this helped increase maternal awareness of the baby's position and increased maternal–fetal attachment. When the procedure is complete, there should be a full discussion of the findings and, if further investigations are required, what they are, and why they are needed. The findings and discussion should be documented in the woman's notes.

The woman will be asked empty her bladder prior to the procedure, as this will be more comfortable for her, and then to lie semi-recumbent on an examining couch or similar firm surface. It is preferable not to lay the woman completely flat because of the risk of aortocaval compression. If for some reason she does need to be flat, a wedge should be placed under her right hip. The woman needs to be comfortable with her arms stretched out and relaxed by her side so that her abdominal muscles relax. This is helped if the room is warm and privacy ensured; she may choose to have family or friends present at this time. The woman will need to reposition her clothes so that access to all of her abdomen is possible.

The midwife should wash and dry her hands before and after touching the woman's abdomen; other standard precautions are usually unnecessary unless contact with body fluids is expected. This may also help to warm the midwife's hands, which is more comfortable for the woman.

Visual appearance of the abdomen

The abdomen is inspected at the beginning of the examination as a lot of information can be gleaned from this.

- The size of the abdomen is considered and this can be affected by maternal obesity, lax abdominal muscles causing a pendulous abdomen, multiple pregnancy, poly- and oligohydramnios, fetal size and lie, uterine fibroids, and gestation period. The enlarging uterus is often seen abdominally from around 12 weeks and will increase in size as the fetus grows and the amount of amniotic fluid increases.
- The shape of the abdomen may give an indication of the fetal position or presentation. For example a dip at the umbilicus can be indicative of an occipitoposterior position; if it appears low and broad, it may indicate a transverse lie. Nulliparous

women may have a more ovoid appearance to their abdomen than multiparous women but this can also be very individual. The abdomen often appears symmetrical in shape.
- Observe for any skin changes such as the linea nigra, stretch marks (new ones, 'striae gravidarum', appear pink/red, while older ones, 'striae albicantes', are silvery-white coloured), signs of previous abdominal surgery (particularly for caesarean section), presence of rashes or itching.
- Fetal movements may be seen.
- Signs of potential domestic abuse, e.g. bruising, may be observed.

Measuring fundal height

Traditionally the fundal height was assessed against landmarks on the maternal body – symphysis pubis, umbilicus, and xiphisternum (Fig. 1.1). This is not an evidence-based practice and at best provides an approximation of gestational age, being affected by the individual shape of the woman. This practice has been superseded by measurement of the fundal height with a tape measure and is not recommended where tape measures are available.

The RCOG (2013) support the measurement of symphysis–fundal height (SFH) measurement from 24 weeks of pregnancy and recommend the result is plotted on a customized chart rather than a population-based chart, as it helps to improve the prediction of a small-for-gestational age (SGA) baby. The customized chart is created by software and is specific for the woman and her current

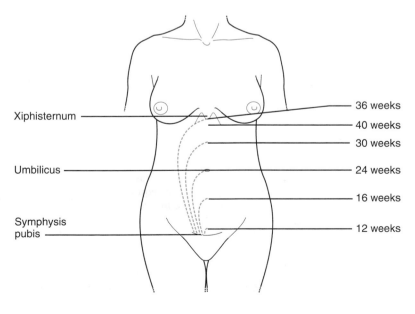

Figure 1.1 Fundal height at different stages of pregnancy using landmarks.

Xiphisternum — 36 weeks
— 40 weeks
— 30 weeks

Umbilicus — 24 weeks

— 16 weeks

Symphysis pubis — 12 weeks

pregnancy, using characteristics such as maternal weight, height, ethnicity, parity, and, if known, the sex of the current fetus to generate a 'term optimal weight' (Gardosi 2012). See www.perinatal.org.uk for more information on customized GROW charts. However, for women where this measurement may be inaccurate (e.g. BMI >35, polyhydramnios, large fibroids), they recommend serial assessment of fetal size via ultrasound. The SFH measurement should ideally be undertaken by the same person each time to reduce interobserver variation (Wright et al 2006). However, Roex et al (2012) found a significantly higher detection rate of SGA by using serial plotting of SFH measurements even when multiple practitioners with varying levels of experience were involved with obtaining these measurements. Peter et al (2012) could only find one randomized controlled trial (from 1990) looking at the use of SFH measurement for detecting babies with intrauterine growth restriction and therefore concluded they did not have sufficient evidence to recommend its universal use. However, they further state they have no evidence to suggest the practice should stop in areas where it is already in practice (Peter et al 2012) and it is not resource-intensive or costly to do.

Detection of babies who are SGA is important as it is a significant factor associated with an increased risk of perinatal mortality in the UK (ONS 2014). In 2012 the perinatal mortality rate for babies over 2500 g was 1.3 per 1000 live births whereas for babies under 2500 g it was 35.2 per 1000 live births (ONS 2014). By detecting these babies early in pregnancy, it is possible to reduce this rate by appropriate management and intervention.

The top of the fundus is palpated as this is the starting point for measuring the SFH. A hand is placed just below the xiphisternum and gentle pressure applied using the length of the fingers to feel for the firmness of the fundus, moving the hand down the abdomen until it is located. The uterus grows with the fetus; thus assessing the change within the fundal height may reflect the growth of the fetus.

The SFH is measured in centimetres and was thought to equate to the weeks of gestation, with a margin of error of ± 2–3 cm. However, Morse et al (2009) caution this is an erroneous assumption as it does not represent a reliable correlation, particularly across the varying maternity population and therefore this practice is not recommended.

A fundal height that is higher than expected may indicate:

- inaccurate dates
- that the fetus is larger than expected
- that the amount of amniotic fluid might be greater than expected – polyhydramnios
- multiple pregnancy
- uterine mass, e.g. fibroid, cyst or tumour
- poor technique.

A fundal height that is shorter than expected may indicate:

- inaccurate dates
- that the fetus is smaller than expected
- that the amount of amniotic fluid is less than expected – oligohydramnios
- abnormal lie, e.g. transverse
- poor technique
- intrauterine death.

PROCEDURE: obtaining the symphysis–fundal height measurement

- Discuss the procedure with the woman and gain her informed consent.
- Encourage the woman to empty her bladder.
- Gather equipment:
  - single-use tape measure
  - sheet, if needed
  - antenatal/labour record.
- Ask the woman to lie semi-recumbent with her arms relaxed at her sides, knees slightly bent and expose her abdomen, using the sheet to cover her legs if necessary and ensuring privacy.
- Wash and dry hands.
- Locate the top of the fundus and place a non-stretchable tape measure face down to avoid observer bias so that 0 cm is on the top of the fundus.
- Keeping the tape measure in contact with the skin, place it along the longitudinal axis of the uterus, without correcting to the midline of abdomen, until the top of the symphysis pubis is reached.
- Note where this is on the tape measure and record the measurement in centimetres.
- The measurement should be only be taken once and documented on the customized growth chart.
- Assist the woman to recover and adopt a comfortable position.
- Wash and dry hands.
- Discuss the findings with the woman and refer as necessary.

The RCOG (2013) recommend the use of ultrasound measurement for fetal size if there is a single SFH below the 10th centile or if serial measurements demonstrate slow or static growth by crossing centiles. This is important as clinical estimation of fetal weight for babies >4.0 kg or <2.5 kg by palpation is not very accurate (Levin et al 2011).

Palpation

As pregnancy progresses, or upon maternal request, a full abdominal palpation comprising a fundal, lateral and pelvic palpation can be undertaken to assess the presentation, lie, and position of the fetus, and, if requested, auscultate the fetal heart sounds. The order of the palpation can vary; however, many midwives begin at the fundus, undertake the lateral palpation and end with the pelvic palpation, whereas others will palpate the fundus, then the pelvic palpation with the lateral palpation last. The order is less important than the technique.

Fundal palpation

This is undertaken to determine which pole is in the upper part of the uterus – usually the breech with a cephalic presentation; although, if the breech is presenting, the head will be felt in the fundus. The woman continues to lie in the position adopted for measuring the SFH. The midwife should be facing the woman so that she can make eye contact and assess verbal and non-verbal communication for signs of discomfort. The midwife places her hand on the top of the woman's abdomen, below the xiphisternum as described above to find the top of the fundus. When the fundus is felt, the palmar sides of the fingers of both hands are placed either side of the fundus and gentle pressure applied as the fingers curve around to palpate what is beneath them (Fig. 1.2). The buttocks often appear broad, irregular, softer, bulkier and difficult to move whereas the head is firm, smooth, more rounded and ballotable; i.e. it can be moved gently from side to side between the hands (this will not happen if there is a breech presentation with extended legs). If no pole is felt in the fundus, it is likely to be due to a transverse lie (Fig. 1.3).

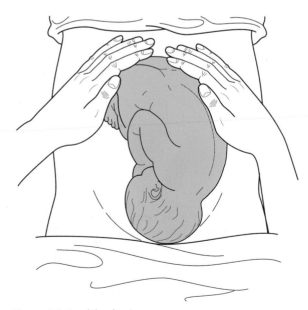

Figure 1.2 Fundal palpation.

Pelvic palpation

The presentation is the part of the fetus lying in the lower segment of the uterus, at or within the pelvic brim. This is determined by pelvic palpation which may also assess the degree of flexion or extension (in conjunction with the lateral palpation), the degree of engagement, and if the presenting part has not engaged, whether or not it is moveable (Fig. 1.4).

There are five main presentations (Fig. 1.5) and two methods of performing a pelvic palpation. Care should be taken to avoid discomfort to the woman; it may be more comfortable for the woman to bend her knees for this procedure:

1. Using both hands, one either side of the presentation and fingers facing towards the woman's feet, press gently inwards and downwards (Fig. 1.4A). The presentation can be felt beneath the hands, as described for fundal palpation and identified according to its features. It is helpful if the woman can take a deep breath and breathe out slowly while the midwife's hands feel deeply around the presentation. At this point, the midwife has her back to the woman but should ensure she is able to look at her face to ensure she is not causing too much discomfort.

2. Pawlik's manoeuvre can also be considered, but this one-handed technique is usually the more uncomfortable procedure of the two. Using one hand with fingers facing the woman's head, the presenting pole is held between the fingers and thumb (Fig. 1.4B). Due to the discomfort encountered, this should only be used if it cannot be avoided.

Engagement

When the widest transverse diameter of the presenting part has passed through the pelvic brim, it is said to have engaged. In a cephalic presentation the widest diameter is the biparietal diameter (9.5 cm). Engagement is generally measured in fifths; for example, a cephalic presentation that is 3/5 palpable has 3/5 of the head palpable out of the pelvis, indicating that 2/5 of the head has passed through the pelvic brim into the pelvis; 1/5 palpable would mean 4/5 has engaged, and so on. When 3/5 of the head has passed through the pelvic brim the presentation is 'engaged'. A non-engaged presentation may be referred to as 'free' or 'at the brim' and may necessitate referral at term, although for some women, particularly multigravida, engagement may not occur until labour.

Lateral palpation

Lateral palpation is undertaken to determine the position of the fetus and will also confirm the lie. It may also provide

Figure 1.3 The lie of the fetus.

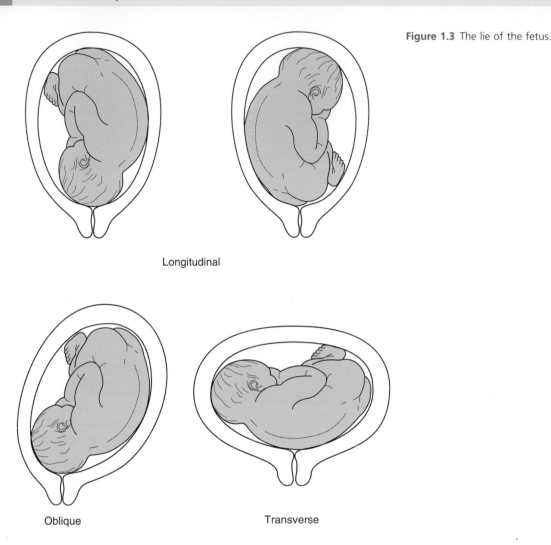

Longitudinal

Oblique

Transverse

information about the fetal size, volume of amniotic fluid, uterine tone, and fetal movements. When undertaking the lateral palpation, the fetal spine is felt for – this is usually firmer and smoother than the less regularly defined limbs palpated on the opposite side, which will also feel softer. There are two methods of undertaking lateral palpation:

1. The hands are placed one on either side of the uterus at about umbilical level: one side of the uterus is supported while the other hand feels down the length of the uterus (Fig. 1.6) and then this side is supported and the other side is palpated in the same way.
2. Alternatively both hands can 'walk' their fingertips across the uterus from side to side, from the fundus to the symphysis pubis (Fig. 1.7).

The lie of the fetus is determined by the relationship of the long axis of the fetal spine to the long axis of the maternal uterus. The lie is normally longitudinal, but can be oblique or transverse (Fig. 1.3).

The position is defined according to the position of the fetal denominator (a fixed point on the presentation, e.g. occiput for cephalic presentation, sacrum for breech presentation) to a pelvic landmark. Figure 1.8 indicates the relevant landmarks on the pelvic brim. For example, if the occiput is in apposition with the iliopectineal eminence of the pelvis, the position is described as occipitoanterior (Fig. 1.9). It is further defined according to whether it is on the maternal left or right. If the occiput is in apposition with the sacroiliac joint, it is described as occipitoposterior. For occipitolateral, the occiput is found midway on the iliopectineal line (Fig. 1.9). The occiput may also be at the front or back of the pelvis – referred to as a direct occipitoanterior or direct occipitoposterior position.

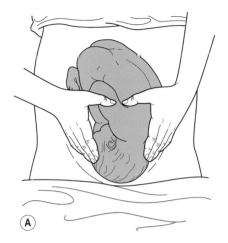

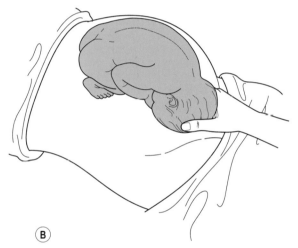

Figure 1.4 A, Pelvic palpation: the fingers are directed inwards and downwards. **B,** Pawlik's manoeuvre.

Abdominal examination in labour

During labour when the uterus is contracting, the abdomen may be more sensitive and thus this may be more uncomfortable for the woman and harder to do, but it is an aspect of care that supports and informs other aspects of care, for example, examination *per vaginam*. The procedure should not be undertaken unnecessarily and should be completed promptly between contractions to minimize discomfort and make it easier to palpate the fetus. Webb et al (2011) found that determining the position, specifically left occipitoanterior, at the onset of labour is not very accurate. Peregrine et al (2007) agree, suggesting the lateral palpation assesses the position of the fetal spine

which does not always correspond to the position of the fetal head.

This procedure requires the woman to be in a semi recumbent position, which is not ideal for labour. Thus the midwife should ensure that the woman is encouraged to adopt a more upright position following the examination, whenever possible. It is undertaken:

- to gain a baseline on which care is provided and subsequent progress assessed, by determining the gestation, lie, position, presentation, engagement, and auscultation of the fetal heart
- to monitor progress in labour by assessing descent and rotation of the presenting part
- prior to auscultation of the fetal heart or commencing monitoring using CTG
- prior to undertaking an examination *per vaginam*
- with multiple births, following delivery of each baby, to determine the lie, position, and presentation of the remaining fetuses.

PROCEDURE: abdominal examination

- Establish the woman's health and wellbeing; discuss her thoughts, e.g. fetal movements, growth, possible position.
- Discuss the procedure with the woman and gain her informed consent.
- Encourage the woman to empty her bladder.
- Gather equipment:
  - single-use tape measure
  - if needed, watch with a second hand, Pinard stethoscope or fetal Doppler with conduction gel and tissues
  - sheet, if needed
  - antenatal/labour record.
- Ask the woman to lie semi-recumbent with her arms relaxed at her sides, knees slightly bent, and expose her abdomen, using the sheet to cover her legs if necessary and ensuring privacy.
- Wash and dry hands.
- Undertake fundal palpation and use the tape measure to assess symphysis-fundal height (see above); undertake lateral and pelvic palpations if gestation >36 weeks or maternal request (see above).
- If requested or indicated, auscultate the fetal heart while simultaneously palpating the maternal radial pulse (described below).
- Assist the woman to replace her clothing and to move into a comfortable position then discuss the findings with her.
- Wash and dry hands.
- Document the findings and act accordingly.

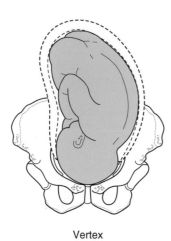

Vertex

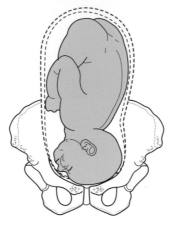

Brow

Figure 1.5 Five presentations of the fetus.

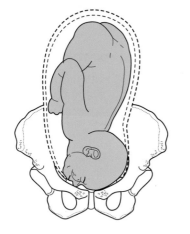

Face

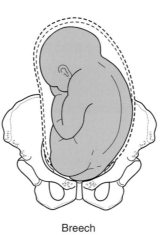

Breech

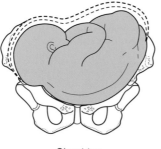

Shoulder

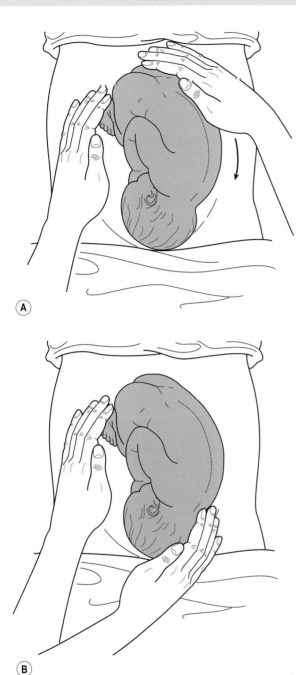

Figure 1.6 Lateral palpation. One side of the uterus is supported as the other hand progresses down the uterus. Both sides are palpated in this way.

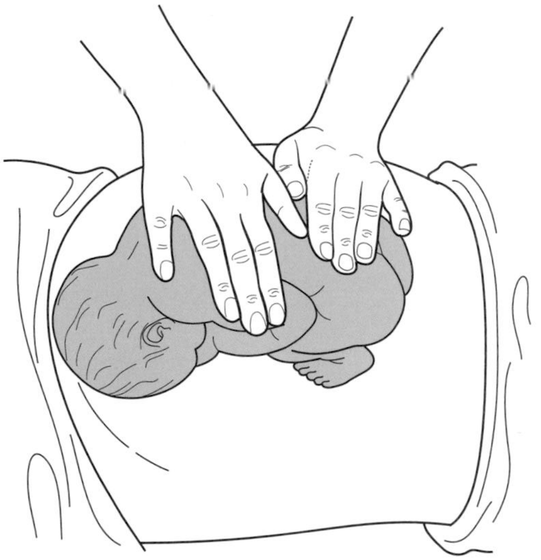

Figure 1.7 'Walking' the fingertips across the abdomen to locate the position of the fetal back.

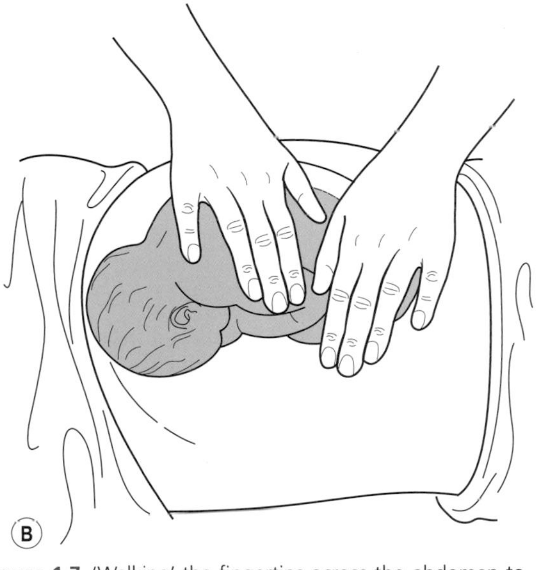

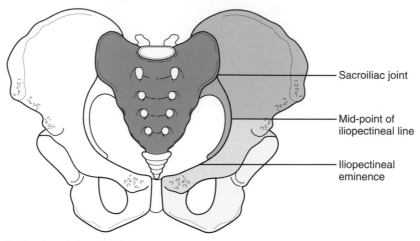

Sacroiliac joint

Mid-point of iliopectineal line

Iliopectineal eminence

Figure 1.8 Relevant landmarks on the pelvic brim.

Auscultation of the fetal heart

In the presence of normal fetal movements, there is limited value in routinely auscultating the fetal heart rate during the antenatal visit. However, auscultation should be undertaken:

* prior to the application of a CTG monitor
* throughout labour to monitor the fetal response to labour
* to determine fetal life in the event of absence of fetal movements
* upon maternal request.

During pregnancy, if there is an indication to auscultate the fetal heart sounds, this can be undertaken using a Pinard stethoscope or with Doppler ultrasound, e.g. sonic-aid device. These may also be used for intermittent auscultation (IA) during labour for low-risk women in established labour or, where continuous monitoring is indicated, through the use of a CTG.

During the first stage of labour, NICE (2014) recommend listening to the fetal heart immediately following a contraction for at least 1 minute and at least every 15 minutes. During the second stage it should be listened to in the same way but every 5 minutes with palpation of the maternal pulse every 15 minutes (NICE 2014). The heart rate should be recorded as a single rate rather than a range and any accelerations or decelerations heard should be noted. In the presence of a fetal heart rate abnormality, e.g. deceleration, bradycardia, the maternal pulse should be palpated to determine whether it is fetal or maternal heart rate sounds heard.

Ideally an abdominal palpation should precede the auscultation as this will assist with locating the best position to listen to the fetal heart. Maternal anxiety will be unnecessarily heightened if the midwife 'guesses' where to place the equipment to hear the fetal heart and has to keep moving it around because an abdominal palpation was omitted. The clearest fetal heart sounds are heard though the fetal shoulder (scapula) although they can sometimes be heard through the fetal chest wall depending on the fetal position. The fetal heart beat is heard as a rapid double beating (often rather like a tapping sound) between 110–160 beats per minute (bpm) with increases in the rate noted with fetal movements.

Use of the Pinard stethoscope

The midwife should be familiar with the use of a Pinard stethoscope as this enables the midwife to confirm it is the fetal heart that has been heard; electrical equipment can confuse the fetal and maternal heart rates. The midwife should palpate the maternal radial pulse while listening to the fetal heart to ensure that it is the fetal and not maternal heart rate being heard. It can be used from 24 weeks' gestation but many midwives would not use one until 28 weeks' gestation. A smaller fetus that is moving significantly can be hard to 'stabilize' and therefore listen to. This is true for any auscultatory equipment. It can be difficult to use the Pinard stethoscope with some labour positions, e.g. all-fours, and as the fetus descends during the second stage of labour. In these instances it is preferable to use Doppler ultrasound.

Using the Pinard stethoscope effectively is a learned and practised skill which improves with practice, but it can be difficult to use to begin with. Wickham (2002) suggests the fetal heart beat is more of a vibration than a sound, similar to listening to the Korotkoff sounds when taking a manual blood pressure. It is harder to hear if there are other external noises competing and it may be easier to hear with closed eyes and hands off the stethoscope. If the fetal heart is not heard where expected the position of the Pinard should be changed but not rotated and if it is still not detected, use the Doppler ultrasound. Midwives with

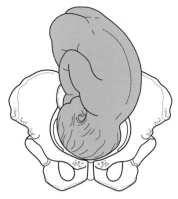

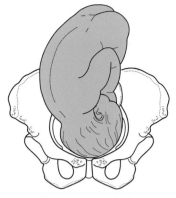

Figure 1.9 Six positions in a vertex presentation.

Left occipitoanterior

Right occipitoanterior

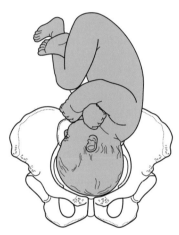

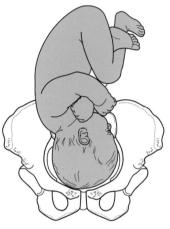

Left occipitolateral

Right occipitolateral

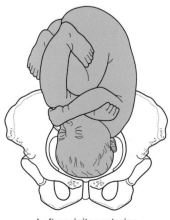

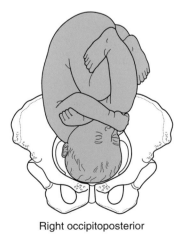

Left occipitoposterior

Right occipitoposterior

hearing difficulties may find it easier to use the Doppler ultrasound.

PROCEDURE: using a Pinard stethoscope

- Discuss the procedure with the woman and gain her informed consent.
- Undertake an abdominal examination to determine the position of the fetus.
- Position the Pinard stethoscope over the area where heart sounds are expected (Fig. 1.10).
- Place the ear over the hole and remove the hand so that the ear, stethoscope and abdomen are in direct contact (this increases the sound variance), applying gentle pressure.
- Listen and count the fetal heart for 1 minute, simultaneously palpating the woman's radial pulse (see Chapter 4) to ensure it is the fetal heart being auscultated.
- Discuss the results with the woman.
- Document the findings and act accordingly.

Use of an ultrasound device

A fetal Doppler ultrasound device (sometimes called a sonicaid after a company that makes them) can also be used to auscultate the fetal heart. These devices emit small, high-frequency sound waves (ultrasound) which reflect from moving objects, in this case the fetal heart, changing the frequency slightly. The Doppler device then changes this into a digital display and or sound that can be heard. This is the advantage of using an ultrasound device for the woman and her family who can hear the sounds, too, which they may find reassuring. The fetal heart rate can be heard at earlier gestations with a Doppler ultrasound compared with a Pinard stethoscope. The midwife should always be alert to the possibility of an absent fetal heart and therefore may choose to confirm its presence with a Pinard stethoscope first. The Doppler ultrasound often needs to be placed directly over the fetal shoulder in order to hear the fetal heart. Less pressure is needed on the abdomen compared with a Pinard and some devices can be used in water. Other sounds (swooshing of uterine vessels, fetal hiccoughs, fetal movements, etc.) can be heard and will need explaining to listening parents.

PROCEDURE: using a fetal Doppler

- Discuss the procedure with the woman and gain her informed consent.
- Undertake an abdominal examination and auscultate the fetal heart using a Pinard stethoscope.
- Lubricate the Doppler ultrasound probe with a suitable conductive gel.
- Position the Doppler probe over the area where heart sounds are expected.
- Count the heart beat for 1 minute while simultaneously palpating the maternal radial pulse (see Chapter 4) to ensure it is the fetal heart that is being listened to.
- Reassure the woman about the other sounds that can be heard.
- Wipe the gel off with a tissue.
- Discuss the results with the woman.
- Document the findings and act accordingly.

CARDIOTOCOGRAPHY

The CTG is a way to undertake continuous monitoring of the fetal heart rate over a specific period of time using Doppler technology. It is also referred to as electronic fetal monitoring (EFM). There will be occasions where it is used during pregnancy; however, its main use is during labour. Nevertheless, NICE (2014) are clear that it should not be offered to low-risk women at all, including 'admission' in labour (Devane et al 2012). During pregnancy it may be undertaken if the woman is reporting reduced or absent fetal movements, but further investigation may be required as the CTG only provides information about the status of the fetal heart at the point in time. A CTG is recommended before and after an external cephalic version for breech presentation (p. 207) and NICE (2008) recommend a CTG should be undertaken twice weekly for gestations >42 weeks and induction of labour has been declined.

If one or more of the following risk factors are present or arise during the course of labour, NICE (2014) recommend continuous EFM:

- oxytocin use
- presence of significant meconium
- suspected chorioamnionitis or sepsis
- temperature ≥38°C
- severe hypertension 160/110 mmHg or above
- fresh intrapartum vaginal bleeding.

It is often used where there are concerns that fetal hypoxia may develop, e.g. fetal growth restriction, abnormalities heard on intermittent auscultation (e.g. bradycardia, tachycardia, decelerations), and preterm labour and, according to NICE (2014), for at least 30 minutes during the establishment of epidural analgesia and following each intermittent bolus administration of 10 mL or more.

Alfirevic et al (2013) caution that while the use of continuous EFM during labour is associated with a reduction in neonatal seizures, there are no significant differences in

Figure 1.10 The approximate points of the fetal heart sounds with a vertex presentation.

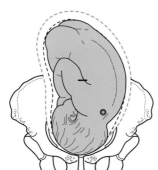

Left occipitoanterior

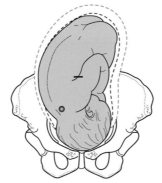

Right occipitoanterior

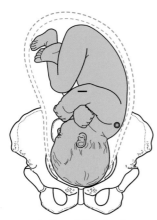

Left occipitolateral

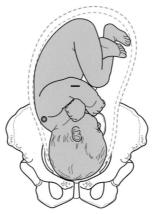

Right occipitolateral

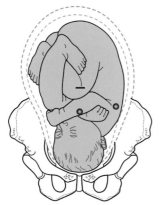

Left occipitoposterior

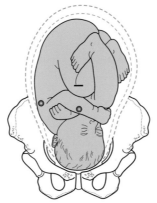

Right occipitoposterior

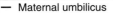

— Maternal umbilicus

● Positioning of sonicaid to hear fetal heart

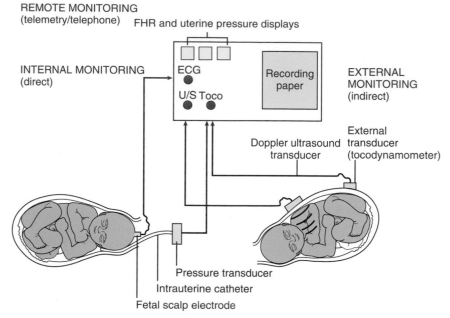

REMOTE MONITORING
(telemetry/telephone)   FHR and uterine pressure displays

INTERNAL MONITORING
(direct)

ECG

U/S Toco

Recording
paper

EXTERNAL
MONITORING
(indirect)

Doppler ultrasound
transducer

External
transducer
(tocodynamometer)

Pressure transducer

Intrauterine catheter

Fetal scalp electrode

Figure 1.11 Cardiotocography monitor.

cerebral palsy incidence, infant mortality rates or other measures of neonatal wellbeing, but there is an increase in both the number of caesarean sections and instrumental deliveries.

The CTG monitor can record the fetal heart and uterine pressure abdominally, with some having the ability to do this internally (Fig. 1.11). There are two transducers, one placed over the fundus to sense the changing pressure of the uterus and one to listen to the fetal heart rate. They are secured in place often with belts wrapped around the woman's abdomen. Internal monitoring of the fetal heart rate requires the application of a fetal scalp electrode (p. 227) and is more invasive. There is the possibility that the maternal pulse rate is detected rather than the fetal heart rate, particularly during the second stage (Nurani et al 2012); thus, it is important to distinguish between the two. Newer machines have a probe that is placed over the woman's finger which will record her pulse rate at the same time. The Medicines and Healthcare Products Regulatory Agency (MHRA, 2010) caution that adverse outcomes are still being reported in the presence of apparently normal CTG traces. They suggest this could be a result of doubling of the maternal heart rate or halving of a very tachycardic fetal heart suggesting a normal baseline rate and cite examples where this has resulted in a stillbirth or a baby requiring extensive resuscitation (MHRA 2010). These examples demonstrate that while CTG can be a useful tool in assessing fetal wellbeing, it is not infallible and confirms NICE (2014) advice that decisions about a woman's care in labour

should not be made on the basis of CTG findings alone. If there is any uncertainty, the fetal heart rate should be auscultated using the Pinard stethoscope or Doppler device. NICE (2014) also recommend this is undertaken before CTG monitoring is commenced, if the fetal heart rate (FHR) has been reassuring and a change occurs, or if the FHR is non-reassuring and then appears to become reassuring.

The readings are printed out on graph paper which should run at 1 cm per minute unless local protocol dictates otherwise. The actual pressure changes in the uterus do not equate exactly with the printed strength of contractions, thus EFM should not replace the regular assessment of uterine activity by the midwife. As the fetus moves loss of contact may occur, which might be accompanied by an increase in the heart rate.

The midwife should remain with the woman for the duration of the CTG, providing one-to-one support and ensuring the focus of the care centres on the woman, not the CTG (NICE 2014). NICE (2014) recommend a documented systematic assessment of the condition of the woman and fetus, which includes an interpretation of the CTG, is undertaken at least hourly. Interpretation of the CTG is a skill that requires regular training and assessment and for many midwives is part of their mandatory annual updating. It is helpful to discuss CTGs with colleagues to maintain knowledge and skills. The midwife should also be trained in the use of the CTG as well as how to clean and store it and is responsible for ensuring it is maintained correctly.

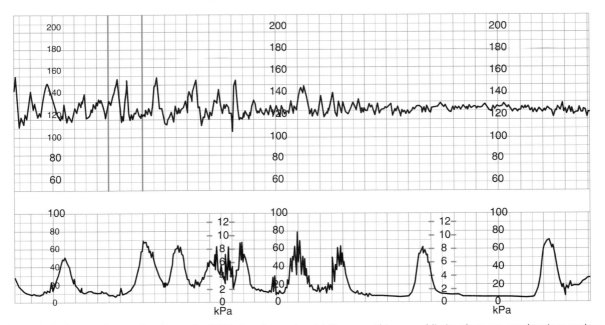

Figure 1.12 A reassuring cardiotocography (CTG): baseline and variability are within normal limits, there are accelerations and no decelerations. This CTG shows a period of fetal activity, followed by sleep.

Cardiotocograph interpretation

CTG interpretation begins with knowledge of the woman's history and current clinical profile and that the monitor has been correctly applied. Any changes of maternal position, vomiting, vaginal examination, epidural analgesia and other such variables should be noted and considered. The presence (or absence) of uterine contractions should be noted for their frequency, strength and length. NICE (2014) recommend three features of the fetal heart tracing are assessed during labour (in conjunction with uterine activity) – baseline rate, baseline variability and decelerations. The absence of accelerations in a normal trace during labour is of unknown significance; thus accelerations become important during an antenatal recording and are seen as an increase from the baseline rate of at least 15 bpm for at least 15 seconds.

NICE (2014) classify each of these three features and the overall trace as being 'normal/reassuring' (Fig. 1.12), 'non-reassuring' or 'abnormal'.

Baseline rate

A normal or reassuring fetal heart rate is between 100 and 160 bpm and is the rate to which the fetal heart returns after accelerations, decelerations or a period of activity. During labour it should be assessed between contractions. It is considered non-reassuring when the rate is 161–180 bpm and abnormal if >180 or <100 bpm (NICE 2014).

Baseline variability

Baseline variability refers to the amount the baseline fetal heart varies over 1 minute; a variation in the heart rate of >5 bpm is normal. Variability reflects the balance between the sympathetic and parasympathetic nervous systems. Normal baseline variability indicates a well oxygenated central nervous system and is considered the most important indicator of fetal wellbeing. Variability may be reduced during fetal sleep periods and with the administration of certain drugs, e.g. magnesium sulphate. According to NICE (2014), it is non-reassuring if baseline variability is <5 bpm for 30–90 minutes and abnormal when it is <5 bpm for >90 minutes.

Decelerations

Decelerations occur when the baseline heart rate decreases at least 15 bpm from the baseline for at least 15 seconds and are classified as early, variable, typical, atypical, and late.

- Early decelerations are usually insignificant and result from head compression. They begin and end with the contraction and can appear as the mirror image of the contraction.

- Variable decelerations vary in their timing and shape and are considered to be typical or atypical:
  - Typical variable decelerations are usually due to cord compression and normal baseline variability is present. The fetal heart rate demonstrates shouldering (a slight elevation in the heart rate before and after the deceleration) and should return to its baseline rate within 2 minutes.
  - Atypical variable decelerations may be associated with intrauterine hypoxia and do not have shouldering but may be accompanied by a slow return to the baseline rate or rebound tachycardia, with reduced or loss of variability. They can take longer for the baseline rate to return to normal.
- Late decelerations can indicate hypoxia; the deceleration begins at or after the peak of the contraction with the lowest point occurring ≥20 seconds after the peak of the contraction. They are usually repetitive and uniform in shape.

A normal/reassuring trace will have either early or no decelerations. NICE (2014) advise that non-reassuring decelerations are:

- variable decelerations of ≤60 bpm lasting ≤60 seconds over a 90-minute period and occurring with >50% contractions OR
- ≥60 bpm lasting over a 30-minute period with >50% contractions OR
- late decelerations for up to 30 minutes with >50% contractions.

Abnormal decelerations are:

- non-reassuring variable decelerations that remain present with >50% contractions 30 minutes after conservative measures have been commenced OR
- late decelerations that have been present for >30 minutes with >50% contractions and are not improving despite the implementation of conservative measures OR
- bradycardia (<100 bpm) or a single prolonged deceleration ≥3 minutes (NICE 2014).

If all three features are normal/reassuring, the CTG is described as normal. When one feature is non-reassuring, the CTG is considered to be non-reassuring, and when one feature is abnormal or two are non-reassuring, the CTG is abnormal.

PROCEDURE: application of the CTG monitor

- Discuss the procedure with the woman and gain and record her informed consent.
- Encourage the woman to empty her bladder.

- Record baseline maternal observations of temperature, blood pressure, and pulse if not already undertaken.
- Perform an abdominal examination and auscultation of the fetal heart using a Pinard stethoscope (p. 10).
- Position the woman in a sitting or semi-recumbent position; this can be changed once the monitor has been applied and is recording well.
- Place the two belts in position behind and around the woman and ensure she is covered sufficiently.
- Apply gel to the ultrasound transducer.
- Place the ultrasound transducer over the area where heart sounds are expected; the signal will indicate when the positioning is good.
- Secure the ultrasound transducer in position using an abdominal belt.
- Palpate the maternal pulse to ensure that the two are different.
- Place the uterine transducer on the fundus of the uterus and secure it with the other abdominal belt.
- When the uterus is relaxed, adjust the setting on the machine to 0 mmHg, unless set automatically or local protocol suggests a different figure.
- Start the paper printing (1 cm per minute) and document the date, time commenced, woman's name and ID number, indication for monitoring, all of the maternal observations and any other relevant details on the trace (e.g. gestation, epidural analgesia, oxytocin); then sign and print name.
- Confirm that any automatic printing of data (e.g. time, date) is correct.
- Encourage the woman to record fetal movements if applicable.
- Discuss what is being looked for on the CTG and the significance of the two printouts, the sounds heard and what to do if loss of contact occurs.
- Document the indication for and commencement of the monitoring in the maternal records with date, time, signature and name.
- Ensure that all who review the CTG tracing records this on the tracing and in the maternal records, including the date, time and findings of the recording.
- The CTG is discontinued when satisfied the tracing is normal or when the baby is delivered if continuous EFM was required during labour.
- Wipe the gel from the woman's abdomen and remove both transducers and belts.
- Sign and correctly store the tracing, record completion of the monitoring and the indications for care.
- If birth has occurred, the date, time, and mode of delivery should also be recorded on the tracing.
- Discuss the results with the woman.
- Clean, restock and store the equipment correctly.

PALPATION OF UTERINE CONTRACTIONS

Assessing uterine activity is the second part of abdominal assessment. Many women experience Braxton Hicks contractions during the latter stages of pregnancy, painless tightenings, which may also be palpated during an abdominal examination. The midwife should be able to distinguish between these and labour contractions, both to reassure the woman and inform clinical care. The midwife should always be alert to the signs of uterine contraction whatever the gestation as women in preterm labour may consider they have backache and not appreciate their uterus is contracting. The midwife uses the information gained from the palpation of contractions during labour to assess progress and inform care, e.g. to aid the appropriate use of Entonox (see Chapter 24).

During a contraction, the muscle fibres of the myometrium contract, causing the uterus to become firm; the contractions begin and end in the fundus, sweeping down over and back up the uterus. Thus the fundus is the best place to detect the contraction occurring and fading away. Contractions are palpated through the abdominal wall; their length and frequency can be determined with relative accuracy (this is a learned skill), although the strength is somewhat more subjective. The resting tone of the uterus can also be observed by assessing the tone of the uterus between the contractions – the abdomen should be soft when the uterus is at rest.

Generally as labour progresses, the length, strength and frequency of contractions increase. The midwife assesses this by palpation of the uterine fundus along with all the other signs of progress seen in the reactions and observations of the woman. As with other examinations, the findings are not taken in isolation, but form part of an overall assessment. CTG may aid some of the observations, i.e. the frequency and length of contractions if the transducer is recording appropriately, but the midwife should still palpate the contractions regularly as the CTG is not infallible. This is particularly true when assessing contraction strength (the monitor may not detect this accurately), if the woman has epidural analgesia and if using oxytocin to induce or augment labour. Excessive contractions (>5 in 10 minutes) usually require a reduction in the amount of oxytocin administered.

Indications

- To assess progress of labour in relation to the length, strength, and frequency of the uterine contractions.
- Correct administration of Entonox (see Chapter 24).

- During the second stage of labour if the woman is being guided when to push, e.g. with epidural analgesia.
- During active management of the third stage of labour to determine if the uterus is contracted prior to undertaking controlled cord traction to deliver the placenta and membranes (see Chapter 32).

Contraindications

- Palpation should be undertaken cautiously when trying to stop a preterm labour or if there is uterine irritability for any other reason, e.g. antepartum haemorrhage or fever, as an incorrect technique may lead to further unnecessary uterine stimulation.
- Excessive interference with the uterine fundus may cause it to have uncoordinated activity as opposed to its usual coordination across the uterus. This is of particular significance during the third stage of labour.

PROCEDURE: assessing uterine contractions

- A watch/clock with a second hand is required to time the contraction.
- Discuss the procedure and gain informed consent.
- Wash, warm, and dry hands.
- Ensure the woman is in a comfortable position, with access to the top of her abdomen, the abdomen can remain covered.
- Place one hand on the top part of the abdomen, over the fundal region of the uterus.
- Keeping the hand still, feel for the contraction along the length of the fingers (not just the fingertips).
- Note the time when the uterus first contracts.
- Observe the length of time the contraction lasts and the extent to which the uterus hardens.
- Keep the hand on the abdomen to await the next contraction, observe the time between contractions to assess frequency and note the relaxed, resting tone of the uterus.
- If the contractions are irregular, palpate the contractions for 10 minutes to calculate the number occurring in a 10-minute period. (This is more intrusive; it might be preferable to ask the woman to note the number of contractions in a 10-minute period, provided she is aware of them.)
- Wash and dry hands.
- Discuss the findings with the woman.
- Document the findings and act accordingly.

ROLE AND RESPONSIBILITIES OF THE MIDWIFE

These are summarized as:

- knowledge and application of current evidence-based practice
- undertaking all procedures correctly
- appropriate CTG trace interpretation and regular update of such skills
- education, advice and support of the woman
- accurate contemporaneous record keeping
- referral for deviations from normal.

SUMMARY

- Abdominal assessment antenatally and in labour is a skill from which significant information can be gained.
- Accurate measurement of the symphysis-fundal height and plotting this on a customized chart can help to detect babies with slow or static growth.
- The midwife has a responsibility to undertake the abdominal examination competently and sensitively, document the findings, and make a referral when necessary. It is more uncomfortable for women when in labour.

- The fetal heart can be auscultated using a Pinard stethoscope, fetal Doppler or CTG monitor. It is always preceded by an abdominal examination.
- CTG monitors should be applied correctly and the trace interpreted accordingly.
- Palpation of uterine contractions in labour assesses the frequency, strength, length, and resting tone of the uterus. It is a significant aspect of labour care.

SELF-ASSESSMENT EXERCISES

The answers to the following questions may be found in the text:

1. Describe the different components of an abdominal examination, discussing the rationale for each aspect.
2. Describe how to measure the symphysis–fundal height.
3. Discuss the different ways the fetal heart rate is auscultated.
4. Describe the procedure when applying a CTG monitor.
5. Discuss which factors the midwife needs to consider when interpreting a CTG tracing.
6. If a CTG tracing was described as 'non-reassuring' what would this mean?
7. Demonstrate how to palpate uterine contractions in labour.
8. Summarize the role and responsibilities of the midwife in relation to abdominal examination and use of electronic fetal monitoring.

REFERENCES

Alfirevic, Z., Devane, D., Gyte, G.M.L., 2013. Continuous cardiotocography (CTG) as a form of electronic fetal monitoring (EFM) for fetal assessment during labour. Cochrane Database Syst. Rev. 5 CD006066. doi:10.1002/14651858.CD006066.pub2.

Blee, D., Dietsch, E., 2012. Women's experience of the abdominal palpation in pregnancy; a glimpse into the philosophical and midwifery literature. N. Z. Coll. Midwives J. 46, 21–25.

Devane, D., Lalor, J.G., Daly, S., et al., 2012. Cardiotocography versus intermittent auscultation of fetal heart on admission to labour ward for assessment of fetal wellbeing.

Cochrane Database Syst. Rev. 2 CD005122. doi:10.1002/14651858.CD005122.pub4.

Gardosi, J., 2012. Customised assessment of fetal growth potential: implications for perinatal care. Arch. Dis. Child. Fetal Neon atal Ed. 97 (5), F314-F317.

Levin, I., Gamzu, R., Buchman, V., et al., 2011. Clinical estimation of fetal weight: is accuracy acquired with professional experience? Fetal Diagn. Ther. 29 (4), 321–324.

MHRA, 2010. Medical Safety Alert Fetal monitor/cardiotocograph (CTG) – adverse outcomes still reported. Available online: <https://www.gov.uk/drug-device-alerts/medical-device-alert-fetal-monitor-cardiotocograph

-ctg-adverse-outcomes-still-reported> (accessed 18 February 2015).

Morse, K., Williams, A., Gardosi, J., 2009. Fetal growth screening by fundal height measurement. Best Pract. Res. Clin. Obstet. Gynaecol. 23, 809–818.

NICE (National Institute for Health and Care Excellence), 2008. Antenatal care. Routine care for the healthy pregnant woman. Available online: <www.nice.org.uk> (accessed 1 March 2015).

NICE (National Institute for Health and Care Excellence), 2014. Clinical Guideline 190 Intrapartum Care. Care of Healthy Women and their Babies during Childbirth. NICE, London. <www.nice.org.uk> (accessed 1 March 2015).

Nishikawa, M., Sakakibara, H., 2013. Effect of nursing intervention program using abdominal palpation of Leopold's maneuvers on maternal-fetal attachment. Reprod. Health 10, 12 doi:10.1186/1742–4755-10–12.

Nurani, R., Chandraharan, E., Lowe, V., et al., 2012. Misidentification of maternal heart rate as fetal on cardiotocography during the second stage of labor: the role of the fetal electrocardiograph. Acta Obstet. Gynecol. Scand. 91, 1428–1432.

ONS (Office for National Statistics), 2014. Statistical Bulletin Childhood, Infant and Perinatal Mortality in England and Wales, 2012. Available online: <http://www.ons.gov.uk/ons/dcp171778_350853.pdf> (accessed 14 February 2015).

Peregrine, E., O'Brien, P., Jauniaux, E., 2007. Impact on delivery outcome of ultrasonographic fetal head position prior to induction of labour. Obstet. Gynecol. 109 (3), 618–623.

Peter, J.R., Ho, J.J., Valliapan, J., Sivasangari, S., 2012. Symphysial fundal height (SFH) measurement in pregnancy for detecting abnormal fetal growth. Cochrane Database Syst. Rev. 7 CD008136. doi:10.1002/14651858.CD008136.pub2.

RCOG (Royal College of Obstetricians and Gynaecologists), 2013. Green-top Guideline No. 31 The Investigation and Management of the Small–for–Gestational-Age Fetus. Available online: <https://www.rcog.org.uk/globalassets/documents/guidelines/gtg_31.pdf> (accessed 14 February 2015).

Roex, A., Nikpoor, P., van Eerd, E., et al., 2012. Serial plotting on customised fundal height charts results in doubling of the antenatal detection of small for gestational age fetuses in nulliparous women. Aust. N. Z. J. Obstet. Gynaecol. 52, 78–82.

Webb, A.A., Plana, M.N., Zamora, J., et al., 2011. Abdominal palpation to determine fetal position at labor onset: a test accuracy study. Acta Obstet. Gynecol. Scand. 90, 1259–1266.

Wickham, S., 2002. Pinard wisdom tips and tricks from midwives, part 2. Pract. Midwife 5 (10), 35.

Wright, J., Morse, K., Kady, S., Francis, A., 2006. Audit of fundal height measurement plotted on customized growth charts. MIDIRS Midwifery Digest. 16 (3), 341–345.

Chapter 2

Principles of abdominal examination: during the postnatal period

LEARNING OUTCOMES

Having read this chapter, the reader should be able to:

- briefly outline the physiology of involution
- discuss the possible deviations from the norm that may be identified when palpating the uterus postnatally
- describe the procedures (verbal and physical) necessary to assess involution of the uterus
- discuss the role and responsibilities of the midwife when undertaking abdominal examination during the postnatal period.

Gale (2008) believes that postnatal care is '… vital because it prepares parents for a lifetime of parenting'. Postnatal morbidity is something for which many women are unprepared, without adequate care it is also something for which mortality is a possibility (NICE 2014). Depending upon other indicators, assessment of the uterus postnatally is one aspect of care that the midwife may undertake as part of holistic and individualized postnatal care. This chapter includes a description of the physiology of uterine involution and a discussion of the ways in which normality is assessed.

PHYSIOLOGY OF INVOLUTION

Involution is the process by which the uterus returns approximately to its prepregnant size, position and tone. This involves a reduction in weight from 1000 to 60 g and reduction in size from $15 \times 11 \times 7.5$ cm to $7.5 \times 5 \times 2.5$ cm. 'Autolysis' refers to the digestion of excess muscle fibres by proteolytic enzymes, a process that is assisted by the continuing contraction and retraction of the uterus that began during labour. As the uterus reduces in size, the decidua is shed within the lochia (the discharges from the vagina following childbirth) and new endometrium begins to grow from the basal layer of the endometrium. New endometrial growth is evident from about the tenth day following delivery; by 6 weeks the endometrium has re-formed. Strong contraction of the muscle fibres occurs in the first 12–24 hours, decreasing in strength and frequency over the next

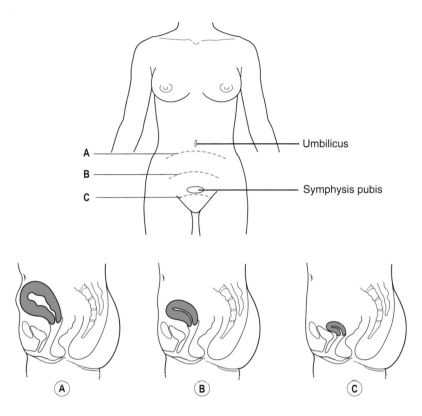

Figure 2.1 The position of the uterus during involution. **A,** Following delivery. **B,** One week following delivery – the fundal height is palpable approximately 5 cm above the symphysis pubis. **C,** Two weeks following delivery – the fundal height is usually not palpable above the symphysis pubis.

few days. They are often stronger and persist for longer in multiparous women (Blackburn 2013). Women recognize these contractions as 'after pains'. The rate at which the uterus involutes is considered to be approximately 1 cm per day. Therefore after 6 days, the fundus is usually about halfway between the umbilicus and the symphysis pubis and should be just palpable by the end of 10 days. For many women, the fundus may not be palpable at this time, and is usually no longer palpable after the twelfth postnatal day (Fig. 2.1).

While most textbooks report the changes described here as standard postpartum physiology, Cluett et al (1997) noted several variations in their assessment of 28 women including several days without uterine involution and uteri palpable at 23 days, both without signs of abnormality. It is considered that subinvolution of the uterus is less likely if breastfeeding (due to the increased action of oxytocin on uterine fibres) but more likely if there has been surgery or trauma. Pathological subinvolution usually relates to endometritis (infection within the uterus), often stemming from retained products. This creates the potential risk of a secondary postpartum haemorrhage (PPH).

Changes in the colour and amount of the lochia reflect the changes occurring within the endometrium and may vary with individual women. During the first 2–4 days following the birth of the baby, the lochia contain blood cells, necrotic deciduae, vernix, lanugo, meconium, and fragments of the amnion and chorion (lochia rubra), and are usually red in colour (initially bright, changing to dark red then brown as the proportion of blood cells within the lochia decreases). From around the third to fourth day, the lochia change to a pinkish-red colour (lochia serosa) and also contain leucocytes, microorganisms, cervical mucous and shreds of decidual tissue. It lasts 2–3 weeks (Blackburn 2013). It then begins to lighten in colour. Lochia alba is a whitish-yellow discharge that contains mainly leucocytes and decidual cells. It continues for another few weeks and so totals the time of lochial loss to 4–6 weeks postnatally (Blackburn 2013).

RATIONALE FOR THE PROCEDURE

The evidence to support the action of uterine palpation (both method and frequency) remains inadequate. NICE (2014) concluded that as a routine assessment abdominal palpation or measurement of the uterus was unnecessary.

However, it also noted that in the presence of other symptoms (fever, excessive or offensive vaginal lochia, abdominal pain) abdominal assessment of the uterus is indicated. If no uterine abnormality is found, other causes for the symptoms should be sought. Davies (2012) found mixed opinions amongst the midwives that she talked to about whether hands-on palpation of the uterus postnatally is necessary. It would seem that if this is not carried out, then other means of assessing normality (see below) should be carefully undertaken. Any deviations from the norm expressed should then lead the midwife to a physical examination. It is clear however, that this will only work if the woman has received guidance on what to realistically expect (and therefore can suggest when there is potentially a deviation from the norm) and if the midwife utilizes good communication skills with open questioning (discussed in detail below).

What is assessed?

- The midwife should know how the woman is feeling generally. Knight et al (2014) are clear that when presented with an unwell woman, firstly practitioners should 'think sepsis', and secondly a full set of vital sign observations should be recorded using a MEOWS chart (p. 66).
- As suggested above, the active 'descent' of the uterus back to a pelvic organ forms the largest part of the assessment. It is considered to reduce by 1 cm per day so that at 10 days postnatally it is just palpable above the symphysis pubis. Bick et al (2009) suggest that an initial palpation of the uterus should be undertaken post-delivery to establish a baseline from which the ueterus is seen to involute thereafter.
- The uterus should be positioned centrally within the abdomen. A full bladder can displace the uterus, causing it to deviate to one side. This can interfere with myometrial contraction, predisposing to postpartum haemorrhage. Thus, when the uterus is deviated, the lochia should be assessed to ensure the woman is not haemorrhaging and she should be encouraged to empty her bladder.
- The tone of the uterus should be firm, indicating a well-contracted uterus. If the tone is poor, the uterus will feel soft, again associated with postpartum haemorrhage. A full rectum, retained products of conception or blood clots can cause the uterus to feel bulky.
- The uterus should not feel tender when palpated but should be comfortable. Discomfort could be indicative of infection.
- The lochia should be observed for its amount, colour, and odour. Scant or malodourous lochia may be

indicative of infection, heavy reddened lochia of haemorrhage.

Palpating after caesarean section

The uterus is often very tender for several days and is slower to involute. While there is less likelihood of retained products, there is a risk of endometritis. In the event of needing to palpate the uterus, the hand should be placed gently over the uterus, the action of feeling the tone of the fundus described below is likely to be too painful. Deaths from haemorrhage do occur after caesarean section (Paterson-Brown & Bamber 2014); the midwife should be alert to uterine tone, heavy loss *per vaginam* and changes in vital signs, especially the pulse rate.

Deviations from the norm

Assessing what the deviation is leads to a plan of care; in almost all instances, the midwife will refer the woman for medical review. Suspected sepsis requires antibiotics promptly, and suspected haemorrhage may require surgery. Other signs of illness, e.g. raised temperature or pulse rate, would require the review to be undertaken quickly. A minor deviation, e.g. signs of normality except for a slower to involute uterus, may cause the midwife to consider the taking of a lower vaginal swab for culture and sensitivity and to be clear about when uterine involution should be assessed again. The woman should be alert to any symptoms that should be reported in the meantime.

Verbal assessment

Initially post-delivery, Bick et al (2009) suggest that the following should be considered:

- Antenatal and delivery records, including antenatal hemoglobin (Hb) and third stage management.
- While palpating the uterus, explanations should be given to the woman as to what is being felt and why. She is then invited to palpate her own uterus.
- Discuss the pattern of her vaginal loss, expected pattern, factors affecting it (e.g. feeding, signs of infection or clots), hygiene and pad changes.
- Visually assess the lochia.

At subsequent assessments it is necessary to discuss:

- Is she feeling well? Are there any signs of pyrexia or pain?
- How much lochial loss is there? Has it changed particularly? What colour is it? Any offensive smell?
- Is there abdominal discomfort? Is it 'after pains' or more continuous?

If the conversation gives the midwife any cause for concern, then the uterus should be palpated.

PROCEDURE: postnatal abdominal palpation of the uterus

- Confirm that palpation is necessary (see above), gain informed consent.
- Ask the woman to empty her bladder if she has not done so recently.
- Wash and dry hands, apply disposable apron and non-sterile gloves.
- Ask the woman to lie down in a recumbent position with her arms by her side.
- Ensure she is comfortable and privacy is maintained.
- Expose the woman's abdomen, note any features that may affect the palpation (e.g. obesity, degree of healing for caesarean section wound).
- Using the outer aspect of one hand, gently depress the abdomen to feel for the fundus. If the fundus is not found, remove the hand and reposition higher or lower and gently press down again.
- When the fundus is felt, use the outer aspect of the hand to estimate the height and position of the uterus. Depress slightly further down into the abdomen to feel over the top of the fundus, assess the uterine tone. A well-contracted uterus is often described as feeling like a cricket ball.
- Note whether the woman displays any non-verbal discomfort or expresses any pain on palpation.
- If not already done so, the lochial loss should be assessed by examining the pad. Check when the pad was last changed to obtain an idea of the extent of the loss. This can be done with the woman in the same position or in left lateral; she may prefer to stand up and remove the pad. If the lochial loss is heavy, the uterus should be palpated at the same time as examining the pad to see if on palpation any clots are expelled from the uterus.
- Assist the woman into a covered and comfortable position. Remove gloves and apron, dispose of them correctly, wash and dry hands.
- Discuss the findings with the woman.
- Document the findings and act accordingly, either with a prompt referral or established plan as to when the next reassessment takes place. NICE (2014) indicate that care plans should be individualized and made in consultation with the woman.

ROLE AND RESPONSIBILITIES OF THE MIDWIFE

These can be summarized as:
- careful communication, undertaking a physical examination correctly if indicated, in line with standard precaution and infection control protocols
- recognizing deviations from the norm and instigating referral
- education, explanations and support of the woman
- appropriate record keeping.

SUMMARY

- It is unnecessary to palpate the uterus routinely postnatally. If a suspected deviation from the norm is revealed on discussion or there are any other clinical signs observed (pyrexia, abdominal pain or offensive lochia) uterine palpation and assessment of lochial loss are then indicated.
- Uterine palpation includes the height, position, tone and comfort of the uterus.
- A deviation from the norm may suggest current or impending haemorrhage or infection. Urgent attention is needed to reduce the morbidity and mortality risks.

SELF-ASSESSMENT EXERCISES

The answers to the following questions may be found in the text:
1. Describe how involution occurs.
2. Based on what information should the midwife palpate the uterus during the postnatal period?
3. What is being assessed for when palpating the uterus during the postnatal period?
4. The lochia may be examined following abdominal palpation. What information may be gained from this in relation to involution?
5. Describe the action that should be taken if sepsis is suspected.

REFERENCES

Bick, D., MacArthur, C., Winter, H., 2009. Postnatal Care Evidence and Guidelines for Management, second ed. Elsevier, Edinburgh, pp. 1–18.

Blackburn, S.T., 2013. Maternal, Fetal and Neonatal Physiology: A Clinical Perspective, fourth ed. Elsevier, Maryland Heights. (Chapter 11).

Cluett, E.R., Alexander, J., Pickering, R.M., 1997. What is the normal pattern of uterine involution? An investigation of postpartum uterine involution measured by the distance between the symphysis pubis and the uterine fundus using a paper tape measure. Midwifery 13 (1), 9–16.

Davies, L., 2012. Care in the postnatal period part 2. Essentially MIDIRS 3 (1), 36–40.

Gale, E., 2008. Throwing the baby out with the bathwater? MIDIRS Midwifery Digest. 18 (2), 277–281.

Knight, M., Kenyon, S., Brocklehurst, P., et al. on behalf of MBRRACE-UK (Eds.), 2014. Saving Lives, Improving Mothers' Care – Lessons Learned to Inform Future Maternity Care from the UK and Ireland Confidential Enquiries into Maternal Deaths and Morbidity 2009–12. National Perinatal Epidemiology Unit, Oxford.

NICE (National Institute for Health and Care Excellence), 2014. Postnatal care CG37. NICE, London. Available online: <www.nice.org.uk> (accessed 5 March 2015).

Paterson-Brown, S., Bamber, J., on behalf of the MBRRACE-UK haemorrhage chapter writing group, 2014. Prevention and treatment of haemorrhage. In: Knight, M., Kenyon, S., Brocklehurst, P., et al. on behalf of MBRRACE-UK (Eds.), Saving Lives, Improving Mothers' Care – Lessons Learned to Inform Future Maternity Care from the UK and Ireland Confidential Enquiries into Maternal Deaths and Morbidity 2009–12. National Perinatal Epidemiology Unit, Oxford, pp. 45–55.

Chapter 3

Assessment of maternal and neonatal vital signs: temperature measurement

LEARNING OUTCOMES

Having read this chapter, the reader should be able to:

- define normal body temperature for the childbearing woman and baby
- describe the factors that influence body temperature and the changes relating to childbearing
- discuss the suitable sites for temperature measurement, highlighting their rationale for use, accuracy, normal temperature ranges and the equipment that can be used
- describe the types of thermometer and how each one is used correctly and safely
- demonstrate taking a baby's temperature
- discuss the midwife's role and responsibilities in relation to temperature measurement, identifying when and how it should be undertaken.

This chapter considers the means and significance of obtaining an 'as accurate as possible' temperature measurement. There is discussion about the different sites for temperature assessment, followed by the equipment available.

BODY TEMPERATURE

Body temperature is the balance between heat gain and heat loss. Humans are homoeothermic; i.e. their core temperature is maintained at 37° Celsius (C) ± 1°C, whatever the external environmental temperature. The hypothalamus acts as the body's thermostat. Humans cannot tolerate extreme changes at either end of the temperature range, should body temperature rise to 40.5°C, cellular damage may begin; temperatures above 42°C may result in brain dysfunction, coma, cardiovascular collapse, and death. Body temperature less than 28°C results in uncoordinated muscle activity and fatigue, unconsciousness, cardiac arrhythmias, and death.

The core temperature refers to the temperature within the brain, abdominal, and thoracic organs, reflecting the warmest parts of the body. Core temperatures are usually reached about 2 cm below the body surface (Hinchliff et al 1996), with two-thirds of body mass maintained at core temperature. The most accurate measurement of the core temperature, the 'gold standard', is found in the pulmonary artery (Board 1995). Maintenance of the body temperature at a constant level is essential to ensure optimal functioning of all cells. Rises in body temperature increase the demands for oxygen and therefore increase the heart rate. This is of significance for the pregnant woman; the nature of oxygen transfer to the fetus means that it is more likely to be compromised if the mother is pyrexial.

The peripheral temperature generated by skin and skeletal muscle is often lower than the core temperature and so helps to regulate the core temperature by assisting with heat loss and gain. Peripheral temperatures reduce proportionally as distances increase from the core. The assessment of body temperature aims to understand core temperature, rather than peripheral temperature.

Normal values

Different body temperature assessment sites have different normal values. These are usually determined according to the nearness of the site to a major blood vessel and the route that it is taking to/from the heart. For example, according to Dubois (1948) the normal oral temperature is set within a range of 35.8–37.3°C; however, each person has a 'normal' oral temperature setting within this range. A rise in core temperature of 1°C may be difficult to detect if a person's normal temperature is 36.0°C orally. It is also widely acknowledged that age affects body temperature, older people have a much lower body temperature, care should be taken when they are ill, a pyrexia may not register, but a 2°C rise in temperature may have occurred, signifying gross infection (Sund-Levander & Grodzinsky 2010, Sund-Levander & Grodzinsky 2013). Davie & Amoore (2010) suggest that many clinicians still regard body temperature to be 37°C without appreciating that normal temperatures are within a range for everyone. The range of normal values for each temperature measurement site is discussed with each site (below). They are taken from Davie & Amoore (2010).

FACTORS INFLUENCING BODY TEMPERATURE

Sensitive neurons in the hypothalamus regulate body temperature to keep it at its 'set point'. If the hypothalamus detects a higher temperature in the blood than the set point, heat loss measures are employed, e.g. sweating. Heat generation mechanisms, e.g. shivering, are employed when the blood is cooler than the set point. Body temperature is influenced by:

- Diurnal variations: circadian rhythms influence both the core and the peripheral temperatures. Body temperature is lowest during the night and peaks in the evening.
- Gender: women have a higher body temperature than men. Fertile women's body temperature is influenced by hormones. Body temperature is lower during the postmenstrual period of the menstrual cycle, increasing by 0.3–0.5°C following ovulation. This rise in body temperature is maintained until progesterone levels decrease prior to the onset of menstruation (Hinchliff et al 1996, Houdas & Ring 1982). This information is commonly used to assess for ovulation, e.g. IVF treatment.
- Age: the young and the old both struggle to maintain body temperature.
- Digestion: a slight increase in temperature of 0.1–0.2°C has been noted to occur with normal digestion.
- Basal metabolic rate: heat is produced as a result of chemical reactions within the body. When the body is at rest, this is referred to as the basal metabolic rate (BMR). The amount of heat produced can be altered by various regulatory mechanisms to ensure the body temperature is maintained within the normal range: the higher the BMR, the more heat is produced, the higher the temperature (Houdas & Ring 1982). BMR decreases with age, with babies having a higher BMR than adults. Certain diseases/disorders will increase the BMR (e.g. hyperthyroidism).
- Exercise: Closs (1987) suggests strenuous exercise may increase the core temperature to 40°C.
- Hot baths: these can raise the body temperature by 0.5–1.0°C for up to 45 minutes.

- Infection: leucocytes release endogenous pyrogens in response to stimulation by pyrogenic substances such as bacterial, viral, and protozoal infection and necrotic tissue. This causes the set point within the hypothalamus to be 'reset' at a higher level. The affected person feels cold and the body attempts to raise the temperature to maintain it within its higher 'normal' range. When the level of endogenous pyrogens decreases, the thermostat returns to its original setting. The person then feels hot, with the body attempting to lower the temperature to its normal setting. Shivering (the response to cold) and rigor (the response to pyrexia/hyperpyrexia) can appear the same clinically, in either instance body temperature should be carefully assessed (Grainger 2013). Other non-pyrogenic disorders can also cause pyrexia. These include malignancy, hyperthyroidism, drug and other allergies, and central nervous system damage, e.g. stroke.
- General anaesthesia: general anaesthetic drugs can interfere with the normal homeothermic mechanisms that assist with heat loss and gain, predisposing to heat loss (Schönbaum & Lomax 1991). Chinyanga (1991) proposes that the greatest decrease in body temperature will occur during the first hour of anaesthesia and that this can induce postanaesthetic shivering.
- Alcohol: Kalant and Lé (1991) conclude from their review of the literature that large amounts of alcohol will lower the body temperature.
- Childbearing: this is discussed in detail below.

The midwife should be aware of these factors so that inappropriate treatments are not commenced or pathologies overlooked.

TEMPERATURE CHANGES RELATED TO CHILDBIRTH

Pregnancy: maternal

During pregnancy, progesterone and a raised metabolic rate increase the amount of heat generated by 30–35%. Although the body attempts to compensate for this by increasing heat loss mechanisms, the maternal temperature can increase by 0.5°C (Blackburn 2013).

Pregnancy: fetal

Intrauterine temperature is determined partly by maternal temperature and partly by the maternal–fetal gradient as the fetus is unable to regulate its own temperature. Generally, the fetal temperature is approximately 0.5°C higher than the maternal temperature (Blackburn 2013). Therefore, a raised maternal body temperature will result in a higher fetal temperature and is associated with intrauterine hypoxia, fetal tachycardia, teratogenesis, and preterm labour (Blackburn 2013).

Labour

During labour, a rise in temperature can be indicative of infection, dehydration or increased muscular activity from uterine contractions. It is often associated with the use of epidural analgesia. A maternal non-infective pyrexia (>38°C) is associated with fetal hypoxia and therefore an increased need to resuscitate the newborn infant (Blackburn 2013).

Postnatal period: maternal

A transient rise in maternal temperature can occur within the first 24 hours following delivery. This may result from the stress of labour and be related to dehydration. Blackburn (2013) suggests that up to 6.5% of women have a rise in temperature up to 38°C in the 24 hours following a vaginal birth. In the majority of cases, this is physiological and resolves spontaneously. Modified Early Obstetric Warning System (MEOWS) scoring would still be used (p. 66) and action would be taken accordingly, particularly if the temperature rise was considered indicative of an infection (e.g. puerperal infection, mastitis, urinary tract infection). An inflammatory response, e.g. the development of a deep venous thrombosis, would also be considered. The temperature may also rise physiologically in breast-feeding women around the second to third day when lactogenesis occurs. This will resolve spontaneously once lactation is established, although it can take several days.

Postnatal period: baby

Babies emerge from the warmth of the uterus (37°C+) to an environment of approximately 21°C, wet and needing to establish several adaptations to extrauterine life simultaneously. Thermoregulation is difficult for the adapting neonate, and is further affected by:

- The large ratio of surface area to body mass with thin layers of insulating subcutaneous fat. This creates an increased opportunity to lose body heat, especially from the head.
- The changeable nature of the environment, especially open doors or windows, fans, cold mattresses etc.
- Factors that predispose to problematic thermoregulation, e.g. prematurity, small for gestational age, delivery by caesarean section, hypoxia, sedation (e.g. maternal use of opioids in labour) and congenital anomaly.

Consequently, babies lose heat by evaporation, especially before thorough drying, by convection when draughts blow over them, by radiation and conduction to nearby items and surfaces. A decrease in temperature of between 1 and 2°C may occur during the first hour after birth; if action is not taken to remedy this, a normal body temperature may not be achieved for 4–8 hours afterwards (Black 1972). Various measures should be taken at birth to protect the baby's temperature. The WHO (1997) call it 'the warm chain'. The room should be warm and draught free. The baby should be dried immediately and thoroughly with a warmed towel. The damp towel should be discarded and a replacement warmed one used to cover the baby. Placing the baby in skin-to-skin contact promotes thermoregulation (amongst other things, see p. 323), alternatively a radiant heater can be placed over the baby or a prewarmed incubator used. A very low birthweight baby's body (<28 weeks' gestation in the UK) can be placed wet into plastic wrapping under the heater, this also provides effective thermoregulation. Items such as weighing scales and X-ray plates should be covered with warmed blankets. Bathing is delayed until the baby's temperature is stable. (See Blackburn (2013) p. 662 for detailed list of further effective actions.) Sensible interventions in the delivery room result in higher neonatal paO$_2$ levels at 1-hour post-birth and therefore reduce levels of morbidity and mortality (Blackburn 2013).

Heat production comes mainly from metabolic processes, moving and shivering both being limited activities for neonates. Warmed external clothing helps, while the stores of brown fat are utilized, along with calories from milk. Metabolism requires both glucose and oxygen; a cold baby rapidly becomes hypoxic and hypoglycaemic and develops serious metabolic acidosis. The problems are compounded significantly if the baby is preterm or small for gestational age. Hyperthermia increases the neonate's demand for oxygen by increasing its metabolic demands. Dehydration and brain damage can occur.

Controlled cooling may take place in neonatal intensive care units as part of the treatment to reduce hypoxic ischaemic encephalopathy. Careful temperature assessment is undertaken in each stage of the process: reducing, cooling and rewarming.

Educating parents to understand the significance of avoiding hypo- and hyperthermia in the newborn and neonate is also an important part of the midwife's role. Blackburn (2013) suggests that thermoregulation is essential for survival and that all necessary measures to maintain it should be taken.

TEMPERATURE ASSESSMENT

A literature search reveals that there is almost only one point on which there is consensus: the pulmonary artery is the 'gold standard' site for temperature measurement. This is highly impractical in day-to-day midwifery, but all other sites and types of equipment used are suspect in their reliability. There are a number of studies published but they are often small, criticize each other for their methodologies and contradict in their conclusions. Smith (2014) illustrates this point well in her discussion regarding neonatal temperature taking. Consequently, it falls to the midwife to:

- keep up-to-date with evaluated current research
- work with the protocols of their employment, influencing these for the better if able
- maintain consistency with temperature measurement, using the same equipment in the same site (documented) for that woman/baby
- not undertake temperature measurement in isolation but as part of a complete clinical assessment.

The taking of a temperature, as for any clinical investigation, may lead to other actions (e.g. further screening with swabs, blood tests or urine specimens; use of antibiotics or other drugs; augmentation of labour if ruptured membranes). Consequently, the result needs to be as accurate as possible. In the normothermic individual, a slightly inaccurate temperature reading does not have the life-threatening consequences that it potentially does in neonates, ill, immunocompromised individuals, and post-operative patients. It can be argued that these groups all have a greater need for accurate assessment using an appropriate site with appropriate equipment (HIS 2012).

Indications

- Pathology: MEOWS (p. 66) assessment includes measurement of the temperature as one of the four vital assessments. This may be undertaken as a baseline reading or for a specific situation, e.g. postoperatively. Scoring may vary (and be either numerical or colour-coded (often traffic lights)), but generally a raised temperature of 38–38.5°C or a lowered temperature of between 35.1 and 36°C scores 1 or amber, while a temperature above and below these figures scores 2 or red. MEOWS scoring is used in many situations but particularly if the woman is looking or feeling unwell, has an existing pathology or has a potentially critical situation evolving, e.g. pre-eclampsia, haemorrhage, sepsis, amniotic fluid or pulmonary embolism. MEOWS charts are still only a guide and should be used in conjunction with other clinical assessments. Care should always be taken if sepsis is suspected or confirmed, hypothermia is very significant, hyperthermia may be disguised by paracetamol or other antipyretics, and raised temperatures can also 'swing' as the hypothalamus readjusts.

- at onset, during and following labour, whatever the gestation (4-hourly when in labour), hourly if in a birthing pool (NICE 2014)
- prelabour rupture of membranes, 4-hourly during waking hours (NICE 2014)
- use of prostaglandin (PGE_2)
- before and during transfusion of blood/blood products.

SITES FOR ADULT TEMPERATURE RECORDING

Choosing a site

Ideally a site would be convenient, pain-free, sensitive, and responsive, defined by a normal temperature range and independent of external effects (Davie & Amoore 2010). However, no one site meets these criteria and therefore the choice is made according to the equipment available and the following:

- known reliability of the site
- accessibility
- ability of the woman to comply
- safety
- local protocol.

These sites are generally readily accessible in adults and therefore are commonly considered:

- oral cavity
- tympanic membrane (ear)
- axilla
- forehead.

These four sites will be discussed in detail below. Other less common sites can also be used:

- Rectum: this is well insulated and considered to correlate with core temperature (approximately 0.5°C higher than the oral normal value) but it is slower to react to changes than other sites. It is less frequently used, being inaccessible and embarrassing for adults. The presence of faeces can create an inaccurate result and care should be taken not to damage the rectal mucosa. This site is generally avoided. The accepted normal temperature range is 34.4 to 37.8°C (Davie & Amoore 2010). Galinstan and electronic thermometers could be used.
- Oesophagus and pulmonary artery: while these may be very good sites, they are only accessible in high dependency care (e.g. intensive care unit), when such accuracy is essential and the readings can be safely obtained. Urinary catheters can also be adapted to accommodate a temperature probe, this also

remains within specialist care rather than everyday practice.
- The groin is considered useful for some circumstances but there is little in the literature to support this and there are no accepted normal values.
- Skin probes are used in environments such as the neonatal intensive care unit.

Oral site

Rationale for use and normal values

The thermometer is placed in one of the sublingual pockets, located on either side of the tongue (Fig. 3.1). A branch of the carotid artery, the sublingual artery, runs beneath the sublingual pocket (Closs 1987) and so, as a site, it can quickly track the changes in body temperature. It is a readily accessible site, with little inconvenience to the woman and minimal contact with body fluids. An acceptable adult oral temperature reading is between 36 and 37.6°C (Davie & Amoore 2010). The temperature in other parts of the mouth is lower than in the sublingual pocket. There is a temperature difference between the right and left sublingual pockets and between the front and back. The temperature in the mouth is also affected by environmental factors: drinking hot fluids and smoking can create an artificially high reading, while mouth breathing, tachypnoea, drinking iced fluids and not placing the thermometer far enough into the mouth can all create a falsely low reading (Sund-Levander & Grodzinsky 2013).

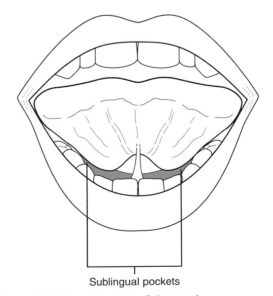

Sublingual pockets

Figure 3.1 Sublingual pockets of the mouth.

Safety and compliance

The woman will be required to hold the apparatus in her mouth with her mouth closed. The oral site should be avoided due to lack of compliance and/or potential danger for:

- labouring women
- anaesthetized, semi-conscious or unconscious women
- women likely to experience seizure, e.g. fulminating pre-eclampsia
- facial or oral impairment/injury
- known oral infection
- nausea or vomiting
- failure to gain consent.

It is therefore only a safe temperature measurement route for a coherent consenting adult.

Suitable equipment

Electronic, Galinstan-in-glass and disposable thermometers (pp. 32 and 33) are all suitable for oral use. Disposable protective covers should be used on galinstan and electronic devices unless using a disposable device. Mercury thermometers have been replaced by galinstan in glass in the UK. This thermometer needs 3 minutes in a sublingual pocket for an accurate result (Garner & Fendius 2011).

Tympanic membrane

Rationale for use and normal values

Advocates of the use of the tympanic membrane for temperature assessment suggest that the internal and external carotid arteries running in close proximity to both the membrane and the hypothalamus can adequately reflect core body temperature (El-Radhi 2013, Sund-Levander & Grodzinsky 2013). However, Davie & Amoore (2010) suggest that the evidence is inconclusive.

The auditory canal is insulated (maintaining the temperature of the site) and it is easily accessible. Tympanic thermometers give a reading (generally) within 3 seconds and so in many places it is the site of choice. Davie & Amoore (2010) suggest that normal values for this site are between 35.6 and 37.4°C, but wish the clinician to be aware that the thermometers themselves are manufactured and calibrated according to data from the clinical trials and therefore are an estimate only.

Suitable equipment

Temperature recordings from the tympanic membrane can only be taken with a specific tympanic thermometer (p. 33). Disposable covers reduce the cross-infection risk but are also integral to the thermometers design and use.

Accuracy

Accuracy is dependent upon the correct positioning of the equipment (user error is often significant (Davie & Amoore 2010)) and the ambient temperature in the ear. Any of the following factors in the ear can affect the validity of the recording:

- presence of moisture, e.g. vernix caseosa, amniotic fluid
- presence of hearing aid within the last 20 minutes (Pullen 2003)
- excessive ear wax
- otitis media
- recent ear surgery
- raised air temperature, e.g. an incubator
- dirty or moist lens on the equipment (45 minutes is needed after cleaning for it to dry before use).

The Medical and Healthcare products Regulation Agency (MHRA 2013) has received several alerts over the last decade with regard to tympanic thermometers. The auditory canal can be 2°C cooler than the tympanic membrane, it is important that the thermometer is placed correctly and takes its reading from the tympanic membrane.

Several studies or reviews (adult and neonatal) now suggest that tympanic thermometers (partly for their ease of use) are the most reliable (Bailey & Rose 2001, Dowding et al 2002, Woodrow et al 2006), but this is not by any means a consistent recommendation (Fawcett 2001, Fountain et al 2008, Scanga et al 2000). Fountain et al (2008) reviewed four studies and considered tympanic thermometers to be unreliable with poor performance, Counts et al (2014) agree. HIS (2012) also suggest in their summary that temporal artery thermometers (while still being questionable) frequently had greater accuracy than tympanic thermometers.

Axilla site

Rationale for use and normal values

Consensus across the literature is that the axilla is a poor choice of site for assessing temperature in adults. It relies on the skin folds meeting in the axilla, something that does not happen for thinner adults. It also often takes longer, is a poor predictor of core temperature, can be affected by sweat and ambient temperature (Davie & Amoore 2010, El-Radhi 2013, McCallum & Higgins 2012, Sund-Levander & Grodzinsky 2013). This contrasts with Fulbrook (1993), who believes that axilla temperatures are closely correlated with core temperature. Davie & Amoore (2010) suggest that the accepted normal values are between 35.5 and 37°C.

Safety and compliance

The axilla is usually accessible by moving clothes slightly and so compliance is good. The woman needs to be mindful of the fact that the thermometer is in the armpit and that mobility is restricted at that time.

Suitable equipment

Disposable, electronic, and galinstan in glass thermometers are all suitable for use in the axilla. Disposable covers should be used for galinstan and electronic thermometers.

Forehead

Rationale for use and normal values

The superficial temporal artery (containing blood from the heart) also stems from the external carotid artery (see oral site, p. 29). It runs up in front of the ear, then bifurcates so that one branch runs along the forehead and the other horizontally above the ear. It is considered to be about 1 mm beneath the skin of the forehead and therefore its 'accessibility' and its ability to represent the core body temperature cause it to be suggested as an appropriate temperature measurement site. However, Sund-Levander & Grodzinsky (2013) suggest that really it is the temperature of the skin that is being assessed and that this is open to large variations. Skin temperature readings can be affected by sweat, make-up, hair (or hats, wigs or bandages – anything that insulates the forehead), position of the device, room temperature, exercise and presence of excess subcutaneous fat. Normal values are suggested to be between 36.1 and 37.3°C.

Suitable equipment

Disposable liquid crystal thermometers and temporal artery thermometers (touch and non-touch) may all be used on the forehead. Temporal artery (TA) thermometers are infrared heat scanners and can generally only be used to scan the temporal artery.

Accuracy

As suggested above, accuracy can be affected by a number of variables. TA thermometers are a relatively new piece of equipment, there are few reliable studies on its accuracy and it is noted that the technology is likely to improve in the coming years.

Safety and compliance

The disruption to the woman when using the forehead is minimal. Liquid crystal thermometers are disposable, some TA thermometers do not touch the skin, while those that do have either disposable covers or an antibacterial coating. The infection risk is therefore small with both.

SITES FOR PAEDIATRIC TEMPERATURE RECORDING

An older, compliant child may be able to cope with any of the recognized sites that are used for temperature measurement (above). However, the newborn infant, or preterm infant nursed in an incubator are very different clinical situations. Booker (2014) suggests that there are problems with all of the potential sites for temperature measurement in babies, as well as potential problems with some of the equipment available.

The rectum has been traditionally used, it is considered to be close to the neonate's core and to be unaffected by environmental factors (Smith 2014). However, defaecation can be stimulated with the thermometer, and this can contribute to fluid loss. Vagal stimulation can occur (Bailey & Rose 2000) and care should be taken to avoid mucosal damage. The act of rectal thermometry is questioned in the light of safeguarding and El-Radhi (2013) questions the comfort, infection risk, and time-consuming nature of this site. Its reliability (as for adults) is also questionable. However, Landry et al (2013) compared continuous rectal thermistor probes with axilla readings for infants undergoing cooling and rewarming. They concluded that rectal measurements were more appropriate than axilla readings.

Temporal artery readings allow for minimal disruption to babies and young children, but their reliability is in doubt (Smith 2014). Tympanic readings can be taken, but accuracy depends on scanning the membrane, rather than the ear canal. Care should be taken to use the correct size of probe. Both these methods can be affected by ambient air temperature and so are not suitable to use for infants in an incubator.

The axilla site is commonly used for babies despite it being considered a poor indicator of core temperature. Generally the skin folds do meet in the axilla of babies and a range of thermometers can be used. It causes minimal disruption and discomfort. There is agreement internationally that the axilla is the site of choice for general temperature taking in neonates, (Asher & Northington 2008, KEMH 2014, Leduc & Woods 2013, NICE 2013) but it is also recognized that rectal is the definitive one. The axilla should be used with caution if pyrexia is present, due to its distance from the core and limited ability to respond quickly. As the body first responds to pyrexia, there is a vasomotor response in the skin; this can reduce peripheral temperature and therefore the axilla route is unlikely to show a pyrexial reading. NICE (2013) recommend that an electronic thermometer is used in the axilla.

Neonatal early warning systems (NEWS) are in use in many parts of the UK. There may be slight variations, but their use is similar to that recommended for adults (p. 28). Often scoring is in the form of traffic light coding (red, amber, green), rather than numerical scores (Roland et al 2010).

TYPES OF THERMOMETER

Choosing the equipment for temperature measurement may depend upon the site chosen and the availability of suitable apparatus. There is again no consensus as to the most accurate piece of equipment to use; Latman et al (2001) had doubts about the whole range of clinical thermometers in use.

Training should be given (and reinforced) and the equipment must always be used according to the manufacturer's instructions. Davie & Amoore (2010) suggest that the biggest variable in obtaining an accurate result is user error, often incorrect positioning of the apparatus. It should also be maintained (calibrated) and cleaned properly. The availability of some of the equipment discussed below may depend upon cost-effectiveness, local protocol, safety, and suitability. Temperature assessment is never made in isolation; how the woman/baby looks and feels is a very important part of this assessment.

Electronic thermometers

These will vary in appearance but are generally available in two designs (Fig. 3.2):
1. a digital reading at the end of the thermometer
2. a digital reading on the hand-held box attached to the temperature probe.

The reading usually occurs within 1 minute and an alarm sounds to indicate that this has happened. Oral, axilla or rectal sites may be used for the adult; the axilla is used for the baby. There is a danger of cross-infection, as the thermometer is often used for more than one woman. Disposable covers must be used and the thermometer must be cleaned and maintained according to the manufacturer's guidelines. Some electronic thermometers have a separate probe for rectal use (often red). Fountain et al (2008) suggest that electronic oral thermometers have a good level of agreement with core body temperature. Depending upon design, the midwife may have to choose which mode to operate the equipment in, predictive or monitoring.

PROCEDURE: electronic thermometer use in oral and axilla sites

- Gain informed consent, establish that temperature assessment is indicated.

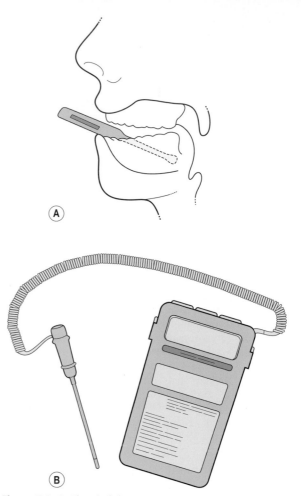

Figure 3.2 A, Electrical thermometer with digital reading; **B,** electrical thermometer with temperature probe.
(Adapted with kind permission from Jamieson et al 1997)

- Apply alcohol handrub.
- Take the thermometer and cover to the woman.
- Clarify if any environmental factors exist that may affect the reading, e.g. a recent hot drink.
- Apply a disposable cover, switch on the thermometer (choose the operating mode, if appropriate), allow it to self-calibrate and when ready insert correctly into the chosen site (posterior sublingual pocket, with mouth closed or placed centrally against chest wall in axilla with arm firmly pressing against it).
- Remove and read when the alarm sounds. Consider whether other vital sign observations need recording at this time also and note whether the reading on the thermometer seems consistent with how the woman is looking and feeling.

- Dispose of the cover correctly.
- Clean the thermometer according to manufacturer's instructions.
- Discuss the findings with the woman.
- Wash and dry hands.
- Document findings and act accordingly.

Summary

- A rapid, easy-to-use (if placed correctly in the site) and easy-to-read thermometer.
- Attention must be paid to the prevention of cross-infection and proper calibration/maintenance.

Tympanic thermometers

Tympanic membrane thermometers scan the tympanic membrane using an infrared scanner to take temperature measurements. Readings are made in less than 30 seconds and are displayed digitally. Clearly, the thermometer is only ever placed in the ear. As discussed earlier, some environmental conditions can affect the accuracy of the result (p. 30). It may be expensive initially and will require regular servicing and calibration. Most models use disposable probe covers, which are both integral to its design (and therefore accuracy) and to prevent cross-infection. The user should be properly instructed in its use, various parts of the auditory canal will be scanned unless the probe is correctly directed to the tympanic membrane, the differences in different parts of the ear canal are widely known (Davie & Amoore 2010).

PROCEDURE: tympanic thermometer use

Due to differences in manufacturers' designs, the reader is encouraged to read the specific instructions with their thermometer. These are general guidelines:

- Gain informed consent.
- Have clean hands and correctly calibrated equipment.
- Cover the thermometer tip with the supplied sheath.
- Switch the thermometer on.
- Aim to use the same ear for each assessment, and document which one.

- When it is ready to scan, insert into the ear canal. Models vary, some require the canal to be straight, (the pinna may be gently pulled upwards and backwards to achieve this (>1 year of age), some need a tight seal to be achieved, others need only a light seal. Mains et al (2008) suggest the tip should be pointing in a horizontal plane, i.e. pointing towards the opposite ear.
- Press the scan button, remove and read the thermometer when the alarm sounds. Note whether the reading on the thermometer seems consistent with how the woman is looking and feeling.
- Remove and dispose of the sheath.
- Switch off the thermometer.
- Wash and dry hands.
- Discuss the findings with the woman.
- Document the findings and act accordingly.

Summary

- A rapid technique causing minimal disruption to the woman, but with a high margin of error if technique is poor.

Disposable (chemical dot) thermometers

Disposable thermometers are widely available. Research into their accuracy is limited; however Fountain et al (2008) noted only non-significant differences between it and an electronic thermometer. El-Radhi (2013) would disagree. They are considered to be cheap, safe, and comfortable to use (Board 1995). They are made of flexible plastic with a series of chemical dots at one end. As the temperature rises, the dots undergo a chemical reaction and colour change (each one is 0.1°C higher than the previous one (Macqueen 2001)). The level to which the colour change has occurred is the point at which the temperature is read (Fig. 3.3). They are suitable for oral and axilla use for the adult, axilla only for the baby. Reliability is impaired if the thermometers are stored above 35°C. The manufacturer's instructions should be read before the thermometer is used.

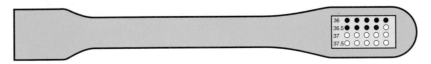

Figure 3.3 Disposable thermometer indicating a reading of 36.8°C.
(Adapted with kind permission from Jamieson et al 2002)

PROCEDURE: disposable thermometer use

The thermometer is used in the same way as an electronic thermometer (p. 32) except that:

- Oral recordings can be made after 1 minute, axilla after 3 minutes (Blumenthal 1992); an accurate time source is needed.
- Orally, it is placed into the posterior sublingual pocket with the dots either facing up or down. The tongue is down over the thermometer and the lips are closed.
- In the axilla, the chemical pads should be placed against the chest wall in a vertical position (Nicol et al 2008).
- The thermometer is given 10 seconds to stabilize before being read (may vary according to manufacturer).
- When reading the thermometer, the first dot on the line is the same as the number next to it. The number is then counted along according to the number of dots that have changed colour (Fig. 3.3 indicates 36.8°C).
- The thermometer is disposed of correctly.

Summary

- Disposable thermometers are easy to use and eliminate the dangers of cross-infection.
- Accuracy may be impaired under certain environmental conditions.

Temporal artery thermometers

These thermometers are used to assess body temperature via the temporal artery. As the equipment moves across the forehead, the scanner takes repeated measurements of the skin and ambient air temperatures. As for electronic thermometers, the result is achieved based on clinical data compiled into algorithms and therefore is an estimate of body temperature. There is a potential margin of error between manufacturers and their different data (Davie & Amoore 2010). Models vary, some (Exergen, Fig. 3.4) control for body sweat by placing the thermometer on the neck behind the earlobe after scanning the forehead and before releasing the scanner. Some models need a probe cover, some may scan other blood vessels in the body, some may be used in temperature-controlled environments like an incubator; in all circumstances the midwife should be fully trained to competently use whichever equipment is available.

PROCEDURE: temporal artery thermometer use

Due to differences in manufacturers' designs, the reader is encouraged to read the specific instructions with their thermometer. These are general guidelines but some thermometers do not touch the skin (and therefore have an even smaller infection control risk) but care would be taken to use it at the correct distance from the skin:

- Gain informed consent.
- Have clean hands, and clean and correctly calibrated equipment.
- Assess for the presence of perspiration; if none, continue.
- Position the sensor on the centre of the forehead, half way between the eyebrows and hair line.

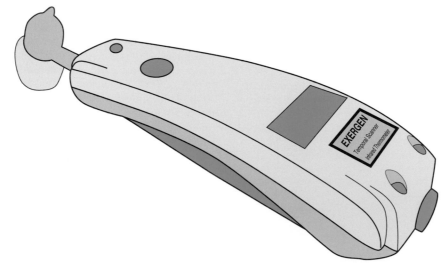

Figure 3.4 Temporal artery thermometer.

- Press and hold the 'scan' button.
- Lightly slide the thermometer to your left (patient's right) across the skin in a horizontal line as far as the edge of the forehead.
- Release the scan button, remove from the head, read the display. Note whether the reading on the thermometer seems consistent with how the woman is looking and feeling.
- The thermometer often switches off automatically. Clean the probe according to the manufacturer's instructions (often using an alcohol swab and left to air dry).
- Wash and dry hands.
- Discuss the findings with the woman.
- Document the findings and act accordingly.

If obvious perspiration is seen on the forehead then the measurement should be delayed until later. Alternatively the thermometer is used to scan the forehead as above, but with the scan button still depressed, it is then placed in the depression behind the right ear. The button is then released and the temperature read (Exergen 2005).

Summary

- A minimally invasive technique with small infection control risks but a questionable level of accuracy, particularly for vulnerable client groups.

Conclusion

When choosing a site for temperature recording in adults, consideration should be given to its accessibility, acceptability, known reliability, and safety. The midwife needs to recognize the strengths and limitations of each site and piece of equipment available in order to make accurate recordings of a temperature. Temperature assessment can provide evidence of the clinical condition and may lead to further investigations and treatment. However, evidence regarding reliability is inconclusive for all sites and equipment currently available in the UK.

TAKING A BABY'S TEMPERATURE

As suggested earlier, NICE (2013) recommend the axilla site, using an electronic thermometer (Fig. 3.5). Technically, disposable thermometers could also be used, and with caution tympanic and temporal artery thermometers, but these are less likely to be used in neonatal practice. The normal values for a neonatal axilla recording are between 36.7 and 37.3 °C.

Indications

- Following birth.
- For any baby for whom the early warning system pathway (NEWS, p. 31) is indicated, e.g. meconium

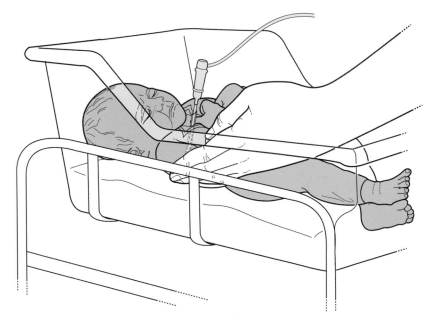

Figure 3.5 Taking a baby's temperature: axilla site using electronic thermometer.

aspiration, if active resuscitation was needed, prolonged rupture of membranes, maternal pyrexia or known infection, small for gestational age, preterm, poor feeding.

- At any time postnatally when the baby looks or feels cool, hot, red, pale, sweaty or unwell, is not feeding or has altered behaviour. Further action would likely follow, e.g. NEWS screening and referral.
- If receiving certain types of phototherapy treatment.

PROCEDURE: taking a baby's temperature (axilla site)

- Ideally, parents should accompany the baby, their informed consent having been gained.
- The thermometer chosen should agree with local policy and be appropriately cleaned and calibrated.
- Wash and dry hands.
- Observe the baby generally, particularly noting its colour, behaviour and other clinical indicators.
- The baby is placed in a safe and warm environment, e.g. in the cot or in the mother's arms.
- Clothing is loosened so that the axilla is accessible; the baby is not allowed to chill, but if respiration is being counted at the same time then the chest may be exposed (Chapter 6).
- The covered thermometer is placed into the axilla and the arm held gently across the chest to keep the thermometer secure (Fig. 3.5).
- After the required length of time (depending on thermometer choice) the thermometer is removed and read. The clothing is replaced and the baby returned to his parents.
- Records are made and action taken according to the findings.

ROLE AND RESPONSIBILITIES OF THE MIDWIFE

These can be summarized as:

- recognizing the significance of an accurate temperature measurement and when to undertake it
- the use of appropriate equipment in the correct sites, recognizing the need for consistency and to reduce user error
- referral or further action, if indicated
- contemporaneous record keeping
- appropriate communication, including patient education, in gaining informed consent.

SELF-ASSESSMENT EXERCISES

The answers to the following questions may be found in the text:

1. Discuss the factors that influence body temperature.
2. What is the normal temperature range for the woman and how does this alter during the ante-, intra- and postpartum periods?
3. Describe the measures that should be taken at delivery to promote neonatal thermoregulation.
4. List the occasions when temperature assessment is undertaken for a childbearing woman and a newborn baby.
5. Discuss the advantages and disadvantages of each of the sites for temperature assessment.
6. What would you say to someone who did not know what a temporal artery thermometer was?
7. Demonstrate taking a woman's temperature using a tympanic thermometer.
8. Demonstrate taking a baby's temperature using the axilla site.
9. Summarize the role and responsibilities of the midwife when undertaking temperature assessment.

REFERENCES

Asher, C., Northington, L., 2008. SPN News. Position statement for measurement of temperature/fever in children. J. Pediatr. Nurs. 23 (3), 234–236.

Bailey, J., Rose, P., 2000. Temperature measurement in the preterm infant: a literature review. J. Neonatal Nurs. 6 (1), 28–32.

Bailey, J., Rose, P., 2001. Axillary and tympanic membrane temperature recording in the preterm neonate: a comparative study. J. Adv. Nurs. 34 (4), 465–474.

Black, L., 1972. Neonatal Emergencies and other Problems. Butterworth Heinemann, Oxford.

Blackburn, S.T., 2013. Maternal, Fetal and Neonatal Physiology: A Clinical Perspective, fourth ed. Elsevier Saunders, Maryland Heights, pp. 657–679. (Chapter 20).

Blumenthal, I., 1992. Should we ban the mercury thermometer? J. R. Soc. Med. 85 (9), 533–555.

Board, M., 1995. Comparison of disposable and mercury in glass thermometers. Nurs. Times 91 (33), 36–37.

Booker, H., 2014. The hypothermic term infant. Br. J. Midwifery 22 (1), 59–64.

Chinyanga, H.M., 1991. Temperature regulation and anaesthesia. In: Schönbaum, E., Lomax, P. (Eds.), Thermoregulation: Pathology, Pharmacology and Therapy. Pergamon Press, New York. (Chapter 9).

Closs, J., 1987. Oral temperature measurement. Nurs. Times 7, 36–39.

Counts, D., Acosta, M., Holbrook, H., et al., 2014. Evaluation of Temporal artery and disposable digital oral thermometers in acutely ill patients. Medsurg Nurs. 23 (4), 239–250.

Davie, A., Amoore, J., 2010. Best practice in the measurement of body temperature. Nurs. Stand. 24 (42), 42–49.

Dowding, D., Freeman, S., Nimmo, S., et al., 2002. An investigation into the accuracy of different types of thermometers. Prof. Nurse 18 (3), 166–168.

Dubois, E.F., 1948. Fever and the Regulation of Body Temperature. C C Thomas, Springfield.

El-Radhi, A., 2013. Temperature measurement: the right thermometer and site. Br. J. Nurs. 22 (4), 208–211.

Exergen, 2005. Temporal artery thermometer instructions for use. Available online: <http://www.exergen.com/medical/PDFs/tat2000instrev6.pdf> (accessed 23 November 2014).

Fawcett, J., 2001. The accuracy and reliability of the tympanic membrane thermometer: a literature review. Emerg. Nurse 8 (9), 13–17.

Fountain, C., Goins, L., Hartman, M., et al., 2008. Evaluating the accuracy of four temperature instruments on an adult oncology unit. Clin. J. Oncol. Nurs. 12 (6), 983–987.

Fulbrook, P., 1993. Core temperature measurement in adults: a literature review. J. Adv. Nurs. 18, 1451–1460.

Garner, A., Fendius, A., 2011. Temperature physiology, assessment and control. Br. J. Neurosci. Nurs. 6 (8), 397–400.

Grainger, A., 2013. Principles of temperature monitoring. Nurs. Stand. 27 (50), 48–55.

Hinchliff, S.M., Montague, S.E., Watson, R., 1996. Physiology for Nursing Practice, second ed. Baillière Tindall, London.

HIS (Health Improvement Scotland), 2012. Temporal Artery thermometers Technologies Scoping Report 11. Available online: <http://www.healthcareimprovementscotland.org/our_work/technologies_and_medicines/earlier_scoping_reports/technologies_scoping_report_11.aspx> (accessed 5 March 2015).

Houdas, Y., Ring, E.F.J., 1982. Human Body Temperature. Plenum Press, New York.

Jamieson, E.M., McCall, J.M., Blythe, R., et al., 1997. Clinical Nursing Practices, third ed. Churchill Livingstone, Edinburgh.

Jamieson, E.M., McCall, J., Whyte, L., 2002. Clinical Nursing Practices, fourth ed. Churchill Livingstone, Edinburgh.

Kalant, H., Lé, A.D., 1991. Effects of ethanol on thermoregulation. In: Schönbaum, E., Lomax, P. (Eds.), Thermoregulation: Pathology, Pharmacology and Therapy. Pergamon Press, New York. (Chapter 15).

KEMH (King Edward Memorial Hospital), 2014. Management of the neonate with a temperature below 36.5°C. Clinical Guideline. Available online: <http://kemh.health.wa.gov.au/development/manuals/O&G_guidelines/sectionb/10/b10.2.7.pdf> (accessed 5 March 2015).

Landry, M., Doyle, L., Lee, K., Jacobs, S., 2013. Axillary temperature measurement during hypothermia treatment for neonatal hypoxic-ischaemic encephalopathy. Arch. Dis. Child. 98 (1), F54–F58.

Latman, N., Hans, P., Nicholson, L., et al., 2001. Evaluation of clinical thermometers for accuracy and reliability. Biomed. Instrum. Technol. 3594, 259–265.

Leduc, D., Woods, S., 2013. Temperature measurement in paediatrics, position statement Canadian Paediatric Society. Available online: <www.cps.ca/documents/position/temperature-measurement> (accessed 5 March 2015).

Macqueen, S., 2001. Clinical benefits of 3M Tempa•DOT thermometer in paediatric settings. Br. J. Nurs. 10 (1), 55–57.

Mains, J.A., Coxall, K., Lloyd, H., 2008. Measuring temperature. Nurs. Stand. 22 (39), 44–47.

McCallum, L., Higgins, D., 2012. Measuring body temperature. Nurs. Times 108 (45), 20–22.

MHRA (Medical and Healthcare Products Regulation Agency), 2013. One liners issue 97 June 2013. Available online: <http://www.mhra.gov.uk/Publications/Safetyguidance/OneLiners/CON286866> (accessed 23 November 2014).

NICE (National Institute for Health and Care Excellence), 2013. Feverish Illness in Children. Assessment and Initial Management in Children

Younger Than 5 Years Clinical Guideline 160. NICE, London. Available online: <www.nice.org.uk> (accessed 5 March 2015).

NICE (National Institute for Health and Care Excellence), 2014. Intrapartum Care: Care of Healthy Women and Their Babies during Childbirth Clinical Guideline 190. NICE, London. Available online: <www.nice.org.uk> (accessed 5 March 2015).

Nicol, M., Bavin, C., Cronin, P., Rawlings-Anderson, K., 2008. Essential Nursing Skills, third ed. Mosby, Edinburgh, pp. 2–7.

Pullen, R., 2003. Using an ear thermometer. Nursing 33 (5), 24.

Roland, D., Madar, J., Connolly, G., 2010. The newborn early warning (NEW)

system: development of an at risk infant intervention system. Infant 6 (4), 116–120.

Scanga, A., Wallace, R., Kiehl, E., et al., 2000. A comparison of four methods of normal newborn temperature measurement. MCN 25 (2), 76–79.

Schönbaum, E., Lomax, P. (Eds.), 1991. Temperature regulation and drugs: an introduction. In: Thermoregulation: Pathology, Pharmacology and Therapy. Pergamon Press, New York. (Chapter 1).

Smith, J., 2014. Methods and Devices of Temperature measurement in the neonate: a narrative review and practice recommendations. Newborn Infant Nurs. Rev. 14 (2), 64–71.

Sund-Levander, M., Grodzinsky, E., 2010. What is the evidence base for the

assessment and evaluation of body temperature? Nurs. Times 106 (1), 10–13.

Sund-Levander, M., Grodzinsky, E., 2013. Assessment of body temperature measurement options. Br. J. Nurs. 22 (16), 942–950.

WHO (World Health Organisation), 1997. Thermal protection of the newborn: a practical guide. Online. Available online: <http://whqlibdoc.who.int/hq/1997/WHO_RHT_MSM_97.2.pdf> (accessed 13 November 2014).

Woodrow, P., May, V., Buras-Rees, S., et al., 2006. Comparing no-touch and tympanic thermometer temperature recordings. Br. J. Nurs. 15 (18), 1012–1016.

Chapter | 4 |

Assessment of maternal and neonatal vital signs: pulse measurement

LEARNING OUTCOMES

Having read this chapter, the reader should be able to:

- discuss factors that influence the heart rate
- discuss the significance of an abnormal rate, rhythm and or amplitude for the woman
- identify the normal range for the childbearing woman and baby
- discuss the midwife's role and responsibilities in relation to pulse assessment, identifying when, where and how it is undertaken
- discuss why manual assessment of the pulse is important.

The pulse is a direct indicator of the action of the heart and provides information about cardiac function and peripheral perfusion (Dearsley 2013); the midwife should recognise the significance of it as an assessor of wellbeing. Assessment of cardiovascular function also includes observing the general appearance of the woman and looking for any signs and symptoms of dysfunction, e.g. cyanosis, pallor, cool skin, temperature (Dearsley 2013). From such a straightforward observation, much information can be gained, and using the correct technique each time increases the reliability of the results. The pulse rate can be visualized with electronic equipment, e.g. electronic blood pressure machine, oxygen saturation monitors. However, these do not take the place of a regular manual assessment by the midwife as they provide no information on rhythm or amplitude. This chapter examines pulse assessment: what it is, how, when and why it is completed. Factors affecting heart rate are also discussed; other means of pulse assessment are discussed briefly. Assessment of the fetal heart is discussed in Chapter 1.

Definition

A pulse is created as the left ventricle contracts causing blood to be ejected into the circulation and a series of pressure waves within the arteries circulate the blood around the body. The pulse can be felt by compressing an artery against a bone or firm tissue and assessed for rate, rhythm and amplitude (volume).

FACTORS INFLUENCING THE HEART RATE

The heart rate is controlled by the conducting system of the heart and the autonomic nervous system. The sinoatrial node within the heart initiates impulses that spread across the conducting system to all areas of cardiac muscle causing atrial then ventricular contraction. The parasympathetic nerve fibres – primarily the vagus nerve – reduce the heart rate while the sympathetic nerve fibres increase the heart rate. Cardiac activity is also affected by chemicals and ions, e.g. adrenaline will increase the heart rate, excess potassium ions decrease the heart's ability to contract (Dearsley 2013).

The following factors increase the rate:

- exercise
- pregnancy and labour (discussed below)
- changes in position, e.g. from sitting to standing
- emotions: stress, anxiety, nervousness, fear, excitement
- gender: females have a slightly higher pulse rate than males
- pain
- infection (with or without changes to other vital signs)
- pyrexia – the pulse can increase 7–10 bpm with each degree the temperature increases
- haemorrhage
- shock
- shortage of red blood cells, e.g. iron-deficiency anaemia
- fluid and/or electrolyte imbalances, including dehydration
- anaphylaxis: causes the pulse to be weak, tachycardic, and irregular
- medications, e.g. salbutamol
- disease, e.g. hyperthyroidism, pulmonary embolism.

The following factors reduce the rate:

- rest and relaxation: calm, controlled breathing can reduce the heart rate
- sleep
- good exercise tolerance: in athletes
- age: heart rate decreases with increasing age
- insult or injury: myocardial infarction or other injury might cause the heart to slow or stop
- hypothermia
- medications, e.g. digoxin
- disease, e.g. hypothyroidism.

NORMAL VALUES

A healthy, non-pregnant female adult has a regular heart rate of approximately 65–85 bpm (Docherty & Coote 2006) (although Edmunds et al (2011) suggest it is 55–90), with the normal range between 60 and 100 bpm.

Tachycardia refers to an abnormally fast pulse rate above 100 bpm and is often one of the first signs of deterioration (Jevon 2010). Churchill et al (2014) advise that a sustained tachycardia above 90 bpm combined with pyrexia, tachypnoea or new onset confusion, OR a heart rate >130 bpm regardless of other signs, is a red flag and warrants prompt referral of the woman for hospital assessment or urgent investigation if she is already an in-patient, due to the association with sepsis.

Bradycardia is a slow heart rate, generally considered to be below 60 bpm, although Higgins (2008) suggests it should be considered bradycardic when the pulse rate is below 50 bpm. Athletes and other physically fit people commonly have a pulse rate below 60 bpm (Dearsley 2013). Bradycardia in an unwell person can indicate poor perfusion (Jevon 2010).

The pulse rhythm should be regular; an irregular pulse (arrhythmia) reflects an irregular pumping action of the heart which may be due to an electrolyte imbalance or damaged cardiac tissue (Dearsley 2013). The amplitude indicates changes in the volume of blood being pumped around the body, the pulse strength and elasticity of the arterial wall. It is subjectively described as 'normal', 'weak' or 'thready' (indicative of poor cardiac output which may be due to hypovolaemia possibly from shock, haemorrhage, cardiac tissue damage), 'rapid', 'full' or 'bounding' (may be due to infection, hypertension, strenuous exercise, strong emotions (Alexis 2010, Dearsley 2013). Where the pulse is so weak it cannot be palpated, it is said to be 'imperceptible' (Dearsley 2013).

A newborn baby has a heart rate of 100–160 bpm (England 2014), although the heart rate varies noticeably with respiration in the newborn; hence it is important to count for 1 minute.

CHANGES RELATED TO CHILDBIRTH

Pregnancy

During pregnancy the maternal heart rate increases gradually and by 32 weeks it is 10–20 bpm higher. The rate declines slightly during the third trimester and in some women it returns to the prepregnancy level at term (Blackburn 2013).

Mild cardiac arrhythmias and murmurs may occur during pregnancy and are usually benign but warrant further investigation (Blackburn 2013). However, the presence of cardiac disease places additional stress on the cardiovascular system of a pregnant woman. Knight et al (2014) report 54 deaths from cardiac disease in childbirth in the UK during the triennium 2010–2012. It was the most common cause of death overall, and the highest number since reporting began. Women with existing cardiac problems or any presenting symptoms need careful combined cardiac and obstetric care from doctors with expertise in cardiac disease in pregnancy.

Labour

During labour each contraction returns 300–500 mL of blood to the circulation increasing cardiac output but the effect on the heart rate is variable and may increase or decrease. An increase in the number and variety of arrhythmias may also be seen during labour (Blackburn 2013).

Postnatal period: maternal

There are changes to the cardiovascular system during the puerperium as it reverts back to its prepregnant state. The heart rate generally reaches its prepregnancy rate by 10 days postpartum (Blackburn 2013)

Postnatal period: baby

Blackburn (2013) advises the baby's heart rate is high for the first hour of life and slowly decreases up to late adolescence.

SITES FOR PULSE MEASUREMENT

A pulse can be felt anywhere in the body where an artery near to the surface can be palpated against something firm, usually bone or tendon. The heart rate can also be heard by using a stethoscope.

The most commonly used site in the adult is the radial artery, being readily accessible; other sites are indicated in Figure 4.1. The radial pulse of the right wrist is best palpated by the midwife's left hand, and vice versa. The right radial pulse is less accurate in assessing amplitude due to its distance from the heart compared to the left radial pulse, but can be used for assessing the rate and rhythm (Docherty & Coote 2006). To find the radial pulse, place the index and middle finger gently in the groove of the woman's wrist that lies beneath the thumb. If a pulsation cannot be felt, the fingers should be moved gently along the groove until the pulse is located. If the pulse is difficult to palpate, exert

more pressure from the middle finger as this can amplify the pulse wave against the index finger. The amount of pressure applied may need to be increased or decreased as well. The thumb should not be used to feel for the pulse as the thumb has a strong pulse which can be mistaken for that of the woman (deWit & O'Neill 2014).

The brachial artery is used in the measurement of blood pressure and is located in the antecubital fossa. The woman should have her arm slightly bent with the palm uppermost and the midwife places her index and middle finger on the inner side of the crease of the elbow. Apply firm pressure for 5 seconds; if no pulsation is felt, begin again in the centre of the crease moving the fingers towards the woman's body.

The carotid or femoral arteries may be palpated in the case of collapse, where cardiac output cannot be detected in the peripheral circulation or with the critically ill person as they reflect the quality of the left ventricular function better than the radial or brachial pulse (Docherty & Coote 2006). The carotid pulse is found by placing 3–4 fingertips against the larynx (at the top of the neck just under the jaw, mid-point between the chin and earlobe), using gentle pressure on one side only. If both sides are compressed the arterial circulation to the brain can be cut off. To locate the femoral pulse, the woman needs to be lying flat with the groin exposed. Three fingers are placed over the superior pubic ramus (near the crease of the groin) and direct downward pressure is applied (this may be quite deep) to feel the pulsation. It may take several attempts to locate and is difficult to find in obese, agitated or confused people (Docherty & Coote 2006). Palpation of the femoral arteries in the baby is also part of the neonatal examination.

Where there is an inconsistency between the heart beat and the peripheral pulse, the two can be counted together (apical and radial) by two midwives. The midwife counting the apical assessment uses the diaphragm side of the stethoscope, placing it in the midline on the left side of the chest between the fifth and sixth ribs. Both midwives should have access to the watch, and agree when to begin and finish the minute's recording so they both record for the same period of time (Jevon 2007). Both readings are recorded using different coloured inks. If the stethoscope being used does not belong to the midwife, the earpieces should be disinfected before and after use, e.g. with an alcohol-impregnated swab (Lippincott et al 2013). The diaphragm and bell should also be disinfected before and after use to reduce the effect of cross-contamination (Campos-Murguia et al 2014).

In the baby, the most usual site of pulse measurement is either apical (which can be heard with a stethoscope or felt) or if this is not accessible, the brachial (Fig. 4.2). Listening to the apical beat has greater reliability and is recommended.

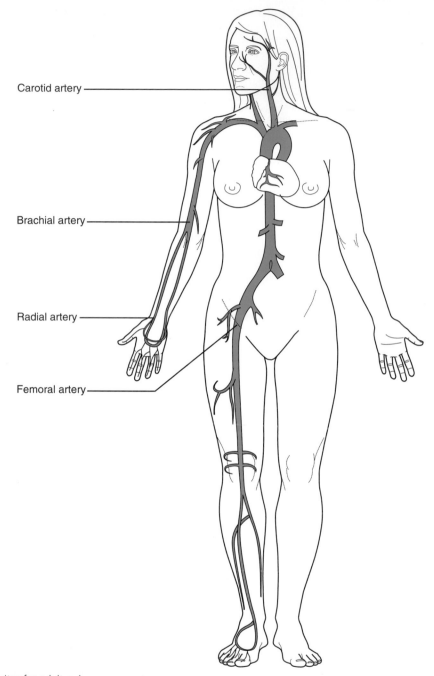

Carotid artery

Brachial artery

Radial artery

Femoral artery

Figure 4.1 Main sites for adult pulse assessment.
(Adapted with kind permission from Thibodeau & Patton 2012)

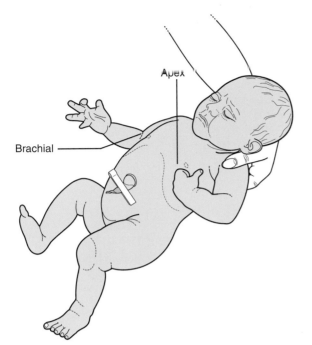

Figure 4.2 Main sites for neonatal pulse assessment.

INDICATIONS

While care should be individual and according to need, indications for pulse assessment are:

Maternal

- On admission, as a baseline recording.
- Any deviation from normal, signs of illness or accident or when the Modified Early Obstetric Warning Score (MEOWS) triggers further investigation and repeat of the vital signs (p. 66).
- Prior to undertaking blood pressure measurements especially when using an electronic sphygmomanometer to ensure there are no irregularities of the pulse (NICE 2011a).
- When auscultating the fetal heart including when applying a cardiotocograph (p. 16).
- During labour – hourly (but not during a contraction) and prior to transfer of care following labour (NICE 2014).
- Following recovery from anaesthesia, NICE (2011b) recommends the pulse should be recorded every half hour for 2 hours, and hourly thereafter provided that the observations are stable. Meakins (2011), however, advises recording the pulse every 15 minutes for the

first 2 hours, then every half hour for 2 hours, followed by 2-hourly for the first 2 days and then 4-hourly for a further 3 days.

- Postnatal assessment, if indicated.
- Prelabour spontaneous rupture of membranes.
- Treatment for preterm labour using tocolytic drugs.
- Following intrathecal or with patient-controlled anaesthesia (PCA) opioid use (according to local protocol).
- Before, during and following a blood transfusion (Chapter 49).

Baby

- At delivery as part of Apgar scoring (p. 294) and resuscitation (see Chapter 56).
- Any signs of cyanosis, irritability or illness.
- As part of vital sign observations for suspected or potential infection, e.g. prolonged rupture of membranes, known maternal *group B streptococcus*, meconium aspiration.

Documentation

Pulse assessment can be written in the woman's/baby's records as prose. However, if repeated observations are undertaken, an overall picture is obtained if the findings are recorded pictorially on an observations chart, particularly the MEOWS chart or partogram. This will show at a glance if there is a pattern emerging or if the condition is changing and triggering further investigation.

PROCEDURE: adult radial pulse

- Obtain informed consent, ensure the woman is comfortable and if possible in the same position as the last assessment.
- Wash and dry hands.
- Locate the radial artery (preferably the left), pressing down using moderate pressure and supporting the woman's wrist and arm across her chest (if the wrist is held too firmly the pulse may be occluded, if held too lightly it is difficult to count).
- Count the pulse for 30 seconds if it is regular, then double it, or 60 seconds if irregular or slow, noting also the rhythm and amplitude.
- Undertake respiration assessment (see Chapter 6) if necessary.
- Discuss the results with the woman, explaining whether and when it will be necessary to re-assess the pulse.
- Wash and dry hands.
- Document the findings and act accordingly.

PROCEDURE: baby

The baby should be peaceful and not crying when undergoing pulse assessment. When using a stethoscope, the bell/diaphragm should be disinfected before and after use and if it does not belong to the midwife, the earpieces should also be disinfected prior to and following use (Campos-Murguia et al 2014).

- Obtain informed consent from the parents, expecting at least one parent to be present throughout.
- Wash and dry hands.
- Loosen the clothing and access the chosen site.
- Place a warmed stethoscope over the apex of the heart (midline, left side of the chest); *or* place index and middle fingers over the apex; *or* place the index and middle fingers over the brachial artery. Count the pulse for 60 seconds, noting amplitude and rhythm.
- Observe the colour, behaviour and general condition of the baby at the same time. Other vital sign observations may also be undertaken, e.g. temperature, respiratory assessment.
- Replace the clothing and ensure comfort.
- Discuss the results with his parents.
- Wash and dry hands and clean the stethoscope if used.
- Document the findings and act accordingly.

Other means of pulse measurement

- ECG (electrocardiogram) monitors give a continuous or single reading, or printout of the heart rate and pattern.
- Automated blood pressure machines may provide a single heart rate reading.
- Pulse oximeters (see Chapter 6) also give a continuous heart rate reading, as do cardiotocograph machines for fetal heart assessment when the finger probe is attached (see Chapter 1).

ROLE AND RESPONSIBILITIES OF THE MIDWIFE

These can be summarized as:
- recognizing what constitutes a normal pulse rate, rhythm and amplitude and identifying deviations
- recognizing when pulse assessment is indicated
- undertaking the assessment correctly
- referral if indicated
- contemporaneous record keeping.

SUMMARY

- Pulse assessment is a straightforward, non-invasive skill of considerable importance.
- An accurate assessment includes the rate, rhythm and amplitude of the pulse.
- Assessment of the general condition of the woman or baby is made simultaneously.

SELF-ASSESSMENT EXERCISES

The answers to the following questions may be found in the text:
1. Discuss the significance of pulse assessment and when it should be undertaken for the childbearing woman.
2. What changes occur to the heart rate during pregnancy and labour and why do they occur?
3. Discuss the factors that increase the heart rate.
4. Summarize the role and responsibilities of the midwife when undertaking pulse assessment.

REFERENCES

Alexis, O., 2010. Providing best practice in manual pulse measurement. Br. J. Nurs. 19 (4), 228–234.

Blackburn, S., 2013. Maternal, Fetal and Neonatal Physiology: A Clinical Perspective, fourth ed. Saunders, St. Louis, pp. 252–296.

Campos-Murguia, A., Leon-Lara, X., Munoz, J., et al., 2014. Stethoscopes as potential intrahospital carriers of pathogenic microorganisms. Am. J. Infect. Control 42 (1), 82–83.

Churchill, D., Rodger, A., Clift, J., Tuffnell, D., on behalf of the MBRRACE-UK sepsis chapter writing group, 2014. Think sepsis. In: Knight, M., Kenyon, S., Brocklehurst, P., et al. on behalf of MBRRACE-UK (Eds.), Saving Lives, Improving Mothers' Care – Lessons Learned to Inform Future Maternity Care from the UK and Ireland Confidential Enquiries into Maternal Deaths and Morbidity 2009–12. National Perinatal Epidemiology Unit, Oxford, pp. 27–43.

Dearsley, A., 2013. Vital signs. In: Koutoukidis, G., Stainton, K., Hughson, J. (Eds.), 2013. Tabbner's Nursing Care, sixth ed. Churchill Livingstone, Chatswood, pp. 301–331.

deWit, S., O'Neill, P., 2014. Fundamental Concepts and Skills for Nursing, fourth ed. Elsevier, St. Louis, p. 348.

Docherty, B., Coote, S., 2006. Monitoring the pulse as part of track and trigger. Nurs. Times 102 (43), 28–29.

Edmunds, S., Hollis, V., Lamb, J., Todd, J., 2011. Observations. In: Dougherty, L., Lister, S. (Eds.), The Royal Marsden Hospital Manual of Clinical Nursing Procedures, eighth ed. Wiley-Blackwell, Oxford, pp. 749–755.

England, C., 2014. Recognising the healthy baby at term through examination of the newborn screening. In: Marshall, J., Raynor, M. (Eds.), 2014 Myles Textbook for Midwives, sixteenth ed. Elsevier, Edinburgh, pp. 591–610.

Higgins, D., 2008. Patient Assessment: part 5 – Measuring Pulse. Nurs. Times 104 (11), 24–25.

Jevon, P., 2007. Cardiac Monitoring part 4: Monitoring the apex beat. Nurs. Times 103 (4), 28–29.

Jevon, P., 2010. How to ensure patient observations lead to effective management of tachycardia. Nurs. Times 106 (3), 16–17.

Knight, M., Nair, M., Shah, A., et al., 2014. Maternal mortality and morbidity in the UK 2009–2012: surveillance and epidemiology. In: Knight, M., Kenyon, S., Brocklehurst, P., et al. on behalf of MBRRACE-UK (Eds.), Saving Lives, Improving Mothers' Care – Lessons Learned to Inform Future Maternity Care from the UK and Ireland Confidential Enquiries into Maternal Deaths and Morbidity 2009-12. National Perinatal Epidemiology Unit, Oxford, pp. 9–26.

Lippincott, Williams, Wilkins, 2013. Lippincott's Nursing Procedures, sixth ed. Wolters Kluwer, Philadelphia, pp. 614–616.

Meakins, S., 2011. Procedures in obstetrics. In: Macdonald, S., Magill-Cuerden, J. (Eds.), Mayes Midwifery, fourteenth ed. Elsevier, Edinburgh, pp. 839–850.

NICE (National Institute for Health and Clinical Excellence), 2011a. Hypertension: management of hypertension in adults in primary care. Available online: <www.nice.org.uk> (accessed 1 March 2015).

NICE (National Institute for Health and Clinical Excellence), 2011b. CG 132 Caesarean Section. Available online: <www.nice.org.uk> (accessed 1 March 2015).

NICE (National Institute for Health and Care Excellence), 2014. CG55 Intrapartum Care: Care of healthy women and their babies during childbirth. Available online: <www.nice.org.uk> (accessed 22 February 2015).

Thibodeau, G., Patton, K., 2012. Structure and Function of the Body, fourteenth ed. Elsevier-Mosby, St. Louis, p. 293.

Chapter | 5 |

Assessment of maternal and neonatal vital signs: blood pressure measurement

LEARNING OUTCOMES

Having read this chapter, the reader should be able to:

- define blood pressure, identifying the difference between systolic and diastolic pressure and the normal range for the childbearing woman and baby
- discuss the midwife's role and responsibilities in relation to the measurement of blood pressure, identifying when and how it is undertaken
- discuss the factors that influence blood pressure including the changes relating to childbearing
- discuss factors that influence the accuracy of blood pressure measurement and how the midwife can minimize these
- describe how central venous pressure is measured using a manual manometer.

Death from hypertensive disease, particularly pre-eclampsia and eclampsia, is the fourth highest direct cause of maternal deaths in the UK and is at its lowest rate since the 1985–87 triennial report (Knight et al 2014). Across the world, it is consistently in the top three causes of maternal mortality. The World Health Organization (WHO) (2011) advise that within Africa and Asia almost 10% of maternal deaths are associated with hypertensive disorders of pregnancy, which is similar to the US rates (CDC 2014), New Zealand (PMMRC 2013), and other developed countries; however, this increases to 25% in Latin America.

The midwife is ideally placed to measure blood pressure in the childbearing woman, confirming normality, detecting deviations from normal and referring the woman for further assessment. It is crucial the midwife carries out this procedure accurately as changes in blood pressure can have serious consequences for both the woman and the fetus/baby. This chapter considers the issues surrounding the accurate measurement of arterial blood pressure, physiology, influencing factors, and changes that occur during childbirth. The equipment used, technique of blood pressure measurement and factors influencing the accuracy of the recording are discussed. The chapter concludes with a discussion of venous blood pressure measurement.

Definition

Blood pressure is the force exerted by the blood on the blood vessel walls. It varies within the different blood vessels, being highest in the large arteries closest to the heart and decreasing gradually within the smaller arteries, arterioles and capillaries. Blood pressure continues to reduce as blood returns to the heart via the venules and veins. Blood pressure measurement usually reflects the arterial blood pressure, although venous pressure may also be measured. The brachial artery is generally used to measure blood pressure in the adult.

Arterial blood pressure

This is the pressure exerted on the arterial walls to facilitate blood flow around the body to ensure adequate oxygenation of the tissues and vital organs. It is not constant, increasing during ventricular contraction (systole) and decreasing when the ventricles relax (diastole). When recording blood pressure, it is important to assess both the highest and lowest levels of pressure as these reflect differing physiological responses of the cardiac cycle. The arterial blood pressure measurement is documented numerically in millimetres of mercury – e.g. systole 130 mmHg and diastole 80 mmHg, pronounced 130 over 80.

Systolic blood pressure (SBP)

This is the pressure exerted on the blood vessel walls following ventricular systole when the arteries contain the most blood and is the time of maximal pressure. SBP is determined by the:

- amount of blood ejected into the arteries (stroke volume)
- force of the contraction
- distensibility of the arterial wall.

An increase in the first two factors or a decrease in the third factor raises SBP, and vice versa.

Diastolic blood pressure (DBP)

This is the pressure exerted on the blood vessel walls during ventricular diastole when the arteries contain the least amount of blood, resulting in the least pressure being exerted on the blood vessel walls. DBP is influenced by the:

- degree of peripheral resistance
- systolic pressure
- cardiac output.

DBP is lower when these are reduced, particularly when the heart rate is slower as there is less blood remaining in the arteries.

Mean arterial pressure (MAP)

The mean arterial pressure is the average pressure required to push the blood through the circulatory system. It provides a sensitive indicator of acute changes in perfusion pressure making it a valuable tool in caring for the critically ill woman (Roberts 2006) and is a better indicator of perfusion than SBP. Perrin & MacLeod (2013) suggest a MAP >60 indicates adequate perfusion. The MAP assists with interpreting changes occurring in blood pressure measurements when the systolic and diastolic pressures alter at different rates. It can be estimated electronically or mathematically using the formula:

$$\text{Mean arterial pressure} = \tfrac{1}{3}\text{ systolic pressure} + \tfrac{2}{3}\text{ diastolic pressure.}$$

Alternatively, it can be calculated quickly by doubling the diastolic pressure reading, adding it to the systolic reading and dividing the total by three. Thus a blood pressure of 110/65 mmHg has a MAP of 80 mmHg while a blood pressure of 150/90 mmHg has a MAP of 110 mmHg.

Pulse pressure

This is the difference between SBP and DBP, a normal SBP is around 40 mmHg higher than the DBP (Lippincott et al 2013). A rise in pulse pressure results from an increased SBP and/or a decrease in DBP due to increased stroke volume, decreased peripheral resistance or both and is associated with infection, pyrexia, exercise and bradycardia. A decrease in pulse pressure is due to a decrease in SBP and/or an increase in DBP resulting from decreased stroke volume, increased peripheral resistance or both and can result from hypovolaemia, e.g. shock and haemorrhage. A narrowing pulse pressure can indicate increasing blood loss (Perrin & MacLeod 2013).

Venous blood pressure

This is the pressure exerted on the walls of the veins, reflecting venous flow to the heart (particularly circulating blood volume) and cardiac function. Central venous pressure (CVP) measures the pressure within the right atrium and is determined by:

- the volume of blood entering the right atrium (venous return)
- right ventricular function
- venous tone
- intrathoracic pressure.

Normal maternal arterial values

Edmunds et al (2011) suggest the normal range for a healthy adult at rest is 110–140/70–80 mmHg, while Dearsley (2013) suggests it is 100–120/60–80 mmHg. Blood pressure varies according to age and other variables. Both the National Institute for Health and Care Excellence (NICE) (2010) and the WHO (2013) define hypertension (raised blood pressure) as an SBP ≥ 140 mmHg and a DBP ≥ 90 mmHg. Lowe et al (2014) agree and specifically apply it to hypertension in pregnancy. NICE (2010) classifies hypertension as 'mild' – SBP 140–149, DBP 90–99; 'moderate' – SBP 150–159, DBP 100–109; and 'severe' – SBP ≥ 160, DBP ≥ 110. NICE (2008) advise that where there is a single DBP ≥110 mmHg or two consecutive readings of 90 mmHg (at least 4 hours apart) and/or significant proteinuria (1+) increased surveillance is required and if the SBP is >160 mmHg on two consecutive readings (at least 4 hours apart), treatment should be considered. Edmunds et al (2011) define hypotension (low blood pressure) as occurring when the SBP is below 100 mmHg. The UK Sepsis Trust (2014) advise that action should be taken if the SBP is <90 mmHg or there is a >40 mmHg fall from baseline as this is indicative of sepsis until proven otherwise.

Blood pressure may vary between the right and left arm; thus it is important to measure the blood pressure using both arms during the first assessment. If there is an inter-arm difference of >20 mmHg, the measurement should be repeated and if the difference remains >20 mmHg, the arm with the highest reading should be used for all subsequent measurements (BHS 2006, NICE 2010, Poon et al 2008). Both Clark et al (2012) and Verberk et al (2011) advise that a failure to recognize an inter-arm difference can result in an underestimation of, and thus undertreatment of, raised blood pressure which can have serious consequences for the woman and her fetus. Furthermore, large inter-arm differences in SBP can be indicative of atherosclerotic plaques or other vascular occlusive disease and are associated with increased cardiovascular risk (van der Hoeven et al 2013). If the woman has had a mastectomy, blood pressure should be recorded on the arm on the opposite side, as Lippincott et al (2013) caution that performing a blood pressure assessment on the arm next to the affected side may decrease an already compromised lymphatic circulation. It can also increase oedema and damage the arm.

BLOOD PRESSURE CHANGES RELATED TO CHILDBIRTH

Pregnancy

Profound haemodynamic changes occur during pregnancy primarily as a result of hormonal and anatomical changes, resulting in an increased blood volume, increased cardiac output and heart rate. In the non-pregnant individual this would result in an increase in blood pressure; however, during pregnancy these changes are counterbalanced by the hormonal effects (e.g. progesterone, prostaglandin) on the blood vessel walls, resulting in decreased peripheral resistance. Pregnancy is not normally associated with significant changes in arterial or venous blood pressure. Blood pressure usually begins to decrease during the first trimester, as the hormonal effects are evident before blood volume has increased to its maximum point in the third trimester. Blood pressure begins to rise gradually from the middle of pregnancy, returning to prepregnancy levels by term. The early decrease in blood pressure is less for SBP than for DBP (Blackburn 2013). Murray & Hassell (2014) propose the SBP decreases by an average of 5–10 mmHg, whereas DBP decreases 10–15 mmHg below the baseline by 24 weeks' gestation. There is a slight increase in the pulse pressure during the third trimester due to the differences between the SBP and DBP.

Venous pressures do not alter significantly during pregnancy, although venous pressure below the uterus does increase with gestation. This may impede venous return to the heart but does not usually create problems. However, up to 8% of women may experience a transient hypotensive episode (supine hypotensive syndrome) due to the weight of the gravid uterus compressing the inferior vena cava decreasing venous return, cardiac output and stroke volume (Blackburn 2013). This occurs more commonly when in a supine position and is quickly rectified by changing to a lateral or semi-recumbent position and it is advisable that women are not laid flat on their back during the second half of pregnancy. If this is required, a wedge should be placed under the woman's right side and hip to provide a lateral tilt.

Labour

Increased anxiety and pain levels can result in a rise in blood pressure, especially in the primiparous woman (Blackburn 2013). Additionally, both systolic and diastolic blood pressures increase during uterine contractions by up to 35 mmHg and 25 mmHg, respectively, as the circulation increases by 300–500 mL during a contraction, increasing cardiac output. Blackburn (2013) advises cardiac output can increase by 10–15% during the first stage and up to 50% during the second stage. Both these increases return to the baseline level once the contraction is over. It is therefore important to measure the blood pressure between contractions.

Postnatal period: maternal

Increased venous return following delivery results in higher venous pressures and cardiac output is 60–80% higher immediately after delivery. A sharp decline follows after 10–15 minutes and cardiac output stabilizes around 1-hour post-delivery (Blackburn 2013). The increased venous return to the heart also results in an increase in the size of the left atria for the first 3 days, increasing CVP (Blackburn 2013). As the blood volume and physiological effects of pregnancy decrease, blood pressure will return to its pre-pregnant level. Heiskanen et al (2011) advise the haemodynamic changes are relatively stable at 12 weeks post-delivery.

Postnatal period: baby

Blood pressure increases with gestational age; blood pressure is lower in the preterm baby than the term baby. A rise in arterial blood pressure occurs during the first few hours to days after birth, with blood pressure, particularly SBP, increasing gradually with age after 4 weeks (Blackburn 2013). Gardner & Hernandez (2011) suggest a SBP of 65–95 mmHg and DBP of 30–60 mmHg is normal during the first 6 hours of life for term babies. Blood pressure increases by 1–2 mmHg/day for the first 3–8 days and then increases by 1 mmHg/week for the next 5–7 weeks, stabilising around 2 months of age (Frost et al 2011).

FACTORS INFLUENCING ARTERIAL BLOOD PRESSURE

A variety of factors influence arterial blood pressure, including:

- Blood volume: a reduction in circulating blood volume (e.g. haemorrhage, shock), resulting in a decrease in both systolic and diastolic blood pressure.
- Heart rate: blood pressure increases with an increasing heart rate providing the circulating blood volume is unaltered.
- Age: blood pressure increases with age due to loss of elasticity of the arterial walls.
- Position: blood pressure is about 10 mmHg higher in standing or sitting positions compared to left lateral, recumbent or supine (Blackburn 2013).
- Position of arm during measurement: an unsupported arm can result in DBP increasing by 10%. Not having the arm at the level of the heart can vary blood pressure by 10 mmHg.
- Talking: if the woman talks while having her blood pressure measured, the DBP can increase by 5.3 mmHg and SBP by 6.2 mmHg (Zheng et al 2012). Dearsley (2013) advises the woman should not speak for at least 1 minute before commencing the procedure as this may increase blood pressure by 10–40%.
- Deep breathing can reduce blood pressure by almost 5 mmHg (Zheng et al 2012).
- Diurnal variations: SBP is highest in the evening, lowest in the morning and changes during rest and sleep periods.
- Season: Blood pressure can vary by 40% depending on the time of day and month of year, with higher measurements occurring during winter months (Thomas et al 2008).
- Weight: overweight people tend to have higher blood pressure.
- Alcohol: a consistently high alcohol intake is associated with higher blood pressure, although alcohol may also lower blood pressure by inhibiting the effects of antidiuretic hormone, resulting in vasodilatation and decreased blood volume.
- Smoking stimulates sympathetic activity resulting in vasoconstriction and the release of norepinephrine and epinephrine, which increase blood pressure, with effects lasting up to 30–60 minutes.
- Eating: blood pressure increases for 30–60 minutes following ingestion of food.
- Stress, fear, anxiety and pain can all raise blood pressure by up to 30 mmHg or more by stimulating the sympathetic nervous system; 'white coat' syndrome refers to anxiety-related hypertension resulting from attending a healthcare setting. O'Brien et al (2003) suggest this may cause an increase in SBP of 50–60 mmHg.
- Exercise increases blood pressure, with effects lasting 30–60 minutes.
- Distended bladder can increase blood pressure, with effects lasting 30–60 minutes.
- Hereditary factors: some people have an inherited predisposition to raised blood pressure; where one parent is hypertensive there is a 10–20% risk of the

offspring developing hypertension with the risk increasing to 25–45% where both parents are hypertensive (Dungan et al 2008).

- Disease: any disease process affecting stroke volume, blood vessel diameter, peripheral resistance or respiration will alter blood pressure.
- Renin: high renin levels cause vasoconstriction and an increase in blood volume (due to increased salt and fluid retention within the kidneys), resulting in a rise in blood pressure.

INDICATIONS

Blood pressure is often recorded as a matter of routine throughout pregnancy and labour, less so during the post-natal period. While the circumstances in which the estimation of blood pressure is undertaken can vary, they include:

- the initial booking history to establish a baseline, ideally by 10 weeks' gestation (NICE 2008)
- at each antenatal visit (NICE 2008)
- during labour, initially and then 4-hourly (NICE 2014)
- following each epidural bolus (see Chapter 25)
- as the clinical condition dictates, e.g. shock and haemorrhage, symptoms such as headaches, visual disturbances, proteinuria or when the Modified Early Obstetric Warning Score (MEOWS) triggers further investigation and repeat of vital signs (p. 66)
- hypertension of any cause
- preterm or sick babies
- before, during and following a blood transfusion (see Chapter 49)
- following recovery from anaesthesia: with other vital sign observations, it should be taken every 30 minutes for 2 hours and then hourly until stable (NICE 2011a), although Meakin (2011) recommends recording blood pressure every 15 minutes for the first 2 hours, then every 30 minutes for 2 hours followed by hourly measurements for 2 hours, 2-hourly measurements for 2 days and 4-hourly measurements for the next 3 days.

EQUIPMENT

Sphygmomanometer

The basis of measuring blood pressure is to exert a measured pressure on an artery usually with a sphygmomanometer, consisting of a manometer (pressure gauge) and an inflatable cuff. As the cuff inflates, the blood flow is occluded, as the pressure is released blood begins to pulsate

and flow through the artery which can be detected via a pressure sensor in the cuff (oscillatory) or the resulting sounds can be heard through a stethoscope (auscultatory) depending on the type of sphygmomanometer used.

Different types of sphygmomanometer are available and can be divided into two categories: auscultatory and oscillatory (electronic). Aneroid and mercury column manometers are the two forms of auscultatory sphygmomanometer available. Auscultatory sphygmomanometers, particularly those that are mercury-based, are considered to be the gold standard for blood pressure measurement (Parati & Ochoa 2012) but are used less in clinical practice because of health and safety concerns should the mercury be spilled. Stergiou et al (2011) suggest that the deflation rates of electronic devices are slightly faster (3.5–4 mm/sec) than the recommended auscultatory rate (2–3 mm/sec), resulting in underestimation of SBP and overestimation of DBP. The sensor and pressure transducer have a limited lifespan and De Greef et al (2010) advise they can be prone to losing calibration over time. Electronic devices may not measure blood pressure accurately if a pulse irregularity exists, emphasizing the importance of palpating either the radial or brachial pulse prior to measuring blood pressure to ensure the most appropriate equipment is used (NICE 2011b). Parati & Ochoa (2012) suggest that oscillatory manometers operate under a completely different principle to auscultatory devices and therefore should not be considered to be a true alternative to mercury devices.

To ensure accurate blood pressure comparisons between different recordings, measurements should be undertaken on similar equipment. It is important to record the type of sphygmomanometer used.

A third type of sphygmomanometer has been developed – a hybrid of the auscultatory and oscillatory devices. It has both automated oscillometric and manual auscultatory features and the user decides which to utilize. It uses an electronic pressure gauge as a substitute for the mercury column but has a visual representation of the column and the blood pressure can be seen to lower, as with the mercury column (Stergiou et al 2012). Parati & Ochoa (2012) and Tasker et al (2010) agree it is a suitable replacement for the mercury sphygmomanometer. Although not widely used at present, it may become more popular.

De Greef et al (2010) found calibration errors with both auscultatory and oscillatory manometers; 25% of devices had an unacceptable calibration error, highlighting the importance that all sphygmomanometers should be maintained properly, with manometers being recalibrated every 6–12 months to maintain accuracy. Parati & Ochoa (2012) advise the calibration should be against mercury sphygmomanometers and Scientific Committee on Emerging and Newly Identified Health Risks (SCENIHR) (2009) recommend mercury sphygmomanometers should be available as reference standards for clinical validation studies of non-mercury manometers until such a time as an internationally recognized alternative is available. Turner et al (2012) suggest that lack of sphygmomanometer calibration can result in both over- and underdetection of hypertension, proposing that systolic hypertension is undetected in 20% of adults but might be falsely detected in 15% of adults. Diastolic hypertension may be undiagnosed in 28% of adults and falsely diagnosed in 31% adults, indicating that some women will be wrongly treated for hypertension and some who should be treated will be missed. The date of the last calibration should be marked on the machine.

The tubing should also be checked regularly for signs of deterioration and replaced accordingly. The control valves should be able to hold a pressure of 200 mmHg for 10 seconds, allowing for a rate of fall of 1 mmHg per second (Jolly 1991); it is important for the control valves to be checked regularly to ensure the free passage of air without undue force.

Aneroid manometers

This type of manometer has a circular gauge encased in glass, with a needle that points to numbers. Pressure variations within the inflated cuff cause metal bellows within the gauge to expand and collapse, moving the needle up and down the gauge. Prior to use, the needle should be set at zero.

These are lightweight, compact and portable but less accurate than mercury column manometers as the metal parts are liable to expand and contract with temperature changes. Aneroid manometers should undergo biomedical calibration on a regular basis to increase accuracy. Skirton et al (2011) suggest further research is needed on the use of aneroid manometers before they can be considered as a replacement for mercury-based manometers.

Mercury column manometers

These have mercury contained within a glass column, with ascending numbers on either side of the column. The mercury should be clearly visible, have no gaps and rest at the zero level. If the mercury is below zero, the reservoir can be topped up. The column of mercury usually needs to be upright and the mercury should be read at eye level as looking up or down at the mercury can result in distorted readings. When examining the manometer, ensure the air vent or filter at the top of the column is clear and clean (oxidation of mercury can make it appear dirty and difficult to read, so columns should be cleaned every year).

Mercury is a highly toxic substance hazardous to health, and should a spillage occur, appropriate steps should be taken to remove the mercury and minimize the risks of contamination. Each NHS Trust should have a policy to deal with this situation. The use of mercury-based equipment is decreasing in Europe due to the associated environmental risks.

Oscillatory manometers

These are electronic machines that measure blood pressure automatically. A cuff is placed around the arm, as with a manual manometer, and is attached to the machine. The machine can be set to record blood pressure on a regular basis, inflating and deflating the cuff at the desired time. A stethoscope is not required. The systolic and diastolic pressures are displayed visibly. The pulse is often counted and recorded at the same time.

Oscillatory manometers can reduce the errors associated with auscultatory sphygmomanometers (e.g. observer bias, end/terminal digit preference, threshold avoidance) and do not require sounds to be listened to and thus can be used by people with hearing difficulties.

Ma et al (2008) measured blood pressure using an automated machine on both bare and sleeved arms and found no significant differences in blood pressure. Thus using an automated machine may be appropriate for women who are unwilling or unable to have a bare arm.

Heinemann et al (2008) found that automated machines consistently recorded lower blood pressure for both systolic and diastolic measurements and concluded that while they can be used with some degree of confidence for recording the systolic pressure, caution should be used with recording the diastolic pressure. Thus it would be sensible to estimate the blood pressure manually on any woman thought to have or be at risk of raised blood pressure.

NICE (2011b) advise that only independently validated automated devices should be used in practice. Automated devices are validated for use against a set of criteria. The European Society of Hypertension (ESH) use the International Protocol (ESH-IP1) which was revised in 2010 (ESH-IP2). To meet the criteria, the device must achieve all the minimum pass requirements, e.g. pressure scale accurate to ±3 mmHg – these are suitable for adults over 25 years but have not been validated for pregnancy (O'Brien et al 2010). The British Hypertension Society (BHS) have a list of validated devices (using IP1, IP2 or their own BHS criteria) on their website at www.bhsoc.org. However, Wan et al (2010) suggest that devices passing a protocol are not necessarily more accurate than devices that fail the protocol and can be inaccurate, particularly in the community setting and in diabetic and older people.

Summary

- Various sphygmomanometers are available for use.
- Aneroid manometers are lightweight and portable; however, there is a tendency to error due to expansion

and contraction of the metal parts with temperature changes.

- The mercury column manometer is considered the gold standard for non-invasive blood pressure measurement.
- Automated manometers reduce errors such as end/terminal digit preference and threshold avoidance and can be used by people with hearing difficulties.
- All manometers should be properly maintained and serviced.

The cuff

The sphygmomanometer has a cuff that is placed around the upper part of the arm, with the lower edge of the cuff positioned 2–3 cm above the point of brachial artery pulsation (Fig. 5.1), or occasionally around the forearm or lower thigh. The cuff is an inelastic cloth that encircles the arm and contains a bladder. Inside the bladder is an inflatable balloon that, when inflated to a pressure higher than the pressure within the artery, occludes the artery. At this point, blood flow ceases and the pulse is no longer palpable. The cuff is held in place either by Velcro fastenings or a long tapering cuff. Tapering cuffs should encircle the arm several

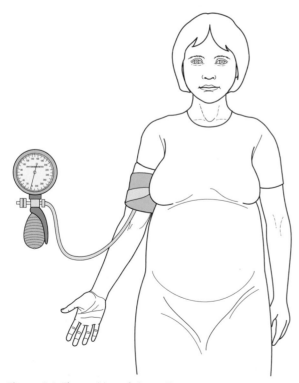

Figure 5.1 The position of the cuff on the upper arm.

times and be securely tucked in. The full length should be 25 cm beyond the end of the bladder, with the taper gradually occurring for a further 60 cm (O'Brien et al 2003). A loose cuff can distort the reading. The bladder is attached to tubing with a bulbous end that is squeezed to inflate the bladder. Edmunds et al (2011) advise the cuff should be placed with the rubber tubing positioned superiorly so that the tubing does not impede the procedure. For cuffs attached to manual sphygmomanometers, a valve on the bulb controls the pressure within the bladder.

If the upper arm cannot be used, the lower arm can be used by placing an appropriately sized cuff centrally above the radial artery, or the lower third of the thigh with the cuff placed above the posterior popliteal artery. Systolic pressure is 20–30 mmHg higher in the leg than in the arm. The lower arm and leg are rarely used in midwifery.

It is important to use the correct cuff size; a cuff that is too small in length or depth can give falsely high readings (cuff hypertension). Conversely, a cuff that is too large can give falsely low readings. Both NICE (2011b) and the BHS (2012) recommend the length of the bladder should be at least 80% of the arm circumference and the depth should be at least 40%. Cuff lengths vary from 22 to 36 cm. The woman should have her mid-arm circumference (MAC) measured at the first visit to ensure the correct size cuff is used. Hogan et al (2011) suggest that if the body mass index (BMI) is accurately measured at the beginning of pregnancy, women with a BMI >34.9 should always be assigned a large cuff. If the BMI is 29.9–34.9, the MAC should be measured as 44% of these women will require a large cuff. The BHS recommends three cuff sizes – small 12 × 18 cm, standard 12 × 26 cm and large 12 × 40 cm – the size refers to the size of the bladder.

Stethoscope

By placing a stethoscope over the artery, the sounds of the blood flow and vibrations in the surrounding tissues can be heard. The level at which the artery is occluded and no sounds heard is equal to the systolic pressure. As the cuff is deflated, the pulse reappears and pulsating sounds are heard with each beat of the heart.

The stethoscope head may be in two parts, with a bell-shaped end and a flat diaphragm side, or it might have just the diaphragm shape. Either side of the stethoscope head can be used for auscultation as similar results are obtained with each (Kantola et al 2005). However, BHS (2012) recommend the use of the diaphragm and it is often easier to hold in this position. Conversely the American Heart Association recommend use of the bell as it is better suited to hearing low-pitch sounds (O'Brien et al 2003).

Care should be taken not to press too hard on the stethoscope head as this compresses the brachial artery, resulting in a misleading murmur and possibly lowering the DBP reading. Bardwell (1995) suggests a pressure of 10 mmHg on the stethoscope significantly reduces the DBP and, of more concern, a pressure of 100 mmHg maintains the sounds until zero, making a recording impossible. It is also important to ensure the stethoscope is not tucked under the cuff edge as this can have the same effect and it should not be touching clothing or the rubber tubing as this can create friction sounds making it difficult to hear the pulse sounds.

Pinar et al (2010) found that the stethoscope can be used over clothing up to a thickness of 2 mm with no effect on blood pressure.

The stethoscope should be in good condition, particularly the earpiece, which should be clean and well fitting. The ear tips should be angled forwards into the external auditory canal as this maximizes hearing (Alexis 2009). Before and following the procedure, the earpieces and diaphragm/bell of the stethoscope should be cleaned, as they can carry microorganisms resulting in cross-contamination to other women or midwives (Campos-Murguia et al 2014).

KOROTKOFF SOUNDS

When assessing blood pressure with a manual sphygmomanometer, a stethoscope is used to listen to the different sounds in the artery when it is occluded and as the blood flow returns. The different sounds heard are named after the man who defined them in 1905 – Korotkoff. He defined the sounds according to five phases, reflecting different stages in the measurement of blood pressure (Table 5.1). SBP is noted when faint tapping sounds are heard initially, and these will increase in intensity as blood flow increases and changes in nature. DBP is noted when the sounds are no longer heard.

Table 5.1 Blood pressure phases and Korotkoff sounds

Phase	Sound
I	Faint tapping sounds that increase in intensity
II	Softening, swishing sounds
III	Crisper sounds with an intense pitch, not as intense as phase I
IV	Abrupt, muffled sounds, which become soft and blowing
V	Silence – no sounds heard

Individual variations can occur in the sequencing of these sounds. In around 5% of hypertensive people, the phase II sounds may be absent, replaced by a short period of silence: the 'auscultatory gap'. This can last through a change of 40 mmHg. Audible Korotkoff sounds may be absent in 20–30% of obese people (Bardwell 1995).

The muffling sounds of phase IV are heard when the pressure gauge is 7–10 mmHg higher than the intra-arterial diastolic pressure. This is due to a loss of transmission of pressure from the cuff to the artery. The absence of sounds associated with phase V is thought to be more closely related to the intra-arterial diastolic pressure. However, phase V sounds may be very low or absent in some adults, particularly during pregnancy.

Whether to use phase IV or phase V sounds to record blood pressure has been the subject of debate, particularly when measuring blood pressure in pregnancy. From their analysis of the evidence, Beevers et al (2001) recommend phase V, as this is 'the most accurate measurement of diastolic pressure' and NICE (2008) agree. However, at times, phase V continues to zero, which occurs in around 15% of women (Action on Pre-eclampsia 2004), thus phase IV should be used and it should be documented that this is the Korotkoff phase used.

PROCEDURE: blood pressure estimation using a manual manometer

- Obtain informed consent.
- Encourage the woman to empty her bladder.
- Disinfect the stethoscope.
- Take the sphygmomanometer and stethoscope to the woman.
- Wash and dry hands.
- If not already done, measure the arm to assess which cuff size is required.
- If the woman has been active, allow her to rest for at least 5 minutes.
- Position the sphygmomanometer so that the base of the manometer is level with the woman's heart, whenever possible.
- Assist the woman into a suitable position, legs uncrossed and feet flat on the ground.
- Ask the woman which arm is used to measure her blood pressure and then expose the correct upper arm, ensuring no constriction from tight clothing.
- Support her arm, and ask the woman to turn the palm of her hand upwards.
- Palpate the brachial artery and position the cuff 2–3 cm above the site of brachial pulsation in the antecubital fossa, with the bladder of the cuff placed centrally above the artery to ensure even distribution

of pressure during cuff inflation, and ensure there is no air in the cuff and the valve is closed.

- Palpate the brachial or radial artery with the fingertips of one hand and, with the other hand, inflate the cuff rapidly by pumping the bulb until the pulse disappears; continue to inflate the cuff 30 mmHg above this.
- Slowly deflate the cuff by opening the valve slightly, taking note of when the pulse reappears; this gives an approximate reading of the systolic pressure and prevents confusion arising from the presence of an auscultatory gap.
- Quickly deflate the cuff by opening the valve fully and wait for 30 seconds then close the valve.
- Place the stethoscope earpieces in your ears and position the head of the stethoscope over the brachial artery.
- Inflate the cuff to a pressure 20–30 mmHg higher than the palpated systolic pressure.
- Slowly deflate the cuff at 2 mmHg per second, listening for the appearance of the first clear sound (Korotkoff I).
- Read the needle position or mercury level (systole) (at eye level) to the nearest 2 mmHg.
- Continue to deflate the cuff slowly until the sounds are absent.
- When the sounds are no longer audible (Korotkoff V), read the needle position or mercury level (diastole) to the nearest 2 mmHg, deflate the cuff rapidly.
- Remove the cuff and assist with readjusting the woman's clothing, if required, and then assist her into a comfortable position.
- Clean the bell, diaphragm and earpieces of the stethoscope with a detergent wipe.
- Wash and dry hands or use alcohol handrub (see Chapter 9).
- Discuss the findings with the woman.
- Document the findings and act accordingly.

FACTORS AFFECTING ACCURACY

Care should be taken throughout to minimize the risk of inaccuracies occurring. Accuracy can be considered under three main headings: technique, equipment and operator.

Technique

Position

The arm should be at the level of the heart (mid-sternum). If above this level, the blood pressure may give a falsely low reading, whereas placing the arm below this level can give a falsely high reading, with differences of up to 10 mmHg (BHS 2006). Blood pressure is altered by 0.49 mmHg (SBP) and 0.47 mmHg (DBP) for each centimetre the arm is above or below the heart (Adiyaman et al 2006). The arm should be horizontal and supported, as an unsupported, extended arm may result in the DBP rising by up to 10% (Edmunds et al 2011).

The woman can adopt any position that is comfortable, although her legs should not be crossed at the knees as this can result in a falsely high recording (Adiyaman et al 2007, Lippincott et al 2013), Edmunds et al (2011) suggest the SBP can increase by 6.6 mmHg when the feet are not flat on the floor and legs are crossed. If the woman changes her position immediately prior to this procedure, it is preferable to wait for a few minutes before recording the blood pressure to avoid erroneous results. Blood pressure should be measured using the same position each time, as blood pressure is higher when standing compared to sitting and supine positions and is lowest in the supine position.

Cuff position

The bladder needs to be over the brachial artery and fitted properly, as discussed earlier.

Deflation of the cuff

Rapid deflation can result in an inaccurate measurement (Edmunds et al 2011, Reinders et al 2006) with the SBP underestimated and DBP overestimated. The measurement should be recorded to the nearest 2 mmHg.

Do not stop the cuff deflating between systolic and diastolic readings or reinflate the cuff to recheck the systolic reading. Blood will begin to flow into the lower arm, increasing the blood volume below the cuff, reducing the intensity and loudness of sounds (Hill 1980).

Rechecking the measurement

If the reading is abnormal, it should be repeated allowing at least 2 minutes to elapse between recordings. If an abnormal blood pressure is found on the initial assessment, it should be estimated in both arms and the arm with the highest reading used for all subsequent measurements (NICE 2010, Poon et al 2008, BHS 2006).

Equipment

- Auscultatory and oscillatory manometers can yield different results.
- Inappropriate cuff size will over- or underestimate blood pressure.

- Equipment not properly maintained, e.g. tubing, or not calibrated regularly may not provide an accurate measurement.

Operator

Operators might have an unconscious bias about what they expect to hear, influenced by knowledge of earlier recordings. If checking a woman's blood pressure that has already been recorded, accuracy is increased if previous findings are unknown.

Manual manometers can only yield results with even numbers, rounding to the nearest five or an uneven number is incorrect and inaccurate. End/terminal digit preference refers to the operator's preference to round the reading to the nearest zero resulting in a reading that is higher or lower than the actual measurement (Ayodele et al 2012).

Accuracy is also influenced by the individual's hearing ability. Song et al (2014) found operators with a hearing loss were more likely to underestimate the SBP and overestimate the DBP.

Summary

- Korotkoff sounds are used to determine blood pressure – Korotkoff I, when the sounds are first heard, represents the systolic blood pressure, and Korotkoff V, when the sounds become absent, represents the diastolic blood pressure.
- There are many factors that can influence blood pressure accuracy, so it is important to undertake the procedure correctly and ensure equipment is properly maintained.

MONITORING BLOOD PRESSURE IN THE BABY

Blood pressure estimation in the baby is of particular significance as babies, especially preterm babies, are unable to tolerate fluctuations in blood pressure, predisposing them to intracranial haemorrhage.

Blood pressure can be read intermittently with a manometer system, using either auscultatory or oscillatory manometers, or continuously, using a transducer attached to an arterial line, connected to an oscilloscope. However, O'Shea & Dempsey (2009) found that non-invasive methods of blood pressure measurement overestimated the mean blood pressure compared with invasive methods. If the manometer system is used, minimal handling is required; oscillatory manometers are preferred. If the cuff is left on between measurements, it should be repositioned every 4–6 hours to reduce the risk of skin damage, nerve palsy or

limb ischaemia. Blood pressure is recorded as for the adult; however, it may be difficult to auscultate the brachial artery with a stethoscope, and thus Doppler stethoscopes are often used. It is important to use the correct cuff size to obtain an accurate measurement; neonatal cuff sizes are available. The cuff can be placed around the arm or leg as values are similar (O'Shea & Dempsey 2009).

Normal range

Blood pressure in the baby varies according to postnatal age, birth weight, body weight, cuff size and state of arousal. It is lowest in babies who are sleeping, increasing during periods of wakefulness, agitation, crying and suckling. While systolic and diastolic pressures can be recorded, it is more usual to record the mean arterial pressure. Normal values have been developed by body weight and postnatal age.

CENTRAL VENOUS PRESSURE

Central venous pressure (CVP) is the pressure within the superior vena cava or right atrium, measured in centimetres of water (cmH_2O) when using a manual manometer and mmHg when monitoring with a pressure transducer. The central venous catheter is inserted via the femoral, brachial, subclavian or internal jugular vein and the catheter tip positioned in the right atrium or upper portion of the superior vena cava (or inferior vena cava if access is via the femoral artery). It is a direct, more accurate measurement of blood pressure and is considered an important determinant of venous return measuring the pressure of blood filling the right atrium and cardiac output. It can be used to inform fluid management in the critically ill woman; however, Marik & Cavallazzi (2013) suggest there are no data to support this widespread practice.

Normal CVP measurements are 5–8 cmH_2O (water manometer) and 2–6 mmHg (Perrin & MacLeod 2013) or 2–8 mmHg (Morton & Fontaine 2013) with a pressure transducer. To convert cmH_2O to mmHg, divide by 1.36; to convert mmHg to cmH_2O, multiply by 1.36.

The position of the woman should always be recorded and ideally the same position used for each measurement; however, this will depend on the woman's condition, for example, if she becomes breathless she might need to alter position from supine to semi-recumbent/upright. The zero point of the manometer should be in line with the base of the woman's right atrium; this is the phlebostatic axis and is located at the fourth intercostal space where it joins the sternum. An imaginary line is extended from here to the side of the chest to intersect with a second imaginary line between the front and back of the chest (Fig. 5.2). This is

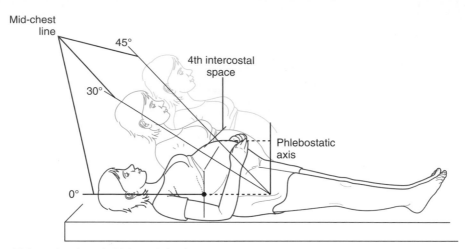

Figure 5.2 The phlebostatic axis and phlebostatic level.

known as the phlebostatic level and the site of intersection is marked on the side of the woman's chest to highlight the place used to obtain the reading.

CVP readings are affected by the amount of blood in the right ventricle prior to systole, the contractility of the right ventricle and the amount of resistance to blood being ejected from the right ventricle. A low CVP reading is associated with haemorrhage, dehydration, hypovolaemia, drug-induced vasodilatation and vigorous diuresis. A high CVP reading is associated with ventricular failure, fluid overload, fluid retention in cardiac and renal disease, pulmonary obstruction, congestion and/or embolism. Increased intrathoracic pressure from coughing, pain or movement can also increase the CVP reading (Edmunds et al 2011).

Equipment

CVP readings can be obtained via a water manometer, suitable for low pressures (<40 cmH$_2$O), or a pressure transducer and oscilloscope. The transducer converts the pressure waves to electrical energy, displayed on the oscilloscope. It is useful when pressures are high or where waveform depiction is required. Water manometers provide intermittent readings, whereas pressure transducers provide continuous readings of a CVP trace with a clear waveform that moves up and down in line with the respiratory pattern.

The CVP line is attached to a three-way tap, allowing for movement of fluid between the central venous line, intravenous infusion (saline, dextrose or dextrose saline), and manometer (Fig. 5.3). This allows for fluid infusion directly into the larger veins, and the tap is usually open to facilitate this. By moving the tap, the fluid can be redirected to an alternative site (e.g. the manometer) or prevented from flowing altogether. It is important to note the position of the tap prior to, during and following CVP measurement.

PROCEDURE: measuring central venous pressure using a manual manometer

- Gain informed consent, gather equipment and ascertain site to be used.
- Wash and dry hands.
- Assist the woman in a supine or semi-recumbent position to allow the baseline of the manometer to be level with the woman's right atrium.
- Place the manometer so that the baseline is level with the woman's right atrium (in line with the mark on the side of the woman's chest).
- Align the base of the manometer with the zero reference point using a levelling device and secure in place.
- Turn off all intravenous infusions running through the same site as the CVP line.
- Turn the three-way tap to open the access from the intravenous infusion to the manometer, allowing the fluid to run slowly into the manometer.
- Allow the manometer to fill several centimetres above the expected reading, without the upper end of the manometer becoming contaminated with fluid, then switch off the infusion line.
- Remove any bubbles in the manometer, as this can distort the reading.
- Turn the three-way tap to direct the fluid from the manometer to the central venous line, allowing the fluid from the manometer to enter the woman's right atrium.
- The column of fluid will fall rapidly and begin to oscillate with respiration between two numbers (usually 1 cmH$_2$O). The pressure in the column of fluid in the manometer is now equal to the pressure in the right atrium.
- Note where the fluid is and read off the higher number.

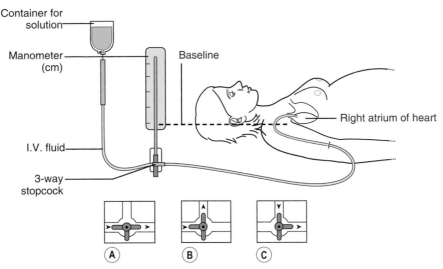

Figure 5.3 Three-way tap on the central venous pressure (CVP) line. **A,** The position prior to reading or between readings, with fluid running from the fluid solution to the woman. **B,** The position at the beginning of the procedure, as the manometer fills with fluid. **C,** The position during the recording.
(Adapted with kind permission from Jamieson et al 1997)

- Turn off the three-way tap to the manometer and recommence the intravenous infusion, adjusting the infusion rate accordingly.
- Assist the woman into a comfortable position, readjusting her clothing.
- Wash and dry hands.
- Document the findings and act accordingly.

Summary

- CVP measurement provides an accurate reading of blood pressure in the critically ill woman.
- The zero point of the manometer should be sited using the mark on the side of the woman's chest indicating the phlebostatic axis.

ROLE AND RESPONSIBILITIES OF THE MIDWIFE

These can be summarized as:
- identifying the need to undertake blood pressure measurement
- completing the procedure correctly and accurately
- recognizing and acting on any deviations from normal
- documenting the findings and acting on them accordingly
- ensuring that any equipment used is properly serviced and maintained.

SELF-ASSESSMENT EXERCISES

The answers to the following questions may be found in the text:
1. What is the difference between systolic and diastolic blood pressures?
2. If a woman has a blood pressure of 130/70 mmHg what are her mean arterial pressure and pulse pressure?
3. Why should blood pressure be recorded between contractions in labour?
4. What cuff size is required for a woman with a mid-arm circumference of 32 cm?
5. If using an oscillatory manometer, how often should it be calibrated?
6. What is the normal blood pressure and how is this altered during:
   a. pregnancy?
   b. labour?
   c. the postnatal period?
7. Identify five factors that can influence blood pressure and discuss why they occur.
8. Discuss five factors that influence the accuracy of the measurement and how the midwife can minimize this.
9. What is the central venous pressure and how can it be measured?

REFERENCES

Action on Pre-eclampsia, 2004. Pre-eclampsia community (PRECOG) guidelines. Available online: <http://action-on-pre-eclampsia.org.uk/wp-content/uploads/2012/07/PRECOG-Community-Guideline.pdf> (accessed 1 March 2015).

Adiyaman, A., Verhoeff, R., Lenders, J.W., et al., 2006. The position of the arm during blood pressure measurement in sitting position. Blood Press. Monit. 11 (6), 309–313.

Adiyaman, A., Tosun, N., Elving, L.D., et al., 2007. The effects of crossing legs on blood pressure. Blood Press. Monit. 12 (3), 189–193.

Alexis, O., 2009. Providing best practice in manual blood pressure measurement. Br. J. Nurs. 18 (7), 410–415.

Ayodele, O., Okunola, O., Akintunde, A., Sanya, E., 2012. End digit preference in blood pressure measurement in a hypertension specialty clinic in Southwest Nigeria. Cardiovasc. J. Afr. 23 (2), 85–89.

Bardwell, J., 1995. For good measure … blood pressure measurement. Nurs. Times 91 (27), 40–41.

Beevers, G., Lip, G., O'Brien, E., 2001. ABC of hypertension. Blood pressure measurement Part 2 – conventional sphygmomanometry: technique of auscultatory blood pressure measurement. Br. Med. J. 322, 1043–1047.

BHS (British Hypertension Society), 2006. Fact file for Health Professionals: Blood pressure measurement. Available online: <http://www.bhsoc.org/files/6813/4398/9702/BHS_BP_Measurement_Factfile_2006.pdf> (accessed 1 March 2015).

BHS (British Hypertension Society), 2012. Blood pressure measurement with manual blood pressure monitors. Available online: <http://www.bhsoc.org/files/9013/4390/7747/BP_Measurement_Poster_-_Manual.pdf> (accessed 1 March 2015).

Blackburn, S., 2013. Maternal, fetal and neonatal physiology: a clinical perspective, fourth ed. Saunders, St. Louis, pp. 252–296. (Ch. 9).

Campos-Murguia, A., Leon-Lara, X., Munoz, J., et al., 2014. Stethoscopes as potential intrahospital carriers of pathogenic microorganism. Am. J. Infect. Control 42 (1), 82–83.

CDC (Centres for Disease Control and Prevention), 2014. Pregnancy Mortality Surveillance System. Available online: <http://www.cdc.gov/reproductivehealth/MaternalInfantHealth/PMSS.html> (accessed 1 March 2015).

Clark, C., Taylor, R., Shore, A., Campbell, J., 2012. The difference in blood pressure readings between arms and survival Primary Care cohort study. Br. Med. J. 344 (e1327), 1–13.

De Greef, A., Lorde, I., Wilton, A., et al., 2010. Calibration accuracy of hospital-based non-invasive blood pressure measuring devices. J. Hum. Hypertens. 24, 58–63.

Dearsley, A., 2013. Vital signs. In: Koutoukidis, G., Stainton, K., Hughson, J. (Eds.), 2013 Tabbner's nursing care, sixth ed. Churchill Livingstone, Chatswood, pp. 301–331.

Dungan, J., Yucha, C., Artinian, N., 2008. Hypertension as a risk factor. In: Moser, D., Riegel, B. (Eds.), Cardiac nursing a companion to Braunwald's heart disease. Saunders, St. Louis, pp. 431–445.

Edmunds, S., Hollis, V., Lamb, J., Todd, J., 2011. Observations. In: Dougherty, L., Lister, S. (Eds.), The Royal Marsden Hospital manual of clinical nursing procedures, eighth ed. Wiley-Blackwell, Oxford, pp. 762–776.

Frost, M.S., Farshaw, L., Hernandez, J., Jones Jnr, M.D., 2011. Neonatal nephrology. In: Gardner, S.L., Carter, B.S., Enzman-Hines, M., Hernandez, J.A. (Eds.), Merenstein & Gardner's handbook of neonatal intensive care, seventh ed. Mosby, St. Louis, pp. 717–747. (Chapter 25).

Gardner, S.L., Hernandez, J.A., 2011. Initial nursery care. In: Gardner, S.L., Carter, B.S., Enzman-Hines, M., Hernandez, J.A. (Eds.), Merenstein & Gardner's handbook of neonatal intensive care, seventh ed. Mosby, St. Louis, pp. 78–112. (Chapter 5).

Heinemann, M., Sellick, K., Rickard, C., et al., 2008. Automated versus manual blood pressure measurement: a randomised cross over trial. Int. J. Nurs. Pract. 14 (4), 296–302.

Heiskanen, N., Saarelainen, H., Karkkainen, H., et al., 2011. Cardiovascular autonomic response to head-up tilt in gestational hypertension and normal pregnancy. Blood Press. 20, 84–91.

Hill, M., 1980. What can go wrong when you measure blood pressure? Am. J. Nurs. 80 (5), 942–946.

Hogan, J., Maguire, P., Farah, N., et al., 2011. Body mass index and blood pressure measurement during pregnancy. Hypertens. Pregnancy 30, 396–400.

Jamieson, E., McCall, J.M., Blythe, R., Whyte, L.A., 1997. Clinical nursing practices, third ed. Churchill Livingstone, Edinburgh.

Jolly, A., 1991. Taking blood pressure. Nurs. Times 87 (15), 40–43.

Kantola, I., Vesalainen, R., Kangassalo, K., Kariluoto, A., 2005. Bell or diaphragm in the measurement of blood pressure. J. Hypertens. 23 (3), 499–503.

Knight, M., Nair, M., Shah, A., et al. on behalf of the MBRRACE-UK, 2014. Maternal mortality and morbidity in the UK 2009–12: Surveillance and epidemiology. In: Knight, M., Kenyon, S., Brocklehurst, P., et al. on behalf of MBRRACE-UK (Eds.), Saving lives, improving mothers' care – lessons learned to inform future maternity care from the UK and Ireland confidential enquiries into maternal deaths and morbidity 2009–12. National Perinatal Epidemiology Unit, Oxford, pp. 9–26.

Lippincott, Williams, Wilkins, 2013. Lippincott's nursing procedures, sixth ed. Wolters Kluwer, Philadelphia, pp. 77–81.

Lowe, S.A., Bowyer, L., Lust, K., 2014. The SOMANZ Guideline for the Management of Hypertensive

Disorders of Pregnancy. Available online: <http://somanz.org/documents/HTPregnancyGuidelineJuly2014.pdf> (accessed 1 March 2015)

Ma, G., Sabin, N., Dawes, M., 2008. A comparison of blood pressure measurement over a sleeved arm versus a bare arm. Can. Med. Assoc. J. 178 (5), 585–589.

Marik, P., Cavallazzi, R., 2013. Does the central venous pressure predict fluid responsiveness? An updated meta-analysis and a plea for some common sense. Crit. Care Med. 41 (7), 1774–1781.

Meakin, S., 2011. Procedures in obstetrics. In: Macdonald, S., Magill-Cuerden, J. (Eds.), Mayes' midwifery, fourteenth ed. Elsevier, Edinburgh, p. 2011.

Morton, P., Fontaine, D., 2013. Essentials of critical care nursing: a holistic approach. Wolters Kluwer, Philadelphia, pp. 97–98.

Murray, I., Hassell, J., 2014. Change and adaptation in pregnancy. In: Marshall, J., Raynor, M. (Eds.), Myles textbook for midwives, sixteenth ed. Churchill Livingstone, Edinburgh, pp. 143–178.

NICE (National Institute for Health and Care Excellence), 2008. Antenatal care routine care for the healthy pregnant woman. Available online: <www.nice.org.uk> (accessed 1 March 2015).

NICE (National Institute for Health and Clinical Excellence), 2010. Hypertension in pregnancy. Available online: <www.nice.org.uk> (accessed 1 March 2015).

NICE (National Institute for Health and Clinical Excellence), 2011a. Caesarean section. Available online: <www.nice.org.uk> (accessed 1 March 2015).

NICE (National Institute for Health and Clinical Excellence), 2011b. Hypertension: management of hypertension in adults in primary care. Available online: <www.nice.org.uk> (accessed 1 March 2015).

NICE (National Institute for Health and Care Excellence), 2014. Intrapartum care of healthy women and their babies during childbirth. Available online: <www.nice.org.uk> (accessed 1 March 2015).

O'Brien, E., Asmar, R., Berlin, L., et al. on behalf of the European Society of Hypertension Working Group on Blood Pressure Monitoring, 2003. European Society of Hypertension recommendations for conventional, ambulatory and home blood pressure measurement. J. Hypertens. 21, 821–848.

O'Brien, E., Atkins, N., Stergiou, G., et al. on behalf of the Working Group on Blood Pressure Monitoring of the European Society of Hypertension, 2010. European Society of Hypertension international protocol revision 2010 for the validation of blood pressure measuring devices in adults. Blood Press. Monit. 15, 23–38.

O'Shea, J., Dempsey, E., 2009. A comparison of blood pressure measurements in newborns. Am. J. Perinatol. 26 (2), 113–116.

Parati, G., Ochoa, J., 2012. Automated-auscultatory (hybrid) sphygmomanometers for clinic blood pressure measurement: a suitable substitute to mercury sphygmomanometer as reference standard? J. Hum. Hypertens. 26, 211–213.

Perrin, K., MacLeod, C., 2013. Understanding the essentials of critical care nursing, second ed. Pearson, Boston.

Pinar, R., Ataalkin, S., Watson, R., 2010. The effect of clothes on sphygmometric blood pressure measurement in hypertensive patients. J. Clin. Nurs. 19, 1861–1864.

PMMRC (Perinatal and Maternal Mortality Review Committee), 2013. Seventh Annual Report of the Perinatal and Maternal Mortality Review Committee: Reporting Mortality 2011. Health Quality and Safety Commission, Wellington.

Poon, L., Kametas, N., Strobl, I., et al., 2008. Inter-arm blood pressure differences in pregnant women. Br. J. Obstet. Gynaecol. 115, 1122–1130.

Reinders, L., Mos, C., Thornton, E., et al., 2006. Time poor: rushing decreases accuracy and reliability of blood pressure measurement technique in pregnancy. Hypertens. Pregnancy 25, 81–91.

Roberts, M., 2006. Blood pressure monitoring: invasive and noninvasive. In: Schell, H., Puntillo, K. (Eds.), Critical care nursing secrets, second ed. Mosby, St. Louis, pp. 36–46.

SCENIHR (Scientific Committee on Emerging and Newly Identified Health Risks) of the European Commission, 2009. Mercury Sphygmomanometers in Healthcare and the Feasibility of Alternatives. Available online: <http://ec.europa.eu/health/scientific_committees/opinions_layman/sphygmomanometers/en/index.htm> (accessed 1 March 2015).

Skirton, H., Chamberlain, W., Lawson, C., et al., 2011. A systematic review of variability and reliability of manual and automated blood pressure reading. J. Clin. Nurs. 20, 602–614.

Song, S., Lee, J., Chee, Y., et al., 2014. Does the accuracy of blood pressure measurement correlate with hearing loss of the observer? Blood Press. Monit. 19 (1), 14–18.

Stergiou, G., Karpettas, N., Kollias, A., et al., 2012. A perfect replacement for the mercury sphygmomanometer: the case of the hybrid blood pressure monitor. J. Hum. Hypertens. 26, 220–227.

Stergiou, G., Lourida, P., Tzamouranis, D., 2011. Replacing the mercury manometer with an oscillometric device in a hypertension clinic: implications for clinical decision making. J. Hum. Hypertens. 25, 691–698.

Tasker, F., De Greef, A., Shennan, A., 2010. Development and validation of a blinded hybrid device according to the European Hypertension Society protocol: Nissei DM-3000. J. Hum. Hypertens. 24, 609–616.

Thomas, C., Wood, G., Langer, R., Stewart, W., 2008. Elevated blood pressure in primary care varies in relation to circadian and seasonal changes. J. Hum. Hypertens. 22, 755–760.

Turner, M., Butlin, M., Avolio, A., 2012. 869 Reliability of the mercury sphygmomanometer as a reference standard for the measurement of blood pressure. J. Hypertens. 30e (Suppl. 1), e254.

UK Sepsis Trust, 2014. Appendix 1: Introducing Red Flag Sepsis. Available online: <http://sepsistrust.org/wp-content/uploads/2015/08/1409314199UKSTAppendix1RFS2014.pdf> (accessed 17 December 2015).

Van der Hoeven, N., Lodestijn, S., Nanninga, S., et al., 2013. Simultaneous compared with sequential blood pressure measurement results in smaller interarm blood pressure differences. J. Clin. Hypertens. 15 (11), 839–844.

Verberk, W., Kessels, A., Thien, T., 2011. Blood pressure measurement method and inter-arm difference: a meta-analysis. Am. J. Hypertens. 24 (11), 1201–1208.

Wan, Y., Heneghan, C., Stevens, R., et al., 2010. Determining which automatic digital blood pressure device performs adequately: a systematic review. J. Hum. Hypertens. 24, 431–438.

WHO (World Health Organisation), 2011. Prevention and treatment of pre-eclampsia and eclampsia. Available online: <http://www.who.int/reproductivehealth/publications/maternal_perinatal_health/9789241548335/en/> (accessed 1 March 2015).

WHO (World Health Organization), 2013. A global brief on hypertension. Available online: <http://www.who.int/cardiovascular_diseases/publications/global_brief_hypertension/en> (accessed 1 March 2015).

Zheng, D., Giovanni, R., Murray, A., 2012. Effect of respiration, talking, and small body movements on blood pressure measurement. J. Hum. Hypertens. 26, 458–462.

Chapter | 6 |

Assessment of maternal and neonatal vital signs: respiration assessment

LEARNING OUTCOMES

Having read this chapter, the reader should be able to:

- define external respiration, identifying the normal ranges for the mother and baby
- discuss when respiration should be assessed and the factors that influence it
- undertake assessment of respiration accurately
- recognize an abnormal respiratory rate, pattern and sounds
- discuss the safe and accurate use of pulse oximetry
- discuss when and why a modified early obstetric warning score (MEOWS) chart should be used.

Changes in the respiratory rate can indicate physiological instability as alterations in the respiratory function are a sensitive indicator of deterioration and an early marker of acidosis (Elliott & Coventry 2012, Jevon 2010, Massey & Meredith 2010). Elliott & Coventry (2012) suggest that even an increase of 3–5 breaths per minute is an early and important sign of respiratory distress and potential hypoxaemia. Breathlessness, particularly when the respiratory rate is above 20, is a red flag that should prompt urgent referral (Oates et al 2011). The respiratory rate is one of the more sensitive markers for identifying patients at risk of deterioration (Carle et al 2013), yet Churchill et al (2014) found the respiratory rate was frequently not recorded in women who died from sepsis. Thus respiration assessment is important for both the woman and baby, and is one of the physiological observations that make up the minimum standard for an early warning score chart (NICE 2007). This chapter considers the effects of childbirth upon the respiratory system, other factors affecting respiration and the midwife's role and responsibilities in completing the observation correctly. Pulse oximetry is also discussed.

Definition

External respiration is the means by which the body gains oxygen (inspiration) and excretes carbon dioxide (expiration).

Assessment of respiration includes observation of the rate (number per minute), depth and regularity of breaths and any associated signs (e.g. skin colour). Breath sounds may also be heard, or the chest felt to rise and fall, as well as being visually observed. Respiration can be consciously controlled (e.g. for swimming, singing, etc.) but is unconsciously determined by definite and precise mechanisms. During quiet, normal breathing (eupnoea) the diaphragm flattens during inspiration and the intercostal muscles pull the ribs upwards and outwards increasing the intra-thoracic volume and pulling 500–800 mL of air into the lungs (Higginson & Jones 2009). Expiration generally lasts twice as long as inspiration allowing a conversation to be held. A quick assessment of respiratory impairment is to ask the woman a question – if she can only speak in short sentences, there is a degree of respiratory distress. Abnormal posture, e.g. sitting up, leaning forwards, may be a compensatory posture designed to improve the mechanics of breathing and should be noted (Massey & Meredith 2010).

Normal values

Automatic control of breathing occurs within the respiratory centres in the brainstem which regulate breathing according to reflex responses and chemical signals (mainly carbon dioxide in the blood), e.g. an excessive carbon dioxide level in the blood (hypercapnia) will cause respirations to increase until it returns to a normal level (Dearsley 2013). There is some debate as to the normal respiratory rate for a healthy adult at rest. Higginson & Jones (2009) and Mooney (2007) suggest this is 12–18 times per minute; Dearsley (2013) and Jevon (2010) prefer 12–20 and Docherty & Coote (2006) propose 10–20. Edmunds et al (2011) advise that when a woman's respiratory rate is greater than 24 breaths per minute, more frequent observations should be performed, and if they are above 27, prompt referral is indicated.

Tachypnoea is an increased respiratory rate above 20 breaths per minute (Churchill et al 2014) although Docherty & Coote (2006) suggest that tachypnoea does not occur until the respiratory rate is above 30 breaths per minute. Tachypnoea is often rapid, shallow breathing and can occur in response to metabolic acidosis, exercise, fear, fever (the rate rises approximately four breaths/minute for each degree the temperature increases), pain and is the most sensitive indicator of an impending adverse event. The UK Sepsis Trust (2014) advise that a respiratory rate >20 is a red flag and when combined with another red flag, action should be taken. However, if the rate is >25, action is taken regardless of the other observations as is it indicative of sepsis until proved otherwise.

Bradypnoea refers to a decreased but regular respiratory rate of below 8 (Docherty & Coote 2006) or, more commonly, 10 breaths per minute (Nelson & Schell 2006).

Dyspnoea denotes difficulty with breathing and the woman may be seen to use some accessory muscles of respiration, e.g. sternomastoid, scalene, abdominal, have nasal flaring and/or pursed lips – typically seen with obstructed lung disease. Pursed lips acts as a physiological positive end expiratory pressure (PEEP) and helps increase intra-airway pressure and prevent expiratory airway closure thus maximizing perfusion by decreasing the respiratory rate and increasing arterial oxygenation. About 60–70% of women experience physiological dyspnoea during pregnancy that can occur at rest or with mild exertion (Blackburn 2013).

Breathing is usually silent; when sounds are present, they are usually the result of narrowed airways or moisture within, or inflammation of, the lungs or pleura:

- Stertorous breathing occurs when respiration is laboured and a snoring sound is heard due to an obstructed airway, e.g. from tracheal secretions.
- Wheezing is due to narrowed airways, particularly the smaller bronchi and bronchioles, e.g. in asthma, and is heard as a high-pitched, squeaking sound.
- Bubbling or gurgling sounds occur as air passes through moist secretions within the respiratory tract.
- Crackles are an abnormal non-musical sound heard on auscultation during inspiration and sounds like hair rubbed together close to the ear.
- Stridor occurs when there is an obstruction or spasm within the trachea or larynx and is heard as a high-pitched musical sound especially during inspiration (Dearsley 2013).

The newborn baby has an erratic periodic breathing pattern that is interspersed with periods of apnoea (10–15 seconds) with a respiratory rate of 30–40 breaths per minute that can increase to 60 (England 2014), although Cameron (2011) suggests the rate is 20–40. Due to the weakness of the intercostal muscles, the baby may appear to be breathing abdominally as the diaphragm is used extensively used (Blackburn 2013). Tachypnoea in the newborn (above 60 breaths per minute) is the earliest sign of respiratory disease and may also indicate other illnesses, e.g. cardiac, metabolic or infectious (Gardner et al 2011). The baby may show other signs of respiratory difficulty when tachypnoeic, such as nasal flaring (where the nares increase in size to decrease the airway resistance up to 40%), grunting (from forced expiration through a partially closed glottis) and using accessory muscles of respiration (the thin chest walls are pulled inwards on inspiration – recession/retraction, usually seen around the sternum, intercostal, subcostal, and supracostal muscles). Grunting acts as a compensatory mechanism to stabilize the alveoli by increasing transpulmonary pressure and delaying expiration which will increase gaseous exchange (Gardner et al 2011).

Babies are mainly diaphragmatic breathers which means their diaphragm moves symmetrically with each breath. Asymmetrical breathing should be investigated particularly following shoulder dystocia as damage to the baby's phrenic nerve may have resulted which is a cause of asymmetrical breathing movement.

CHANGES RELATED TO CHILDBIRTH

Pregnancy

When supporting both the fetus and the woman, the body's oxygen demands are high. The function and anatomy of the respiratory tract alters. Breathing is largely diaphragmatic, with the diaphragm being displaced up to 4 cm upwards as the lower ribs flare. The transverse diameter of the chest increases 2 cm from widened subcostal angles countering the effect of the enlarging uterus and elevated diaphragm, leaving pulmonary function altered but not compromised (Grindheim et al 2012).

Labour

Oxygen consumption increases 40–60% and inadequate oxygenation can increase the severity of pain which in turn can result in hyperventilation. The number and strength of contractions affect the pattern and depth of respiration during labour. Breath holding should be discouraged as it increases $PaCO_2$ levels which in turn results in compensatory hyperventilation in an effort to lower $PaCO_2$ levels. Maternal hyperventilation can also lead to dizziness, tingling and decreased fetal oxygenation (Blackburn 2013). Deep slow breathing between contractions should be encouraged to maintain oxygenation amidst considerable muscular activity.

Postnatal period: maternal

Respiration returns swiftly to its prepregnant rate, volume, and pattern once labour is completed. This is due to the decrease in intra-abdominal pressure that allows increased movement of the diaphragm and the decrease in progesterone. Anatomical changes revert to their prepregnant state by 24 weeks post-delivery (Blackburn 2013).

Postnatal period: baby

Lung development and growth occurs throughout pregnancy and continues for the first 2–3 years of life. Although terminal air sacs appear by 24–26 weeks, blood vessels, lung surface area and volume do not increase sharply until 30 weeks. The number of air spaces increases from 240 000 at 24 weeks, to four million at 32–36 weeks and 50–150 million at term. The alveolar develop further from 36 weeks with about 20% formed by term. Surfactant levels also increase significantly towards term. Thus a baby born preterm is likely to experience respiratory difficulties. Additionally the baby's lungs are fluid-filled, and the fluid has to be removed at birth and replaced with air for effective ventilation to occur.

Respiration is initiated as the baby is born and the fetal circulation adapts to the extrauterine circulation, but the process begins before birth. Lung fluid absorption begins during early labour and fluid is expelled through the baby's nose and mouth as the thorax is squeezed during the baby's journey through the birth canal. At birth there is approximately 35% of the original lung fluid volume remaining that has to be removed (Blackburn 2013).

The first diaphragmatic breath occurs within 9 seconds of delivery and generates high positive intra-thoracic pressures (70 cmH_2O). As the pressure begins to decrease (30–40 cmH_2O), air enters the lungs. Subsequent breaths require less pressure as the smaller airways and alveoli remain open due to the action of surfactant.

Respiration is initiated by a number of factors:

- stimulation (light, tactile and temperature)
- compression and decompression of the chest as it passes through the vagina
- stimulation of chemoreceptors
- hypoxaemia and hypercapnia
- changes within the cardiovascular system to perfuse the lungs.

FACTORS INFLUENCING NORMAL RESPIRATION

- Exercise: an increase in oxygen demand causes an increase in respiration.
- High altitude increases respiration.
- Emotions: the respiration rate and depth can be consciously controlled, which can be useful, e.g. breathing patterns in labour. Anxiety, nervousness, stress, excitement, fear and other emotions can also affect respiration.
- Pain: hyperventilation is a physiological response to pain.
- Insult or injury: complications such as pulmonary embolism can cause infarction of lung tissue and respiration may cease.
- Prematurity: the preterm infant may have an immature respiration centre in the brain or structural/physiological deficiencies, e.g. lack of surfactant.
- Infection: when infection impairs lung function the lungs work harder to oxygenate the body. Fever also increases the body's oxygen demands.

- Reduced number of red blood cells: anaemia or haemorrhage reduces the oxygen-carrying capacity of the blood. To overcome this hypoxia, the respiration rate increases to supply the body with extra oxygen.
- Acidosis/alkalosis: respiration adjusts automatically to maintain acid–base balance in conjunction with other body systems. Changes in respiration can shift the balance, e.g. hyperventilation creates alkalosis. Hypercapnia results in increased respirations.
- Medications: opioids depress respiration; they are unlikely to have this effect in a healthy woman receiving small doses (e.g. pethidine) but transplacental passage of the opioid occurs and there is a risk of respiratory depression for the baby at birth. The woman undergoing a general anaesthetic will require mechanical ventilation as paralysis of her respiratory function is induced.
- Sleep decreases both rate and depth of respiration.

INDICATIONS

Respiration assessment: maternal

- As part of baseline observations.
- Whenever other vital signs are recorded, particularly when completing a MEOWS chart (p. 66).
- Admission to hospital particularly with any respiratory complaint (e.g. asthma, chest infection), chest pain, breathlessness, cyanosis, after a road traffic accident or with any serious disorder (e.g. major haemorrhage, thromboembolism, haemorrhage).
- Prior to commencing resuscitation (see Chapter 55).
- After recovery from anaesthesia – half hourly for 2 hours, then hourly if stable (NICE 2011).
- Following intrathecal opioids: hourly for 12 hours if diamorphine has been used and 24 hours when morphine has been administered (NICE 2011).
- Patient-controlled analgesia or epidural with opioids: hourly monitoring throughout and for at least 2 hours following discontinuation of the treatment (NICE 2011).
- Any signs of altered breathing pattern.

Respiration assessment: baby

- At birth, as part of the Apgar score (p. 292).
- Whenever vital signs are being recorded, e.g. after meconium-stained amniotic fluid, maternal prolonged rupture of membranes, known maternal

group B streptococcus, administration of naloxone at delivery, hypothermia and hypoglycaemia.
- Any signs of cyanosis, sternal recession, nasal flaring, noisy breathing (e.g. grunting) or increased work of breathing, where the baby is using more energy to breathe.
- During resuscitation (see Chapter 56).

PROCEDURE: assessment of maternal respiration

This is probably the only procedure when the consent of the woman is not sought as making her aware of the action of counting her respirations may cause her to think about them and thus give a false reading. A respiration assessment is made at the same time as counting the pulse (see Chapter 4): if the wrist is supported across the woman's chest, it is possible to count the pulse and then to either feel the rise and fall of the chest, or observe it, counting respiration. Other factors (e.g. sound, depth, regularity, symmetry of both sides of the chest) are observed at the same time, along with the woman's colour, behaviour (shortage of oxygen can result in confused behaviour and speech), level of consciousness and condition. Central cyanosis (due to prolonged hypoxia) might be seen in the mucous membranes (e.g. lips, tongue, nail beds); peripheral cyanosis usually results from vasoconstriction occurring from a physiological response to a cold environment or a pathological cause, e.g. hypovolaemia. Signs of increased respiratory effort should be noted: nasal flaring, pursed lips, use of accessory muscles (e.g. shoulder/neck) and any audible cough/wheeze. All findings should be documented. The respiration rate should be counted for 60 seconds if irregular otherwise for 30 seconds, then doubled (Lippincott et al 2013). Records are completed and the result should be acted on accordingly. As for pulse assessment, the findings can be recorded pictorially on an observations chart such as a MEOWS chart or written in prose. The findings are discussed with the woman.

PROCEDURE: assessment of baby's respiration

Informed consent must be gained from the parent(s). A crying or excited baby should be calmed before respiration can be counted accurately. When assessing the respiration rate of a baby, it is better to expose the chest and abdomen, and observe/feel, listen and count for 1 minute, due to the irregularity of respiration. Signs of increased respiratory effort should be noted – nasal flaring, grunting, sternal, subcostal or supracostal recession/retraction. Record the findings, discuss them with the baby's parent(s) and act on the findings accordingly.

PULSE OXIMETRY

Pulse oximetry is used in conjunction with respiration assessment, particularly when a woman is seriously ill or after surgery, for the baby with increased work of breathing or during neonatal resuscitation (see Chapter 56). Approximately 98–99% of the oxygen breathed is carried by the haemoglobin in the blood to the body tissues and organs (arterial haemoglobin saturation: SaO_2). The other 1–2% is dissolved in the plasma and is known as the partial pressure of oxygen (PaO_2). Pulse oximetry measures arterial saturation, referred to as SpO_2. Arterial oxygen saturation is a common component of the MEOWS assessment and has been a useful predictor of the need for admission to the Intensive Care Unit (Carle et al 2013).

Pulse oximetry uses two light-emitting diodes of different wavelengths and sensors that measure the amount of light emerging from the tissues. Oxygenated blood absorbs red light at a wavelength of 640 mm and deoxygenated blood absorbs infrared light at 940 mm. The ratio of oxygenated and deoxygenated haemoglobin is calculated and converted to a percentage to give the saturation reading (Frank et al 2013, Kelly 2006). The use of pulse oximetry can detect hypoxaemia before visible cyanosis is evident, which may not occur until the SpO_2 <80% (Frank et al 2013, Ramjattan & Allen 2013).

Pulse oximetry is straightforward to use and is extremely precise regardless of location of the sensor (Frank et al 2013). Kelly (2006) suggests the monitors are accurate within 2–4% of oxyhaemoglobin levels measured in arterial blood gas samples and that the machines maintain this accuracy rate within the SpO_2 range 70–100%; below 70%, the reliability is poor, although Frank et al (2013) suggest it is extremely accurate when the reading is 85–100%. Docherty & Coote (2006) advise that saturation levels of 95% or above are acceptable for an adult. Babies have lower saturation levels at birth and should not receive supplemental oxygen unless they do not meet the lower limit of normal, e.g. 60% at 60 seconds of age (Kattwinkel et al 2010).

Pulse oximetry is being used in hospitals around the world to increase early detection of critical congenital heart disease (CCHD) in babies and is undertaken at 24–48 hours of age or close to discharge if less than 24-hours old (Andrews et al 2014, Ewer et al 2013). These babies can deteriorate suddenly, making treatment more difficult and early prevention improves the long-term outcome (Ramjattan & Allen 2013). Although there are false positives and negatives, it is generally viewed as a useful screening tool as the routine newborn examination does not usually detect serious CCHD, as the babies are rarely exhibiting signs at this time (Prudhoe et al 2013). Murmurs are not

the greatest indicator of heart disease and Frank et al (2013) caution that CCHD should not be ruled out if no murmurs are heard. Ramjattan & Allen (2013) advise the screening should be undertaken when the baby is in a quiet, alert, awake state. During periods of crying, feeding and sleeping the baby can have periods of desaturation <95% and when the baby is in the active, alert state, motion artefact can create falsely low readings. Readings are taken from the right foot and the right hand – if both are ≥95% or the difference between them is ≤3% the screen is negative, if both are <90%, the screen is positive and the baby is referred for further tests. If the readings are 90–<95% or the difference is above 3% the screen is repeated in 1 hour and the screen may be negative or positive as above. If the same results occur, it is repeated again in 1 hour. If the same reading persists, the screen is positive.

Informed consent is gained. For adults, the monitor (Fig. 6.1) is placed over a finger, toe or earlobe; for babies, a hand, wrist or foot is the most likely site for the probe. The light should pass from the top of the probe to the bottom of the probe (switch on and check direction before applying the monitor).

Accuracy and safety

- Accuracy and safety are maintained only if the right type of probe is applied correctly, hence the need to understand the different manufacturers' instructions.
- Accuracy also depends on blood flow through the light being adequate, e.g. poor circulation, too much extraneous light (poorly fitted probe).
- Results can be misleading in the presence of anaemia as the SpO_2 may be normal despite a lowered potential to carry oxygen (Dearsley 2013, Tollefson 2010).
- Accuracy is also affected by movement, e.g. shivering/tremors/seizures, dirt, vasoconstriction, bright or fluorescent lighting and an inaccurately sized probe.
- Studies conflict on the effect of nail polish. Yamamoto et al (2008) found that it had limited effect in mildly hypoxic patients but results were less accurate when the patient was very hypoxic. While clear and red nail polish and acrylic nails gave accurate results, Desalu et al (2013) found that black and brown nail polish was more likely to produce an inaccurate result. Villaflor et al (2013) found that acrylic gel nail art did not affect the results.
- Hypoventilation will not be reliably detected if the woman is receiving supplemental oxygen (Iscoe et al 2011).
- Neonatal probes are supplied with their fixative (tape or Velcro); applying additional tape can also affect the results.
- Pulse oximetry is unaffected by natural skin colour (Moyle 1999).

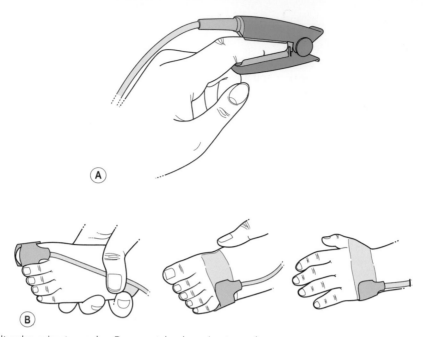

Figure 6.1 A, Adult pulse oximetry probe. **B,** neonatal pulse oximetry probe.
(Adapted with kind permission from Jamieson et al 2002)

- There is disagreement as to whether jaundice affects results, Moyle (1999) reports it does not but Mahle et al (2009) disagree.
- Thermal damage, which can cause necrosis, may occur in the baby if a probe is left in one position for too long. It is therefore advisable to resite the probe every 4 hours.
- The midwife must be familiar with the equipment, noting correct storage, use, and maintenance, and knowing when to refer.
- Pulse oximetry should not be used on someone who has had dye treatments, e.g. methylene blue, as results are unreliable.
- Pulse oximetry use and findings must be documented.

THE MODIFIED EARLY OBSTETRIC WARNING SCORE

The seventh report on confidential enquiries into maternal deaths in the UK made a recommendation that all hospitals, including all departments that provide care for pregnant women, e.g. Emergency Department, Gynaecology, should use an Early Warning Scoring (EWS) system until a national obstetric EWS chart is available (Lewis 2007). It

was again a 'top ten' recommendation in the eighth report (McClure et al 2011) to assist with identifying and managing very sick women; Mhyre et al (2014) suggest that delays in recognition, diagnosis and management precede the majority of deaths from infection, hypertension, venous thromboembolism and haemorrhage. This chart allows important physiological recordings of blood pressure, pulse rate, temperature, respiratory rate and urinary output to be charted, in addition to maternal response, to give a pictorial overview of the woman's condition and facilitate more timely recognition, referral and treatment of women who have or who are developing a critical illness as physiological abnormalities often precede critical illness (Singh et al 2011). The chart is colour coded to highlight abnormal findings and act as a red flag/trigger. The UK Sepsis Trust (2014) advises that action should be taken if two red flags are present – temperature >38.3°C or <36.0°C, tachycardia >90 bpm (the Royal College of Obstetricians and Gynaecologists (RCOG 2012) suggest this should be >100 bpm in pregnancy), respiratory rate >20 (counted over 1 minute), new onset of mental confusion or altered mental state – or if one of the following red flags is present – systolic blood pressure <90 mmHg or a >40 mmHg fall from baseline, tachycardia >130 bpm, oxygen saturations <91%, if the woman only responds to voice or pain or if she is unresponsive (abnormalities of blood glucose, lactate, and white cell levels are also highlighted as triggers). Clutton-Brock (2007) suggests the respiratory rate is the most important of the variables recorded for assessing the clinical condition, yet it is also the one that is recorded the least. Each of the results are given a score between 0–3 and the scores should be totalled each time the MEOWS is used. The chart contains information on what pathway to take with each totalled score and it is important the midwife takes the appropriate action. In particular, it should identify who to call and how (so timely response occurs), and how and when the clinical chain of command should be contacted (Mhyre et al 2014). The MEOWS chart can be used for pregnant women from 20 weeks' gestation and can be modified to include postnatal factors up to 6 weeks (Cole 2014).

McGlennan & Sherratt (2013) discuss the National Early Warning Score (NEWS), which was implemented in 2012, and the recommendation by the NEWS Development and Implementation Group that NEWS should not be used within obstetrics because it does not take into account the physiological changes associated with childbirth. The MEOWS chart does take these changes into account and thus should be more sensitive in detecting changes to the pregnant woman's condition. However, Clutton-Brock (2007) advises MEOWS can only be part of the solution, as it is the response to the abnormal score that determines whether there will be any real change to the outcome. Mhyre et al (2014) suggest that this form of monitoring is the cornerstone of timely diagnosis and treatments and that it should detect abnormality and trigger a response. Singh et al (2011) found that women who had triggered were more likely to develop or already have morbidity and conclude that MEOWS is a simple bedside screening tool for maternal morbidity. McGlennan & Sherratt (2013) suggest the use of MEOWS has improved the recording of 4-hourly postoperative observations and recognize it may assist in the early detection of pre-eclampsia or sepsis and facilitate earlier detection of maternal illness. There is not yet a national MEOWS chart but a definite need for one (Carle et al 2013).

ROLE AND RESPONSIBILITIES OF THE MIDWIFE

These can be summarized as:

- recognizing the significance of respiration assessment, when it is indicated and when other interventions such as pulse oximetry are required
- recognizing normal respiration rates, depths, patterns, and sounds and identifying deviations from normal for both the woman and the baby
- undertaking the assessment correctly
- using pulse oximetry appropriately
- completing the MEOWS chart accurately and identifying and acting on any triggers found.

SUMMARY

- Assessing respiration in an adult should be undertaken discreetly.
- A baby's respiratory rate can be observed or felt and should be counted for 60 seconds.
- Respiration assessment includes rate, depth, regularity, sound and posture.
- The general condition of the woman or baby is assessed simultaneously.
- Pulse oximetry is an accurate, non-invasive technique that measures oxygen saturation via a correctly fitted peripheral probe and can be used as a screening tool for critical congenital heart disease in the newborn.
- A MEOWS chart should be used for pregnant and postnatal women who have or are at risk of developing deviations from the normal.

SELF-ASSESSMENT EXERCISES

The answers to the following questions may be found in the text:

1. Discuss how pregnancy, labour, and the puerperium affect respiration. What would be the accepted normal values during these times?
2. Identify five factors that may increase respiration.
3. Why is a preterm baby more likely to develop respiratory problems than a term baby?
4. Describe when the midwife is likely to complete a respiration assessment:
   a. for a woman
   b. for a baby.
5. Which factors affect the accuracy of pulse oximetry?
6. Summarize the role and responsibilities of the midwife when undertaking respiration assessment.
7. What is a MEOWS chart and why should it be used for a woman following a caesarean section?

REFERENCES

Andrews, J., Ross, A., Salazar, M., et al., 2014. Smooth implementation of critical congenital heart defect screening in a newborn nursery. Clin. Paediatr. 53 (2), 173–176.

Blackburn, S., 2013. Maternal, Fetal and Neonatal Physiology: A Clinical Perspective, fourth ed. Saunders, St. Louis, pp. 297–355. (Chapter 10).

Cameron, J., 2011. Respiratory and cardiac disorders. In: Macdonald, S., Magill-Cuerden, J. (Eds.), Mayes' Midwifery, 14th ed. Elsevier, Edinburgh, pp. 659–674. (Chapter 10).

Carle, C., Alexander, P., Columb, M., Johal, J., 2013. Design and internal validation of an obstetric early warning score: secondary analysis of the intensive care national audit and research centre case mix programme database. Anaesthesia 68, 354–367.

Churchill, D., Rodger, A., Clift, J., Tuffnell, D., on behalf of the MBRRACE-UK sepsis chapter writing group, 2014. Think Sepsis. In: Knight, M., Kenyon, S., Brocklehurst, P., et al. on behalf of MBRRACE-UK 2014 (Eds.), Saving Lives, Improving Mothers' Care – Lessons Learned to Inform Future Maternity Care from the UK and Ireland Confidential Enquiries into Maternal Deaths and Morbidity 2009–12. National Perinatal Epidemiology Unit, Oxford, pp. 27–44.

Clutton-Brock, T., 2007. Critical Care. In: Lewis, G., 2007 The confidential enquiry into maternal and child health (CEMACH) (Eds.), Saving Mothers' Lives: Reviewing Maternal Deaths to Make Motherhood Safe – 2003–2005. The Seventh Report on Confidential Enquiries into Maternal Deaths in the UK. CEMACH, London, pp. 238–247. (Chapter 19).

Cole, M.F., 2014. A modified early obstetric warning system. Br. J. Midwifery 22 (12), 862–868.

Dearsley, A., 2013. Vital Signs. In: Koutoukidis, G., Stainton, K., Hughson, J. (Eds.), 2013 Tabbner's Nursing Care, sixth ed. Churchill Livingstone, Chatswood, pp. 301–331.

Desalu, I., Diakparomre, O.I., Salami, A.O., Abiola, A.O., 2013. The effect of nail polish and acrylic nails on pulse oximetry reading using the lifebox oximeter in Nigeria. Niger. Postgrad. Med. J. 20 (4), 331–335.

Docherty, B., Coote, S., 2006. Respiratory assessment as part of track & trigger. Nurs. Times 102 (44), 28–29.

Edmunds, S., Hollis, V., Lamb, J., Todd, J., 2011. Observations. In: Dougherty, L., Lister, S. (Eds.), The Royal Marsden Hospital Manual of Clinical Nursing Procedures, eighth ed. Wiley-Blackwell, Oxford, pp. 776–786.

Elliott, M., Coventry, A., 2012. Critical care: the eight vital signs of patient monitoring. Br. J. Nurs. 21 (10), 621–625.

England, C., 2014. Recognising the healthy baby at term through examination of the newborn screening. In: Marshall, J., Raynor, M. (Eds.), 2014 Myles Textbook for Midwives, sixteenth ed. Elsevier, Edinburgh, pp. 591–610.

Ewer, A., Granell, A., Manzoni, P., et al., 2013. Pulse oximetry screening for congenital heart defects. Lancet. 382 (Sep 7), 856–857.

Frank, L., Bradshaw, E., Beekman, R., et al., 2013. Screening for Critical Congenital Heart Disease using Pulse Oximetry. J. Pediatr. doi:10.1016/j/peds.2012.11.020.

Gardner, S.L., Enzman-Hines, M., Dickey, L.A., 2011. Respiratory Diseases. In: Gardner, S.L., Carter, B.S., Enzman-Hines, M., Hernandez, J.A. (Eds.), Merenstein & Gardner's Handbook of Neonatal Intensive Care, seventh ed. Mosby, St. Louis, pp. 581–677. (Chapter 23).

Grindheim, G., Toska, K., Estensen, M., Rosseland, L., 2012. Changes in pulmonary function during pregnancy: a longitudinal cohort study. Br. J. Obstet. Gynaecol. 119, 94–101.

Higginson, R., Jones, B., 2009. Respiratory assessment in critically ill patients: airway and breathing. Br. J. Nurs. 18 (8), 456–461.

Iscoe, S., Beasley, R., Fisher, A., 2011. Supplementary oxygen for nonhypoxemic patients: O_2 much of a good thing? Crit. Care 15, 305.

Jamieson, E., McCall, J., Whyte, L., 2002. Clinical nursing practices, fourth ed. Churchill Livingstone, Edinburgh.

Jevon, P., 2010. How to ensure patient observations lead to prompt identification of tachypnoea. Nurs. Times 106 (2), 12–14.

Kattwinkel, J., Perlman, J.M., Aziz, K., et al., 2010. Part 15: Neonatal Resuscitation: 2010 American Heart Association guidelines for cardiopulmonary resuscitation and emergency cardiovascular care. Circulation 122, S909–S919.

Kelly, P., 2006. Pulse oximetry and capnography. In: Schell, H., Puntillo, K. (Eds.), Critical Care Nursing Secrets, second ed. Mosby, St. Louis, pp. 284–290.

Lewis, G., The Confidential Enquiry into Maternal and Child Health (CEMACH) (Eds.), 2007. Saving Mothers' Lives: Reviewing Maternal Deaths to Make Motherhood Safe – 2003–2005. The Seventh Report on Confidential Enquiries into Maternal Deaths in the UK. CEMACH, London.

Lippincott, Williams, Wilkins, 2013. Lippincott's Nursing Procedures, sixth ed. Wolters Kluwer, Philadelphia, pp. 617–619, 629–631.

Mahle, W.T., Newburger, J.W., Matherne, G.P., et al., 2009. Role of pulse oximetry in examining newborns for congenital heart disease: A scientific statement from the AHA and AAP. Pediatrics 124 (2), 823–836.

Massey, D., Meredith, T., 2010. Respiratory Assessment 1: Why do it and how to do it. Br. J. Cardiac Nurs. 5 (11), 537–541.

McClure, J.H., Cooper, G.M., Clutton-Brock, T.H., on behalf of the Centre for Maternal and Child Enquiries, 2011. Saving mothers' lives: reviewing maternal deaths to make motherhood safer: 2006–8: a review. Br. J. Anaesth. 107 (2), 127–132.

McGlennan, A.P., Sherratt, K., 2013. Charting change on the labour ward. Anaesthesia 68, 333–342.

Mhyre, J.M., D'Oria, R., Hameed, A.B., et al., 2014. The Maternal Early Warning Criteria. Obstet. Gynecol. 124 (4), 782–786.

Mooney, G. 2007 Respiratory assessment. Available online: <http://www.nursingtimes.net/ntclinical/respiratory_assessment.html> (accessed 1 March 2015).

Moyle, J., 1999. Pulse oximetry. J. Neonatal Nurs. 5 (2), 24–26.

Nelson, C., Schell, H., 2006. Respiratory assessment. In: Schell, H., Puntillo, K. (Eds.), Critical Care Nursing Secrets, second ed. Mosby, St. Louis, pp. 241–246.

NICE (National Institute for Health and Care Excellence), 2007. CG50 Acutely ill patients in hospital: recognition of and response to acute illness in adults in hospital. Available online: <www.nice.org.uk> (accessed 1 March 2015).

NICE (National Institute for Health and Clinical Excellence), 2011. CG 132 Caesarean section. Available online: <www.nice.org.uk> (accessed 1 March 2015).

Oates, M., Harper, A., Shakespeare, J., Nelson-Piercy, C., 2011. Back to basics. Br. J. Obstet. Gynaecol. 118 (Suppl. 1), 16–21.

Prudhoe, S., Abu-Harb, M., Richmond, S., Wren, C., 2013. Neonatal Screening for Critical Cardiovascular Anomalies using Pulse Oximetry. Arch. Dis. Child. Fetal Neonatal Ed. 98, F346–F350.

Ramjattan, K., Allen, P., 2013. Pulse Oximetry Screening for Critical Congenital Heart Disease in the Newborn. Pediatr. Nurs. 39 (5), 250–256.

RCOG, (Royal College of Obstetricians & Gynaecologists), 2012. Green-top Guideline No. 64a. Bacterial Sepsis in Pregnancy. Available online: <https://www.rcog.org.uk/globalassets/documents/guidelines/gtg_64a.pdf> (accessed 28 January 2015).

Singh, S., McGlennan, A., England, A., Simons, R., 2011. A validation study of the CEMACH recommended modified early obstetric warning system (MEOWS). Anaesthesia 67, 12–18.

Tollefson, J., 2010. Clinical Psychomotor Skills: Assessment Tools for Nursing Students, fourth ed. Cengage, Melbourne.

UK Sepsis Trust, 2014. Appendix 1: Introducing Red Flag Sepsis. Available online: <http://sepsistrust.org/wp-content/uploads/2015/08/1409314199UKSTAppendix1RFS2014.pdf> (accessed 17 December 2015).

Villaflor, C., Morean, C., Lim, N., Foo, K., 2013. Effect of acrylic gel nail art on pulse oximetry readings. Singapore Nurs. J. 40 (4), 38–41.

Yamomoto, L., Yamomoto, J., Yamomoto, J., et al., 2008. Nail Polish does not significantly affect pulse oximetry measurements in mildly hypoxic subjects. Respir. Care 53 (11), 1470–1474.

Chapter | 7 |

Assessment of maternal and neonatal vital signs: neurological assessment

LEARNING OUTCOMES

Having read this chapter, the reader should be able to:

- describe the different components of the Glasgow Coma Scale (GCS)
- discuss how the midwife can complete the GCS
- identify the other observations that should be undertaken in conjunction with the GCS to gain a thorough neurological assessment.

Neurological assessment may be undertaken when there are concerns about actual or possible alterations in a woman's level of consciousness (e.g. post-seizure, magnesium toxicity, meningitis, head injury). Initially a doctor with neurological experience will complete the neurological assessment evaluating level of consciousness, pupillary reaction, motor (including reflexes), sensory and cerebellar function and vital signs. A reduced assessment of level of consciousness, motor signs (limb movement), pupillary assessment in conjunction with vital signs – respiration, heart rate, blood pressure, temperature and oxygen saturation – can be undertaken by the midwife. The midwife must be appropriately trained to enable her to complete a neurological assessment competently and safely, as it provides invaluable information regarding the woman's condition. The Modified Early Obstetric Warning Scoring (MEOWS) chart may contain some of the components of neurological assessment, e.g. alertness, response to stimulation (p. 66) This chapter focuses on the principles of neurological assessment and the midwife's role in relation to undertaking this assessment.

FREQUENCY OF OBSERVATIONS

NICE (2014) recommend that neurological observations should be completed every 30 minutes until the GCS is 15, when they can then be recorded hourly for 4 hours, then every 2 hours, reverting to 30-minute assessments if the condition deteriorates.

GLASGOW COMA SCALE

The GCS was developed in 1974 and revised in 1979 to provide a quick and objective assessment of eye opening, verbal response and motor ability, enabling the level of consciousness to be monitored effectively and is accepted as the 'gold standard' assessment tool (Palmer & Knight 2006). Each of these three categories has four to six different responses and each response is scored. The three scores are totalled to score between 15 (fully conscious) and 3 (no response) to provide a rapid assessment of the woman's condition and response to treatment. NICE (2014) state that a GCS >12 indicates a normal or minimally impaired level of consciousness. The score should be recorded as a fraction using 15 as the denominator (e.g. 10/15). NICE (2014) recommend that information about the three separate GCS responses should also be recorded, e.g. a score of 12/15 based on scores of 3 on eye opening, 4 on verbal response, and 5 on motor ability should be recorded as E3, V4, M5.

Eye opening

Eye opening is the first GCS measurement of consciousness, as without this cognition does not occur; however, it does not indicate the neurological system is intact (Iankova 2006). Okamura (2014) states it is assessing the integrity of the reticular activating system found in the brainstem. It cannot be used if there has been damage to the eyes resulting in swelling, as it is unlikely the eyes will open easily, rendering this aspect of the assessment unreliable until the swelling subsides. Jevon (2008) recommends recording this as 'C'.

The midwife should look at the woman to see if her eyes are opening spontaneously (score 4). If the eyes remain closed, the midwife should speak to the woman, which should provoke the eyes to open (score 3). Waterhouse (2009) suggests a greater response is achieved by asking the woman if she 'wants a cup of tea' rather than saying her name.

If the eyes continue to remain closed, a painful peripheral stimulus is used – this may be a gentle shake but if no response a deeper stimulus is needed. Pressure is applied using a pen positioned just below the lateral outer aspect of the second or third interphalangeal joint for 10–15 seconds (Iankova 2006, Okamura 2014, Waterhouse 2009) (score 2). Painful stimulation should be applied slowly up to a maximum of 15 seconds. Pressure should not be applied to the nail bed because of the risk of bruising (Edmunds et al 2011).

If there is no response using a painful peripheral stimulus, a central painful stimulus is used. Central stimulation involves the application of a noxious painful stimulus to the core of the nervous system via the cranial nerves to elicit a complete motor response (Waterhouse 2009). However, the woman may grimace while keeping her eyes closed, and so it is not generally used unless the midwife has been appropriately trained. It is important to use the same stimulus on each assessment. A score of 1 is given if the eyes remain closed.

Jevon (2008) recommends squeezing the trapezium muscle using a thumb and two fingers and Edmunds et al (2011) advise twisting 3–5 cm of muscle from where the neck and shoulders meet for up to 30 seconds to stimulate

the spinal accessory nerve (XI), although this is difficult on large or obese women. Waterhouse (2009) considers this to be the safer technique for inexperienced staff. Alternatively the supraorbital nerve, part of the trigeminal nerve (V), can be stimulated by applying pressure to the supraorbital ridge provided there is no suspected or confirmed facial fracture or glaucoma (Palmer & Knight 2006) but bradycardia may occur. This is achieved by placing the thumb into the indentation below the eyebrow, close to the nose, and applying gradual pressure for up to 30 seconds (Okamura 2014). Sternal rubs are used with caution because they can cause bruising and the flat of the hand should be used, not the knuckles. It should not be used for repeated assessments (Edmunds et al 2011).

Waterhouse (2009) recommends central painful stimulus, rather than peripheral pain stimulus, is used as it can result in both an eye opening response and assess motor ability. The type and site of the stimulus used should be documented.

Verbal response

Assessing the verbal response is an assessment of the integrity of the higher, cognitive and interpretive centres of the brain (Okamura 2014). The midwife should ascertain the level of verbal response by asking questions that require answers to show clarity and understanding – What is your name? Where are you? What day is it? – an accurate answer scores 5. If the woman is able to speak using full sentences but the answers are incorrect, a score of 4 is given. If only words and incomplete sentences are given, the score is 3, regardless of whether the words are appropriate. A score of 2 is given if incomprehensible sounds (e.g. grunts, groans) are made. If no sound is made in response to verbal or painful central stimuli, 1 is scored.

It is important to take into account the language spoken by the woman; if she does not speak English, an interpreter should be used.

Motor ability

The response of the upper limbs is tested to determine the integrity of the motor strip within the cerebral cortex (Okamura 2014), as the lower limbs can also be affected by spinal function. The midwife should ask the woman to bend then hold out her arms and squeeze the midwife's hands with both of her hands. The midwife can then determine that both arms can be moved and the elbows flexed, the power and release of grip from each hand can be noted.

A score of 6 is given if the woman is able to complete these movements and 1 if there is no response despite painful central stimuli. Scores of 2–5 are given according to the degree of movement and flexion occurring as a result of painful stimulus: the arm moving towards the stimuli to try to remove it (5), arm bends at the elbow without rotation of the wrist (4) or with wrist rotation and forearm rotation (3), the arm extends at the elbow while the wrist flexes (2).

Pupillary assessment

While this is not part of the GCS, it is a separate and important component of the neurological assessment. The size and shape of each pupil and reaction to light are assessed. The midwife should look at the pupils to determine if they are the same shape and whether the eyes are working together. The diameter of each pupil is then measured – the normal range is 2–6 mm (Dawson 2000) – and they are usually equal in size (unequal pupils are a late sign associated with raised intracranial pressure, but may be of little significance if the woman is alert and orientated and small differences in pupil size are often normal). Pupil reaction is assessed by shining a bright light from a pen torch into one eye, then the other – approach from the side rather than directly in front. The pupils should decrease in size and the speed at which this occurs is recorded. If there is no response, the pupil is fixed and suggests the midbrain may be suffering from pressure as constriction and dilation of the pupils is controlled by the oculomotor nerve (cranial nerve III). Pupils that are slow to respond or which dilate suddenly and unequally indicate that cerebral oedema or haematoma is worsening (Waterhouse 2005). The level of sedation administered to the woman will affect pupil reaction – pupils measuring 1–2 mm can occur when barbiturates or opiates have been used. Edmunds et al (2011) suggest that if the pupil size is equal but they are pinpoint in size, opiates or a Pontine lesion may be the cause whereas when they are equal but small and reactive, there be metabolic encephalopathy, equal-sized and fixed may be due to a midbrain lesion and equal, mid-sized pupils may be caused by a metabolic lesion. They also advise that when pupils are unequal, dilated, and unreactive, a cranial nerve III palsy may be responsible and unequal, small, reactive pupils may be a result of Horner's syndrome (Edmunds et al 2011).

The findings of the neurological assessment should be recorded on a neurological observation chart (Fig. 7.1) in conjunction with the MEOWS, vital signs including temperature (see Chapter 3), pulse (see Chapter 4), blood pressure (see Chapter 5), and respiratory rate (see Chapter 6). Blood oxygen saturation should also be monitored (NICE 2014) (see p. 65). While the total GCS score is recorded, it is also important to record separately the scores of the three different categories, as each one is assessing different areas of the brain. A decreasing score indicates the woman's condition is deteriorating and referral is indicated.

The doctor should be informed if there is a severe or increasing headache, persistent vomiting, new or evolving neurological signs and symptoms (e.g. pupil inequality), a reduction to 3 or less points in eye opening or verbal responses or 2 in motor responses, agitation or abnormal behaviour as these can indicate deterioration of the woman's neurological status.

PROCEDURE: Neurological assessment

* Gather equipment and take to the bedside:
  * pencil torch
  * observation chart
  * thermometer
  * sphygmomanometer
  * pulse oximeter.
* Wash and dry hands.
* Inform the woman of the procedure and gain consent if conscious and responsive.
* Complete vital signs: temperature, blood pressure, pulse, respiration and arterial oxygen saturation.
* Assess level of consciousness by talking with the woman and asking her who she is, what day it is and where she is; use peripheral or central painful stimulus if no response.
* Assess motor function by asking the woman to bend and lift her arms and to squeeze both your hands.
* Assess the size and shape of the pupils and movement of the eyes.
* Assess pupillary reaction by:
  * darkening the room if necessary
  * holding one eyelid open, move the pen torchlight towards and across the eye, moving the light from side to side
  * assess the degree and speed at which the pupil constricts
  * repeat with the other eye
  * then with both eyelids held open, shine the light into one eye – the pupil in the other eye should also be observed to constrict
  * repeat with the other eye.
* Ensure the woman is covered and comfortable.
* Document all findings on the observation chart.
* Wash and dry hands.
* Act on findings accordingly.

ROLE AND RESPONSIBILITIES OF THE MIDWIFE

These can be summarized as:
* ensuring appropriate training in assessing neurological observation has been undertaken prior to performing the neurological assessment
* undertaking a competent examination in which all of the information is gained
* recognizing deviations from normal and instigating referral
* appropriate record keeping.

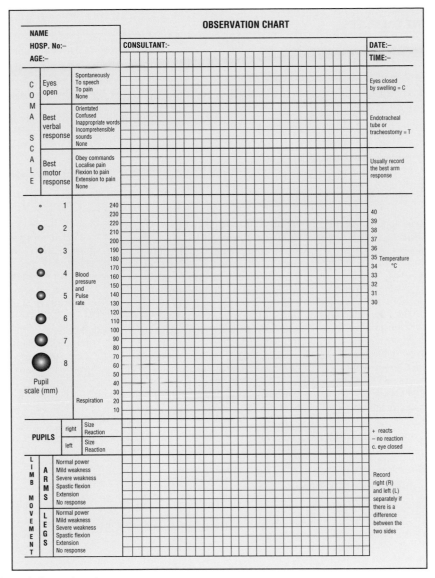

Figure 7.1 Neurological observation chart.
(Adapted with kind permission from Jamieson et al 2002)

SUMMARY

- Neurological assessment is undertaken where there are actual or potential altering levels of consciousness.
- The GCS determines the level of consciousness by assessing the woman's response to the three categories of eye opening, verbal response and motor ability.
- The midwife who has been appropriately trained can undertake the GCS and recording of vital signs as part of the woman's neurological assessment to determine any changes to her condition.
- Additionally, the doctor will evaluate motor and sensory function as required.

SELF-ASSESSMENT EXERCISES

The answers to the following questions may be found in the text:

1. What are the three categories of the Glasgow Coma Scale?
2. What observations should you undertake in conjunction with the Glasgow Coma Scale?
3. How does the midwife assess eye opening?
4. If there is no response, how is central stimuli applied?
5. How can the midwife determine the verbal response?
6. How does the midwife assess motor response?

REFERENCES

Dawson, D., 2000. Neurological care. In: Sheppard, M., Wright, M. (Eds.), Principles and practices of high dependence nursing. Baillière Tindall, Edinburgh, pp. 145–182.

Edmunds, S., Hollis, V., Lamb, J., Todd, J., 2011. Observations. In: Dougherty, L., Lister, S. (Eds.), The Royal Marsden Hospital manual of clinical nursing procedures, eighth ed. Wiley-Blackwell, Oxford, pp. 699–802.

Iankova, A., 2006. The Glasgow coma scale. Emerg. Nurse 14 (8), 30–35.

Jamieson, E., McCall, J., Whyte, L., 2002. Clinical nursing practices, fourth ed. Churchill Livingstone, Edinburgh.

Jevon, P., 2008. Neurological assessment part 3 – Glasgow Coma Scale. Nurs. Times 104 (29), 28–29.

NICE (National Institute for Health and Care Excellence), 2014. CG 176 Head injury triage, assessment, investigation and early management of head injury in infants, children and adults. Available online: <www.nice.org.uk> (accessed 2 March 2015).

Okamura, K., 2014. Glasgow coma scale flow chart: a beginner's guide. Br. J. Nurs. 23 (20), 1068–1073.

Palmer, R., Knight, J., 2006. Assessment of altered conscious level in clinical practice. Br. J. Nurs. 15 (22), 1255–1259.

Waterhouse, C., 2005. The Glasgow coma scale and other neurological observations. Nurs. Stand. 19 (33), 56–64, 66–67.

Waterhouse, C., 2009. The use of painful stimulus in relation to the Glasgow Coma Scale observations. Br. J. Neurosci. Nurs. 5 (5), 209–214.

Chapter | 8 |

Principles of infection control: standard precautions

LEARNING OUTCOMES

Having read this chapter, the reader should be able to:

- discuss the nature and significance of standard precautions, indicating the midwife's role and responsibilities

- identify specific situations in which personal protective equipment (PPE) should be used
- describe source and protective isolation nursing.

Healthcare professionals are widely exposed to large numbers and varieties of microorganisms. This poses a threat both to the practitioner and to the women and babies in her care. The term 'standard precautions' (previously having incorporated 'universal precautions') refers to the measures taken universally, i.e. by all health professionals for all women and babies, all the time, (whatever the clinical environment, whether infection is known or suspected or not) to achieve mutual protection. The ultimate aim of standard precaution use is to prevent the transfer of infection. As an important area of care, the reader is required to keep up-to-date with developing protocols. The cost of infection to individuals (service users and staff), the NHS, and the community as a whole is large and the increasing incidence of healthcare-associated infections (HCAIs) all mean that the use of standard precautions has to be correct every time. This chapter reviews the nature and use of standard precautions and the principles of isolation nursing.

STANDARD INFECTION CONTROL PRECAUTIONS

Childbearing women are considered to be in a high-risk category for standard precaution use because:

- unprotected sexual intercourse is likely to have taken place
- there is exposure to large amounts of blood and body fluid during episodes of care.

Applying standard precautions to everyone maintains safety and prevents any individual feeling isolated or 'singled out'. In the UK the NHS encourages service users to be aware

75

of, and involved in, the infection control issue with campaigns such as 'It's ok to ask' (NPSA 2011), giving permission for women to ask midwives and doctors if they have washed their hands. Confidentiality may be compromised if some procedures are perceived to be used for some women and not for others. While there may be times when wearing protective clothing is potentially disruptive to the relationship that a midwife has built up with a woman, the midwife must consider the significance of protection, both for the woman and midwife, and that of other women, too. Simple explanations to the woman are usually sufficient and reassuring.

Standard precautions should be used when there is or expected to be contact with blood, vaginal and seminal secretions, urine or faeces, amniotic fluid, cerebrospinal fluid, saliva, breast milk or any other bodily fluid. Sweat is the only exception. While the principles need to be applied correctly, the midwife needs to be alert to these situations:

- examination *per vaginam*, use of amnihook, fetal scalp electrodes, etc.
- childbirth, of whichever type
- theatre work, including suction/aspiration of body fluids
- disposal of administration sets, blood transfusion sets, etc.
- specimens, including neonatal capillary sampling and urinalysis
- injections
- newborn babies prior to bathing
- postnatal observations of lochia and perineum
- perineal repair
- cannulation and venepuncture.

PRINCIPLES OF STANDARD PRECAUTIONS

Hand decontamination

This is discussed in detail in Chapter 9; this is a summary.

- It should be practised routinely and thoroughly using approved liquid soap and running water at a comfortable temperature.
- Good-quality paper towels should allow the hands to dry with one or two of them and a hands-free clinical waste bin should be immediately available.
- There are five moments (WHO 2009 pp. 93–94, 113) when hand decontamination is necessary, Chapter 9 expands further on this. In summary, handwashing and drying must be undertaken (WHO 2009 p. 113):
  1. before every episode of direct contact or care
  2. after every episode of direct contact or care
  3. before an aseptic procedure

4. immediately after contact with body fluids, mucous membranes and non-intact skin
5. immediately after contact with objects/equipment in the immediate patient environment and also when putting on and taking off gloves, prior to handling food, when hands are visibly soiled, after going to the toilet and after several applications of handrub.

- Alcohol handrub can be used but only if the hands are clean, i.e. not contaminated with body fluids or visibly dirty and if the woman being cared for is free from enteric infection (diarrhoea or vomiting-type illnesses) (Loveday et al 2014).
- Cuts or abrasions on the skin should be covered with a waterproof dressing that is an effective barrier to viruses and bacteria.
- Arms should be bare below the elbows.

Personal protective equipment

Personal protective equipment (PPE) is that which aims to protect healthcare practitioners from being infected and to stop the potential transfer of infection from one client to another via staff members. Such items include gloves, gowns, aprons, masks, goggles, visors, caps and theatre footwear. Wyeth (2013) suggests that there can be inappropriate and overuse of such items, this agrees with Wilson & Loveday (2014) who found that staff wanted to protect themselves and their families from the threat of infection. This has a safety and a cost implication.

The appropriate items should be selected following a risk assessment:

- What is the likelihood of transmission of microorganisms to the woman or midwife?
- What is the risk of the midwife/midwife's clothing being contaminated by any of the woman's body fluids?
- Is the equipment suitable for the proposed use? (Loveday et al 2014).

Determining the risk will aid the midwife in their choice of protection. The items should all be readily available at the point of use. Care should also be taken to **remove** PPE correctly and in the correct order:

1. Gloves (added last, removed first)
2. Apron
3. Eye protection
4. Masks
5. Wash and dry hands.

Gloves

Gloves should be selected according to the task that is to be undertaken and according to size. Wearing the wrong-sized gloves can affect dexterity and cause muscle fatigue and sweatiness (RCN 2012). Gloves should be stored correctly and used within the expiry date. For many routine tasks, gloves are not required, e.g. vital sign observations; non-sterile gloves (examination gloves, ambidextrous) should be worn when handling body fluids, e.g. emptying catheter bags, removing vomit, urine testing, while sterile gloves (surgical gloves, clearly marked right and left) are worn for childbirth, surgery, and any procedures in which an Aseptic Non Touch Technique (ANTT) causes the hands to be in close proximity to Key-Sites or Key-Parts (Chapter 10) (WHO 2009, p. 128). As a general rule, gloves should be selected and worn:

- for invasive procedures and those with actual or potential risk of exposure to blood or body fluids
- when in contact with aseptic sites, non-intact skin or mucous membranes
- when handling sharps or contaminated devices (Loveday et al 2014).

Gloves are also worn to protect the hands from repeated exposure to particular chemicals/situations, e.g. use of surface wipes to clean trays and trolleys. The hands are decontaminated on glove removal as for any other procedure. Gloves should be worn once only, removed as soon after use as possible, removed correctly and disposed of in the clinical waste.

How to remove gloves (WHO 2009, p. 129)

- Use the dominant hand to grasp the outside wrist of the other glove, pull it off so that it becomes inside out.
- Keep hold of it with the gloved hand then slide the ungloved thumb inside the cuff of the other glove.
- Remove the glove, turning it inside out. As this happens both gloves become contained, inside out, within the second glove.
- Decontaminate hands.

Removing gloves in this way (whether sterile or non-sterile) prevents the hands from being contaminated from the gloves and contains contamination within the gloves. Gloves that are just 'ripped off' spread contamination into the air and onto nearby surfaces. Wilson & Loveday (2014) suggest that gloves put on too early or removed too late add to the transmission of microorganisms.

Gloves offer some measure of protection but hand contamination still occurs and gloves perforate; consequently Hubner et al (2013) suggest that after 15 minutes the hands should be washed and new gloves applied. Double gloving is not recommended (RCN 2012).

Plastic aprons

Disposable plastic aprons should be worn when close contact with a woman or any materials or equipment is anticipated that risks contaminating the midwife's clothing (Loveday et al 2014). Like gloves, they are single-use items, worn for one task and then removed. Hart (2008) indicates that an apron should not touch the hair when being put on and it should be worn loosely. At the end of the procedure it should be removed after the gloves (see above), by breaking the cleaner parts, e.g. neck ties and sides, it is then folded 'in' so that the potentially contaminated area does not touch the clothing. Hand decontamination should then be undertaken. Different-coloured aprons are worn for different tasks.

Full-body gowns

Gowns are usually worn for surgical procedures, including perineal repair and siting epidurals. They are sterile, fluid repellent, single-use and designed to protect the whole body/clothing of the practitioner. They are folded in such a way that they are put on without touching the outside that will be nearest to the woman. Martirani & Weaving (2011, p. 98) illustrate this.

Masks and eye protection

Masks (fluid repellent) and eye protection are necessary when body fluids can be splashed, e.g. during surgical procedures. If used, they are removed after gloves and aprons and are always removed by handling the ties/frame at the sides and back of the head, rather than touching the front that is likely to be contaminated.

Sharps

A sharps injury is one that occurs as a result of the skin being broken by a medical sharp – needles, scalpels, stitch cutters, etc. It is a common but preventable injury that has significant cost financially and in human terms. New legislation affecting the UK (NHS EO 2013) requires employers to inform and train employees and to provide safety-engineered sharps wherever practical, to reduce the risk and incidence of sharps injuries. A protocol must also exist so that in the event of an injury, staff know what action to take and how prophylactic exposure treatment can be accessed.

The handling of sharps must be kept to a minimum. This means that in practice:

- Used needles must never be resheathed; needle protection devices should be fitted and used.
- All sharps should be placed directly into an approved sharps box at the point of care by the person who used it. The sharps box should only be filled to the indicated level then secured and disposed

of correctly. It should be temporarily closed between each use.

- A neutral zone should be used so that sharps are never passed hand to hand, e.g. in theatre.

Isolation

Isolation for known infections is necessary, this will be according to local protocol. It is discussed in greater detail below.

Infection control protocols

The control of infection is also undertaken at service provider level. Protocols exist locally (and are regularly updated) to cover issues such as cleanliness of the environment, equipment hygiene, sterile supplies, prevention of overcrowding or excessive transferring of clients between areas, disposal of clinical waste, managing accidents and spillages (discussed below), and postexposure prophylaxis, all of which the reader needs to be familiar with. However, Loveday et al (2014) suggest that some of these issues, e.g. environmental and equipment hygiene, are in fact the responsibility of us all. All equipment should be decontaminated correctly after use, clinical waste should be disposed of properly in hospitals and at home, and the cleanliness of the environment is something that all practitioners contribute to.

MANAGEMENT OF SPILLS OR ACCIDENTS

A specific protocol will be available in each area. These are general guidelines:

- Skin that is accidentally exposed should be washed immediately with soap and water.
- If the conjunctiva or any mucous membrane is splashed the areas should be irrigated with copious amounts of water. Avoid swallowing if the splash is into the mouth, then rinse several times with cold water.
- In the event of a needlestick injury (or other percutaneous injury, e.g. a bite) the area should be encouraged to bleed (but do not suck the wound) under running water for at least 5 minutes (Boyle 2000). It should then be washed thoroughly (but not scrubbed) with soap and water and covered with a waterproof dressing (NHS 2013). The agreed local protocol should be followed; this is likely to include reporting the incident to a manager and to occupational health, completing an incident form

and being involved in a risk assessment/incident investigation.

- Spillages of body fluids should be cleared up using gloves, an apron, and disposable wipes as soon after the event as possible. The local protocol will suggest which detergents are to be used, often chlorine-releasing granules are used which need to be left in place for at least 2 minutes before being cleared away.

ISOLATION NURSING

Source isolation

Standard precautions aim to contain any infections, restricting their transmission between individuals. Sometimes, for specific infections, e.g. hepatitis B, tuberculosis, *Salmonella*, or MRSA (methicillin-resistant *Staphylococcus aureus*), stricter isolation is necessary. The decision to isolate someone needs a multidisciplinary risk assessment that considers these factors:

- the known pathogen
- suitability of the environment, with specific regard to hygiene and domestic services support
- the anticipated length of time of the isolation
- the immune status of other ward occupants (Hart 2008).

A scoring system can be implemented to aid with single-room prioritization, e.g. Breathnach et al (2010). Standard precautions and PPE are indicated as for any other clinical situation, but additional measures, depending upon the causative organism and its mode of transmission, will be included. For example, droplet infections (meningococcal meningitis, tuberculosis) require the wearing of a mask and, for certain procedures, eye protection. The woman may find isolation daunting, lonely, and stressful. Her understanding and cooperation are needed to achieve the desired outcome. Barratt et al (2011) also note that sometimes in isolation women received substandard care.

General principles

- In a hospital environment the use of an en suite side room is the most likely means of isolation; it is helpful if it has an anteroom where necessary items can be kept. The room should ideally have negative pressure ventilation, i.e. air is drawn in from the ward but leaves the room externally, away from the ward (Cutter & Dempster 1999).
- The room should be equipped with all the essential but minimum materials required, e.g. sphygmomanometer, washing equipment, water jug

and glass, sharps box, antibacterial soap and disposable towels, dissolvable linen sack (red in the UK), clinical waste sack, Pinard stethoscope, etc. The refuse sack is sealed in the room and then removed, but otherwise none of the equipment is removed from the room until cleaned or disposed of appropriately after the woman's departure. Unnecessary furniture is removed and a visible indication is placed on the door – often a colour-coded sign – to remind all staff. Instructions should be given to friends and relatives as to how to maintain the isolation principles.

- A trolley outside the room contains items that are needed when entering the room, e.g. gloves, disposable gowns, masks, goggles, overshoes, plastic aprons and antibacterial handrub. This should not cause an obstruction.
- The midwife should recognize the value of the multidisciplinary team: the infection control nurse, microbiologist, obstetrician, and midwife will all need to work in close communication and partnership to provide appropriate care for the woman. The woman may also remain in her side room for delivery and additional precautions should be instigated accordingly.
- Ideally, specific members of staff may be assigned to care for infected women; they should then have restricted access to other women, especially any that may be considered vulnerable to infection.

PROCEDURE: entering, attending the woman, and leaving the room

- Gather any necessary additional equipment.
- Wash and dry hands, apply apron and any other necessary protective clothing necessary for the procedure. Use alcohol handrub (apply gloves only if expecting to handle body fluids).
- Knock, enter the room, and close the door.
- Complete the necessary care, containing all of the tasks within the room:
  - crockery may be brought out of the room, providing that it will be decontaminated in a dishwasher
  - domestic services are required to clean the room and bathroom daily using approved cleansers and including a thorough damp dusting; other spillages should be cleaned according to standard precaution guidelines. Cleaning cloths etc. remain in the room for the duration of the stay and are only used in that room
  - used linen should be placed in the dissolvable sack in the room. This must be sealed before

leaving the room. Clinical waste is managed in the same way.
- On preparing to leave the room, remove gloves (if worn) and apron, place in the clinical waste. Decontaminate hands.
- Close the door on leaving; use antibacterial handrub once outside the room (unless enteric infection, see p. 82).
- On discharge the room is thoroughly cleaned using approved solutions; steam cleaning may be required. All furniture and equipment is washed and dried, curtains are sent to the laundry; carpeted floor should be steam cleaned.

Protective isolation

This involves protecting an individual from infection because they are in some way vulnerable or immunocompromised. The midwife is less likely to be involved in this type of care. All unnecessary visitors are prohibited and extreme care is taken to ensure that no infection is taken into the room. A positive pressure environment is needed where clean air is drawn into the room from outside and forced out into the general ward area. Clearly, the ventilation systems need to be properly understood so that the opposite does not happen (Cutter & Dempster 1999) Hands are decontaminated and protective clothing is applied before entering and removed after leaving the room.

ROLE AND RESPONSIBILITIES OF THE MIDWIFE

These can be summarized as:
- recognizing the significance of standard precautions and PPE, risk assessing and utilizing them appropriately on every occasion and documenting their use accordingly
- the ability to adapt them to each area of work, maintaining safety for all
- the need to be familiar with up-to-date reports and protocols
- universal use to protect dignity and confidentiality
- the need to report and act on spillages or incidents.

SUMMARY

- Standard precautions aim to protect all staff, women, babies and visitors from potentially serious infections.

79

They use a range of measures including hand hygiene and PPE use. It is an important aspect of the midwife's role.

- The midwife works with a high-risk client group and should include a risk assessment for standard precautions and PPE use in every clinical situation.
- Source isolation aims to contain infection by carrying out all procedures within the woman's single room, keeping all equipment and materials within that room.
- Protective isolation prevents infection from entering the room by use of protective measures before entering and after leaving; visitors are restricted.

SELF-ASSESSMENT EXERCISES

The answers to the following questions may be found in the text:

1. Describe what constitutes standard precautions.
2. In which situations is a risk assessment necessary to appreciate which of the standard precautions or PPE are indicated?
3. Describe how to correctly apply a plastic apron.
4. Demonstrate how to remove soiled gloves, apron, and goggles.
5. Discuss the principles of source and protective isolation nursing.

REFERENCES

Barratt, R., Shaban, R., Moyle, W., 2011. Patient experience of source isolation: lessons for clinical practice. Contemp. Nurse 39 (2), 180–193.

Boyle, M., 2000. Blood borne infections. Pract. Midwife 3 (7), 48–50.

Breathnach, A., Zinna, S., Riley, P., Planche, T., 2010. Guidelines for prioritization for single room use: a pragmatic approach. J. Hosp. Infect 74 (1), 89–91.

Cutter, M., Dempster, L., 1999. Cover notes. Nurs. Times 95 (31), 25–27.

Hart, S., 2008. Barrier Nursing. In: Doughty, L., Lister, S. (Eds.), The Royal Marsden Hospital Manual of Clinical Nursing Procedures Student Edition. Wiley Blackwell, Oxford, pp. 117–204.

Hubner, N., Goerdt, A., Mannerow, A., et al., 2013. The durability of examination gloves used on intensive care units. BMC Infect. Dis. 13 (226), 1471–2334.

Loveday, H., Wilson, J., Pratt, R.J., et al., 2014. epic3: National Evidence-Based Guidelines for Preventing Healthcare – Associated Infections in NHS Hospitals in England. J. Hosp. Infect 86 (Suppl. 1), S1–S70.

Martirani, R., Weaving, A., 2011. Infection prevention & control. In: Doughty, L., Lister, S. (Eds.), The Royal Marsden Hospital Manual of Clinical Nursing Procedures, eighth ed. Wiley Blackwell, Chichester, (Chapter 3). pp. 79–128.

NPSA (National Patient Safety Agency), 2011. It's ok to ask. Available online: <http://www.npsa.nhs.uk/cleanyourhands/about-us/faqs/> (accessed 5 March 2015).

NHS EO (National Health Service European Office), 2013. Protecting healthcare workers from sharps injuries Briefing 13. The NHS Confederation, Brussels.

NHS (National Health Service), 2013. NHS Choices: What should I do if I injure myself with a used needle? Available online: <http://www.nhs.uk/chq/Pages/2557.aspx?CategoryID=72> (accessed 23 January 2015).

RCN (Royal College of Nursing), 2012. Tools of the trade. RCN, London. Available online: at <www.rcn.org.uk> (accessed 5 March 2015).

WHO (World Health Organisation), 2009. WHO Guidelines on Hand Hygiene in Health Care. WHO, Geneva, pp. 101, 102, 123, 140, 141.

Wilson, J., Loveday, H., 2014. Does glove use increase the risk of infection? Nurs. Times 110 (39), 12–15.

Wyeth, J., 2013. Hand hygiene and the use of personal protective equipment. B. J. Nurs 22 (16), 920–925.

Principles of infection control: hand hygiene

LEARNING OUTCOMES

Having read this chapter, the reader should be able to:

- discuss why hand hygiene is important
- discuss the principles of general hand care
- discuss the benefits of alcohol handrub and when it should be used
- identify the occasions when the midwife should undertake hand decontamination and what should be used
- describe the main differences between 'medical/ social' and 'surgical' scrub
- discuss the role and responsibilities of the midwife in relation to hand hygiene.

This chapter focuses on the principles of hand hygiene, an important means of infection control. Hand hygiene encompasses both hand care and hand decontamination; hand decontamination includes both handwashing and the use of alcohol handrub (NICE 2014). Hand hygiene is the most effective, least expensive way to prevent healthcare-associated infections (HCAIs) and one of the most important approaches to patient care (Kilpatrick et al 2013, Spruce 2013).

Transient microorganisms colonize the superficial layers of the skin; usually they do not multiply, although they occasionally survive and multiply but can be removed by hand decontamination. Colony forming units (CFUs) of bacteria on the hands range from $3.9 \times 10^4 - 4.6 \times 10^6$ CFU/cm^2 but can be much higher in the perineal and inguinal areas (WHO 2009). Up to 10^6 skin squames containing viable microorganisms can be shed each day from normal skin causing contamination of clothes, bedding, furniture, etc.; thus it can be easy to contaminate hands during 'clean' procedures such as taking vital signs, assisting with changing clothes. Microorganisms survive for differing time periods on the hands in the absence of hand decontamination, e.g. only 50% of *Escherichia coli* are killed in 6 minutes (WHO 2009). WHO (2009) advise that microorganisms such as staphylococci, enterococci, and *Clostridium difficile* are more resistant to desiccation and thus more likely to be the cause of contamination. Resident flora are attached to the deeper layers of the skin and are more resistant to removal but are also less likely to be a cause of a HCAI. Cross-contamination can also occur from hands to paper, including medical records (Hübner et al 2011).

Approximately 30% of the population is colonized with *Staphylococcus aureus* on their skin or in their nose with no ill effects. However 3% of the population has the methicillin-resistant *Staphylococcus aureus* (MRSA) strain of this microorganism which is difficult to treat because of its antibiotic resistance. MRSA is spread by direct contact with a contaminated surface/material or skin-to-skin and its spread is reduced with handwashing and the use of alcohol handrub (AHR). *Clostridium difficile,* another bacterial source of HCAIs, lives in the intestine of approximately 3% of the population. Usually the normal gut bacteria prevent *C. difficile* from affecting the person. However, if these are destroyed by antibiotics, *C. difficile* multiplies, producing toxins that can cause diarrhoea. Their spores are not killed by AHR use. MRSA and *C. difficile* were the underlying cause or contributory factor in approximately 9000 deaths in hospitals in England during 2007 (NICE 2012).

Healthcare-associated infections are infections acquired as a result of healthcare intervention; they are caused by a wide variety of microorganisms, many of which are commensals. HCAIs are troublesome to those affected because they are likely to have to stay in hospital three times longer than those who are unaffected and require longer-term follow-up and care (Gould et al 2007). Up to 300 000 patients per year in England, 1:10 according to Moore et al (2013), develop a HCAI as a result of receiving care in the NHS (NICE 2012), costing the NHS approximately one billion pounds each year. In the USA, there are approximately 1.7 million HCAIs per year, with 99 000 deaths and costing an additional $33.8 billion each year (Patrick & Van Wicklin 2012, Spruce 2013). Hand hygiene can reduce the incidence of HCAI.

GENERAL HAND CARE

- Hands should be examined daily for cuts, grazes, and torn cuticles as these increase the risk of infection to the midwife and should be covered with a waterproof dressing (NICE 2012).
- Nails should be kept short and filed smoothly as long or ragged nails can scratch women and babies or tear gloves. Dirt and secretions, which can harbour microorganisms, may be found under fingernails. The ideal length of nails is under debate – Loveday et al (2014) advise 'short', Fagernes and Lingaas (2010) advise <2 mm, WHO (2009) <5 mm, and the CDC (2002) <6.3 mm. Regardless of which of these are correct, when looking at the palmar side of hands, the nails should not be visible (Patrick & Van Wicklin 2012).
- Apply an emollient hand cream/moisturizer, which is compatible with the antiseptics and barrier products used, to the hands on a regular basis to prevent them from drying out and cracking. The product should list

water as its first ingredient and contain no anionic-based chemicals or petroleum.

- Be bare from the elbows down when providing direct patient care (Loveday et al 2014, NICE 2012). Long sleeves can be easily contaminated and make handwashing less effective (Martirani & Weaving 2011, NICE 2012). If exposure of the forearms is unacceptable for religious reasons, the sleeve should not be loose or dangling and must be rolled/pulled back securely during handwashing and direct patient care (NICE 2012).
- Rings, bracelets, and watches should not be worn (Loveday et al 2014). Rings (particularly stoned rings) increase the number of microorganisms found on the hand; jewellery and watches also make it difficult to clean the hands thoroughly, apply AHR and put gloves on (Hautemaniere et al 2010, Khodavaisy et al 2011). Hautemaniere et al (2010) suggest that wearing a flat band wedding ring does not interfere with hand decontamination, a view supported by Al-Allah et al (2008) who found that the wearing of a flat band wedding ring did not provide a source of increased bacterial load following a surgical scrub and suggest they may be kept on for this form of hand decontamination.
- False nails or nail extensions should not be worn as microorganisms can flourish in the ridge that appears as the nail grows. Additionally, Ward (2007) suggests the percentage of Gram-negative bacteria found on false nails is higher than on natural nails.
- Patrick & Van Wicklin (2012) suggest that nail polish can be worn as long as it is not cracked, crazed, or chipped. However the majority of hand hygiene and uniform policies exclude the wearing of nail polish, recognizing that it can chip easily.

HAND DECONTAMINATION

Handwashing refers to both social and clinical situations where hands are washed. Social handwashing is generally ineffective in removing/killing microorganisms due to incorrect washing technique or inappropriate cleansing agents used. Hand decontamination is a more accurate term that refers to the removal of blood, body fluids, microorganisms and their debris by mechanical means or their destruction (Loveday et al 2014).

Cleansing agents

The use of soap and water removes almost all transient microorganisms but does not significantly reduce the number of resident microorganisms. While this is acceptable in non-invasive situations with a low-risk population, there are many situations where the resident microorganisms also need to be reduced (e.g. aseptic procedures). Antiseptics (e.g. chlorhexidine) reduce the transient and resident microorganisms at the time of application, with some residual activity keeping bacterial counts low over several days as the chlorhexidine binds to the stratum corneum (the top layer of the superficial skin layer) (Gould et al 2007). Loveday et al (2014) reviewed the effectiveness of different handwashing preparations and concluded that soap was as effective as antiseptic agents.

Both soap and antiseptics usually involve the use of running water following one of two procedures: the 'medical/social' or the 'surgical' scrub. The former is used for normal handwashing and prior to aseptic techniques, whereas the latter is used when scrubbing for an operative procedure; this is a lengthier procedure involving the hands and arms.

Alcohol handrub

Products containing alcohol are inexpensive, have very good bactericidal activity and are effective against most Gram-negative and Gram-positive bacteria (Gould et al 2007). There is a theoretical fire risk with AHR, thus they should not be placed within 6 inches/15 cm of electrical switches or outlets (Patrick & Van Wicklin 2012). AHRs are used without water and require only 3–5 mL rubbed over the hands and wrists for 20–30 seconds (CDC 2002). This is much quicker than handwashing as the handrub often dries within 15 seconds; however, the action of the handrub is short-lived, has no effect on spores and some enteroviruses, and has no detergent effect. Thus, AHRs are recommended for use only when the hands are visibly clean and when the woman is not vomiting and has no diarrhoeal illness (Loveday et al 2014) as they do not remove organic material or dirt. When used effectively, AHRs remove transient microorganisms and significantly reduce the number of resident microorganisms but are not effective against some microorganisms such as *C. difficile* and noroviruses (Jabbar et al 2010, Loveday et al 2014).

Alcohol handrubs are as effective as aqueous scrubbing in preventing surgical site infections; chlorhexidine gluconate-based aqueous scrubs are more effective than povidone–iodine-based aqueous scrubs as they result in fewer bacteria on the cleaned hands (Tanner et al 2008). Tanner et al (2008) found no evidence regarding the use of brushes and sponges for the surgical scrub. However, Hsieh et al (2006) suggest that frequent and prolonged use of a brush/sponge might cause deterioration in skin condition, removal of the outer layer of epidermis and lead to potentially undesirable changes in colonizing skin flora such as increased colonization with Gram-negative bacteria. They further suggest the use of an AHR was more

effective in reducing microbial counts than the more traditional surgical scrub of 6 minutes using chlorhexidine gluconate.

Irritated skin can become chafed and cracked which not only causes pain but the damage to the protective barrier of the skin that results encourages colonization. This risk can be reduced if the AHR contains an emollient to reduce skin damage, dryness, and irritation (Patrick & Van Wicklin 2012, Visscher et al 2010). Ahmed-Lecheheb et al (2012) and Chamorey et al (2011) found no deterioration in skin condition when AHR was used and suggest there may be a protective effect. This is important, as Visscher et al (2010) suggest that irritant contact dermatitis can lead to the development of allergic contact dermatitis. Wyeth (2013) suggests that 25% of nurses develop symptoms associated with dermatitis. For example, nurses with irritated hands were significantly more likely to be colonized with a number of potentially harmful bacteria, including *Staphylococcus aureus* (Cook et al 2007). Hand irritation is also a commonly cited reason among nurses for not washing their hands as often as recommended (Carrico et al 2013).

Some people may object to using AHR on religious grounds (WHO 2009). Sikhism prohibits the use of alcohol, and if used it may be considered an offence requiring a penance. Islam also forbids the use of alcohol as it may cause mental impairment but the Qur'an permits the use of any man-made substance that is used to alleviate illness or contribute to better health. Hinduism also prohibits the use of alcohol for the same reason. Buddhism forbids the killing of a living being which includes microorganisms. However, Buddhists may consider the life of the human to be more valuable than the microorganism and use AHR (WHO 2009).

INDICATIONS FOR HAND DECONTAMINATION

- Immediately before and after every episode of direct patient contact or care, including aseptic procedures.
- Immediately after any exposure to body fluids.
- Immediately after any other activity or contact with a patient's surroundings that could potentially result in hands becoming contaminated.
- Prior to putting on and immediately after removal of gloves particularly as gloves provide a warm moist environment (Kilpatrick et al 2013, NICE 2012). Fuller et al (2011) found the rate of hand hygiene compliance was significantly lower before and after glove wearing.
- Prior to handling food.
- When visibly soiled.

- After going to the toilet (postnatal women should be advised to wash their hands before and after going to the toilet and when changing sanitary towels to reduce the risk of sepsis (Harper 2011).
- After several consecutive applications of handrub.

PRINCIPLES OF HAND DECONTAMINATION

- Consider all equipment as being contaminated: minimal handling of taps, soap dispenser, sinks, drying equipment, especially after washing; the use of foot-operated pedal bins and elbow taps is advised. Sinks should not have plugs as they can be difficult to clean and can act as a reservoir for microorganisms, e.g. *Pseudomonas*.
- Use running water at a comfortable temperature. Water temperature for handwashing is often recommended to be 'warm' or 'hot' but hot water opens the pores predisposing to skin irritation. It can also be drying to the skin which in turn can result in the skin being less resistant to bacterial colonization (Carrico et al 2013). Carrico et al (2013) discuss water temperature and found having the water at a temperature that is comfortable encourages more frequent handwashing for longer periods and lower water temperatures makes no difference to the effectiveness of removal of microorganisms.
- The flow of the water should be regulated to avoid splashing water, especially over clothes, as microorganisms can be transferred and multiply in moisture.
- Hands should be wet before applying liquid soap (NICE 2012).
- Use appropriate antimicrobial liquid soap and work up a lather as the soap will emulsify fat and oil and lower the surface tension, making cleaning easier.
- Use a circular motion, encouraging rubbing and friction which loosens and removes dirt and transient microorganisms.
- Rinse hands thoroughly to reduce the risk of irritant hand dermatitis.
- Hand drying is an important component of hand hygiene as hands that retain moisture after handwashing have more microorganisms remaining than very dry hands. Loveday et al (2014) suggest that good-quality disposable paper towels are better at removing microorganisms because of the friction used during drying compared with hot air driers and

towels, a view supported by Besta et al (2014). Huang et al (2012) agree and also suggest that rubbing hands under a hot air drier to speed up drying leads to an increased number of microorganisms, possibly by causing microorganisms to move from the hair follicles to the skin surface as well as airborne dispersal. The used paper towel should be disposed of correctly as microorganisms will transfer from the hands to the paper towel during drying.

PROCEDURE: medical/social scrub

- Remove all jewellery (except for plain gold band), including wrist watch (however, these should not be worn as the midwife should be 'bare below the elbows').
- Turn the taps on and adjust the flow and water temperature to warm, taking care not to splash the water, and wet the hands (Fig. 9.1A).
- Using an appropriate cleansing agent, rub the palms together vigorously (Fig. 9.1B), then rub the palm of one hand along the top of the other hand and along the fingers, using the fingers on the top hand to rub along the edge of the lower hand; repeat for the other hand (Fig. 9.1C).
- Wash the fingers by interlacing together, rubbing them back and forth, ensuring the inner aspects of both sides of all the fingers are rubbed together (Fig. 9.1D).
- Wash the fingertips of one hand by rubbing them against the palm of the other hand; repeat for the other hand (Fig. 9.1E).
- Wash the thumb of one hand by using the fingers of the other hand wrapped around it, washing in a circular motion; repeat for the other thumb (Fig. 9.1F).
- Grasp the left wrist with the right hand, rubbing around the wrist; repeat for the right wrist (Fig. 9.1G).
- Rinse all the surfaces of the hand and wrist with warm running water.
- Repeat handwashing if hands are heavily contaminated.
- Dry each hand and wrist separately with a paper towel, do not 'rub'; rather, use a patting motion.
- Turn off the taps using elbows or the paper towel.
- Dispose of the towel using a foot-operated or automatic pedal bin.
- If an AHR is used, application follows the steps in Figure 9.1B-G with hands rubbed until the hands and wrists are dry.

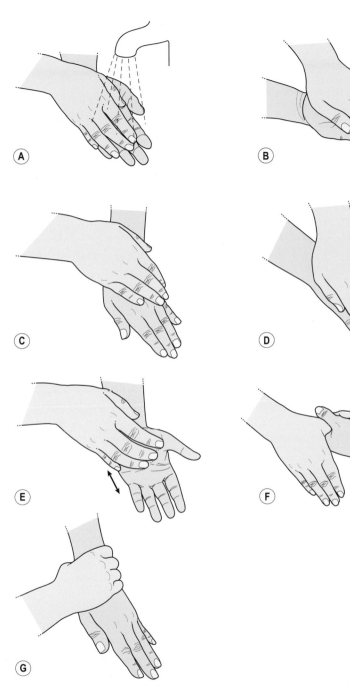

Figure 9.1 Medical/social scrub. **A,** Rinsing with water. **B,** Washing the palms. **C,** Washing the top surfaces of the fingers and hand. **D,** Interlacing the fingers. **E,** Washing the fingertips. **F,** Washing the thumbs. **G,** Washing the wrists.

PROCEDURE: surgical scrub

This involves washing the hands and forearms to remove as many transient and resident microorganisms as possible from these areas and maintain the lowest possible microbial count throughout the surgical procedure; washing should take at least 3–5 minutes (Spruce 2013).

- Remove all jewellery (except for plain gold band), including wrist watch (however these should not be worn as the midwife should be 'bare below the elbows').
- Turn the taps on and adjust the water flow and temperature to warm, taking care not to splash the water.
- Keeping the hands above the level of the elbows, wet the hands and forearms to the elbows.
- Using an antiseptic soap, e.g. 4% chlorhexidine solution, povidone–iodine, wash fingers and hands as for medical scrub and extend washing to include forearms (this may require several applications of antiseptic soap) using brush/sponge if it is the first surgical scrub of the day.
- Rinse the soap from hands and elbows, keeping the hands above the level of the elbows, allowing the water to run from the fingertips down to the elbows.
- Turn off the taps using elbows.
- Dry each hand and arm separately with a disposable towel, drying from the fingertips towards the elbows, keeping the hands above waist level.
- Dispose of the towel using a foot-operated pedal bin.

ROLE AND RESPONSIBILITIES OF THE MIDWIFE

These can be summarized as:
- recognizing the importance of correct hand hygiene
- following the principles of hand care
- recognizing when and how hand decontamination should be undertaken
- reducing the risk of contamination to self and others through appropriate hand hygiene.

SUMMARY

- Hand decontamination is an important means of infection control.
- The use of soap and water will remove almost all transient microorganisms, blood, body fluid and dirt but does not significantly reduce the number of resident microorganisms.
- Healthcare professionals involved in direct patient care should be 'bare below the elbows'.
- Alcohol handrubs remove almost all transient microorganisms and significantly reduce the number of resident microorganisms but do not remove blood, body fluid, dirt, and spores, e.g. from *C. difficile*.
- Disposable paper towels should be used to dry hands.
- A 'medical/social scrub' involves washing for a minimum of 15 seconds.
- A 'surgical scrub' involves washing for at least 3–5 minutes, with the hands above the elbows.

SELF-ASSESSMENT EXERCISES

The answers to the following questions may be found in the text:
1. Why is hand hygiene important?
2. What are the general principles of hand care and why are they important?
3. In what situations would the midwife use an AHR?
4. When should the midwife undertake hand decontamination?
5. What are the principles of hand decontamination?
6. What are the main differences between a 'medical/social' and a 'surgical' scrub?

REFERENCES

Ahmed-Lecheheb, D., Cunat, L., Hartemann, P., Hautemaniere, A., 2012. Prospective observational study to assess hand skin condition after application of alcohol-based handrub solutions. Am. J. Infect. Control 40 (2), 160–164.

Al-Allah, A., Sarasin, S., Key, S., Morris-Stiff, G., 2008. Wedding rings are not a significant source of bacterial contamination following surgical scrubbing. Ann. R. Coll. Surg. Engl. 90 (2), 133–135.

Besta, E.L., Parnella, P., Wilcox, M.H., 2014. Microbiological comparison of hand-drying methods: the potential for contamination of the environment, user, and bystander. J. Hosp. Infect. 88 (4), 199–206.

Carrico, A.R., Spoden, M., Wallston, K.A., Vandenbergh, M.P., 2013. The environmental cost of misinformation: why the recommendation to use elevated temperatures for handwashing is problematic. Int. J. Consum. Stud. 37 (4), 433–441.

CDC (Centres for Disease Control and Prevention), 2002. Guideline for

Hand Hygiene in Health-Care Settings: Recommendations of the Healthcare Infection Control Practices Advisory Committee and the HICPAC/SHEA/APIC/IDSA Hand Hygiene Task Force. Available online: <www.cdc.gov/mmwr/pdf/rr/rr5116.pdf> (accessed 2 March 2015).

Chamorey, E., Marcy, P.-Y., Dandine, M., et al., 2011. A prospective multicenter study for evaluating skin tolerance to standard hand hygiene technique. Am. J. Infect. Control 39 (1), 6–13.

Cook, H.A., Jeannie, M.P.H., Cimiotti, P., et al., 2007. Antimicriobial resistance patterns of colonizing flora on nurses' hands in the neonatal intensive care unit. Am. J. Infect. Control 35 (4), 231–236.

Fagernes, M., Lingaas, E., 2010. Factors interfering with the microflora on hands: a regression analysis of samples from 465 healthcare workers. J. Adv. Nurs. 67 (2), 297–307.

Fuller, C., Savage, J., Besser, S., et al., 2011. The dirty hand in the latex glove: A study of hand hygiene compliance when gloves are worn. Infect. Control Hosp. Epidemiol. 32 (12), 1194–1199.

Gould, D.J., Hewitt-Taylor, J., Drey, N.S., et al., 2007. The clean your hands campaign: Critiquing policy and evidence base. J. Hosp. Infect. 65 (2), 95–101.

Harper, A., 2011. Sepsis. In: Centre for Maternal and Child Enquiries (CMACE). Saving Mothers' Lives: reviewing maternal deaths to make motherhood safer: 2006–08. The eighth report on confidential enquiries into maternal deaths in the United Kingdom. Br. J. Obstet. Gynaecol. 118 (Suppl. 1), 85–96.

Hautemaniere, A., Cunat, L., Diguio, N., et al., 2010. Factors determining poor practice in alcoholic hand gel rub technique in hospital workers. J. Infect. Public Health 3 (1), 25–34.

Hsieh, H., Chiu, H., Lee, F., 2006. Surgical hand scrubs in relation to microbial counts: systematic literature review. J. Adv. Nurs. 55 (1), 68–74.

Huang, C.L., Ma, W., Stack, S., 2012. The hygienic efficacy of different hand-drying methods: a review of the evidence. Mayo Clin. Proc. 87 (8), 791–798.

Hübner, S.-O., Hübner, C., Kramer, A., Assadian, O., 2011. Survival of bacterial pathogens on paper and bacterial retrieval from paper to hands: preliminary results. Am. J. Nurs. 111 (12), 30–34.

Jabbar, U., Leischner, J., Kasper, D., et al., 2010. Effectiveness of alcohol-based hand rubs for removal of Clostridium difficile spores from hands. Infect. Control Hosp. Epidemiol. 31 (6), 565–570.

Kilpatrick, C., Hosie, L., Storr, J., 2013. Hand hygiene – when and how should it be done? Nurs. Times 109 (38), 16–18.

Khodavaisy, S., Nabili, M., Davari, B., Vahedi, M., 2011. Evaluation of bacterial and fungal contamination in the health care workers' hands and rings in the intensive care unit. J. Prev. Med. Hyg. 52 (4), 215–218.

Loveday, H.P., Wilson, J.A., Pratt, R.J., et al., 2014. epic3: National evidence-based guidelines for preventing healthcare-associated infections in NHS hospitals in England. J. Hosp. Infect. 86 (Suppl. 1), S1–S70.

Martirani, R., Weaving, A.P., 2011. Infection prevention and control. In: Dougherty, L., Lister, S. (Eds.), The Royal Marsden Hospital Manual of Clinical Nursing Procedures, eighth ed. Wiley-Blackwell, Oxford, pp. 93–154.

Moore, G., Dunhill, C., Wilson, A., 2013. The effect of glove material upon the transfer of methicillin-resistant *Staphylococcus aureus* to and from a gloved hand. Am. J. Infect. Control 41, 19–23.

NICE (National Institute for Health and Care Excellence), 2012. Infection: prevention and control of healthcare-associated infections in primary and community care. Available online: <www.nice.org.uk> (accessed 2 March 2015).

NICE (National Institute for Health and Care Excellence), 2014. Infection prevention and control Quality Standard 61. Available online: <www.nice.org.uk> (accessed 23 February 2015).

Patrick, M., Van Wicklin, S., 2012. Implementing AORN recommended practices for hand hygiene. AORN J. 95 (4), 492–509.

Spruce, L., 2013. Back to basics: hand hygiene and surgical hand antisepsis. AORN J. 98 (5), 449–460.

Tanner, J., Swarbrook, S., Stuart, J., 2008. Surgical hand antisepsis to reduce surgical site infection. Cochrane Database Syst. Rev. (1), Art. No.: CD004288, doi:10.1002/14651858.CD004288.pub2.

Visscher, M., Said, D., Wickett, R., 2010. Stratum corneum cytokines structural proteins and transepidermal water loss: effect of hand hygiene. Skin Res. Technol. 16, 229–236.

Ward, D., 2007. Hand adornment and infection control. Br. J. Nurs. 16 (11), 654–656.

WHO (World Health Organisation), 2009. Guidelines on Hand Hygiene in Health Care. WHO, Geneva.

Wyeth, J., 2013. Hand hygiene and the use of personal protective equipment. Br. J. Nurs. 22 (16), 920, 922–925.

Chapter 10

Principles of infection control: principles of asepsis

LEARNING OUTCOMES

Having read this chapter, the reader should be able to:

- discuss the principles of asepsis, including equipment used, non-touch technique, and establishing an aseptic field
- summarize the role and responsibilities of the midwife.

Asepsis – the absence of sepsis or infection – is a critical component of care. Healthcare-associated infections (HCAIs) are costly in monetary and human terms and are often preventable. The risk of litigation is also real (Pratt 2014). Preventing sepsis is a multi-faceted issue, the epic3 guidelines (Loveday et al 2014) place significance on hospital environmental hygiene, hand hygiene, use of personal protective equipment, and the safe use and disposal of sharps, while the Department of Health (2010) also place it within the context of the whole of health care provision, e.g. appropriate prescribing, laboratory and mortuary services, food provision, etc.

It is the principles of asepsis that midwives need to understand in order to then apply them across a range of care situations. This chapter should be read in conjunction with several others including hand hygiene, obtaining swabs, intravenous medicines, epidural analgesia, wound care, etc. This chapter reviews the principles of aseptic practice, particularly with regard to the ANTT (Aseptic Non Touch Technique) framework (Rowley et al 2010).

THE ANTT PRACTICE FRAMEWORK

The ANTT Practice Framework (www.antt.org) (Rowley & Clare 2011a) provides a standardized way in which any Key-Site on the woman can be protected from the introduction of bacteria by using appropriate sterile equipment and fluids. The approach utilizes three strands:

1. education for practitioners
2. standardized ANTT guidelines
3. audit to assess implementation.

In the UK the DH (2010) require that healthcare providers have a standardized and auditable approach to asepsis management. The ANTT framework has been endorsed by the epic3 guidelines (Loveday et al 2014) and is now widely adopted internationally also (Rowley & Clare 2011a). It moves away from defining terms such as 'clean' or 'sterile' techniques into recognizing the importance of achievable and well-defined terminology forming a common and meaningful practice language. ANTT is based on a concept of Key-Part and Key-Site Protection for all invasive procedures that involve a risk of infection for the woman. The aim is freedom from infection – asepsis (Rowley et al 2010).

HOW IS IT ACHIEVED?

A clear differentiation is made between Standard-ANTT and Surgical-ANTT. Surgical-ANTT is typically used in operating theatres, e.g. laminar air flow, surgical hand scrub, full protective gowning, gloving, etc. and uses an extensive and Critically Managed Aseptic Field. However, Surgical-ANTT is also used in other clinical settings for complicated invasive procedures (such as central line insertion). Standard-ANTT generally uses a smaller aseptic field that is managed differently to Surgical-ANTT. It relies more heavily on a non touch technique and therefore may use non-sterile gloves. The practitioner considers their level of competency and the technical difficulty of maintaining asepsis of Key-Parts and Key-Sites. As a rough guide, if a procedure is likely to take 20 minutes or less, be technically simple due to involving few and relatively small Key-Parts and Key-Sites, then Standard-ANTT is used. Not only is this safe, it is more efficient. Examples of this include:

- venepuncture and peripheral cannulation
- urinary catheterization
- examination *per vaginam*
- childbirth, of whichever mode
- perineal suturing
- siting of epidural analgesia
- wound dressing.

If, however, the procedure is more complex, will take longer, or involves larger Key-Sites or many Key-Parts, then Surgical-ANTT is appropriate. Sometimes ANTT-specific risk assessment may determine that a procedure could come into either category due to the competency of the practitioner or the technical difficulty of maintaining Key-Part/ Site protection. On occasion, a modified approach may be used, some Standard-ANTT procedures may warrant the introduction of sterile gloves based on this risk assessment, e.g. peripheral cannulation (Rowley et al 2010). However, the emphasis, whichever approach is used, is on the *non touching* of Key-Sites and Key-Parts (see below). Non touch may refer to the literal non touching of Key-Parts or the necessary (non) touching of Key-Parts by using sterile gloves.

ANTT is built on 10 principles, some of which are summarized above. Others include (Rowley & Clare 2011b):

- Healthcare professionals – do they understand that they are the risk? Do they know how to establish and maintain asepsis? Aseptic technique should be standardized. Staff should receive appropriate training and assessment.
- Key-Sites are any portal of entry on the woman that could be infected, e.g. any wound, insertion, or puncture site (Rowley & Clare 2011a). If inserting a urinary catheter, for example, the Key-Site is the urethra, if undertaking venepuncture, it is the

skin/puncture site. Key-Parts are any items (equipment or fluids) that have direct or indirect contact with the Key-Sites, e.g. the peripheral cannula and the insertion point of any connections into it are both Key-Parts. Thereafter Key-Parts, e.g. needleless ports, should also be disinfected before use. When cleaning an item, e.g. bottle top, needleless port, or sampling port, friction should be generated and scrubbing, with different parts of the wipe, should take place for at least 20 seconds. Key-Sites, e.g. skin cleansing prior to venepuncture, should be cleaned for 30 seconds using the right-to-left and up-and-down approach. The locally approved cleanser is often 70% alcohol/2% chlorhexidine.

- Using a non touch technique to protect Key-Parts and Key-Sites from contamination. Even when wearing sterile gloves, try not to touch Key-Parts directly if practically possible.
- Establishing an aseptic field. The main aseptic field in Surgical-ANTT is managed 'critically'. Only sterile equipment must be placed onto it. Its therefore called a Critical Aseptic Field. The main aseptic field in Standard-ANTT is managed 'generally', and clean but not necessarily sterile equipment may be placed onto it. It is therefore promoting asepsis. On a General Aseptic Field, Key-Parts are protected by individual caps and covers which are said to be Micro Critical Aseptic Fields. The available equipment, e.g. plastic tray or dressings trolley, is cleansed, with decontaminated hands, using the locally approved cleanser. Sterile items, e.g. dressings pack, are then removed from their outer packaging and placed onto the cleansed area. Care is taken to open the pack using only the corners so that the inside of the pack remains an aseptic field. Other items are then added aseptically to the field. This is shown in Figure 10.1.
- Other contributory factors, e.g. hand decontamination, environmental conditions. The ANTT guidelines (www.antt.org) show clearly when hand decontamination should take place. This is always before commencing the procedure and always on completing it, but often during also. For example, after removing a wound dressing and before applying the new one, the hands should be decontaminated. Handwashing and drying should be effective (see Chapter 9).
- Care is taken to control the environment; nearby people coughing, using commodes or making beds can increase airborne pathogens.

Equipment

Equipment that is sterilized centrally is usually autoclaved. The colour change on the packet indicates sterility but the

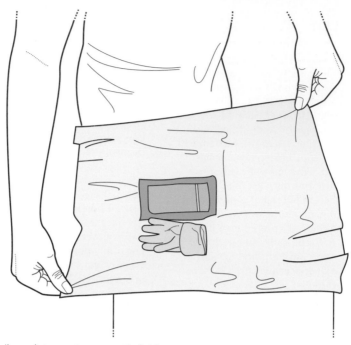

Figure 10.1 Opening a sterile pack to create an aseptic field.
(Adapted with kind permission from Nicol et al 2000)

pack should be inspected to ensure that it has not been damaged or wet in the meantime. Sterile items should be used within their expiry date. Sterile lotions, syringes, cannulas, etc. are all supplied for single-use only (unless otherwise stated) and are disposed of after use. Increasingly a system operates that allows sterile packs to be traced through the system, from central sterilizing through to which operator used them for which woman. A label (or something similar) is placed in the woman's record after the equipment has been used and the same verification returns to the sterile supplies department.

Many packs contain a disposal bag. This can be used over the hand (like a glove) to remove wound dressings. It is then inverted (so that the dressing remains in the bag) and is attached to the trolley for other waste. It is placed on the side of the trolley nearest to the woman so that waste materials are not taken across the aseptic field but are disposed of immediately.

The use of an assistant

Frequently in practice the midwife will undertake aseptic procedures alone. However Hart (2007) notes that the use of an assistant is helpful in maintaining the asepsis. The assistant needs to:

- have decontaminated hands
- handle/open the external wrappers and pass the sterile contents to the aseptic field or directly to the midwife (see Fig. 10.2) if asked
- aid the woman to be comfortable and 'uncovered' at the correct time
- appreciate the presence of an aseptic field around the woman, taking care not to decontaminate it
- be prepared to collect additional items if necessary.

UNDERTAKING THE PROCEDURE

- Check the identity of the woman, ensure that she has given consent and is in an appropriate place for the procedure.
- Decontaminate hands, locate a clean trolley/tray, clean it with the locally approved wipes.
- Gather the equipment needed, checking for sterility, expiry date, etc. Place on the lower shelf of the trolley.
- Take the trolley to the woman, position her accordingly, keeping her covered until ready.
- Decontaminate hands and put on an apron.

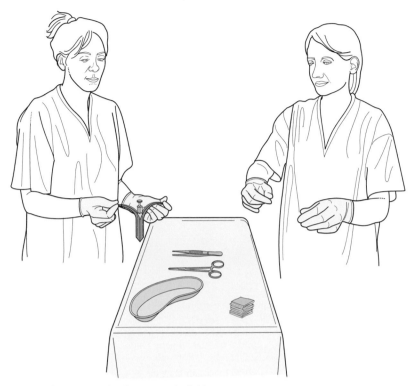

Figure 10.2 Assistant passing items to maintain an aseptic field.

- Taking hold of the outer wrapper of the sterile pack (whatever sort it is), open it carefully (not touching any part of the inner wrapper) onto the cleansed trolley top.
- Open out the sterile inner wrapper by using only the corners or edges of the paper to create an aseptic field (Fig. 10.1).
- Slide or 'drop' on all other items needed without them touching anything else.
- Decontaminate hands with handrub, than apply chosen gloves.
- Ensure that the woman is comfortable, ask her to remove any covers etc. Establish an aseptic field around her, placing the drapes appropriately.
- Undertake the procedure using a non touch technique for all Key-Sites and Key-Parts.
- Once this is completed and the woman is made comfortable, the equipment is disposed of correctly. The aseptic field is disposed of by wrapping the remaining contents (if disposable) in the paper and placing them into the disposal sack.
- Gloves and apron are removed and put into the clinical waste and hands are washed and dried.
- The trolley is cleaned using the locally agreed wipes, the non-disposable items are prepared for return to the sterile supplies department in the agreed format.
- Decontaminate hands and complete the woman's records.

ROLE AND RESPONSIBILITIES OF THE MIDWIFE

These can be summarized as:
- appreciating the significance and principles of aseptic practice and undertaking the procedure thoroughly and consistently. The ANTT framework uses a non touch technique for all Key-Sites on the woman and Key-Parts of the equipment/fluids. Practice should be regularly updated and assessed as competent
- working in a team allows the midwife to seek support if unsure and to challenge any other examples of poorer practice. Staff should protect themselves as well as the clients
- document all care given contemporaneously
- educating the woman when caring for herself and her baby, in the light of available evidence.

SUMMARY

- The principles of asepsis should be included (adapted if necessary) for every invasive procedure in which body defences are breached. The process will differ according to the degree of technical difficulty. ANTT offers a standardized technique. When undertaking an aseptic procedure, the midwife should not touch the Key-Site or the Key-Parts. These are different for each procedure. When touching Key-Parts or Key-Sites is unavoidable, sterile gloves should be used.
- Effective hand hygiene is essential before and after every patient contact, and often during procedures also.

SELF-ASSESSMENT EXERCISES

The answers to the following questions may be found in the text:
1. Give four examples of the circumstances in which aseptic practice is indicated.
2. Suggest examples of Key-Parts and Key-Sites.
3. Demonstrate opening a sterile pack including preparation of the aseptic surface used.
4. Summarize the role and responsibilities of the midwife when undertaking an aseptic procedure.

REFERENCES

DH (Department of Health), 2010. The Health and Social Care Act 2008. DH, London.

Hart, S., 2007. Using an aseptic technique to reduce the risk of infection. Nurs. Stand. 21 (47), 43–48.

Loveday, H., Wilson, W., Pratt, R.J., et al., 2014. Epic3: national evidence-based guidelines for preventing healthcare – associated infections in NHS hospitals in England. J. Hosp. Infect. 86 (Suppl. 1), S1–S70.

Nicol, M., Bavin, C., Bedford-Turner, S., et al., 2000. Essential Nursing Skills, second ed. Mosby, Edinburgh.

Pratt, R.J., 2014. Epic3: an evidence-based approach for protecting patients and saving lives. Br. J. Healthcare Manage. 20 (9), 418–422.

Rowley, S., Clare, S., Macqueen, S., Molyneux, R., 2010. ANTT v2: An updated practice framework for aseptic technique. Br. J. Nurs. 19 (5), S5–S11. Intravenous supplement.

Rowley, S., Clare, S., 2011a. ANTT: a standard approach to aseptic technique. Nurs. Times 107 (36), 12–14.

Rowley, S., Clare, S., 2011b. ANTT: an essential tool for effective blood culture collection. Br J Nurs 20 (14), S9–S14. Intravenous supplement.

Chapter 11

Principles of infection control: obtaining swabs

LEARNING OUTCOMES

Having read this chapter, the reader should be able to:

- describe how a swab is obtained from the eye, ear, nose, throat, groin, umbilicus, vagina, wound and placenta
- discuss the role and responsibilities of the midwife in relation to obtaining swabs.

Swabs may be obtained when infection is suspected so that the correct antibiotics are administered which are specific to the infecting microorganism or for screening purposes to help inform care, e.g. methicillin-resistant *Staphylococcus aureus* (MRSA) screening, history of vaginal *group B streptococcus* (GBS). Increasingly pre-admission screening, often with nasal and groin swabs, is being undertaken prior to elective surgery, e.g. caesarean section, to detect MRSA and reduce the incidence of surgical site infections. While screening for MRSA seems to be acceptable to the 'patients', it is important they are aware of the implications of a positive result and that screening is undertaken with sufficient time for treatment to avoid delaying surgery (Currie et al 2013). Early recognition and treating of infection is essential to avoid genital tract infection which was the second highest cause of direct maternal deaths in 2010–2012 (Knight et al 2014). *Group A streptococcus* (GAS) is a common microorganism involved in maternal infection particularly in early pregnancy and the postnatal period (Churchill et al 2014). It is a common cause of sore throats, particularly in children, and is often a community-acquired infection. Strict adherence to hand hygiene, particularly before and after changing sanitary pads may help to reduce the incidence of infection (Harper et al 2011). When obtaining a swab because of suspected uterine or perineal infection, it is best to do so before antibiotics are used. This chapter focuses on obtaining swabs from the more common sites of the eye, ear, nose, throat, groin, umbilicus, vagina, wound and placenta.

GOOD PRACTICE

Good practice for the taking of all swabs should include:

- Correct identification of the woman (asking her to state her name and date of birth) and the granting of consent. Some swabs require the woman to take more action than others. In each instance she needs to understand what is being tested, why and how the swab is obtained.

- Clinical assessment – is the swab necessary? Is it appropriate to the current clinical condition, in what way will the result impact care?
- Is this a repeat swab? Taking swabs unnecessarily is costly and can be stressful for the woman. Will a repeat swab add to her plan of care?
- Is it being collected at the right time, in the right way (avoiding contamination) using the correct equipment, the correct swab, and transport medium, and labelled as per locally agreed policy? Failure at any of these stages wastes resources and can lose patient confidence in the service.
- Is the swab being taken in a manner that protects all staff including the midwife, transportation, and laboratory services? Is it sealed and labelled 'high risk' if appropriate? Has adherence to standard precautions and infection control protocols been upheld?
- Can the swab be dispatched or stored correctly so that it reaches the laboratory as it should and in the correct time frame?
- Has it been documented in the correct places and will the results be located and acted upon in a timely manner?

OBTAINING THE SWAB

Sterile swabs are usually made of cotton or rayon attached to a long stick and when obtained they are placed whole into a transport medium. It is vital that the swab stick used is sterile and in date, as this can affect the results. The lid should be firmly tightened and correctly labelled, including the woman's name, hospital number, date of birth, specimen taken, and time and date, all of which should correspond with the pathology form (this should also indicate if the woman is taking antibiotics and any signs or symptoms). The swab is then placed in a transport bag that is sealed to prevent spillage and contamination with the pathology form and taken to the laboratory as soon as possible, as microorganisms can multiply when kept at room temperature. If delay is anticipated, refrigeration may be necessary (although some swabs can be kept at room temperature); it is therefore important the midwife is aware of how to store swabs and specimens when they cannot be transported quickly. In high-risk situations, the swab may need to be double-wrapped and labelled accordingly.

The laboratory test requested is usually 'microscopy, culture and sensitivity' (MC&S) which involves a microscopic examination for a quick initial report of the microorganism(s) present, culture of the microorganism(s) to identify which microorganisms are present, a microbial count to determine if they are the result of colonization or infection and an analysis of sensitivity to antibiotics that can be administered to prevent further growth and replication.

When taking the swab, it is important that the microorganisms coat the swab all over to increase the chances of identifying the infecting microorganism and this is best achieved by rotating the swab over the site of swabbing. An Aseptic Non Touch Technique (Chapter 10) should be used to avoid cross-contamination and only the affected area should be swabbed (Dimech et al 2011). In some situations, a sample of pus, exudate, moisture, etc. from the woman or baby (e.g. from the umbilical stump) may need to be collected. While they can be collected via a swab stick, it may be more appropriate to use a sterile syringe to collect pus/exudate. Standard precautions, including hand hygiene, should be followed when obtaining a swab (Chapters 8, 9). Where swabs are required from more than one site (e.g. both eyes, ears), a separate swab should be used for each site to reduce the risk of cross-infection from an infected to a non-infected area. However, usually only one swab is required from the area that appears most affected.

There are a variety of transport mediums as different microorganisms can thrive or die in certain mediums, thus it is important that the correct swab and transport medium are used for the suspected microorganism, for example, *Trichomonas vaginalis*, *Chlamydia* spp. and *Bordetella pertussis* require charcoal-based swabs and medium. If the midwife is unsure of which swab and transport medium to use, she should ask a doctor or microbiologist who should be able to advise.

The midwife should record in the notes which swabs have been taken and the time and date. This will ensure that all staff are aware the swabs have been obtained and will serve as a reminder to check the results as soon as they are ready. The woman should also be aware of why the swab/s are undertaken and how soon she can expect to have the result.

Eye

When obtaining an eye swab from a woman, she should be sat up, with her head supported and the woman asked to look upwards to prevent corneal damage (Dimech et al 2011). If the swab is from a baby, he should be supported with his head held steady. The lower eyelid should be pulled down gently. The swab is held parallel to the cornea and rubbed very gently against the conjunctiva in the lower eyelid moving from the inner canthus to the outer canthus. If *Chlamydia* is the suspected microorganism, apply slightly more pressure when swabbing (Dimech et al 2011). It is important to avoid touching the eyelid borders or eyelashes with the swab. Usually just one swab is sufficient. If *Gonococcus* is the suspected organism, the swab should not be refrigerated as there will be no recovery of the *Gonococcus* organism and a false negative will be reported.

Ear

It is important to withhold medication administered via the ears for 3 hours prior to obtaining the swab as the medication can interfere with the growth of the microorganism. To obtain a swab from the ear, the woman should be sat up with her head tilting to the unaffected side. When taking a swab from a baby, one of the parents or another midwife can hold the baby with the head up, tilted to one side. If the baby is too ill to be moved, lay the baby on the unaffected side. For both the woman and the baby, straighten the external canal by gently pulling the pinna upwards and backwards, the swab is inserted gently into, and rotated around the walls of the external canal. If necessary, the external canal can be cleaned with a moistened swab to remove any debris and/or crust before inserting the swab. A charcoal medium may be required to transport the swab.

Nasal swab

When taking a nasal swab, the woman should be sitting up or lying in a supine position with her head tilting back. If the swab is from a baby, he can be cradled in someone's arms or laid on his back. The procedure may be easier if there is someone to hold the baby's arms; alternatively wrap the baby in a blanket. The end of the swab should be moistened with sterile water and inserted gently into the nose, moving it upwards towards the tip of the nose, into the anterior nares (HPA 2013) while rotating it. Repeat the procedure using the same swab in the other nostril. Self-swabbing does not appear to compromise the specimen integrity and may be more comfortable for the woman (Akmatov et al 2012).

Throat

The woman should be sitting or lying facing a strong light source and asked to open her mouth widely and say 'Ah' as she sticks out her tongue (deWit & O'Neill 2014). The tongue should be depressed using a disposable spatula and the swab inserted to the back of the throat. The swab is then rotated quickly around the back of the throat around the tonsillar area and/or the posterior pharynx (HPA 2014), this is likely to make the woman gag. When removing the swab, ensure it does not come into contact with any part of the mouth, uvula, tongue, or saliva. A charcoal medium may be required to transport the swab.

Groin

Because the skin of the groin is dry, it is important to moisten the end of the swab with sterile normal saline. The swab is then rolled along the groin, using the area of skin along the inside part of the thigh that is nearest the genitalia.

Umbilicus

The baby should be positioned to allow easy access to the umbilicus (e.g. cradled in someone's arms or lying in a cot) and undressed to expose the umbilicus. The swab is moved gently around the umbilicus and rotated. The baby should be redressed following the procedure.

High vaginal swab

Using an aseptic procedure, a speculum is inserted and opened inside the vagina (Chapter 28). The swab should be inserted through the speculum to the top of the vagina and rotated around. When the procedure is completed the speculum should be removed and the woman assisted into a comfortable position.

Low vaginal swab

Self-swabbing does not appear to compromise the specimen integrity and is less embarrassing for the woman (Eperon et al 2013, Page et al 2013). The swab is inserted into the lower vagina for 2–4 cm and rubbed firmly around the front, side, and back walls of the vagina while rotating the swab.

Wound

It is important to obtain the wound swab correctly. If only microorganisms from the wound surface are obtained and not those that penetrate the soft tissue, a false positive result may ensue as the microorganisms found on the wound surface are frequently different to the microorganisms responsible for the infection (Angel et al 2011, Kingsley 2003). Prior to obtaining a wound swab Pattern (2010) recommends using a gentle stream of normal saline to irrigate the wound to remove surface contamination, e.g. slough, necrotic tissue, eschar, using an Aseptic Non Touch Technique (Chapter 10). Allow 1–2 minutes to pass before taking the swab. If the wound is dry, the swab should be moistened with sterile saline or transport medium.

The swab should be rotated across a 1 cm^2 area of the wound (Levine's technique) for at least 5 seconds using sufficient pressure to release exudate or fluid from the wound (Gardner et al 2006). If the wound is large, swab as much of the wound as possible. The Levine technique is considered more reliable than the zigzag method of obtaining a wound swab (Angel et al 2011). If there is a sinus or pocket in the wound a separate swab should be used. Care should be taken to ensure the swab does not come into contact with the wound edge. The swab should be kept in room air and taken to the laboratory within 4 hours (Cooper 2010).

Placental swab

There are several ways of obtaining a placental swab so it is important that the midwife is aware of which surfaces require swabbing – the fetal surface, maternal surface, or between the membranes. If a swab of the fetal and or maternal surface is required, the swab should be moved around the surface(s) in a zigzag direction. Pettker et al (2007) found little correlation between placental swabs and the infectious and inflammatory status of the amniotic fluid.

If sampling is required between the membranes, this can be obtained by cutting through the chorion at the base of the umbilicus (using a sterile scalpel) and swabbing the chorion-amnion interface on the underside of the amnion (Kraus 2011) or between the membranes at the edge of the placenta. Care must be taken not to cross-contaminate by touching the surface of the placenta or outer side of the membranes.

PROCEDURE: obtaining a swab

- Discuss the procedure and obtain informed consent.
- Gather equipment:
  - non-sterile gloves and apron (if required)
  - sterile swab and appropriate transport medium
  - speculum and lubricating jelly, e.g. KY Jelly® (high vaginal swab only)
  - sterile water (nasal swab only)
  - sterile normal saline (groin or wound swab)
- Wash and dry hands and apply apron and gloves.
- Position the woman or baby appropriately and obtain the swab specimen.
- Insert the swab into the transport medium and seal securely.
- Label the container with the name, hospital number and date of birth of the woman or baby, date and time the swab was obtained, nature of specimen, whether right or left (if applicable), and signature. Place into transport bag.
- Assist the woman or baby into a comfortable position.

- Remove and dispose of gloves and apron.
- Wash and dry hands.
- Arrange transportation of the specimen to the pathology laboratory.
- Document findings and act accordingly.

ROLE AND RESPONSIBILITIES OF THE MIDWIFE

These can be summarized as:
- recognizing the need for a swab to be taken
- using the correct swab and transport medium
- ensuring the procedure is undertaken correctly, with minimal discomfort to the mother or baby and with the use of appropriate standard precautions/personal protective equipment
- follow-up of swab results and instigating referral/ treatment as necessary
- correct documentation.

SUMMARY

- Obtaining a swab is a significant, simple, but invasive procedure that may be undertaken on either the woman or the baby.
- It is important to take the swab correctly and avoid contamination from adjoining structures/debris to avoid false positive/negative results.

SELF-ASSESSMENT EXERCISES

The answers to the following questions may be found in the text:
1. How would the midwife obtain a swab from:
   a. the ear of a baby?
   b. the eye of a baby?
   c. the nose of a woman?
   d. the throat of a woman?
2. How is an umbilical swab obtained?
3. Describe how a wound swab is obtained from a small wound.
4. What are the differences in procedures for obtaining high and low vaginal swabs?

REFERENCES

Alkmatov, M., Gatzemeier, A., Schugart, R., Pessler, F., 2012. Equivalence of self- and staff-collected nasal swabs for the detection of viral respiratory pathogens. PLoS ONE 7 (11), 1–7.

Angel, D., Lloyd, P., Carville, K., Santamaria, N., 2011. The clinical efficacy of two semi-quantitative wound-swabbing techniques in identifying the causative organism(s) in infected cutaneous wounds. Int. Wound J. 8 (2), 176–185.

Churchill, D., Rodger, A., Clift, J., Tuffnell, D., on behalf of the MBRRACE-UK sepsis chapter writing group, 2014. Think sepsis. In: Knight, M., Kenyon, S., Brocklehurst, P., et al. on behalf of MBRRACE-UK (Eds.), Saving Lives, Improving Mothers' Care – Lessons Learned to Inform Future Maternity Care from the UK and Ireland Confidential Enquiries into Maternal Deaths and Morbidity 2009–12. National Perinatal Epidemiology Unit, Oxford, pp. 27–43.

Cooper, R. 2010. Ten top tips for taking a wound swab. Wounds Int. 1 (3), 1–4.

Currie, K., Knussen, C., Price, L., Reilly, J., 2013. Methicillin-resistant staphylococcus aureus screening as a patient safety initiative: using patients' experiences to improve the quality of screening practices. J. Clin. Nurs. 23, 221–231.

deWit, S., O'Neill, P., 2014. Fundamental Concepts and Skills for Nursing, fourth ed. Elsevier, St. Louis, pp. 400–409, 424.

Dimech, J., Dougherty, L., Fernandes, A., et al., 2011. Interpreting diagnostic tests. In: Dougherty, L., Lister, S. (Eds.), 2011 The Royal Marsden Hospital Manual of Clinical Nursing Procedures, eighth ed. Wiley-Blackwell, Oxford, pp. 617–697.

Eperon, I., Vissilakos, P., Navarria, I., et al., 2013. Randomized comparison of vaginal self-sampling by standard vs. dry swabs for Human papillomavirus testing. BMC Cancer 13, 353.

Gardner, S.E., Frantz, R.A., Saltzman, C.L., et al., 2006. Diagnostic validity of three swab techniques for identifying chronic wound infection. Wound Repair Regen. 14 (5), 548–557.

Harper, A., 2011. Sepsis. In: Centre for maternal and child enquiries (CMACE). Saving Mothers' Lives: reviewing maternal deaths to make motherhood safer: 2006–08. The eighth report on confidential enquiries into maternal deaths in the United Kingdom. Br. J. Obstet. Gynaecol. 118 (Suppl. 1), 85–96.

HPA (Health Protection Agency), 2013. Investigation of Nose Swabs. Available online: <http://www.hpa.org.uk/ ProductsServices/Microbiology Pathology/UKStandardsFor MicrobiologyInvestigations/ TermsOfUseForSMIs/AccessTo UKSMIs/SMIBacteriology/ smiB05InvestigationofNoseSwabs/> (accessed 5 March 2015).

HPA (Health Protection Agency), 2014. Investigation of skin, superficial and non-surgical wounds swabs. Online. Available online: <https:// www.gov.uk/government/ publications/smi-b-11-investigation-of-skin-superficial-and-non-surgical-wound-swabs> (accessed 5 March 2015).

Kingsley, A., 2003. Audit of wound swab sampling: why protocols could improve practice. Prof. Nurse 18 (6), 338–343.

Knight, M., Nair, M., Shah, A., et al. on behalf of the MBRRACE-UK, 2014. Maternal mortality and morbidity in the UK 2009–12: surveillance and epidemiology. In: Knight, M., Kenyon, S., Brocklehurst, P., et al. on behalf of MBRRACE-UK (Eds.), Saving Lives, Improving Mothers' Care – Lessons Learned to Inform Future Maternity Care from the UK and Ireland Confidential Enquiries into Maternal Deaths and Morbidity 2009–12. National Perinatal Epidemiology Unit, Oxford, pp. 9–26.

Kraus, F., 2011. Examination of the placenta, membranes and cord: Basic examination. In: Kay, H., Nelson, M., Wang, Y. (Eds.), 2011 The Placenta: From Development to Disease. Wiley-Blackwell, Oxford, pp. 111–112.

Page, C., Mounsey, A., Rowland, K., 2013. Is self-swabbing for STIs a good idea? J. Fam. Pract. 62 (11), 651–653.

Pattern, H., 2010. Identifying Wound Infection: Taking a Swab. Wound Essentials 5, 64–66.

Pettker, C., Buhimsch, I., Magloire, L., et al., 2007. Value of placental microbial evaluation in diagnosing intra-amniotic infection. Obstet. Gynaecol. 109 (3), 739–749.

Chapter | 12 |

Principles of hygiene needs: for the woman

LEARNING OUTCOMES

Having read this chapter, the reader should be able to:

• discuss the ways in which the midwife facilitates personal hygiene
• describe the ways in which vulval and oral toilets are undertaken
• identify the principles applied for the making of an occupied or unoccupied bed
• discuss the midwife's role and responsibilities in relation to each of these aspects of care.

This chapter considers the skills required to meet the complete range of hygiene needs of the woman. Cleanliness and attention to physical appearance can be significant in promoting psychological wellbeing, as well as physical health. The principles of bed making are considered as well as personal, vulval, and oral hygiene.

PERSONAL HYGIENE

Cleanliness is a basic human right. It is something for which individuals will set their own standards. Downey & Lloyd (2008) suggest that it is inappropriate for health professionals to apply their own standards to the women that they care for. However, the Healthcare Commission (2007) found that approximately one-third of the complaints received related to failures in meeting personal hygiene and standards of privacy for inpatients in NHS Trust hospitals.

Meeting hygiene needs

Midwives work with women for whom their level of independence is generally sufficient for them to care for their own hygiene needs. The occasions when the midwife may need to give assistance include:

• immobility – epidural or spinal analgesia, surgery or existing mobility problem
• intensive or high dependency care
• prescribed bed rest, e.g. antepartum haemorrhage.

Maintaining personal hygiene affects several aspects of care. Psychologically most people feel 'better' when clean, particularly to know that there are no offensive odours around them. This particularly applies to postnatal women and their perineal care. The skin itself is the largest body organ and needs to be kept free from breaks and infection in order to protect the inner organs. Where a wound does exist, good standards of hygiene are often the means of preventing colonization and so aiding healing. Perineal trauma is one such example (Steen 2007). Vulval toilet is discussed below. Pressure area care (Chapter 53) (particularly when incontinence is also an issue) is an important aspect of care that maintains the skins integrity and is hindered by poor hygiene.

In ensuring that the woman's hygiene needs are met, the midwife should consider facilitating as much independence as is possible. Many people will feel embarrassed to have someone else undertaking very personal aspects of care; mobility is also encouraged (when appropriate) in order to reduce the thromboembolic risks that accompany childbearing (Chapter 54). Consequently these measures are often preferable to being bathed in bed:

- assisting a woman to sit with a bowl, or at the sink, midwife assisting as necessary
- assisting a woman into a bath or shower, remaining with her or returning after a few minutes to assist as required.

When assisting a woman to facilitate her own needs, care should be taken to ensure that all that she needs is with her (clean clothes, toiletries, pads, etc.) and that she has access to a call bell. The need for analgesia should be considered prior to these tasks being undertaken and it should be recognized that in some circumstances the woman may find washing and dressing very tiring.

Assisting with hygiene needs (in whatever way) does necessitate some risk assessment. The use of infection control strategies (standard precautions and personal protective equipment) and moving and handling guidelines should be employed accordingly (Pegram et al 2007). Consideration should also be given to upholding individual preferences and dignity with privacy.

BED BATHING

Bed bathing aims to meet the complete hygiene needs of a woman if she is confined to bed, but Baker et al (1999) indicate that bed bathing is the least effective method of patient hygiene. If it is required, it is a task that can bring psychological wellbeing from the period of uninterrupted individualized care. It is also a time in which holistic care is completed; these aspects of care should accompany a bed bath:

- observation of consciousness and levels of pain (on both resting and moving)
- observation of the skin, particularly areas of pressure (see Chapter 53), inflammation, infection or allergy

- general health and nourishment, oral intake of diet and fluids
- ante- or postnatal examination
- assessment of vital signs
- wound care
- catheter or bladder care, vulval toilet
- bowel care
- attention to circulation, passive or active exercises, observations for varicosities or oedema, prevention of complications associated with immobility (see Chapter 54)
- care of intravenous infusion and fluid balance
- oral hygiene
- hair washing, pedicure, or manicure
- therapeutic touch, communication, education
- attention to a safe and aesthetic environment including changes of sheets and bedding.

Principles

- Ideally the midwife is assisted by another practitioner; this enables the woman to be exposed for a shorter time and reduces the moving and handling risks.
- The procedure should be carried out in a warm environment. Informed consent is obtained. All equipment that is needed should be gathered before commencing in order to reduce the risks of interruption.
- Own or single-use toiletries should be used and areas such as the perineum should be cleansed using disposable cloths. Attention is paid to changes in water so that dirty water (after cleansing the perineum) is not then used for cleaner areas, e.g. the feet.
- A coordinated approach is used so that there is minimal exposure of the body. Washing and drying the areas nearest to each practitioner prevents leaning over the woman and dampening areas that have already been dried (Pegram et al 2007).
- A nearby linen skip allows for the correct disposal of the used sheets once the bed has been changed, without soiled linen contaminating anything else.
- All care and observations are documented contemporaneously.

Modified bed baths

If the woman is able, a modified bed bath allows her to wash as much as she can, with the midwife completing any outstanding areas afterwards. If the woman is seriously ill or too uncomfortable, a partial bed bath may be performed,

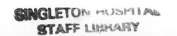

using the same principles, but washing only the hands, face, axillae, and genital area.

Vulval toilet

This is particularly appropriate for women in the early postnatal period. The majority of women who experience a vaginal birth experience perineal trauma (Bick & Bassett 2013). There are specific risk factors, these include nulliparity, instrumental delivery, prolonged second stage, epidural, and induction (Steen 2012), but whether injury is sustained or not (caesarean section), heavy lochial loss post-delivery necessitates good perineal hygiene. Good hygiene contributes to the prevention of infection and to the promotion of healing (Steen 2012). It can also act as a soothing analgesic. Plain warm water is used; Sleep and Grant (1988) indicated that water was comparable to salt or Savlon in its soothing and healing effects. Soaps and other substances can be irritants to the delicate tissues of the perineum.

The midwife records this aspect of care as for any other and adheres to standard precaution and infection control protocols. The midwife may carry out the procedure or advise the woman how to undertake it herself. Informed consent is gained.

There are three methods of vulval toilet:

1. Assist the woman onto a bedpan, pour warm water over the vulva and perineum, and pat dry with disposable wipes.
2. Sit the woman on the toilet and pour warm water over the vulva and perineum from a jug.
3. Sit the woman on the bidet (facing either direction depending upon her mobility and the comfort of her perineum). It is important that:
   a. the water is warm, not hot
   b. the sprinkle rather than jet is used, gently, so that water does not enter the vagina
   c. the perineum is dried carefully afterwards using disposable wipes.

Care of the traumatized perineum

Steen (2012) suggests that the majority of perineal wounds heal well. Women do need to understand what to expect, how to care for a damaged perineum and the signs and symptoms of an infected perineal wound (Bick & Bassett 2013). Current care recommends:

- Use of maternity sanitary towels (softer with less friction generated).
- Regular changing of sanitary towels using decontaminated hands, and washing and drying hands afterwards (Harper 2011).

- Regular cleansing of the perineum, bathing or showering.
- Use of systemic and topical analgesia. The use of heat or cold is debated, both may have value. Steen & Marchant (2007) advocate the use of cooling gel packs, while anecdotal evidence (Davies 2012) suggest that heat is soothing. Care should be taken; however, wound cooling can impede the healing process (Chapter 52); Boyle (2006) recommends cooling methods should only be used for short periods of time and not after 24–48 hours.
- Other alternative therapies, e.g. use of lavender oil, may be considered (Davies 2012) but this should only be within the midwife's professional sphere of practice if trained accordingly.
- Careful diet (increase in protein, vitamins and fibre) can aid healing and prevent constipation.
- Resumption of pelvic floor muscle exercises.
- Being alert to the possibility of wound infection: failure to heal, persistent/increased pain, discharge (often offensive).

(Adapted from Bick & Bassett 2013)

ORAL HYGIENE

The majority of clients that the midwife works with will attend to their own oral hygiene without assistance or prompting. However, the oral cavity houses commensal microorganisms that live happily without causing the host harm or benefit (Dickinson 2012) until something disrupts this relationship. Commonly illness, dietary problems, poor oral health, smoking, and excessive drinking all potentially trigger a response that ultimately leads to dental decay. Dental decay is not just a localized problem but can cause septicaemia, heart attacks, endocarditis, and stroke (Dickinson 2012). Anon (2012) reports a halving in the incidence of pneumonia on an intensive care unit because of an improved mouth care regime.

For the pregnant woman specifically, changes in saliva pH and fluid retention within the gums can predispose women to dental caries. Existing gingivitis can worsen. Keirse & Plutzer (2010) cite studies which suggest that poor maternal dental health can reduce fetal weight and increase the incidence of preterm birth. Keirse & Plutzer (2010) found that of 649 women, only 35% of them had seen a dentist in pregnancy. Their study suggests that maternal dental health has a relationship with children's dental health and that women should take oral care seriously for themselves.

Physically an unclean mouth is unpleasant, it can also affect how the woman feels psychologically. Halitosis is a social problem that damages relationships (Wilson 2011). If a woman is unable to attend to her own oral hygiene, for whatever reason, the midwife must carry out this aspect of care with her. Informed consent is gained. Likely occasions when the midwife will need to assist include:

- when nil by mouth:
  - pre- or post-surgery
  - nasogastric tube *in situ*
  - unconscious, receiving intensive or high-dependency care
- nausea and vomiting
- oxygen therapy
- mouth breathing, e.g. labour; use of inhalational analgesia
- if affected by mouth drying/unpleasant tasting medicines.

Undertaking oral hygiene

For oral hygiene, essential equipment includes:

- a toothbrush, soft with a small head
- toothpaste, fluoride, pea-sized amount
- water for rinsing, paper towels for drying, receiver for spitting (if not at the sink).

Depending on the woman's position and degree of alertness, covering for her clothing may be needed. Ideally the woman is positioned in an upright position, but if this is not possible suction may be needed. The unconscious or semi-conscious woman will benefit from the use of a specific suction toothbrush (Stout et al 2009).

When cleaning the teeth the brush is held at a 45° angle (bristles pointing towards the roots of the teeth) and moved gently, slightly from side to side, systematically around the top and then the lower jaw, on all surfaces of the teeth. Electric toothbrushes should be held over the tooth being cleaned for 10 seconds, and then moved onto the next tooth. The need to 'scrub' the teeth is not necessary when the brush head is revolving itself. The tongue and gums can also be gently brushed (Wilson 2011) and the mouth should be rinsed thoroughly to prevent any burning sensations from the toothpaste residue (Turner 1996). Foam sticks are considered to be less effective than a toothbrush, but may be useful in situations where the mouth is sore. Mouthwash is also an alternative to brushing, but only on a short-term basis. Moisturizer may be applied to dried lips (Wilson 2011).

This aspect of care is documented contemporaneously as for any other aspect of care. In some instances an oral assessment chart may be maintained, oral assessment is undertaken using a torch and disposable spatula, often on admission to hospital and as clinical changes dictate.

BED MAKING

Changing sheets or remaking a bed is indicated if the sheets are soiled, sweaty, or dishevelled. The aim is to ensure that the bed is crease free, protecting skin integrity, and increasing comfort. It is a difficult and time-consuming procedure to complete alone. Standard precautions use and correct disposal of used linen both reduce the risks of infection transmission. The timing of bed making should fit in with the individualized plan of care. This is particularly important if a wound is to be redressed (Chapter 52) as the disturbance of used sheets in the environment increases atmospheric microorganisms. The babies of postnatal women also often have contact with the woman's bed clothes, e.g. use of pillows when breastfeeding; this also necessitates that bed linen is changed frequently and that babies are exposed to minimal sources of potential cross-infection.

Principles

- All equipment needed should be gathered before commencing. The bed should be at a suitable working height for both practitioners and should be easily accessible.
- If in any way contaminated, the mattress is cleaned according to the agreed protocol before the bed is made.
- Care is taken to ensure that none of the bedding touches the floor, the pillows or other items that will be reapplied to the bed should be carefully stacked on an empty chair or the shelf (it pulls out) at the end of the bed.
- Working in a coordinated way, e.g. lifting the mattress at the same time, allows the sheets to be anchored correctly.
- The woman's preference is considered when deciding how many layers of bedding are added.
- A linen skip is kept to hand so that soiled linen can be put straight in.

Making an occupied bed

This is generally undertaken by moving the woman from one side of the bed to the other side, and back again while the sheet is changed underneath her. An assistant is required and, if able, the woman helps too. Care is taken to maintain her temperature and dignity. She needs to be aware of what will happen and of the fact that at some point there will be a linen 'lump' to ease over. Analgesia may be required prior to this. Any appliances, catheters, drains, infusions, etc. should all be handled with care.

The woman is assisted to roll onto her side facing the assistant. The old sheet is untucked from the bed and rolled up next to the woman's back. The new sheet is tucked in at the top, bottom and side of the bed. It is then also rolled up next to the woman's back. The woman is assisted to roll over the 'lump' to now face the midwife on her other side. The assistant removes the old linen, unrolls the new and tucks it in. The woman is repositioned.

ROLE AND RESPONSIBILITIES OF THE MIDWIFE

These can be summarized as:
- completing the procedures safely with the maintenance of dignity and privacy, applying infection control and moving and handling protocols
- ensuring informed consent is gained and working within current evidence based practice offering an individualized approach, encouraging independence and mobility where possible
- contemporaneous record keeping.

SUMMARY

- Attention to all types of hygiene benefits the physical and psychological wellbeing of the woman. Generally,

hygiene contributes to less infection and improved wound healing.
- The midwife should adapt care according to the individual woman's needs and level of dependence.
- Vulval hygiene may be both cleansing and soothing, particularly after a vaginal birth.
- Toothbrush and paste are the recommended cleaning agents for oral hygiene.

SELF-ASSESSMENT EXERCISES

The answers to the following questions may be found in the text:
1. Discuss the significance of personal hygiene.
2. Identify the ways in which a woman may be assisted to wash when mobility is restricted.
3. Describe the different ways that a vulval toilet may be completed.
4. Discuss the advice given to a woman regarding the care of her traumatized perineum.
5. Demonstrate bed making – occupied and unoccupied.
6. Describe how to complete an oral toilet.
7. Summarize the midwife's responsibilities in relation to the complete hygiene needs of the woman.

REFERENCES

Anon (Anonymous), 2012. News: Pneumonia in ICU halved by oral regime. Nurs. Times 108 (27), 6.

Baker, F., Smith, L., Stead, L., 1999. Giving a blanket bath – 1. Nurs. Times 95 (3), 4.

Bick, D., Bassett, S., 2013. How to provide postnatal perineal care. Midwives 16 (2), 34–35.

Boyle, M., 2006. Wound Healing in Midwifery. Radcliffe, Oxford, p. 75.

Davies, L., 2012. Care in the postnatal period part 2. Essentially MIDIRS 3 (1), 36–40.

Dickinson, H., 2012. Maintaining oral health after stroke. Nurs. Stand. 26 (49), 35–39.

Downey, L., Lloyd, H., 2008. Bed bathing patients in hospital. Nurs. Stand. 22 (34), 35–40.

Harper, A., 2011. Sepsis. In: CMACE (Centre for Maternal and Child Enquiries) 2011 Saving Mothers' lives:

reviewing maternal deaths to make motherhood safer: 2006–2008. The eight report on confidential enquiries into maternal deaths in the United Kingdom. Br. J. Obstet. Gynaecol. 118 (Suppl. 1), 85–96.

Healthcare Commission, 2007. State of Healthcare 2007: Improvements and Challenges in England and Wales. Commission for Healthcare Audit and Inspection, London.

Keirse, M., Plutzer, K., 2010. Women's attitudes to and perceptions of oral health and dental care during pregnancy. J. Perinat. Med. 38 (1), 3–8.

Pegram, A., Bloomfield, J., Jones, A., 2007. Clinical skills: bed bathing and personal hygiene needs of patients. Br. J. Nurs. 16 (6), 356–358.

Sleep, J., Grant, A., 1988. Routine addition of salt or Savlon bath concentrate during bathing in the immediate postpartum period: a

randomised controlled trial. Nurs. Times 84 (21), 55–57.

Steen, M., 2007. Perineal tears and episiotomy: how do wounds heal? Br. J. Midwifery 15 (5), 273–280.

Steen, M., 2012. Risk, recognition and repair of perineal trauma. Br. J. Midwifery 20 (11), 768–772.

Steen, M., Marchant, P., 2007. Ice packs and cooling gel pads versus no localized treatment for relief of perineal pain: a randomised controlled trial. Evid. Based Midwifery 5 (1), 16–22.

Stout, M., Goulding, O., Powell, A., 2009. Developing and implementing an oral care policy and assessment tool. Nurs. Stand. 23 (49), 42–48.

Turner, G., 1996. Oral care. Nurs. Stand. 10 (28), 51–54.

Wilson, A., 2011. How to provide effective oral care. Nurs. Times 107 (6), 14–15.

Chapter 13

Principles of hygiene needs: for the baby

LEARNING OUTCOMES

Having read this chapter, the reader should be able to:

- discuss the role and responsibilities of the midwife in meeting the hygiene needs of the baby
- discuss the structure of the stratum corneum at birth and the factors that affect its barrier function
- discuss the rationale for the use of soap or bath additives
- discuss the principles of bathing and washing the baby
- describe the methods used for applying a non-disposable nappy.

The midwife has a pivotal role in educating and advising new parents on the care of their baby while helping them adjust to their new roles. Sadly though, Wray (2006) found that two-thirds of women (50% were primiparous women) were not shown how to change their baby's nappy or undertake a 'top and tail' and 34% were not shown how to bathe their baby. While this may not be a requirement for all women, primiparous women may not be confident with caring for babies and this might add to their anxieties and insecurities of becoming a new mother. This chapter focuses on the hygiene needs of the baby: bathing and washing, cleaning the genital area, the cord stump and the eyes. Oral hygiene can be important for an unwell baby but it is rarely needed for the healthy baby and is not discussed.

NEWBORN SKIN

Afsar (2009a) advises that epidermal development of the skin is complete by 34 weeks' gestation but some authors are now suggesting this process continues for the first year of life (Blume-Peytavi et al 2009, Garcia-Bartels et al 2010, Lavender et al 2012). The stratum corneum is the outer layer of the epidermis, the barrier layer and is composed of keratinocytes embedded in a lipid- (ceramides) rich matrix of cholesterol, ceramides, and fatty acids (Blackburn 2013, Sarkar et al 2010). The stratum corneum of the newborn term baby is thinner and less hydrated than that of an adult, which makes the baby vulnerable to microorganisms and infection, contaminants that can lead to trauma and increased fluid loss (Furber et al 2012, Lavender et al 2012), these risks are greatly increased for the preterm baby (Blackburn 2013).

The skin of the newborn baby is more permeable to topical substances and microorganisms than an adult's skin, with permeability decreasing with increasing gestational age (Blackburn 2013). This can predispose the baby to the development of allergic and irritant reactions occurring from contact with chemicals; the risk escalates with damaged skin (Atherton 2005, Blackburn 2013, Hale 2007, Trotter 2006). The stratum corneum contains natural moisturizing factors (NMFs) which act as lubricants and humectants to assist the skin retain moisture (Blackburn 2013). Blackburn (2013) and Visscher et al (2011) advise that skin hydration is reduced immediately after birth and increases as the stratum corneum adjusts to extrauterine life.

Trans-epidermal water loss (TEWL) is higher in the term baby than the adult – 25 g/m/hr in the baby compared to 7 g/m/hr in the adult (Lavender et al 2012) and even higher in the preterm baby. Afsar (2009a) suggests the TEWL in a baby at 25 weeks' gestation is 15-fold higher than a baby of 40 weeks' gestation, which he advises results in significant morbidity due to dehydration, electrolyte imbalance and thermal instability.

Immediately after delivery, the skin pH of the newborn baby increases from the fetal pH of 5.5–6.0 and gradually decreases to 5.0–5.5 during the first week, reaching adult values around 3–4 weeks (Blackburn 2013). Garcia-Bartels et al (2010) and Blume-Peytavi et al (2012) suggest the skin pH at birth is close to neutral at 6.2–7.5. A high skin pH is associated with increased bacterial proliferation and increased proteolytic enzymes which Blume-Peytavi et al (2012) suggest are detrimental to good skin barrier function whereas Afsar (2009a) advises that a pH of 5.0–5.5 encourages commensal colonization and discourages the growth of pathological microorganisms. The 'acid mantle' which helps to protect the skin is created from the stratum corneum, sweat, sebum, superficial fat, metabolic by-products of keratinization and external substances such as amniotic fluid (Blackburn 2013). Trotter (2013) refers to it as a 'very fine film' resting on the skin surface; as such, this barrier is easily disturbed. Blume-Peytavi et al (2012) suggest that each time the skin is washed the outer layer is removed and it takes 120 minutes for the skin to recover.

Vernix caseosa is a white biofilm that covers the baby *in utero* to provide insulation, acts as an emollient, and minimizes friction at delivery (Blackburn 2013). It is composed of water, sebaceous secretions, and desquamated skin cells; is rich in triglycerides, fatty acids, ceramides, cholesterol and unsaponified fat; and has microbial properties (Blackburn 2013, Ness et al 2013, Sarkar et al 2010, Trotter 2013). Afsar (2009b) and Ness et al (2013) consider it has an important hydration, thermoregulation and bacterial and wound protection function and should not be removed. Sarkar et al (2010), however, suggest the function of vernix caseosa after birth is debatable. Visscher et al (2011) suggest that when vernix caseosa is not removed there is a significant increase in skin hydration at 24 hours than when it is removed. They also found the pH of the stratum corneum was more acidic when vernix caseosa was not removed. Trotter (2013) agrees vernix caseosa should not be removed, rather it should be left to be absorbed naturally. Ness et al (2013) concur, suggesting it should not be removed until the baby is bathed.

Some babies, particularly when postmature, have dry skin which can crack. Although there is a temptation to rub in substances such as emollients or olive oil in an attempt to 'moisturize' the skin, Trotter (2004) cautions against this practice as she suggests the dry layer will peel off within a few days revealing a healthy layer of skin underneath, which will regain its protective barrier in 2–4 weeks. It may therefore be advisable to avoid the use of emollients or creams on the skin during the first 2–4 weeks. Blume-Peytavi et al (2009) disagree and suggest the use of an emollient on a dry skin can help protect the integrity of the stratum corneum and consider it may be of benefit in babies at risk of developing atopic dermatitis. Ness et al (2013) support this view suggesting topical emollients not only protect the stratum corneum but can also potentially enhance the maturation and repair of the skin barrier. They advise using an emollient with a physiological balance of lipids (3:1:1:1 molar ration of cholesterol, ceramides, palmitate and linoleate) and to avoid using lanolin alcohol due to the risk of sensitivity occurring. They also advise against the use of mustard oil, which is used in some of the developing countries, due to its effect of slowing the recovery of the skin barrier and increasing TEWL but suggest sunflower oil has been shown to accelerate the skin barrier recovery (Ness et al 2013). Sunflower oil has low levels of oleic acid and also has high levels of linoleic acid, which Cooke et al (2011) recommend, as it can repair/enhance the skin barrier. Trotter (2013) agrees on the use of sunflower oil but recommends no skin care products for the first month and avoiding nut oils because of the risk of sensitization. Olive oil is used as a traditional emollient in some countries and cultures, e.g. Turkey (Erenel et al 2010) but Trotter (2013) and Cooke et al (2011) caution against the use of olive oil, as it is high in oleic acid which can damage the skin barrier. Hugill (2014) warns it may be implicated in the development of atopic eczema and other skin conditions.

SKIN CLEANSERS/BATH ADDITIVES

There is a lot of debate around the use of skin cleansers and bath additives, the effect they have on skin pH and the risk of absorption creating an allergic or irritant reaction. Current skin care practices for babies vary among populations, tradition, ethnicity and culture (Blume-Peytavi et al 2009). NICE (2014) advise that cleansing agents should not be added to bath water, or medicated wipes or lotions used when cleaning the baby during the first 2–4 weeks. Trotter (2013) cautions against using anything that contains sulphates SLS/SLES, parabens, phthalates, artificial colours, and perfume. Brennan (2010) agrees, arguing that because the newborn skin is thinner and metabolizes chemicals differently, the skin surface area : weight ratio is higher and because the liver and kidneys are immature the baby is at increased risk for a toxic reaction. Blume-Peytavi et al (2012) suggest the risk is small as the German Cosmetic Toiletry, Perfumery and Detergent Association report an average of one adverse effect per million products sold and the American Food and Drug Administration report they receive one to three adverse effect reports per million products sold. However, it is possible that this is underreported.

The purpose of skin cleansing is to clean the skin without changing the pH, affecting the skin microbiota or removing the surface lipids that protect the skin (Hugill 2014). Water is effective at removing much of the matter that has accumulated on the baby's skin but may not remove it all, particularly where there is faecal soiling; thus parents may want to use a cleanser or bath additive at times (Furber et al 2012, Garcia-Bartels et al 2012, Lavender et al 2012, Lavender et al 2013). Furber et al (2012) found that parents allocated to a 'water only' group for cleansing of the genital and perianal area were less likely to clean the baby's skin when only urine was in the nappy than parents allocated to use of a wipe, which is concerning. However, when diaper dermatitis (DDM) (nappy rash) was present, those using wipes were more likely to change to water only but parents using just water were unlikely to change to using wipes to eliminate the DDM. Thus in some situations, e.g. DDM, parents may prefer the use of water only.

Lavender et al (2012) advise that the pH of tap water is 7.9–8.2 which compromises the acidic environment of the skin. Lavender et al (2013) also suggest water may increase the pH of skin to 7.5 which will increase skin protease activity and inhibit lipid synthesis leading to a breakdown of the skin barrier. Blume-Peytavi et al (2009) suggest that washing with tap water alone can have a drying effect on the skin which may be heightened in areas of hard water. Hard water can have an effect on the development of dermatitis (Hugill 2014) thus bathing babies in hard water may increase the risk of eczema occurring. Adam et al (2009) are concerned that water has no buffering capacity, which means it is unable to neutralize external influences to maintain the pH level and that it does not solubilize lipophilic substances.

Liquid cleansers are designed to interact with surface 'soil' and remove harmful substances such as faecal enzymes without damaging the skin (Blume-Peytavi et al 2009). Many also contain an emollient. The bulk of the cleanser is comprised of surfactants which act to decrease the surface tension between water and air and also have a foaming action which assists with the removal of fat-soluble substances (Sarkar et al 2010). Surfactants however can have a deleterious effect on the barrier function of the baby's skin and may increase the skin pH. Trotter (2006) cautions the use of surfactants also have a risk of trauma occurring to the skin surface which can result in allergic and/or irritant dermatitis. Sarkar et al (2010) advise that the higher the foaming power, the higher the risk of skin damage as excessive lipids can be removed from the stratum corneum. However, products being developed now may be less damaging to the skin than just using water.

Soap may have an alkali or acid/neutral pH. Syndets are synthetic detergents with a pH that is acidic or neutral, the lauryl sulphate of traditional soap has been replaced with natural fats and oils. Ness et al (2013) and Sarkar et al (2010) suggest syndets are milder and less irritating than traditional soaps and that they do not alter the skin pH or alter the microflora. They further suggest that a moisturizer be added to avoid excessive dryness. Traditional alkali soaps have a pH around 10, alter the skin pH and affect the barrier function in terms of TEWL, and are drying and irritant to the skin (Blume-Peytavi et al 2009, Furber et al 2012, Ness et al 2013). Blackburn (2013) and Sarkar et al (2010) suggest it takes at least 1 hour for the pH to return to its pre-wash level whereas Blume-Peytavi et al (2012) advise 30 minutes. Thus the best advice is to not use alkaline soap.

Baby wipes are popular with many parents but may contain chemicals that are irritant to the baby's skin. Trotter (2013) suggests that wipes should not be used during the first month of life and if they are to be used, they should be free from alcohol, parabens, phthalates, artificial colours, and perfumes. Furber et al (2012) consider that the modern, high-quality wipes used today are not associated with a higher incidence of DDM in healthy newborns. In support of this view, Garcia-Bartels et al (2012) found that neither baby wipes nor water hampered hydration and that wipes did not harm the acid mantle barrier during the first 4 weeks. Lavender et al (2012) tested wipes with a pH of 4.9 and found the hydration effects on the buttocks to be the same as using water and cotton wool. They found no evidence of differences on skin pH, TEWL, erythema, and microbial skin contaminants.

Although shampoo is not necessary it is often used during bathing. Ness et al (2013) recommend the shampoo does not contain cocamidopropyl betaine and MIDA-laureth sulphate, as they are allergens. To reduce the risk further of developing irritant dermatitis, Sarkar et al (2010) advise using the minimal time of contact between the shampoo and the scalp and using a shampoo that is free from fragrance and anti-infective agents. Trotter (2013) suggests that shampoo should not be used for the first year of life.

Ness et al (2013) recommend that if using a cleanser, use it sparingly and only on soiled areas and ensure it is completely rinsed off. It seems sensible that if cleansers, wipes, or soaps are to be used, they should have a neutral/acidic pH, with no perfume or dye added and be specifically designed for babies (never use an adult product).

BABY BATHING

Blume-Peytavi et al (2012) suggest that routine bathing poses no risk to the baby and is superior to washing or sponge bathing. However the timing of the first bath is contentious and varies between different traditions and cultures. It is important that the baby is healthy and has thermal stability. Ness et al (2013) do not advocate bathing shortly after birth but suggest it should be delayed until the cardio-respiratory status has been stable for 2–4 hours, and not within the first 6 hours of life because of the risk of hypothermia, respiratory distress, increased oxygen consumption, unstable vital signs, and behavioural disruption. Sarkar et al (2010) argue bathing should be delayed 2–6 hours after birth provided the baby weighs >2500 gm. The World Health Organization (WHO 2013) suggest bathing should be delayed for 24 hours but if the baby has to be bathed, he should be at least 6 hours old. Trotter (2013) advises the bath is delayed until the cord has separated so that the microorganisms at the base of the cord are not disturbed, which she suggests may hamper the natural processes involved with cord separation. Blume-Peytavi et al (2012) found that bathing immediately after birth does not appear to affect cord healing and separation but also advise that there is no clear evidence about the effect of regular bathing on cord separation.

Parents should be involved as much as possible with the care of their baby and be given the opportunity to bath their baby if they choose to, or be shown how to bath their baby if they have not had prior experience. Parents with little or no experience of handling babies may not feel confident to bath them initially; thus it is important that the midwife considers the needs of the parents and supports them accordingly. A concern of parents may be that they may drop the baby in the water. If they express

this concern, the midwife should ask them what they would do if this happened. Invariably the response will be 'I'd pick the baby up'. This can then lead to a discussion of how to bath the baby safely and help the parents recognize what they would do if something unexpected occurred.

It is not necessary to bath babies every day, nor is it necessary to wash the baby's hair with each bath. For some parents, daily bathing may be an easier and more pleasurable option than washing the baby. Immersing a baby in water, may cause the superficial layers of the skin to hydrate and thicken with an associated reduction in cellular cohesion. Thus, skin that is overhydrated from frequent or prolonged bathing becomes more fragile increasing the risk of trauma occurring to it (Hale 2007). Blume-Peytavi et al (2009), Lavender et al (2013) and Sarkar et al (2010) recommend that immersion in the bath should last no longer than 5 minutes.

While there is no right or wrong way to bath a baby, it is important to adhere to certain principles:

- keep the baby warm
- keep the baby secure and safe
- use warm water: the temperature should be neither too hot (which risks scalding the baby) nor too cold.

Keeping the baby warm

Heat loss occurs quickly in babies who are undressed or wet, thus both the room and water temperature should be warm and the baby bathed quickly, without unnecessary exposure. Closing windows, keeping doors closed, and switching off fans to stop draughts can minimize convective heat loss. Conductive heat loss is lessened by warming clothes, towel and surfaces (e.g. changing mat). Evaporative heat loss can be reduced by drying the baby quickly, particularly the head and ensuring the baby is not bathed and dressed close to cold surfaces such as windows minimizes heat loss via radiation.

Security and safety

Cold water should be used to fill the bath initially, as this prevents the bottom of the bath from becoming too hot and reduces the risk of other children scalding themselves should they play with the bath water as it is filling. The bath should not be more than half full; Blume-Peytavi et al (2012) recommend the water should reach the level of the baby's hips when he is sitting, approximately 5 cm. The baby should never be left unattended and should always be held to prevent the head from submerging. A woman with epilepsy should place the bath on the floor rather than

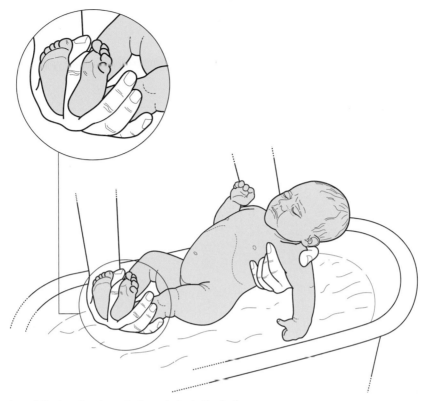

Figure 13.1 Positioning of the hands when placing a baby in the bath.

on a stand and should not be alone. Following a caesarean section, the woman will have difficulty lifting the baby and equipment and will require assistance. It may be advisable to use a jug to fill and empty the bath as lifting even a small bath half full with water may result in muscular damage.

To wash the face and hair, wrap the baby securely in a towel and hold under the non-dominant arm, secured between the arm and body, with his head and neck supported by the non-dominant hand. When ready for bathing, remove the towel. Place the baby in the bath while supporting his head and neck across the forearm and wrist of the non-dominant hand and encircling the top of his arm with the forefinger and thumb. The dominant hand grasps the ankles to lift the baby in and out of the water (Fig. 13.1). The baby can be sat up to wash his back by supporting his head across the wrist or forearm of the dominant hand (Fig. 13.2), then returning him to the original position.

Water temperature

Garcia-Bartels et al (2010) suggest the water temperature should be 37–38°C while Sakhar et al (2010) suggest a higher range of 38–40°C. This can be tested using the inner aspect of the wrist or the elbow. It is inadvisable to use fingers to test the heat of the water, as fingers are able to tolerate quite hot water and so are less sensitive to heat. Alternatively a bath thermometer can be used.

Equipment

The bath and any bath toys are a potential source of microbial contamination and should be cleaned following use (Blume-Peytavi et al 2009). Flannels and sponges are often used during the bath but Blume-Peytavi et al (2009), Ness et al (2013) and Trotter (2013) advise against the use of a flannel or washcloth to rub the skin because of the risk of epidermal injury and suggest a sponge is gentler. However Blume-Peytavi et al (2009) point out that sponges can also be a source of contamination and so recommend not using them. If a sponge or flannel is used, it should be used only for the baby and cleaned regularly and a separate one used if the water is contaminated with faeces.

- Baby bath: a large bowl will suffice provided it is only used for bathing the baby; the bath or sink can be

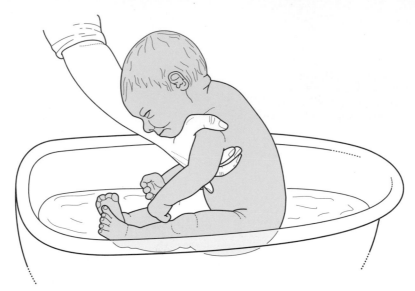

Figure 13.2 Positioning of the hands when washing the back of the baby in the bath.

used, although the latter may be more tiring for the woman's back.

- Towel: some towels have an integral hood, useful for drying the baby's head (if using an ordinary towel, fold over about 25 cm of towel lengthways; this can then be pulled up to dry the head).
- Sponge (optional).
- Nappy-changing equipment and nappy.
- Baby clothes.
- Plastic apron (non-slip).
- Non-sterile gloves, if necessary.

PROCEDURE: bathing a baby

Although this procedure is written as if the midwife is bathing the baby, it can also be used as the basis for instructing the parents on how to bath their baby:

- Discuss the procedure and gain informed consent from the parents.
- Gather equipment and prepare room.
- Wash and dry hands and apply apron (put on gloves if contact with bodily fluids is likely).
- Fill the bath using cold water first then hot and check the water temperature.
- Undress the baby, leaving the nappy on, and wrap the baby in the towel.
- Wash the baby's face with plain water, if using a sponge wipe over the face in a gentle patting motion avoiding the eyes.
- Dry the face with the towel, using gentle patting motions.

- Wash the hair if required with water, rubbing gently over the baby's hair, rinse thoroughly and dry.
- Remove the nappy, cleaning the genitalia if necessary (p. 111).
- Place the baby in the water as discussed earlier, using the dominant hand to gently wash the body and limbs with water.
- Wash the baby's back.
- Lift the baby out of the water using both hands, taking care as the baby may be slippery.
- Wrap the baby in the towel.
- Dry the baby quickly using gentle patting motions, with particular attention to skin folds.
- Put on a clean nappy (see below) and dress the baby.
- Give the baby to one of the parents, or place in the cot on his back.
- Empty the bath water and dispose of equipment.
- Wash and dry hands.
- Document the findings and act accordingly.

NAPPY CHANGING

Ness et al (2013) recommend the nappy is changed every 3–4 hours or when soiling occurs. When urine encounters faeces, the ureases in the faecal microbes create ammonia which increases the skin pH. This causes a reactivation of the digestive enzymes which degrades the lipids and proteins within the stratum corneum, breaking down the skin barrier (Adam et al 2009, Lavender et al 2012, Ness et al 2013). Additionally, the presence of the excretory by-products of microbial proliferation in the skin folds act as irritants and sensitizers (Hale 2008).

The skin should be cleaned at this time with either warm water or a baby wipe/mild cleanser to minimize the risk of the skin becoming excoriated and diaper dermatitis/nappy rash occurring (Atherton 2005, Trotter 2006). Nappy rash is generally a result of irritant contact dermatitis rather than infection (Blincoe 2006). It is important that the midwife can demonstrate to the parents how to change the baby's nappy, using whichever method the parents will use at home.

Nappies

Nappies are either reusable or disposable. Reusable nappies are usually made of towelling or cloth, in a variety of styles. The traditional terry towelling nappy is square shaped, requiring folding prior to use. A nappy liner can be used to line the nappy to reduce the amount of urine and faeces coming into contact with the skin and reduce the risk of DDM. Manufacturers' instructions should be followed when disposing of nappy liners; they should be used once only and not disposed of down the toilet. Waterproof over-pants may be used to prevent urine and faeces seeping onto the baby's clothes. Alternatives are the all-in-one reusables (self-fastening fitted cloth nappies, covered with a waterproof shell), two-piece reusables (cloth nappies that fit into special waterproof pants with self-adhesive fastenings) and wrap-around nappies (cloth nappies with ties, used in conjunction with waterproof overpants). All reusables require laundering. A thin layer of a barrier cream can be used to protect the genitalia and buttocks and reduce the risk of DDM, but may be contraindicated with some nappy liners.

There are three ways to fold a towelling nappy: the triangle, the kite, and the triple-fold method. The triple-fold is useful for boys as it provides extra thickness and absorbency at the front of the nappy where urination is likely to occur.

1. The triangle method (Fig. 13.3)

- Place the nappy in a diamond shape (A), fold in half to make a triangle shape with the longest side at the top and the point at the bottom (B).
- Place the baby on the nappy and bring up the top layer between the baby's legs (C).
- Wrap one side of the nappy across the baby, then the other side (C).
- Bring up the lower layer of the nappy between the baby's legs and secure with a safety pin (D, E).

2. The kite method (Fig. 13.4)

- Place the nappy in a diamond shape (A); fold the outer two points to the centre to make a kite shape (B).
- Fold the top corner down and the bottom corner up towards the centre; the latter fold can be adjusted to suit the length of the baby (C).
- Place the baby on the nappy, bring up the nappy between the baby's legs (D).
- Wrap one side of the nappy across the baby, then the other side and secure with two safety pins (D, E).

3. The triple-fold method (Fig. 13.5)

- Place the nappy in a square shape and fold into half lengthways from top to bottom (A).
- Fold in half again, from left to right, to make into a four-layer-thick square shape (B).
- Take hold of the bottom right hand corner of the first layer of the nappy and open it to the left (C, D).
- Turn the nappy over carefully, keeping the layers in position so that the point lies to the left (E).
- Take hold of the next two layers forming the square shape and fold the outer third over towards the centre and then in half, creating a triangle shape with an extra thick pleat in the centre (E, F).
- Place the baby on the nappy and bring up the nappy between the baby's legs (G).
- Wrap one side of the nappy across the baby, then the other side and secure with a safety pin (G, H).

Disposable nappies

Disposables are paper nappies (made from fluffed wood pulp) containing absorbent crystals that form a gel when they become wet from urine. Many use super-absorbent polymers to increase their absorbency, resulting in the nappies staying drier against the baby's skin for longer and consequently less incidence of DDM (Hale 2007). Breathable nappies, which allow more airflow around the baby's skin regardless of whether the skin is wet or dry, are also available; this inhibits the growth of *Candida albicans*, reducing the risk of DDM (Hale 2007). Some nappies have nappy liners impregnated with a barrier cream (e.g. petroleum) which Hale (2007) suggests is another way of reducing the incidence of DDM. The barrier cream is hydrophobic and transfers from the nappy to the baby's skin in response to the warmth of the skin and movement by the baby to serve as a protective barrier.

Disposable nappies have an outer plastic layer, fitted elasticated leg bands and sticky tapes at the sides to fasten the nappy. Some have elasticated waists; some have a hole for the umbilical cord, to allow it to remain dry. They come in a variety of sizes, from newborn to toddler size.

109

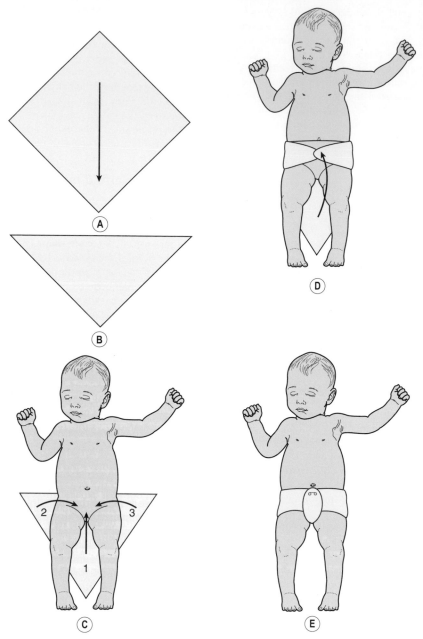

Figure 13.3 Triangle method of nappy folding.

Disposables are used once only and should not be disposed of down the toilet.

Use of barrier creams

Ness et al (2013) recommend the use of a barrier cream as a preventative measure for DDM and suggest it should be preservative free and zinc oxide– or petrolatum-based. Hale (2007) supports this view and Sarkar et al (2010) recommend these be used when DDM is present. Ravanfar et al (2012) suggest the barrier cream should contain zinc oxide, titanium dioxide and starch or dexpanthenol to prevent contact between skin and faeces, avoid humidity and minimize TEWL. The barrier cream is applied thinly following

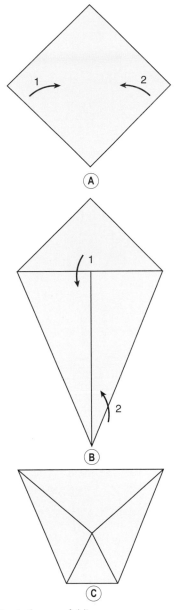

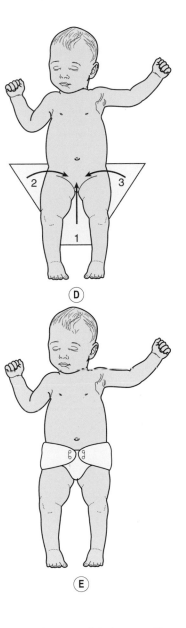

Figure 13.4 Kite method of nappy folding.

each nappy change and always after handwashing or use of alcohol handrub to reduce the risk of cross-contamination (see Chapter 9). Bacterial preparations are unnecessary as DDM is not caused by infection and they may interfere with the resident skin flora.

Barrier cream used as a protective layer should:

- allow the transfer of fluid from the skin to the nappy
- prevent the transfer of fluid from the nappy to the skin

- contain no antibiotics, steroids, perfumes or preservatives.

PROCEDURE: changing a nappy

- Gain informed consent from the parents.
- Gather equipment:
  - non-sterile gloves and apron
  - changing mat or towel

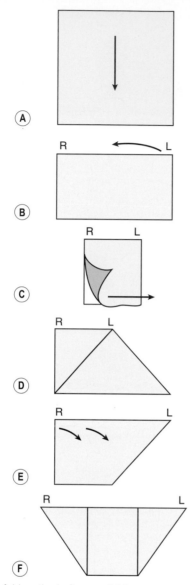

Figure 13.5 Triple-fold method of nappy folding.

- small bowl and cotton wool balls or dry wipes/baby wipes
- nappy bag or nappy bucket and disposable bag for used nappy and wipes
- clean nappy
- nappy liner (optional)
- barrier cream (optional)
- alcohol handrub
- Wash and dry hands, put on apron and gloves.
- Put warm water into the bowl if using water.

- Lay the baby on a safe, flat surface (e.g. cot mattress, changing mat), with the towel under the baby if required.
- Undress the baby sufficiently to gain access to the nappy.
- Remove the dirty nappy and put to one side.
- Using the non-dominant hand, hold the baby securely around the ankles enabling the legs to be straightened then slightly raise the buttocks to facilitate cleansing of the genital area.

- With the dominant hand, using either a cotton wool ball or wipe moistened with water or a baby wipe, clean the genitalia from front to back before the perianal area to reduce the risk of infection and taking care not to drag the skin:
  - females: wipe gently one side of the labia then the other, moving from front to back
  - males: wipe gently around the penis, towards the scrotum.
- Place the used cotton wool ball/wipe in the nappy bag and repeat on the other side until the genitalia is clean.
- Clean gently between the folds of the groin and thigh, then the buttocks.
- Pat the area dry with the towel or dry cotton wool balls/wipes
- If a barrier cream is used, remove gloves, apply alcohol handrub and put on clean gloves then apply a thin layer to the genitalia and buttocks.
- Place the nappy under the baby and secure, ensuring a boy's penis points down and the cord is outside the nappy.
- Redress the baby.
- Dispose of equipment correctly.
- Remove gloves and apron, wash and dry hands.
- Document the findings and act accordingly.

CLEANING THE EYES

To minimize the risk of trauma and infection, the baby's eyes should not be cleaned unless they are discharging. 'Sticky' eyes are commonly due to blocked tear ducts and usually are not infected; the discharge is a yellowish colour and may be seen as crusting on the eyelid. Infection can cause a profuse, offensive, or different-coloured discharge which may be accompanied by erythema and localized oedema of the eye. If infection is suspected, a swab may be taken (see Chapter 11), referral made and topical antibiotics commenced. To reduce the risk of cross-infection, each eye is cleaned separately; the cotton wool ball is used to wipe the eye once from the inner part outwards and then disposed of. While sterile water can be used if available, cooled boiled water will suffice. This procedure can be demonstrated to the parents to enable them to clean their baby's eyes.

PROCEDURE: cleaning the baby's eyes

- Gain informed consent from the parents.
- Gather equipment:
  - non-sterile gloves
  - cotton wool balls
  - clean container and cooled boiled/sterile water
  - paper towel/bag or disposable tray
- Wash and dry hands, apply gloves.
- Pour the water into the container.
- Using a cotton wool ball moistened with water, wipe from the inner edge of the eye outwards, using the cotton wool ball once only.
- Dispose of the used ball and repeat with another cotton wool ball.
- Repeat until the eye is clean then undertake for the other eye.
- Dispose of the equipment correctly.
- Remove gloves, wash and dry hands.
- Discuss ongoing care with the parents, e.g. when to repeat the procedure, signs to be aware of.
- Document the findings and act accordingly.

CORD CARE

The umbilical cord is usually clamped after birth to leave 2–5 cm of umbilical cord that has no further function. The cord vessels fibrose, the Wharton's jelly dries and the cord separates by a process of dry gangrene (it will dry, harden, shrivel, and blacken); finally, it detaches (this may occur more quickly with a lotus birth, see Chapter 33). During this process, polymorphonuclear leucocytes infiltrate the base of the cord between the drying cord and the abdominal wall creating a pus-like appearance with separation between 5–15 days (Imdad et al 2013). Although this can be mistaken for pus, it is part of the normal physiological process of cord separation and not due to infection (although omphalitis can also occur). The cord stump and surrounding skin are colonized soon after birth primarily by non-pathogenic microorganisms, e.g. coagulase-negative staphylococci and diphtheroid bacilli (Ness et al 2013) and pathogenic microorganisms can also colonize the cord stump. The umbilical cord is a favourable medium for colonization because of the necrotic tissue (Erenel et al 2010). Imdad et al (2013) suggest *Staphylococcus aureus* colonizes 99.7% of cords in the USA, whereas in Bangladesh the predominant flora is gram-negative *Escherichia coli*, *Klebsiella pneumoniae*, and *Pseudomonas* spp. – all of which can track up the cord and cause infection – omphalitis – a significant cause of morbidity and mortality in developing countries.

Practices surrounding cord care vary across the world. WHO (2013) recommend the use of daily chlorhexidine applied to the umbilical cord stump during the first week of life for newborns born at home in settings with a high neonatal mortality rate (≥30 deaths per 1000 live births) but in low-mortality settings they advocate keeping the cord clean and dry. Imdad et al (2013) support the use of chlorhexidine in high-mortality settings and suggest it reduces the risk of death by 23%, although it does delay cord separation by 1–7 days. Karumbi et al (2013) found the use of 4% chlorhexidine within the first 24 hours reduced neonatal mortality in community settings for topical cord care in Kenya. Suliman et al (2010) report on the use of triple dye (brilliant green, crystal violet, proflavine hemisulphate) with and without rubbing alcohol several times a day until separation. While this may be advantageous in reducing colonization with *Staphylococcus aureus*, it does increase cord separation times. Erenel et al (2010) caution against the use of triple dye as animal studies suggest it may have toxic and carcinogenic effects.

The current management for babies not at high risk of infection, including those who have had a lotus birth, continues to revolve around scrupulous hand hygiene, keeping the cord clean and dry, and using water when bathing or nappy changing.

ROLE AND RESPONSIBILITIES OF THE MIDWIFE

These can be summarized as:

- keeping up-to-date with the changes to cleansers and baby wipes
- completing the procedures safely and correctly
- recognizing deviations from normal and taking appropriate action
- educating the parents
- correct documentation.

SUMMARY

- Meeting the hygiene needs of the baby is an important skill for the midwife, who not only undertakes this but also educates the parents on how to do this.

- Evidence relating to the use of bath additives, shampoos, emollients and baby wipes is constantly evolving and the midwife must keep up-to-date with these changes.
- The baby does not need to be bathed every day.
- Shampooing the hair is not necessary during each bathing.
- Bathing the baby can be an enjoyable process for all involved but attention must be paid to keeping the baby warm, safe and secure.
- The use of alkaline soaps and bath additives disrupts the acid mantle of the skin, predisposing to infection; the use of plain water is recommended.
- The baby's eyes should not be cleaned unless discharging.
- Nappies may be disposable or reusable, with three ways of folding the latter.
- The cord should not be cleaned routinely in low-mortality settings as this can delay separation and increase the risk of infection.

SELF-ASSESSMENT EXERCISES

The answers to the following questions may be found in the text:

1. What advice can a midwife provide to parents who are enquiring which cleansing agent to use?
2. How can the midwife ensure the safety of the baby during bathing?
3. Describe how a baby bath is undertaken.
4. What advice can a midwife provide to parents who are unsure whether to use baby wipes or just water?
5. Demonstrate the different ways to apply a reusable nappy.
6. When would the midwife clean the baby's eyes and how is this done?
7. What advice can be given regarding cord care?

REFERENCES

Adam, R., Schnetz, B., Mathey, P., et al., 2009. Clinical demonstration of skin mildness and suitability for sensitive infant skin of a new baby wipe. Pediatr. Dermatol. 26 (5), 506–513.

Afsar, F., 2009a. Physiological skin conditions of preterm and term neonates. Clin. Dermatol. 35, 346–350.

Afsar, F., 2009b. Skin care for preterm and term infants. Clin. Exp. Dermatol. 34, 855–858.

Atherton, D., 2005. Maintaining healthy skin in infancy using prevention of irritant napkin dermatitis as a model. Community Pract. 78 (7), 255–257.

Blackburn, S., 2013. Maternal, Fetal and Neonatal Physiology: A Clinical

Perspective, fourth ed. Saunders, St. Louis, pp. 496–505. (Chapter 14).

Blincoe, A., 2006. Protecting neonatal skin: cream or water? Br. J. Midwifery 14 (12), 731–734.

Blume-Peytavi, U., Cork, M., Faergemann, J., et al., 2009. Bathing and cleansing in newborns from day 1 to first year of life:

recommendations from a European round table meeting. J. Eur. Acad. Dermatol. Venereol. 23, 751–759.

Blume-Peytavi, U., Hauser, M., Stamatas, G., et al., 2012. Skin care practices for newborns and Infants: Review of the Clinical Evidence for Best Practices. Pediatr. Dermatol. 29 (1), 1–14.

Brennan, G., 2010. Should baby toiletries get The Yellow Card? MIDIRS Midwifery Digest 20 (2), 235–239.

Cooke, A., Cork, M.J., Danby, S., Lavender, T., 2011. Use of oil for baby skincare: A survey of UK maternity and neonatal units. Br. J. Midwifery 19 (6), 354–362.

Erenel, S., Vural, G., Efe, S., et al., 2010. Comparison of Olive Oil and Dry-Clean Keeping Methods in Umbilical Cord Care as Microbiological. Matern. Child Health J. 14, 999–1004.

Furber, C., Bedwell, C., Campbell, M., et al., 2012. The challenges and realities of diaper area cleansing for parents. J. Obstet. Gynecol. Neonatal Nurs. 41, E13–E25.

Garcia-Bartels, N., Scheufele, R., Prosch, F., et al., 2010. Effect of standardized skin care regimens on neonatal skin barrier function in different body areas. Pediatr. Dermatol. 27 (1), 1–8.

Garcia-Bartels, N., Massoudy, L., Scheufele, R., et al., 2012. Standardized diaper care regimen: A prospective, randomized pilot study on skin barrier function and

epidermal IL-1α in newborns. Pediatr. Dermatol. 29 (3), 270–276.

Hale, R., 2007. Newborn skin care and the modern nappy. Br. J. Midwifery 15 (12), 784–787.

Hale, R., 2008. Maintaining healthy infant skin. Br. J. Midwifery 16 (6), 403–406.

Hugill, K., 2014. Neonatal skin cleansing revisited: Whether or not to use skin cleansing products. Br. J. Midwifery 22 (10), 694–698.

Imdad, A., Bautistak, R., Senen, K., et al. 2013 Umbilical cord antiseptics for preventing sepsis and death among newborns. Cochrane Database Syst. Rev. (5), Art No:CD008635 doi:10.1002/14651858.CD0086535.pub2.

Karumbi, J., Mulaku, M., Aluvaala, J., et al., 2013. Topical umbilical cord care for the prevention of infection and neonatal mortality. Pediatr. Infect. Dis. J. 32 (1), 78–83.

Lavender, T., Furber, C., Campbell, M., et al., 2012. Effect on skin hydration of using baby wipes to clean the napkin area of newborn babies: assessor blinded randomized controlled equivalence trial. BMC Pediatr. 12 (59), 1–9.

Lavender, T., Bedwell, C., Roberts, S., et al., 2013. Randomized, controlled trial evaluating a baby wash product on skin barrier function in healthy term neonates. J. Obstet. Gynecol. Neonatal Nurs. 42, 203–214.

Ness, M., Davis, D., Carey, W., 2013. Neonatal skin care: a concise review. Int. J. Dermatol. 52, 14–22.

NICE (National Institute for Health and Care Excellence), 2014. Clinical Guideline 37 Postnatal Care. NICE, London. Available online: <www.nice.org.uk> (accessed 3 March 2015).

Ravanfar, P., Wallace, J., Pace, N., 2012. Diaper dermatitis: a review and update. Curr. Opin. Pediatr. 24 (2), 472–479.

Sarkar, R., Basu, S., Gupta, P., 2010. Skin care for the newborn. Indian Pediatr. 47 (July 17), 593–598.

Suliman, A., Watts, H., Beiler, J., et al., 2010. Triple dye plus rubbing alcohol versus triple dye alone for umbilical cord care. Clin. Pediatr. (Phila) 49 (1), 45–48.

Trotter, S., 2004. Care of the newborn: proposed new guidelines. Br. J. Midwifery 12 (3), 152–157.

Trotter, S., 2006. Neonatal skincare: why change is vital. RCM Midwives 9 (4), 134–138.

Trotter, S., 2013. Why no baby skincare product should be advertised or promoted as 'suitable for newborn skin'. MIDIRS Midwifery Digest 23 (2), 217–221.

Visscher, M., Utturkar, R., Pickens, W., et al., 2011. Neonatal skin maturation – vernix caseosa and free amino acids. Pediatr. Dermatol. 28 (2), 122–132.

WHO (World Health Organisation), 2013. Postnatal Care of the Mother and Newborn. WHO, Geneva.

Wray, J., 2006. Seeking to explore what matters to women about postnatal care. Br. J. Midwifery 14 (5), 246–254.

Chapter 14

Principles of elimination management: micturition and catheterization

LEARNING OUTCOMES

Having read this chapter, the reader should be able to:

- define micturition, describing the adult normal urine volumes
- discuss the changes to the urinary tract that child-bearing brings
- describe how to facilitate normal micturition, including the correct use of a bedpan
- describe, with rationale, the equipment chosen for urinary catheterization
- describe how to insert and remove a urethral catheter.

Care of the urinary tract, supporting normal micturition, or using a catheter is an important aspect of care for the childbearing woman. This chapter reviews the factors that influence micturition, the direct effects of childbearing on the urinary tract, the safe use of bedpans, urinary catheterization, and correct (short-term) indwelling catheter care.

MICTURITION

Micturition is the voiding of urine from the bladder via the urethra. It requires a correctly functioning renal system as well as coordination between the brain and the nervous system. Inability (for whatever reason) to pass urine is an acute emergency, acute urinary retention is very painful and can cause complications such as renal failure. The urinary system consists of the bladder (a pelvic organ but displaces out of the pelvis when full), two ureters that connect the bladder to the kidneys, two kidneys that (among other things) are responsible for urine formation and filtration and one urethra that carries urine out of the body from the bladder. The bladder fills at approximately 0.5 mL/kg/hr, the sensation of needing to empty the bladder occurs in adults at a 200–400 mL volume. An adult normally voids 800–2000 mL per day. An understanding of fluid balance (Chapter 48) is also fundamental to appreciating elimination care.

Various factors influence micturition, these include:

- anxiety/stress
- personal habits: distraction (e.g. reading), privacy, time, etc.
- poor muscle tone due to damage or increasing age
- pain
- position
- disease
- urinary infection
- obstruction: e.g. compression from the enlarging uterus, presenting part, faecal impaction
- damage to the nervous pathway due to trauma, disease, or age
- surgery
- childbirth (discussed below) (Dolman 2007), particularly poor bladder care in labour (Blackburn 2013)
- stress incontinence
- drugs: anticholinergics (e.g. atropine), antihypertensives (e.g. methyldopa), antihistamines (e.g. pseudoephedrine), beta-adrenergic blockers (e.g. propranolol), uterotonics (e.g. oxytocin).

Changes related to childbirth

Pregnancy

During pregnancy, a number of structural and functional changes occur within the renal system, some of which continue into the postnatal period. Blackburn (2013) summarizes the changes, some of which are discussed below.

Early in pregnancy there is an increase in blood flow to the kidneys, this results in an increase in urine production (and therefore voids per day) and an increase in the ability of the kidneys to remove products of metabolism from the circulation (Doyle & Birch 2011). Also during the first trimester, the renal calyces, renal pelvis and ureters begin to enlarge, resulting in physiological hydroureter and hydronephrosis becoming more pronounced during the second half of the pregnancy. During the last trimester, the enlarging uterus displaces the ureters laterally; they elongate, becoming more tortuous. The volume of the ureters increases, possibly up to 25 times, resulting in up to 300 mL of urine being stored in the ureters (Blackburn

2013). This has implications for the accuracy of 24-hour urine collections and increases the risk of urinary tract infection (UTI).

Progesterone relaxes the smooth muscle of the bladder, resulting in decreased tone, oestrogen predisposes vesi-courethral valve incompetence (and therefore reflux of urine) and the glomerular filtration rate increases by 40–60% (Blackburn 2013). Bladder capacity doubles by term, holding up to 1000 mL. The bladder mucosa becomes more oedematous, predisposing it to trauma or infection. McCormick et al (2008) cite that the incidence of UTI in pregnancy is 8%. NICE (2008) suggest all women should be routinely offered midstream specimen of urine (MSU) screening in early pregnancy (initial booking visit) to screen for asymptomatic bacteriuria. UTI in pregnancy affects morbidity and can lead to premature rupture of membranes and preterm labour (SIGN 2012).

The enlarging uterus in the first trimester compresses the bladder, increasing the desire to micturate, resulting in urinary frequency. During the second trimester, the bladder is displaced upwards, allowing bladder capacity to return to normal. However, during the third trimester, pressure from the presenting part, particularly following engagement, can once again result in urinary frequency or stress incontinence. As the bladder is displaced into the abdomen the urethra is elongated and bladder emptying is affected. Nocturia may also occur during pregnancy due to increased excretion of sodium and water occurring when the woman lies down (Blackburn 2013).

Labour

Pressure may be exerted on the sacral plexus by the presenting part during its descent through the pelvis, resulting in increased frequency or retention of urine; this is contributed to by carrying the fetus in an occipitoposterior position.

Retention of urine occurs when the pressure on the sacral plexus results in inhibition of impulses. The bladder fills but there is no associated desire to void urine, compounded by the distension-inhibiting nerve receptors within the bladder wall. Pressure from the descending presenting part is exerted on the bladder and urethra, particularly at their junction. The resulting compression prevents the passage of urine, even with the desire to void. Lack of privacy and poor posture also contribute to retention of urine. Women should be encouraged to void urine every 1–2 hours during labour to minimize these risks, and particularly at the onset of second stage. The bladder is displaced upwards in labour making it physiologically an abdominal organ. This means that palpation of the bladder is an unreliable sign of the presence of urine (Doyle & Birch 2011).

Decreased awareness of the need to void urine occurs if regional anaesthesia is used (e.g. epidural or pudendal block), as the drugs temporarily block the nerves supplying the bladder.

A full bladder may be traumatized in labour and may also affect the course of labour in several ways:

- delayed descent of the presenting part (Simkin & Ancheta 2011)
- reduced efficiency of uterine contractions (Walsh 2004) and therefore delayed cervical dilatation. May worsen a postpartum haemorrhage (PPH), preventing the uterus contracting efficiently (Begley 2014)
- increased/unnecessary pain (Simkin & Ancheta 2011)
- dribbling of urine during expulsive second-stage contractions (Verralls 1993)
- delayed delivery of the placenta (Gee & Glynn 1997).

Postnatal period

During the early postnatal period, a marked diuresis occurs. Between the second and fifth postnatal days, up to 3000 mL of urine may be produced daily, with 500–1000 mL being voided at a time (Blackburn 2013). Proteinuria may be evident as a result of autolysis (Abbott et al 1997). The structural changes that occurred during pregnancy slowly return to normal during the puerperium, although in some women this may take longer (up to 16 weeks).

Women should pass urine within 6 hours following delivery (Blackburn 2013). However, some women may experience a delayed sensation to void urine. The risk of partial or complete inability to void urine is increased in the presence of:

- trauma to the bladder or urethra – sometimes in the form of oedema or sphincter spasm
- decreased bladder sensation arising from the use of regional anaesthesia, catheter use, or an overdistended bladder
- continued physiological distension of the abdominal wall (until uterine involution increases over the following week, and muscle tone is regained) resulting in reduced intra-abdominal pressure
- haematoma formation within the genital tract (Blackburn 2013).

Incomplete emptying of the bladder and urinary stasis increase the risk of urinary tract infection. NICE (2014a) advocate that if no void has occurred 6-hours post-delivery measures should be taken to assist (see below). If urine has still not been passed, the bladder should be assessed and catheterization considered. A displaced uterus is often caused by a full bladder.

Stress incontinence may also occur following delivery as a result of damage to the perineal branches of the pudendal nerves (Abbott et al 1997). If this persists beyond the puerperium, medical attention should be sought.

An important part of the midwife's role and responsibilities is record keeping, especially if the woman is experiencing difficulty with micturition (dysuria). Postnatally particularly, records should show the time, amount of urine passed, and the frequency, with any symptoms associated with dysuria, e.g. stinging.

The baby

A baby's bladder is an abdominal organ, it being too large for the small pelvis to accommodate it. Consequently a full bladder can compress the diaphragm and affect respiration. For the baby, micturition is an involuntary process with no control over when and where to void urine. Babies usually pass urine within the first 48 hours of life, 95% of them in the first 24 hours (Blackburn 2013). It is important the midwife records that the baby has passed urine following birth and helps the parents to understand the expected urine output in the days that follow (Chapter 38). Neonates from mothers who received magnesium sulphate are at higher risk of urinary retention. Urinary output is variable, depending on gestational age, fluid and solute intake, the ability of the kidneys to concentrate urine and perinatal events. It increases during the neonatal period, e.g. breastfed babies pass around 20 mL of urine during the first 24 hours, increasing to 200 mL by the 10th day (Johnston et al 2003).

FACILITATING NORMAL MICTURITION (ADULTS)

Given that the changes to the urinary tract and the effects of childbirth are significant, the midwife has a responsibility to ensure good bladder care for all women. Wherever possible the woman should be encouraged to void normally, namely, on the toilet. However, at times the use of a bedpan is indicated and urinary catheters, in particular circumstances, are also used. Catheterization of the bladder is not without risks and so should be used only when there is a clinical indication. The midwife should facilitate normal micturition wherever possible; three factors influence this:

1. stimulating the micturition reflex
2. maintaining elimination habits
3. maintaining adequate fluid intake.

Stimulating the micturition reflex

Position

- An upright position, leaning forwards with feet on the floor, facilitates contraction of the pelvic and intra-abdominal muscles, forced glottis expiration, bladder contraction, and sphincter control.

- This is difficult to achieve in bed; use of a bedpan or commode by the bedside or use of the toilet should be encouraged.

Reduce anxiety

- Anxiety can cause a sense of urgency and frequency, resulting in voiding small amounts of urine and the bladder may not empty completely, as the abdominal and perineal muscles and external urethral sphincter do not relax. Anxiety can result from lack of privacy, embarrassment, fear of passing urine, and the use of cold bedpans.
- Staying with a woman while she attempts to pass urine may inhibit micturition; if she feels unsteady she may prefer someone with her; her needs should be ascertained. Warming the bedpan prior to use encourages relaxation.
- Use of the toilet can increase the sense of privacy.
- Allowing sufficient time to relax and pass urine is also important.
- Warm water poured over the perineum may help the woman to relax (measure amount of fluid first if recording fluid balance).

Use of sensory stimuli

- Thompson (2015) recommends the sound of running water, using the power of suggestion. If the woman is embarrassed by the noise made during micturition, particularly if others are close by, the sound of running water may mask the sound of her passing urine.
- Stroking the inner aspect of the woman's thigh, placing her hand in warm water, or offering a drink may stimulate the sensory nerves to stimulate the micturition reflex (Thompson 2015).

Reduce fear of pain

- Pain, or fear of pain, often has an inhibitory effect on micturition. This is not unusual following delivery with perineal trauma. Concentrated urine may increase pain; additional fluid intake should be encouraged.
- Strategies to minimize actual pain should be used, e.g. analgesia, cooling gel packs for perineal pain (Chapter 12).

Encourage regular emptying of the bladder

- This is important, especially in the absence of the desire to void (caused by prolonged use of an indwelling catheter, damage to the nervous pathways, following surgery, use of drugs, etc.).

Encourage muscle tone

- Weakness of the pelvic floor muscles (e.g. following vaginal birth), indwelling catheter or severe constipation can affect micturition.
- Dolman (2007) recommends undertaking regular pelvic floor exercises to increase muscle volume. This increases the maximum urethral closure pressure, promoting stronger reflex contractions that follow a rise in intra-abdominal pressure.
- Prevent severe constipation that can obstruct the flow of urine.

Maintaining elimination habits

Supporting the woman to adopt the position and routine (including habits such as reading) that she is used to can assist with micturition.

Maintaining an adequate fluid intake

Normal renal function requires approximately 2000 mL per day and the midwife should encourage a regular fluid intake.

BEDPANS

The majority of women would prefer not to use a bedpan; the embarrassment factor and difficult issues concerned with its use (discussed above) mean that sensitive care is required for those that will need to use one. There are two main types of bedpan (Fig. 14.1), standard (deeper) and slipper (smaller and shallower). While cardboard liners are available, local infection control protocols are upheld whichever type of pan is used.

PROCEDURE: use of a bedpan

- Gain informed consent, prepare the environment to facilitate micturition (discussed above) and gather equipment:
  - bedpan
  - non-sterile gloves and apron
  - liner (if used)
  - bedpan cover
  - toilet paper
  - sanitary towel disposable bag and clean sanitary towel (if required)
  - handwashing facilities

119

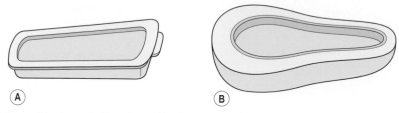

Figure 14.1 Different types of bedpan. **A,** Non-disposable slipper; **B,** Bedpan with disposable lining.

- Wash and dry hands, apply apron and gloves.
- If possible, warm the bedpan prior to administration.
- Consider moving and handling issues (bed at correct height, need for second midwife, etc.).
- Take the bedpan to the woman and ensure privacy.
- Help the woman to remove her underwear and sanitary towel.
- Place the bedpan under the woman, assisting her into a comfortable, preferably upright position. Lying on her side and then rolling back onto the bedpan may be easier for some women. Her legs should be slightly apart.
- Stay with the woman if necessary; otherwise supply call bell.
- When she has finished, allow time for her to wipe between her legs.
- Remove and cover the bedpan.
- Assist the woman with replacing her sanitary towel and knickers, ensuring she is comfortable.
- Remove gloves and wash and dry hands.
- Provide facilities for the woman to wash her hands.
- Remove the bedpan to the sluice, apply non-sterile gloves, undertake urinalysis and measure urine if required.
- Place bedpan/liner into disposal unit or washer.
- Dispose of remaining equipment correctly.
- Remove apron and gloves and wash and dry hands.
- Document findings and act accordingly.

URINARY (URETHRAL) CATHETERIZATION

Definition

A sterile catheter is inserted aseptically into the bladder in order to drain it of urine. The most common catheterization is urethral (via the urethra), for which the catheter may be secured in the bladder (indwelling) or inserted and immediately removed (intermittent).

An indwelling catheter can drain urine continually via a urine bag, or a catheter valve can be inserted into the end of the catheter that allows the bladder to be emptied intermittently. The bladder can also be catheterized through the abdominal wall (suprapubic), but this is seen infrequently within the maternity setting.

Indications

While a straightforward procedure, catheterization is undignified and not without risks: trauma, pain and infection being the three most likely. Consequently it should only be undertaken when clinically indicated and with full consent from the woman. Clinical indicators include:

- Prior to caesarean section or other abdominal surgery.
- Prior to instrumental delivery.
- If unable to pass urine during labour, e.g. use of epidural analgesia.
- During the third stage of labour when a full bladder may be impeding normal uterine activity, e.g. during postpartum haemorrhage or retained placenta.
- Inability to pass urine, e.g. post-surgery or postnatal retention.
- For diagnostic purposes, e.g. postnatal incontinence.
- Accurate monitoring of fluid balance when acutely ill or in shock e.g. pre-eclampsia, major haemorrhage.
- On each occasion the clinical decision is made as to whether an indwelling or intermittent catheter is the most appropriate.

Contraindications

In the UK nearly one-fifth of healthcare-associated infections are urinary tract infections. Of these, approximately half will be a catheter-associated urinary tract infection (CAUTI) (Loveday et al 2014). The effects of this on both the woman and healthcare provision are significant. Catheters can also block, urine can bypass and bladder spasms can be very uncomfortable. The urinary tract can be traumatized or inflamed, urinary stones can form, and body image and sexual function can be affected.

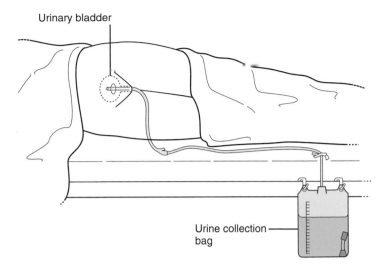

Figure 14.2 Closed drainage system – no breaks or open entry points from bladder to drainage tap. *(Adapted with kind permission from Jamieson et al 2002)*

Prevention of infection

The infection risk increases according to the susceptibility of the woman, type and length of time the catheter is *in situ*, and the quality of catheter care. The risk is higher for women than for men, due to the close proximity of the urethra to the anus, and the shorter length of the female urethra. Catheterization is often a short term measure in maternity (<28 days); this reduces the risk of infection.

Infection reducing measures (largely adapted from Loveday et al 2014):

- Document the indication (as well as other details, see below), review (and document) daily, removing the catheter as soon as possible.
- Strict hand decontamination before and after any aspect of catheter care and the correct use of personal protective equipment.
- An Aseptic Non Touch Technique (ANTT, Chapter 10) for insertion using sterile equipment. Loveday et al (2014) advocate the cleansing of the meatus with sterile 0.9% sodium chloride. NICE (2014b) suggest that the perineum is cleansed with tap water prior to vaginal examination. Where the two procedures are likely to take place at a similar time, the local protocol regarding meatal cleansing should be followed.
- The use of a sterile lubricant reduces trauma, discomfort, and infection. Baston (2011) suggests that anaesthetic gel provides both pain relief and lubrication; care should be taken if there is any break in the mucous membranes or if contact with the fetus/neonate is likely, bradycardia may ensue.

- Comprehensive catheter care, including maintaining a sterile closed drainage system that does not allow entry to bacteria (Fig. 14.2). Clean non-sterile gloves should be worn over decontaminated hands for every aspect of catheter care. Specimens should be obtained aseptically using the sampling port and care should be taken when emptying the drainage system to avoid contamination between the tap and the container.
- The drainage bag should be supported at a level lower than the bladder (max. 30 cm) to allow free drainage and prevent backflow of the urine. A catheter stand is used to both keep the bag away from the floor and to reduce trauma to the urethra. Drainage bags should be changed after the manufacturers' agreed number of days.
- The bag should be emptied when two-thirds full. Occluding or kinking the catheter (e.g. in the knicker leg) can cause stasis of urine in the bladder and subsequent UTI. Ongoing catheter care includes observing the amount, colour, clarity and smell of the urine, in conjunction with the woman's vital signs and clinical signs of illness or UTI. Advice regarding all aspects of catheter care must be given to the woman.
- Attendance to daily personal hygiene, Leaver (2007) suggests that showering is preferable to bathing.
- Choice of equipment (discussed below).
- General health of the woman. While largely unresearched, a daily oral fluid intake of 2L per day is considered to flush the urinary tract and limit the chances of UTI (Getliffe & Fader 2007).
- Trained and competent staff.

Choice of equipment

Catheter choice should consider reducing:

- tissue inflammation and trauma to the urethra (also improves comfort)
- mineral deposits that may cause the catheter to block
- bacterial growth.

Sterile polytetrafluroethylene (PTFE) latex catheters have a lifespan of 7–21 days and so are often the catheters of choice for maternity use. Caution must be taken to ensure that there is no latex allergy on the part of the recipient. A standard length catheter (40–45 cm) is used for larger women, otherwise a female catheter (23–26 cm) is acceptable. The lumen should be large enough to drain adequately without overdistending the urethra, a size 12 Ch is suitable for most women.

Indwelling catheters are retained in the bladder by a balloon inflated with a maximum (in adults) of 10 mL of water (Foley catheter) (Loveday et al 2014). Catheters vary; some have a self-inflating balloon or a prefilled sterile syringe. The sterile water is squeezed from the external balloon or syringe to the internal balloon (and clamped) when the catheter is in the bladder. Catheters for intermittent use are generally made from PVC plastic with holes at the tip (no balloon). All catheters are singly wrapped, sterile, and with an expiry date. Correct storage – out of sunlight, heat, and humidity; in original cardboard; and without elastic bands (Winder 1999) – protects the quality of the catheter. Valves, drainage bags, and catheter packs (containing swabs, gallipot, and receivers) are also sterile and for single-use only.

Analgesia

It's noted that it's difficult to anesthetize the length of the female urethra, but nevertheless efforts should be made to reduce the pain and the discomfort/trauma of catheter insertion. Usually preprepared 6 mL lidocaine (lignocaine) 2% gel is used but with caution (as above). It takes effect after 3–5 minutes.

Documentation

As well as the clinical indication for the catheterization, these details also need to be recorded in the woman's record:

- date of insertion
- the catheter – type, length, size, manufacturer, batch number, expiry date and number of millilitres in balloon (sometimes a label is supplied with the catheter for sticking into the woman's records)
- cleansing solution and lubricant used, complete medicine administration chart also

- any problems encountered with the insertion
- plan of care including duration/expected removal time
- specimen taken and sent (if needed)
- drainage system used
- name and signature of midwife.

PROCEDURE: female urethral catheterization using an indwelling catheter

This is based on the ANTT guidelines (Chapter 10), working from a suitable height and using a dressings trolley. The procedure is adapted according to the working environment. It is helpful to have an assistant while setting up for catheterization. If one is not available, the procedure is adapted using additional hand hygiene episodes.

- Confirm identification, gain informed consent, and ensure privacy.
- Wash and dry hands, obtain dressings trolley, put on non-sterile gloves, and clean the trolley with the locally approved wipes.
- Gather equipment onto lower shelf:
  - sterile Foley catheter (likely size 10–12 Ch) (a second one may be helpful)
  - sterile drainage bag and stand
  - 2 pairs of sterile gloves and a plastic apron
  - sterile catheter pack (sterile receiver will also be needed if not contained in this pack)
  - sterile anaesthetic gel
  - sterile sachet sodium chloride 0.9% or other approved skin cleanser
  - disposable sheet
  - good light source
  - 10 mL sterile water and sterile 10 mL syringe and sterile drawing up needle (not needed if catheter has a self-inflating balloon).
- Take trolley to the woman. Position the woman (removing sanitary towels and underwear) on a disposable sheet, in a semi-recumbent position, ankles together, knees apart. Keep the woman covered while the remainder of the preparations are made.
- Apply apron and decontaminate hands, open the outer layer of the catheter pack, sliding the inner part onto the trolley. Open the inner wrapper handling only the corners (Fig. 10.1 p. 90)
- Open the gloves, catheter (syringe and needle if needed), drainage bag, and anaesthetic gel onto the sterile field. Ask the assistant to pour in the sodium chloride and to hold the vial while drawing up the sterile water. Protect all Key-Parts.
- Decontaminate hands and put on sterile gloves. Ask the assistant to lift the covers off the woman.

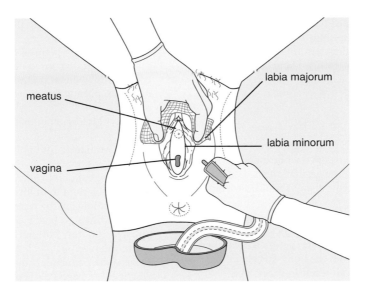

Figure 14.3 Female catheterization.
(Adapted with kind permission from Nicol et al 2000)

- Establish an aseptic field by placing a sterile drape beneath the woman's buttocks and one over her abdomen.
- Using the non-dominant hand, separate the labia with gauze swabs (this minimizes pressure on the labia, increases visibility, and makes catheter insertion easier, Fig. 14.3), cleanse the vulva using each swab once only, cleaning front to back, beginning with the labia majora, then to the labia minora, and then centrally.
- Locate the urethra, insert the anaesthetic gel, and wait for this to take effect (3–5 minutes).
- Remove gloves, wash and dry hands, put on second pair of sterile gloves.
- Place the receiver on the sterile field between the woman's thighs, expose the tip of the catheter, hold it using only the plastic wrapper (Fig. 14.3)
- Use the non-dominant hand to part and hold the labia with a gauze swab while the dominant hand passes the catheter gently and smoothly in an upwards and backwards direction into the urethra until urine begins to flow. Maintain asepsis by pulling back the plastic wrapper as the catheter is advanced. If the urethra is difficult to visualize, ask the woman to take a deep breath in; on expiration the urethra is easier to see (the pelvic floor relaxes).
- Once urine is seen, the catheter should be inserted a further 5 cm to ensure the balloon is in the bladder.
- If the woman is very uncomfortable or there is resistance at any stage, stop and seek experienced assistance.
- Inflate the balloon by squeezing the fluid from the external balloon or syringe, apply the clamp/remove the syringe. If there is great discomfort, the balloon may be in the urethra, and the catheter would need to be advanced further into the bladder before the balloon is inflated.
- Fully remove the plastic wrapper, attach the drainage bag.
- Clear the area, remove gloves, decontaminate hands, and apply non-sterile gloves if necessary. Assist the woman to replace her sanitary towel and underwear as required, and to adopt a comfortable position.
- Attach the catheter bag to the stand, securing it to the side of the bed. Additional support can be provided by taping the catheter to the leg, this reduces trauma to the urethra.
- Discuss ongoing care, e.g. principles of infection control, sufficient mobility, and oral fluids, avoiding constipation.
- Undertake urinalysis if necessary (using the sample gained when the catheter was inserted).
- Dispose of equipment correctly in the clinical waste bin in the room, remove gloves, and wash and dry hands. Take the trolley to the dirty utility room, clean using non-sterile gloves with approved cleanser.
- Decontaminate hands.
- Document findings and act accordingly.

ANTT summary: Key-Parts and Key-Sites

The urethral opening (Key-Site) is cleansed using sterile normal saline that has been poured into a sterile gallipot on an aseptic field, using sterile gauze by hands decontaminated and in sterile gloves (all Key-Parts). New sterile gloves are applied to decontaminated hands in order to place the sterile catheter (all Key-Parts) into the urethra (Key-Site). The balloon is inflated (unless self-inflating) using sterile water drawn up in a sterile syringe using a sterile needle (all Key-Parts). A sterile drainage bag (Key-Part) is attached to the catheter (Key-Part).

Precautions

- In the event of mistakenly placing the catheter into the vagina, it should be retained while a new one is placed into the urethra. The vaginal one is then removed. A contaminated catheter should *never* be placed into the urethra.
- If a urine specimen is needed for culture and sensitivity it should be taken from the catheter before the drainage bag is attached. A sterile specimen pot is used.
- Excessive loss of fluid from the body quickly in one episode, i.e. up to 1 L, can result in shock. The immediate drainage of urine should be observed and the flow halted with a clamp, if the volume is approaching 1 L.

INTERMITTENT CATHETERIZATION

The procedure is exactly the same as inserting an indwelling catheter, except that the catheter is a sterile single-use residual one, which is removed once the urine has been drained. It is also an ANTT procedure and the receiver should be both sterile and large enough to hold the expected volume of urine.

REMOVING A URETHRAL INDWELLING CATHETER

Catheter removal should occur as soon as the woman's condition allows. Depending on local protocol, a catheter specimen of urine (CSU) may be obtained before removal to screen for infection. Traditionally catheters are removed early in the morning. However, Kelleher (2002) suggests that removal at midnight allows the woman to rest and begin a normal voiding pattern in the morning. The reader is encouraged to be aware of the evolving research on this issue.

PROCEDURE: removing an indwelling catheter

- Gain informed consent and ensure privacy.
- Gather equipment:
  - disposable receiver
  - 10 mL syringe (depending on catheter design) (check insertion documentation)

- non-sterile gloves and plastic apron
- disposable sheet
- equipment for perineal cleansing (p. 100), depending on chosen method.
- Position the woman on the disposable sheet, as for insertion, placing the receiver between her legs; keep covered.
- Apply apron, decontaminate hands, and apply gloves.
- Ask the woman to lift up the sheet that is covering her.
- Deflate the balloon by removing the clamp and allowing the fluid to drain into the external balloon or by withdrawing the water using the syringe.
- Ask the woman to take a deep breath, remove the catheter smoothly but quickly as she exhales, placing it into the receiver.
- Cleanse the perineum using one of the methods described on page 100. Remove gloves and decontaminate hands.
- Assist the woman to replace her sanitary towel and underwear as required and to adopt a comfortable position.
- Provide explanations regarding:
  - possible frequency and urgency of micturition due to urethral irritability, or mild haematuria due to urethral trauma
  - the need to pass urine within 6 hours, with output matching input over the next 24 hours
  - possible urinary retention
  - a fluid intake of 2 L to wash out any bladder debris.
- Measure and record the drained urine if fluid balance is being monitored.
- Dispose of equipment correctly, wash and dry hands.
- Document findings and act accordingly, ensuring the next urine output is measured and recorded.

ROLE AND RESPONSIBILITIES OF THE MIDWIFE

These can be summarized as:
- understanding and applying the measures necessary to facilitate normal micturition, including advising and educating the woman
- undertaking all the clinical procedures described correctly, particularly in relation to prevention of infection
- recognizing deviations from the norm, managing them, and if necessary referring
- correct documentation of all care.

SUMMARY

- All aspects of childbearing can affect and be affected by the urinary tract.
- Micturition can be influenced in three main ways: stimulating the micturition reflex, maintaining normal habits and ensuring adequate fluid intake.
- Catheterization of the bladder is indicated in certain clinical circumstances. Infection is one of the greatest risks; the midwife must be aware of all the care that contributes towards reducing the risk.

SELF-ASSESSMENT EXERCISES

The answers to the following questions may be found in the text:

1. Which factors influence micturition?
2. Describe how childbearing affects micturition and therefore the measures that the midwife can undertake to promote good urinary care.
3. Describe the advantages and disadvantages of bedpan use.
4. List the situations in which a midwife is likely to undertake catheterization for a childbearing woman.
5. Discuss the similarities and differences between indwelling and intermittent catheterization.
6. Which is the most likely complication to occur from catheterization and how may this be prevented in all stages of care?

REFERENCES

Abbott, H., Bick, D., MacArthur, C., 1997. Health after birth. In: Henderson, C., Jones, K. (Eds.), Essential Midwifery. Mosby, London, pp. 285–318.

Baston, H., 2011. Female bladder catheterisation: step by step. Pract. Midwife 14 (1), 26–28.

Begley, C., 2014. Physiology and care during the third stage of labour. In: Marshall, J., Rayner, M. (Eds.), Myles Textbook for Midwives, sixteenth ed. Elsevier, Edinburgh.

Blackburn, S.T., 2013. Maternal, Fetal and Neonatal Physiology: A Clinical Perspective, fourth ed. Elsevier, Maryland Heights. (Chapter 11).

Dolman, M., 2007. Mainly women. In: Getliffe, K., Dolman, M. (Eds.), Promoting Continence: A Clinical and Research Resource, third ed. Elsevier, Edinburgh. (Chapter 3).

Doyle, P., Birch, L., 2011. Urine elimination in pregnancy: indications for catheterization. Br. J. Midwifery 19 (9), 550–556.

Gee, H., Glynn, M., 1997. The physiology and clinical management of labour. In: Henderson, C., Jones, K. (Eds.), Essential Midwifery. Mosby, London, pp. 171–202.

Getliffe, K., Fader, M., 2007. Catheters and containment products. In: Getliffe, K., Dolman, M. (Eds.), Promoting Continence: A Clinical and Research Resource, third ed. Elsevier, Edinburgh. (Chapter 10).

Jamieson, E.M., McCall, J., Whyte, L., 2002. Clinical Nursing Practices, fourth ed. Churchill Livingstone, Edinburgh.

Johnston, P.G.B., Flood, K., Spinks, K., 2003. The Newborn Child, ninth ed. Churchill Livingstone, Edinburgh.

Kelleher, M., 2002. Removal of urinary catheters: midnight vs. 0600 hours. Br. J. Nurs. 11 (2), 84–90.

Leaver, R.B., 2007. The evidence for urethral meatal cleansing. Nurs. Stand. 21 (41), 39–42.

Loveday, H., Wilson, J., Pratt, R., et al., 2014. epic3: National evidence-based guidelines for preventing healthcare associated infections in NHS hospitals in England. J. Hosp. Infect. 86 (Suppl. 1), S1–S70.

McCormick, T., Ashe, R., Kearney, P., 2008. Urinary tract infection in pregnancy. Obstet. Gynaecol. 10 (3), 156–162.

NICE (National Institute for Health and Care Excellence), 2008. Antenatal care Routine care for the healthy pregnant woman CG62. NICE, London. Available online: <www.nice.org.uk> (accessed 6 March 2015).

NICE (National Institute for Health and Care Excellence), 2014a. Postnatal Care NICE clinical guideline 37. NICE, London. Available online: <www.nice.org.uk> (accessed 6 March 2015).

NICE (National Institute for Health and Care Excellence), 2014b. Intrapartum Care: care of healthy women and their babies during childbirth. NICE clinical guideline 190. NICE, London. Available online: <www.nice.org.uk> (accessed 6 March 2015).

Nicol, M., Bavin, C., Bedford-Turner, S., et al., 2000. Essential Nursing Skills, second ed. Mosby, Edinburgh, p. 185.

SIGN (Scottish Intercollegiate Guidelines Network), 2012. SIGN 88 Management of suspected bacterial urinary tract infection in adults. Health Improvement Scotland,

Edinburgh. Available online: <http://www.sign.ac.uk/pdf/sign88.pdf> (accessed 9 January 2015).

Simkin, P., Ancheta, R., 2011. The Labor Progress Handbook, third ed. Willey Blackwell, Chichester.

Thompson, D., 2015. Urinary elimination. In: Potter, P.A., Perry, A.G., Stockert, P., Hall, A. (Eds.), Essentials for Nursing Practice, eighth ed. Elsevier, St Louis. (Chapter 34).

Verralls, S. (Ed.), 1993. Anatomy and Physiology Applied to Obstetrics, third ed. Churchill Livingstone, Edinburgh.

Walsh, D., 2004. Care in the first stage of labour. In: Henderson, C., Macdonald, S. (Eds.), Mayes Midwifery: A Textbook for Midwives, thirteenth ed. Baillière Tindall, London, pp. 428–457.

Winder, A., 1999. Female urinary catheterisation. Community Nurse 5 (10), 33–34, 36.

Chapter | 15 |

Principles of elimination management: urinalysis

LEARNING OUTCOMES

Having read this chapter, the reader should be able to:

- recognize the components of 'normal' urine and gain some understanding of the significance of the abnormal findings of urinalysis
- discuss the midwife's role and responsibilities in relation to urinalysis, identifying when and how it is undertaken.

Urinalysis is a screening tool commonly used by midwives to identify when further testing is required. While urinalysis may be an effective screening tool, it should not be used in isolation when considering whether or not treatment is required (Steggall 2007). Urinalysis is not sensitive and specific enough to screen routinely for asymptomatic bacteriuria (Awonuga et al 2011); a midstream specimen of urine (MSU) (p. 139) should be obtained for diagnostic purposes if required. This chapter considers the components of 'normal' urine, the significance of abnormal findings and the procedure for undertaking urinalysis. Although pregnancy tests can also be undertaken using a specimen of urine, this is not discussed within this chapter.

Definition

Urinalysis is the testing of both the physical characteristics and the composition of freshly voided urine and is undertaken for the purposes of:

- screening: for systemic and renal disease
- diagnosis: of a suspected condition
- management and planning: as a baseline and for planning and monitoring care.

In addition to assessing the physical characteristics of colour, clarity, and odour of urine, urinalysis can be undertaken by laboratory testing or, more commonly and for immediate results, by using a chemical reagent strip. Urine should not be tested if it has stood for 15 or more minutes, as its characteristics may have changed (deWit & O'Neill 2014); thus it is better if the sample is produced at the antenatal clinic rather than bringing one in from home. Leucocytes and erythrocytes tend to precipitate on the bottom of the container and if the sample is not mixed or is left too long the results may be inaccurate.

THE PHYSICAL CHARACTERISTICS OF URINE

- Colour: urine is coloured by urochrome, a by-product of haemoglobin breakdown and varies from pale straw to amber colour, depending on its concentration. Urine voided in the morning is usually more concentrated and darker than urine voided throughout the day when fluids are taken in.
- Clarity: freshly voided urine is usually transparent.
- Odour: urine has a characteristic inoffensive odour.

COMPOSITION OF URINE

Urine has a pH of 4.5–8, specific gravity of 1.005–1.030 and is mainly water (96%) with 4% dissolved substances:

- urea (2%)
- uric acid, creatinine, sodium, potassium, phosphates, sulphates, oxalates and chlorides
- cellular components, e.g. epithelial cells, leucocytes
- protein and glucose are present in negligible amounts, normally undetectable by routine testing.

Normal occurrences during childbirth

- Pregnancy: changes in renal tubular function make glycosuria and proteinuria more common (Blackburn 2013).
- Labour: ruptured membranes or contamination by a vaginal discharge or the operculum can give the appearance of proteinuria and or haematuria.
- Ketonuria: may occur and, provided it is mild, is insignificant.

INDICATIONS FOR URINALYSIS

- At each antenatal visit.
- On admission to hospital for any reason, as a baseline observation.
- Specific maternal disorders or treatment, e.g. hypertensive disease, diabetes mellitus, anticoagulant therapy.
- Clinical symptoms, e.g. dysuria, raised blood pressure.
- Altered micturition.

SIGNIFICANCE OF FINDINGS

Colour

The colour of urine varies with the specific gravity: concentrated urine is dark yellow in colour whereas dilute urine can appear pale. Urine that is very dark amber or brown–green in colour may contain bilirubin and this should also be suspected if, when shaken, the urine develops yellow foam. Haematuria also alters the colour: dark red if bleeding is within the kidneys or ureters, bright red if bleeding is from the bladder or urethra. Diet and drugs can also influence the colour – rhubarb and beetroot change the urine to a deep red colour, sulfasalazine can result in orange-coloured urine. *Pseudomonas* infection can give the urine a green colour and dyes such as methylene blue will also alter the colour of the urine (Edmunds et al 2011).

Clarity

Urine is usually transparent or slightly cloudy but when left to stand for several minutes urine becomes cloudy (turbid) due to precipitation of some of the dissolved substances (e.g. uric acid). Proteinuria, bacteriuria and infection may also cause the urine to appear cloudy (Piljic et al 2010). Foamy urine may be due to bilirubin or protein and infection may make the urine seem thick.

Odour

The odour of urine becomes stronger as its concentration increases. Stagnant urine smells of ammonia due to the breakdown of urea into ammonium carbonate. A sweet odour may be indicative of ketones, a by-product of fat metabolism. Infection may cause the urine to smell offensive. The ingestion of fish, asparagus, curry, and other strongly flavoured food can also affect the smell of urine. Phenylketonuria causes the urine to smell musty while a smell of maple syrup could be a result of a congenital defect in protein metabolism (Thibodeau & Patton 2012).

Specific gravity

This reflects the kidneys' ability to concentrate or dilute urine, a healthy adult has a specific gravity of 1.005–1.030 (deWit & O'Neill 2014, Thibodeau & Patton 2012). Low levels are associated with diuresis, hypercalcaemia and hypokalaemia, high levels with dehydration, proteinuria and glycosuria.

pH

The pH of urine varies between 4.5 and 8. Urine is usually more acidic in the morning and becomes more alkaline as food is ingested. A low pH indicates the urine is more acidic and can predispose to the formation of calculi (stones) within the bladder or kidney. Diet can influence pH values with a protein-rich diet causing the urine to become more acidic while one with a high intake of vegetables or dairy products can result in the urine becoming more alkaline (Steggall 2007). Stale urine will have a high pH (Wilson 2005). The presence of urea-splitting organisms that convert urea into ammonia can render the urine more alkaline (Edmunds et al 2011).

Bilirubin: bilirubinuria

This is due to hepatic or biliary disease, particularly if the flow of bile into the duodenum is obstructed and may be found in conjunction with urobilinogen. A false-positive result may occur when certain drugs are taken (e.g. chlorpromazine) and a false-negative result if the urine is stale, particularly if the sample is exposed to sunlight, as it is unstable in light and at room temperature (Edmunds et al 2011).

Blood: haematuria

Blood should not appear in the urine and its presence could be indicative of infection, trauma, tumour or calculi, or may be due to contamination by blood from another part of the body (e.g. vaginal discharge, haemorrhoids). A positive result warrants further investigation. Haematuria is either visible or non-visible. Visible haematuria refers to urine that is pink or red in colour (Bagnall 2014).

Glucose: glycosuria

Glucose appears in the urine when blood glucose levels rise (hyperglycaemia), if renal absorption lowers and when the body is under stress (Edmunds et al 2011). It may be indicative of diabetes mellitus or, less commonly, acute pancreatitis or Cushing syndrome. It may also reduce the pH due to glucose metabolism by microorganisms within the urine (Edmunds et al 2011).

Ketones: ketonuria

Ketones are a by-product of fatty acid metabolism and are not commonly found in urine, as they are usually completely metabolized. In situations where there is disruption of carbohydrate metabolism, metabolic imbalances and ketone production (as a by-product of fat metabolism) can occur. This may be due to starvation, malabsorption, the inability to metabolize carbohydrates (e.g. diabetes mellitus), or frequent vomiting. Some drugs, e.g. captopril, may give a false-positive result. Ketonuria in labour is not uncommon and usually does not require treatment.

Leucocytes

Leucocyte esterase is an enzyme that is not usually found in urine (Edmunds et al 2011), their presence is suggestive of pyuria, indicating a urinary tract infection (UTI). However, the urinalysis test is less sensitive than microscopy and the specimen may be contaminated by leucocytes from an alternative source (e.g. vaginal discharge). Thus a positive test does not diagnose UTI, although when found with nitrites it makes the diagnosis more probable. Equally, a negative result does not exclude UTI as pyuria is not always present with a UTI. False-negative results can occur with high levels of protein, glucose, oxalic acid and ascorbic acid and with a high specific gravity.

Nitrites

Dietary nitrates are converted to nitrites in the presence of bacteria, particularly Gram-negative bacteria (e.g. *Escherichia coli*) and are indicative of a UTI. An MSU specimen should be sent for laboratory analysis. A false-negative result can occur if the bacteria have had insufficient time to convert the nitrates; for example, if the woman is experiencing frequent micturition (common with cystitis). The urine should be in the bladder for at least 4 four hours prior to obtaining a sample. Additionally, if the urinary reagent strip has been exposed to air, the nitrite test can become inactive causing a false-negative result and hyperbilirubinaemia may give a false-positive result (Watts et al 2007).

Protein: proteinuria

Protein is usually only present in very small amounts, as the molecule is too large to pass through the glomerular filtration membrane in the kidneys. Proteinuria is indicative of an increased permeability of the filtration membrane which can occur during disease or as a result of injury, raised blood pressure, or irritation of the kidney cells (Tortora & Derrickson 2012). Proteinuria may also be the result of a contaminated specimen, e.g. vaginal discharge. Transient positive tests are usually insignificant; to detect larger amounts of protein an early morning specimen is required. To exclude infection an MSU specimen should be obtained, tested and sent for laboratory analysis (if necessary). A false-positive test result may occur if the urine is very alkaline or if the strip is left in the urine for too long. Nelson-Piercy et al (2014) state that proteinuria should be quantified so that further investigation is initiated if it is significant. Twenty-four-hour urine collections may be undertaken if there is concern about the amount of protein in the urine, particularly if blood pressure is elevated. NICE (2010) recommend obtaining a spot urinary protein:creatinine ratio if 1+ or more protein is found when testing with a urine chemistry analyser.

Urobilinogen: urobilinogenuria

Bile is converted to urobilinogen by intestinal bacteria and most of the urobilinogen is excreted in faeces or reabsorbed and transported back to the liver to be converted back into bile. However the remaining urobilinogen, approximately 1% of the total, is excreted in the urine. Thus urobilinogen is normally present in small quantities but larger amounts may be indicative of liver abnormalities or excessive haemolysis. A false-negative result may occur if the sample is not fresh, has been exposed to ultraviolet light, with certain drugs, e.g. rifampicin, and with ingestion of high amounts of ascorbic acid, as vitamin C inhibits the reaction. A false-positive may occur if the woman is taking phenothiazines.

EQUIPMENT FOR URINALYSIS

Urinary reagent strips or 'dipsticks' are the current method used for testing the composition of urine. They are plastic strips impregnated with chemicals that react to abnormal substances in the urine and change colour. The results are given as a semi-quantitative value, e.g. trace, 1+, 2+, 3+. They are quick and easy to use with good reliability, particularly for detecting proteinuria (Craver & Abermanis 1997), although Walerstein (2005) considers them to be unreliable and recommends 24-hour urine collection for hypertensive pregnancies. Accuracy for detecting glycosuria increases as the plasma glucose level increases (Li & Huang 1997); glycosuria may not be detected when hyperglycaemia is mild. It is important to check the results at the correct time specified by the manufacturer – different sub-stances will require different times to react. Use of a urine chemistry analyser reduces observer error and increases the sensitivity of the reagent strips, resulting in a more accurate analysis (Cronin 2008, Patel et al 2005).

The reagent strips can degenerate with time, compounded by storage at temperature extremes or exposure to excessive humidity. Storage should be according to the manufacturer's instructions, in a cool, dry, dark area. The lid should be tight and the desiccant should not be removed from the bottle. The expiry date and condition of the reagent strip should be checked before use to ensure it is suitable to use.

PROCEDURE: urinalysis

- Obtain a fresh specimen of urine for testing (if refrigerated, allow it to warm to room temperature prior to testing and invert the sample to ensure even distribution of constituents).
- Gather equipment:
  - reagent strips (ensure they are still in date and suitable for use)
  - non-sterile gloves
  - apron (if contact with urine is likely)
  - watch with second-hand if reading manually.
- Wash and dry hands, put on apron if required and gloves.
- Observe the colour, clarity, and odour of the urine.
- Insert the reagent strip into the urine to cover the reagent areas, remove immediately.
- Tap the edge of the strip against the side of the urine container to remove excess urine, keeping the strip horizontal to avoid urine running down the strip and mixing the colours.
- When reading the reagent strip manually, follow the manufacturer's instructions for timing, hold the strip close to the colour charts and read the results in good lighting (alternatively a urine chemistry analyzer may be used in accordance with the manufacturer's instructions and the results printed off).
- Dispose of urine and equipment correctly.
- Wash and dry hands.
- Discuss the findings with the woman.
- Document the findings and act accordingly.

ROLE AND RESPONSIBILITIES OF THE MIDWIFE

These can be summarized as:
- undertaking the procedure correctly, using an appropriate urine specimen
- recognizing deviations from normal and their significance, referring if necessary
- correct documentation.

SUMMARY

- Urinalysis may be undertaken for the purpose of screening, diagnosis or assessment and management.
- Changes in pregnancy may predispose the pregnant woman to have abnormal substances in her urine with no ill effects.
- It is quick and easy to do, with instantaneous results, detecting abnormal constituents in the urine.
- False-negative and false-positive results may occur; these can be minimized if the correct procedure is followed.

SELF-ASSESSMENT EXERCISES

The answers to the following questions may be found in the text:
1. What are the normal constituents of urine?
2. For what reasons might urinalysis be undertaken?
3. What observations are undertaken on urine prior to urinalysis and why?
4. List the abnormal substances that may be found on urinalysis and discuss the significance of each.

REFERENCES

Awonuga, D., Fawole, A., Dada-Adegbola, H., et al., 2011. Asymptomatic bacteriuria in pregnancy: evaluation of reagent strips in comparison to microbiological culture. Afr. J. Med. Med. Sci. 40 (4), 377–383.

Bagnall, P., 2014. Haematuria: classification, causes and investigations. Br. J. Nurs. 23 (20), 1074–1078.

Blackburn, S., 2013. Maternal, Fetal and Neonatal Physiology: A Clinical Perspective, fourth ed. Saunders, St. Louis, pp. 356–360. (Chapter 11).

Craver, R., Abermanis, J., 1997. Dipstick only urinalysis screen for the pediatric emergency room. Paediatr. Nephrol. 11 (3), 331–333.

Cronin, M., 2008. Automated urinalysis technology improves efficiency and patient care. Med. Lab. Obs. 40 (10), 30–31.

deWit, S., O'Neill, P., 2014. Fundamental Concepts and Skills for Nursing, fourth ed. Elsevier, St. Louis, pp. 409–411.

Edmunds, S., Hollis, V., Lamb, J., Todd, J., 2011. Observations. In: Dougherty, L., Lister, S. (Eds.), The Royal Marsden Hospital Manual of Clinical Nursing Procedures,

eighth ed. Wiley-Blackwell, Oxford, pp. 699–802.

Li, K., Huang, H., 1997. Comparing urinary reagent strips for detecting glycosuria in patients with diabetes mellitus. Lab. Med. 28 (6), 397–401.

Nelson-Piercy, C., MacKillp, L., Williamson, C., Griffiths, M., on behalf of the MBRACCE-UK Medical Complications Chapter Writing Group, 2014. Caring for women with other medical complications. In: Knight, M., Kenyon, S., Brocklehurst, P., et al., on behalf of MBRRACE-UK (Eds.), 2014. Saving Lives, Improving Mothers' Care – Lessons Learned to Inform Future Maternity Care from the UK and Ireland Confidential Enquiries into Maternal Deaths and Morbidity 2009–12. National Perinatal Epidemiology Unit, Oxford, pp. 81–87.

NICE (National Institute for Health and Clinical Excellence), 2010. Hypertension in Pregnancy: The Management of Hypertensive Disorders during Pregnancy CG107. NICE, London. Available online: <www.nice.org.uk> (accessed 3 March 2015).

Patel, H.D., Livsey, S.A., Swann, R.A., Bukhari, S.S., 2005. Can urine

dipstick testing for urinary tract infection at point of care reduce laboratory workload? J. Clin. Pathol. 58 (9), 951–954.

Piljic, D., Piljic, D., Ahmetagic, S., et al., 2010. Clinical and laboratory characteristics of community-acquired urinary tract infections in adult hospitalized patients. Bosn. J. Basic Med. Sci. 10 (1), 49–53.

Steggall, M., 2007. Urine samples and urinalysis … clinical skills: 29. Nurs. Stand. 22 (14–16), 42–45.

Thibodeau, G., Patton, K., 2012. Structure & Function of the Body, fourteenth ed. Elsevier, St. Louis, p. 1095.

Tortora, G., Derrickson, B., 2012. Principles of Anatomy and Physiology, thirteenth ed. Wiley, Hoboken, p. 399.

Walerstein, S., 2005. Review: point of care dipstick urinalysis has low accuracy for detecting proteinuria in pregnancy. Evid. Based Med. 10 (1), 25.

Watts, S., Bryan, D., Marill, K., 2007. Is there a link between hyperbilirubinemia and elevated urine nitrite. Am. J. Emerg. Med. 25 (1), 10–14.

Wilson, L., 2005. Urinalysis. Nurs. Stand. 19 (35), 51–54.

Chapter | 16 |

Principles of elimination management: defaecation

LEARNING OUTCOMES

Having read this chapter, the reader should be able to:

- describe the physiology of defaecation
- discuss the factors that influence defaecation
- discuss the ways in which the midwife can promote defaecation.

During pregnancy and the postnatal period, women can experience a number of changes with their bowel habits that might lead them to feel constipated or have loose stools, both of which can be uncomfortable and embarrassing. The midwife plays an important role in promoting normal bowel habits and preventing complications. This chapter focuses on defaecation for the adult: the passage of faeces through the anal sphincter. Relevant physiology, factors influencing defaecation and a discussion on how the midwife promotes defaecation are all included.

PHYSIOLOGY

Faeces contain 70% water and are normally semi-solid in consistency. The remaining constituents are the end-products of digestion – residue of unabsorbed food, bile pigments, epithelial cells, mucous, bacteria, cellulose, and some inorganic material. Peristalsis propels the faeces through the large intestine to the sigmoid colon while up to 2 L of water is absorbed from them (Brown et al 2011). The longer the faeces remain in the large intestine, the greater the amount of water absorbed, the harder the faeces become, and vice versa. Faeces usually stay in the sigmoid colon until the stimulus for defaecation occurs.

The presence of faeces in the sigmoid colon initiates the stimulus to defaecate as they pass into the rectum. This stimulus can vary from person to person, e.g. two to three bowel movements per day to three or four bowel movements per week (Tortora & Derrickson 2012). The rectum is very sensitive to changes in pressure and, as the faeces enter the rectum, the longitudinal rectal muscles contract which shortens the rectum and the pressure rises 2–3 mmHg (Brown et al 2011, Tortora & Derrickson 2012). As the rectal walls distend, the internal anal sphincter relaxes, reducing anal pressure and creating an awareness of the need to defaecate. If it is appropriate to defaecate, the diaphragm, abdominal and levator ani muscles contract and the glottis closes. Breath holding can assist by increasing intra-abdominal pressure up to four to five times the normal pressure (Dempsey et al 2014). This results in a rise in pressure within the rectum and a decrease in pressure exerted by the internal and external sphincters. The pelvic floor lowers as the puborectalis muscle relaxes, increasing the anorectal angle, facilitating the passage of faeces into the anal canal by peristalsis. The posture adopted can assist this process by increasing the action of the abdominal muscles and pushing the walls of the sigmoid colon and rectum inwards. If defaecation is assisted by the person 'bearing down' (Valsalva manoeuvre) the increased intra-abdominal and intrathoracic pressure that results causes a reduction in blood flow to the heart, temporarily reducing cardiac output. When bearing down ends, the pressure reduces and a larger than normal amount of blood returns to the heart which may cause a dangerous rise in blood pressure, particularly in a hypertensive individual (Dempsey et al 2014).

This reflex stimulus can be ignored and inhibited by adults as the external anal sphincter is under voluntary control. When ignored, the external anal sphincter contracts, increasing the anal pressure. As a result, rectal pressure decreases and the puborectalis muscle contracts. The anorectal angle is reduced as the rectum is pulled backwards and the faeces return from the anal canal to the rectum and sigmoid colon (retroperistalsis). The stimulus then disappears until the next wave of mass peristalsis moves the faeces back into the rectum (Tortora & Derrickson 2012). If the stimulus continues to be inhibited, suppression of the reflex occurs and constipation ensues.

If it is inconvenient to defaecate, impulses pass to the cerebral cortex to inhibit defaecation. In babies and young children this ability is absent, and defaecation becomes a reflex response to faeces in the rectum.

Once passed, faeces are often referred to as 'stools' and can vary in appearance between individuals and even within the individual. For further description of stools, refer to the Bristol stool classification (see Fig. 17.2).

CONSTIPATION

Tortora & Derrickson (2012) define constipation as infrequent or difficult defaecation caused by decreased intestinal motility and affects up to 27% of the general population (Brown et al 2011). Thibodeau & Patton (2012) advise that if the faeces remain in the large intestine for longer than 5 days more water is absorbed making the faeces hard, dry, and more difficult to pass. Prolonged constipation can lead to faecal impaction where the faeces become a large, hardened mass which are very painful to expel (Brown 2013) and faecal incontinence, which Hurnauth (2011) describes as the 'involuntary release of bowel products or gas through the anus'. NICE (2007) suggest that 10% of the general population are affected by faecal incontinence, a condition that is poorly understood. Constipation may also indirectly predispose to haemorrhoids developing. Flatus (gas) can

accumulate with reduced or absent peristalsis and can lead to abdominal distension and pain (deWit & O'Neill 2014).

Blackburn (2013) states that 10–30% of women will experience constipation in pregnancy which is worse in the first and second trimesters, although Murray & Hassell (2014) and Jefferson & Croton (2013) suggest the figure is higher at 40%. Progesterone relaxes the smooth muscle of the intestines which decreases intestinal motility and results in a prolonged transit time allowing more water and electrolytes to be absorbed. This may be compounded by progesterone inhibiting motilin release. The enlarging uterus compressing the rectosigmoid area may also contribute to constipation (Blackburn 2013).

Constipation in pregnancy causes discomfort and may result in damage to the pudendal nerve and impair the supportive function of the pelvic floor musculature (Jefferson & Croton 2013). Haemorrhoids occur in 85% of women in late pregnancy as a result of a rise in intra-abdominal pressure and the effect of the enlarging uterus impeding venous return from the lower limbs resulting in stagnation of blood and arteriovenous shunting within the compressed rectal veins (Murray & Hassell 2014). Postnatally 15–20% women experience constipation (Jackson 2011) which can be associated with haemorrhoids, perineal pain, and anal fissures.

While constipation is not life threatening, it causes pain, discomfort and distress. Other associated symptoms the woman may experience include fatigue, malaise, cramps, nausea, vomiting, confusion, restlessness, headaches and halitosis (Brown et al 2011). Constipation requires forceful abdominal compression, which if repeated can cause perineal stress (Amselem et al 2010). Straining, particularly using the Valsalva manoeuvre of forced exhalation against a closed glottis, should be avoided as it can result in an increase in both intrathoracic and central venous pressure. It may also result in a temporary reduction in vision with subconjunctival haemorrhage which may occur as a result of transient sub-clinical retinal oedema (Connor 2010). Thus it is important to treat constipation and encourage comfortable defaecation.

Factors inhibiting defaecation, predisposing to constipation

- Poor habits and constantly delaying defaecation.
- Diet, e.g. inadequate bulk, high intake of processed cheese, lean meat, eggs, and pasta (Dempsey et al 2014).
- Dehydration.
- Lack of exercise or immobility.
- Pelvic floor damage – Amselem et al (2010) found a higher incidence of pelvic floor damage amongst patients with constipation compared to those without.

- Changes to normal lifestyle and routines, e.g. hospitalization, as this causes interruption to the normal gastrocolic reflex.
- Pregnancy.
- Psychological: unfavourable conditions (e.g. lack of privacy, shared toilet facilities, bedpans), fear of damaging a sutured perineum.
- Pain: may be associated with haemorrhoids and fissures.
- Drugs, e.g. opiates, iron supplements, antidepressants, calcium channel blockers, aluminium antacids.
- General anaesthesia.
- Obstruction, e.g. faecal impaction.
- Disease, e.g. hypothyroidism.
- Psychiatric disorders, e.g. depression. Zhou et al (2010) advise that depressive emotion could decrease rectal sensitivity.

DIARRHOEA

Diarrhoea is an increase in the frequency, volume, and fluid content of the faeces resulting from increased motility of the intestines (Tortora & Derrickson 2012). Consequently there is also decreased absorption of water, nutrients and electrolytes and the faeces will be semi-formed or liquid. Diarrhoea may also lead to temporary faecal incontinence (deWit & O'Neill 2014). Diarrhoea can be classed as acute or chronic depending on the cause and how long it lasts. Acute diarrhoea is common and usually self-limiting within 2 weeks, chronic diarrhoea lasts longer than 2 weeks and may be the result of an underlying disease. Women presenting with acute diarrhoea may need to be put into 'Source Isolation' (see Chapter 8) until infection is ruled out as a cause. Fluid and electrolyte replacement and maintenance of a fluid balance chart should be considered, as the woman may be dehydrated with an electrolyte imbalance.

Factors increasing defaecation, predisposing to diarrhoea

- During the onset and early part of labour (this could result in defaecation being delayed in the first 48 hours after delivery).
- Infection, e.g. helminths.
- Diet: excessive intake of certain foods, e.g. fruit, alcohol, coffee, chocolate (Dempsey et al 2014), or food intolerance, e.g. lactose intolerance.
- Stress.
- Drugs, e.g. antibiotics, iron supplements, laxatives.
- Disease, e.g. irritable bowel syndrome, diverticulitis.

- Damage: lax pelvic floor muscles provide little support for the anal sphincter; as the abdominal pressure rises, faeces will be forced down the anal canal and pass out through the sphincter.

PRINCIPLES: PROMOTING DEFAECATION

Posture

Sitting forwards in a crouched position with the forearms supported on parted knees which are higher than the hips allows the diaphragm to move down and facilitates the action of the contracted abdominal muscles. The abdomen should bulge out, the spine straightened; the glottis closed, the jaw relaxed, lips open, and teeth apart. The use of a footstool to raise the legs may facilitate this position. This posture is difficult to achieve when sitting on a bedpan which, accompanied by embarrassment, can inhibit defaecation (Dempsey et al 2014).

Diet

NICE (2008) recommend that the midwife inform the pregnant woman who is constipated about diet modification such as bran or wheat supplementation to promote normal defaecation but do not specify the amount of fibre needed. Added bulk in the diet will increase pressure on the intestinal wall creating the stimulus for peristalsis and moving the intestinal contents more quickly so that less water is absorbed (Dempsey et al 2014). Wheat bran is a good dietary source of fibre, iron, B vitamins, zinc, and magnesium and it has a high capacity to absorb water (each gram of wheat bran will absorb more than five times its weight in water) and so provide bulk to the faeces (Jefferson & Croton 2013) and is found in many whole wheat and wholemeal foods. Qui et al (2008) propose a positive side effect from increasing dietary wheat bran is a reduced risk of pre-eclampsia. It may also help control blood glucose in pregnancy (Zhang et al 2006). Although the UK does not have a recommendation for the daily amount of fibre required in pregnancy, the USA, Australia, and New Zealand advise 28 g for pregnancy and 29–30 g for lactation as opposed to 25 g for the non-pregnant adult female (Jefferson & Croton 2013). Increasing the amount of fibre in the diet may initially cause bloating, abdominal distention and flatulence, but this is self-limiting and the symptoms will reduce (Brown et al 2011). To avoid this, a gradual increase in fibre is advisable. An increasing high-fibre diet with an adequate fluid intake will prevent the stools becoming too firm to pass. Dempsey et al (2014) advise a daily fluid intake of 2–3 L when eating a high-fibre diet.

Other measures include:

- Conditioning: sitting on the toilet following a meal may help bowel habits be relearned, especially after breakfast, as Dempsey et al (2014) suggest this is when the gastrocolic and duodenocolic reflexes cause mass propulsive movements within the large intestine.
- Privacy, so that the sounds and smell of defaecation are not noticed – wherever possible allow the woman to use the toilet rather than a commode or bedpan.
- Education: advice on care of the perineum and likelihood of causing damage to a sutured perineum; reassurance of expected changes and return to normal bowel function following birth.
- Use of soft toilet paper, as this may help psychologically.

- Increasing mobility: constipation is associated with decreased mobility, so mild exercise will help.
- Easy access to clean toilet facilities: avoid using the bedpan which increases straining and oxygen consumption.
- Treating haemorrhoids.
- Using a suitable barrier cream to prevent anal excoriation.
- Use of oral laxatives, but these should not be the first course of action.
- Suppositories and microenemas (see Chapter 22) may provide immediate but short-term relief of constipation; the cause of constipation should also be treated.

ROLE AND RESPONSIBILITIES OF THE MIDWIFE

These can be summarized as:

- asking the woman about her bowel habits as part of the antenatal and postnatal examination; this should be undertaken in such a way so as not to embarrass the woman
- any difficulties with defaecation should be discussed and advice given to promote defaecation
- a record of any problems, advice given and evaluation of the advice should be recorded in the woman's case notes

- any drugs given to assist defaecation should be in accordance with the standards for medicine management (NMC 2007)
- if difficulties with defaecation do not resolve, the midwife should refer the woman for further investigation.

SUMMARY

- Defaecation is primarily under conscious control (in the adult).
- Inhibition of defaecation can lead to constipation.
- Defaecation can be promoted by a number of different factors.

SELF-ASSESSMENT EXERCISES

The answers to the following questions may be found in the text:

1. Describe the physiology of defaecation.
2. What factors influence the ability to defaecate?
3. How can the midwife promote defaecation?

REFERENCES

Amselem, C., Puigdollers, A., Azpiroz, F., et al., 2010. Constipation: a potential cause of pelvic floor damage? Neurogastroenterol. Motil. 22 (2), 150–153.

Blackburn, S.T., 2013. Maternal, Fetal, & Neonatal Physiology, fourth ed. Elsevier, Maryland Heights, p. 402.

Brown, H., Crisford, M., Fernandes, A., et al., 2011. Elimination. In: Dougherty, L., Lister, S. (Eds.), The Royal Marsden Hospital Manual of

Clinical Nursing Procedures, eighth ed. Wiley Blackwell, Oxford, pp. 239–320.

Brown, S., 2013. Bowel Elimination. In: Koutoukidis, G., Stainton, K., Hughson, J. (Eds.), Tabbner's Nursing Care. Theory and Practice, sixth ed. Churchill Livingstone, Chatswood, pp. 696–717.

Connor, A., 2010. Valsalva-related retinal venous dilation caused by defaecation. Acta Ophthalmol.

88 (4), e149. doi:10.1111/j.1755-3768.2009.01624.x.

Dempsey, J., Hillege, S., Hill, R., 2014. Fundamentals of Nursing and Midwifery A Person-Centred Approach to Care, second ed. Australian and New Zealand edn. Lippincott, Williams & Wilkins Pty Ltd, Sydney, pp. 1132–1168.

deWit, S., O'Neill, P., 2014. Fundamental Concepts and Skills For Nursing, fourth ed. Elsevier, St. Louis, pp. 570–571.

Hurnauth, C., 2011. Management of faecal incontinence in acutely ill patients. Nurs. Stand. 25 (22), 48–56.

Jackson, P., 2011. Morbidity following childbirth. In: McDonald, S., Magill-Cuerden, J. (Eds.), Mayes' Midwifery, fourteenth ed. Elsevier, Edinburgh.

Jefferson, A., Croton, J., 2013. Using wheat bran fibre to improve bowel habits during pregnancy – a call to action. Br. J. Midwifery 21 (5), 331–341.

Murray, I., Hassell, J., 2014. Change and adaptation in pregnancy. In: Marshall, J., Raynor, M. (Eds.), Myles Textbook for Midwives, sixteenth ed. Elsevier, Edinburgh, pp. 163–164.

NICE (National Institute for Health and Care Excellence), 2007. Faecal Incontinence: The Management of Faecal Incontinence in Adults CG 49. NICE, London. Available online: <www.nice.org.uk> (accessed 3 March 2015).

NICE (National Institute for Health and Care Excellence), 2008. Antenatal Care CG 62. NICE, London. Available online: <www.nice.org.uk> (accessed 3 March 2015).

NMC (Nursing and Midwifery Council), 2007. Standards for medicines management. Available online: <http://www.nmc-uk.org/Publications/Standards/> (accessed 3 March 2015).

Qui, C., Coughlin, K., Frederick, I., et al., 2008. Dietary fibre in early pregnancy and risk of subsequent preeclampsia. Am. J. Hypertens. 21 (8), 903–909.

Thibodeau, G., Patton, K., 2012. Structure & Function of the Body, fourteenth ed. Elsevier Mosby, St. Louis, p. 365.

Tortora, G., Derrickson, B., 2012. Principles of Anatomy and Physiology, thirteenth ed. Wiley, Hoboken, p. 1040.

Zhang, C., Liu, S., Solomon, C., Hu, F., 2006. Dietary fiber intake, dietary glycemic load and the risk for gestational diabetes mellitus. Diabetes Care 29 (10), 2223–2230.

Zhou, L., Lin, Z., Lin, L., et al., 2010. Functional constipation: implications for nursing interventions. J. Clin. Nurs. 19, 1838–1843.

Chapter | 17 |

Principles of elimination management: obtaining urinary and stool specimens

LEARNING OUTCOMES

Having read this chapter, the reader should be able to:

- describe the procedure for obtaining a catheter specimen, a midstream specimen and a neonatal specimen of urine
- describe how a 24-hour urine collection is taken
- describe how a stool specimen is obtained
- summarize the midwife's role and responsibility in relation to specimen collection.

If specimens are taken in the correct manner and are dispatched promptly with the correct request form, their results can be considered to have greater validity than if any of these steps have been compromised. Midwives take a large number of urine specimens; this chapter reviews the correct way to do this. Stool specimens are also discussed.

GOOD PRACTICE

Good practice for the taking of all specimens should include:

- Correct identification of the woman (asking her to state her name and date of birth) and the granting of consent. Some specimens require the woman to take more action than others. In each instance, she needs to understand what is being tested, why and how the specimen is obtained.
- Clinical assessment: is the specimen necessary? Is it appropriate to the current clinical condition? In what way will the result impact care?
- Is this a repeat specimen? Taking specimens unnecessarily is costly and can be stressful for the woman. Will a repeat specimen add to her plan of care?
- Is it being collected at the right time, in the right way (avoiding contamination) using the correct equipment, the correct sample pot and labelled as per locally agreed policy? Failure at any of these stages wastes resources and can lose patient confidence in the service.
- Is the specimen being taken in a manner that protects all staff including the midwife, transportation and laboratory services? Is it sealed and labelled 'high risk' if appropriate? Has adherence to standard precaution and infection control protocols been upheld?

- Can the specimen be dispatched or stored correctly so that it reaches the laboratory as it should and in the correct time frame?
- Has it been documented in the correct places and will the results be located and acted upon in a timely manner?

CATHETER SPECIMENS OF URINE (CSU)

Urine may be taken from a catheterized woman for the purposes of urinalysis or infection screening, but occasionally a catheter may be inserted (often intermittent, p. 124) to obtain an uncontaminated specimen (e.g. protein urinalysis when pre-eclamptic). This section focuses on obtaining a catheter specimen from an indwelling catheter.

It is important that the following principles are applied:

- all of the good practice points above
- asepsis: this improves the accuracy of the result and prevents infection entering the closed drainage system

- maintaining a closed drainage system means that only the drainage port should be used and that specimens should only be taken when absolutely necessary
- fresh urine is screened.

The type of catheter or urinary drainage bag (depending upon which manufacturer) will determine the way in which the specimen is taken:

- a resealing rubber 'window' port in the tubing
- a needleless port in some part of the tubing or drainage bag (Fig. 17.1).

In maintaining an aseptic technique, the port should be cleansed with a locally approved wipe, often 70% alcohol/2% chlorhexidine, and allowed to dry. Aseptic Non Touch Technique (ANTT) (Rowley & Clare 2011) advocates using four corners of a wipe and the middle, each for approximately 5 seconds, generating friction. This is the recommendation for intravenous ports (p. 89); it would seem sensible to apply the same practice to urinary catheter ports. Loveday et al (2014) also state that non-sterile gloves should be worn before any manipulation of a catheter.

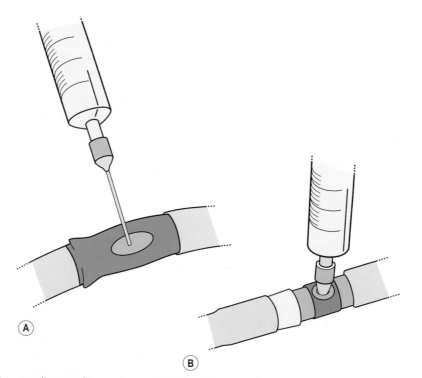

Figure 17.1 A, Rubber resealing needle sampling port; **B,** Needleless sampling port.

PROCEDURE: catheter specimen of urine

- Gain informed consent, confirm identity and gather equipment:
    - sterile specimen pot (correct one for the nature of the test required)
    - non-sterile gloves and disposable plastic apron × 2
    - 20 mL sterile syringe (and 25 g sterile needle if it is a resealing port, with portable sharps box)
    - locally approved equipment wipe
    - gate clamp.
- Ensure privacy, wash and dry hands, put on apron and gloves.
- Examine the tubing for fresh urine; if none present apply the gate clamp below the level of the port and wait a few minutes for urine to collect. Remove gloves and apron, and wash and dry hands. If urine is present proceed to taking the specimen ('Wipe the 'port...' below).
- Return to the woman, wash and dry hands, and apply apron and gloves.
- Wipe the port with the wipe for at least 20 seconds as described above and allow to dry for 30 seconds.
- Resealing port:
    - connect the syringe and needle using an ANTT, insert the needle into the rubber port taking care not to pierce out through the other side
    - withdraw the required amount of urine (10–20 mL usually)
    - discard the needle straight into the sharps box.
- Needleless port:
    - insert the syringe firmly into the port using an ANTT
    - withdraw the required amount of urine (10–20 mL usually).
- Place urine carefully into the specimen pot. Wipe the port for at least 20 seconds with a swab as before. Dispose of syringe correctly.
- Remove the clamp.
- Remove gloves and apron and wash and dry hands.
- Label the specimen correctly and dispatch to the laboratory with the request, often within 1 hour; this will depend on the nature of the test (if delayed, refrigeration at 4°C is sometimes acceptable).
- Document the findings and act accordingly.

MIDSTREAM SPECIMENS OF URINE (MSU)

The urethra is contaminated with microorganisms from the vagina and gastrointestinal tract. If a urine specimen is to be specifically screened for infection, it is important that as much bacterial contamination as possible is excluded. Consequently, the middle part of a urine specimen is collected, with the initial voiding clearing the urethra of debris and microorganisms. The woman is required to contract her pubococcygeal muscle to 'stop and start' the urine flow, something that may be harder to achieve in late pregnancy. NICE (2008) recommend that all women are offered screening for asymptomatic bacteriuria in early pregnancy, culturing the urine from an MSU.

Meatal cleansing remains debatable. Lifshitz & Kramer (2000) suggest that in females, cleansing makes no difference to contamination rates but that if personal hygiene is poor or faecal contamination is suspected, then meatal cleansing is recommended (Gilbert 2006). However, a strong urine flow would appear to flush out the urethra when first voiding and so Leaver (2007) recommends ensuring that the bladder is at least half full prior to taking an MSU. Dolan & Cornish (2013) and Dimech et al (2011) both recommend meatal cleansing, in both cases it is unclear which is the solution of choice: soap and water, 0.9% sodium chloride, or some other skin disinfectant. The reader is encouraged to understand their local protocol. Any cleansing is completed by wiping from front to back, away from the urethra, rather than towards it.

Equipment may vary, in some places sterile bowls or funnels are used, in others the urine is voided directly into the specimen pot. Whatever the system is, care is taken to maintain asepsis and avoid all contamination.

PROCEDURE: midstream specimen of urine

- Confirm identity. Explain the procedure to the woman and gain her consent, ensure that her bladder is at least half full. If dexterity is a problem, the midwife may need to wear an apron and non-sterile gloves to assist.
- Gather equipment:
    - sterile specimen pot (correct for the investigation)
    - sterile receiver/funnel
    - sterile gauze and approved skin cleanser.
- Ask the woman to wash and dry her hands and part the labia.
- Using the gauze and skin cleanser, wipe down the labia minora once on the left, discard the wipe, then repeat the process for the right and then centrally over the urethra.
- Ask the woman to void the first part of the urine into the toilet, halt the flow, void again to collect the specimen using either the funnel with the pot, or the receiver, then complete the voiding into the toilet, washing her hands when finished.

- Transfer the urine from the receiver to the pot, if necessary (wear non-sterile gloves to do this).
- Dispose of equipment and wash and dry hands.
- Label the specimen and dispatch to the laboratory immediately.
- Document the findings (including the time of specimen) and act accordingly.

24-HOUR URINE COLLECTION

The entire amount of urine passed in 24 hours is sent for analysis, usually for protein. It is important that every drop is sent; if a sample is missed, the test is invalid and should be recommenced. It is important to have the correct specimen container. Some tests require the presence of nitric acid; the amount may be subtracted from the total volume on completion; local protocols will guide on this. The woman needs to have a good level of understanding and compliance to complete this test correctly.

- The collection is started in the morning and is completed and sent the following morning.
- Urine is passed and discarded, the exact time noted and the collection begins.
- The woman is supplied with a sterile jug and asked to void into the jug then transfer the urine into the correct specimen container. If urinalysis is required, this is done using the specimen in the jug prior to its transfer to the container.
- Twenty-four hours later the woman is asked to pass urine as near to finishing time as possible. Once the last collection is added, the container(s) are sent directly to the laboratory with the request card.
- Any other specimens required are taken before or after the 24-hour collection.

URINE SPECIMENS FROM THE BABY

There are several possible ways of obtaining a urine specimen from a baby:

- A clean catch: aiming to catch the specimen in a sterile bowl or pot. This can be tricky, unreliable, and time consuming, but remains the method of choice.
- Use of a sterile adhesive specimen bag. This can cause excoriation to the skin and can be contaminated by faeces.
- Use of urine collection pads. Placed in the nappy, they too can be contaminated.

- Suprapubic aspiration. A sterile needle and syringe are used to aspirate urine from the bladder via the abdominal wall.

Herreros Fernandez et al (2013) identify that none of these methods are ideal and so report on a new technique. Firstly the baby is fed. Twenty-five minutes later non-nutritive sucking is offered, then the baby is supported in an upright position under his armpits. A second practitioner then taps gently suprapubically (over the baby's bladder) at a frequency of 100 times per minute. This is followed by 30 seconds of gentle circular massage over the baby's lower back. If micturition has not taken place the cycle of suprapubic tapping and lower back massage is repeated. The authors report a success level that has allowed them to dispense with urine bags and to use this as their primary method of urine collection.

OBTAINING STOOL SPECIMENS

For childbearing women, stool specimens are likely to be screened for:

- gastrointestinal (GI) infection, e.g. infective diarrhoeas
- presence of occult blood
- helminth infection, e.g. hookworm.

If the woman necessitates stool specimens sending, it is important to understand the timing and frequency of the tests; some infections require repeated sampling several days running. Some infective agents cannot survive for long outside of the body so the specimen needs to be dispatched promptly. Stool specimens should be assessed for their colour, consistency, odour, and frequency, and the information recorded. The Bristol stool chart (Fig. 17.2) describes the seven main types of stool classification.

PROCEDURE: stool specimen (adult)

- Confirm identity, explain the procedure to the woman and gain informed consent.
- Gather equipment:
  - clean bedpan or disposable liner
  - stool specimen pot with integral scoop or spatula
  - non-sterile gloves and apron.
- Ask the woman to defaecate into the bedpan, but not to urinate. (If incontinent, take specimen from soiled pads, without urine contamination, if possible).
- Wash and dry hands, apply apron and gloves.

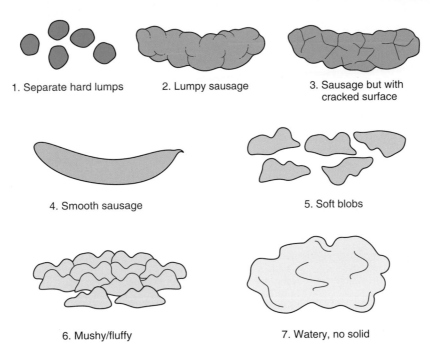

Figure 17.2 Bristol stool classifications. Type 1, separate hard lumps; type 2, lumpy sausage; type 3, sausage but with cracked surface; type 4, smooth sausage; type 5, soft blobs; type 6, mushy/fluffy; type 7, watery, no solid.

- Using the scoop, place the stool sample in the specimen pot, filling approximately one-third of the container, and seal the lid.
- If any parasite is visible, aim to place all of it in the pot.
- Dispose of equipment, wash and dry hands, label and dispatch specimen, document findings (including stool classification) and act accordingly.

PROCEDURE: stool specimen (baby)

- Gain parental consent
- Observe the baby for signs of straining (to obtain a fresh specimen).
- Decontaminate hands, using non-sterile gloves, fill one-third (if possible) of the stool specimen pot with the stool taken from the baby's nappy. Avoid contamination with urine if possible.
- If the stool is too wet and has been absorbed, efforts should be made to catch the sample in a sterile foil bowl on the next evacuation.
- Remove gloves, wash and dry hands.
- Label and dispatch specimen (immediately for some screenings), indicating whether contamination with urine was likely.
- Document findings and act accordingly.

ROLE AND RESPONSIBILITIES OF THE MIDWIFE

These can be summarized as:

- explaining the procedure and gaining consent
- ensuring correct specimen collection and dispatch
- knowledge and application of infection control and standard precaution protocols
- correct documentation and action on results.

SUMMARY

- Specimens should be obtained, labelled and dispatched correctly.
- A catheter specimen is taken from the recognized port using an aseptic technique, causing minimal disruption to the closed drainage system.
- An MSU is the middle part of the voided urine, the bladder should be at least half full before collecting the specimen.
- Urinary specimens from babies may be obtained using a specimen bag, a 'clean catch', sterile suprapubic aspiration or a newer bladder stimulation technique.
- Stool specimens from the woman are obtained from a clean bedpan; from the baby, they are obtained from the baby's nappy.

SELF-ASSESSMENT EXERCISES

The answers to the following questions may be found in the text:

1. Discuss at least six considerations that form good practice for specimen collection.
2. Describe how a catheter specimen of urine is obtained.
3. Why is a midstream specimen of urine so named? Describe how one is collected.
4. List the ways a urine specimen may be obtained from a baby.
5. Describe how a stool specimen is obtained from a woman.
6. Summarize the role and responsibilities of the midwife in relation to specimen collection.

REFERENCES

Dimech, A., Dougherty, L., Forsythe, C., et al., 2011. Doughty, L., Lister, S. (Eds.), The Royal Marsden Hospital Manual of Clinical Nursing Procedures, eighth ed. Wiley Blackwell, Chichester, pp. 618–622, 684–690. (Chapter 11).

Dolan, V., Cornish, N., 2013. Urine specimen collection: how a multidisciplinary team improved patient outcomes using best practices. Urol. Nurs. 33 (5), 249–256.

Gilbert, R., 2006. Taking a midstream specimen of urine. Nurs. Times 102 (18), 22–23.

Herreros Fernandez, M., Merino, N., Garcia, A., et al., 2013. A new technique for fast and safe collection of urine in newborns. Arch. Dis. Child. 98 (1), 27–29.

Leaver, R.B., 2007. The evidence for urethral meatal cleansing. Nurs. Stand. 21 (41), 39–42.

Lifshitz, E., Kramer, L., 2000. Outpatient urine culture. Arch. Intern. Med. 160 (16), 2537–2540.

Loveday, H., Wilson, J., Pratt, R.J., et al., 2014. epic3: National Evidence-Based Guidelines for Preventing Healthcare – Associated Infections in NHS Hospitals in England. J. Hosp. Infect. 86 (Suppl. 1), S1–S70.

NICE (National Institute for Health and Care Excellence), 2008. Antenatal Care Routine Care for the Healthy Pregnant Woman. CG 62. NICE, London. Available online: <www.nice.org.uk> (accessed 4 March 2015).

Rowley, S., Clare, S., 2011. ANTT: an essential tool for effective blood culture collection. Br. J. Nurs. (Intravenous supplement) 20 (14), S9–S14.

Chapter 18

Principles of drug administration: legal aspects, pharmacokinetics and anaphylaxis

LEARNING OUTCOMES

Having read this chapter, the reader should be able to:

- discuss the responsibilities of the midwife in relation to drug administration, particularly identifying the legal framework that the midwife works within and the autonomous administration of medicines under Midwives Exemptions
- identify the classifications of drugs and discuss briefly the implications of using them 'off label'
- discuss the nine 'rights' of safe medicine administration and the full information required for a correct prescription
- describe the safe administration of controlled and all other classified medicines (in this text: known as non-controlled drugs)
- highlight the process for the supply, storage, and surrender of controlled drugs in the hospital and community settings
- discuss briefly the issues that should be considered when women self-medicate
- understand how drugs are absorbed, distributed, metabolized, and excreted, for both pregnant women and neonates
- recognize the signs and symptoms of anaphylaxis and discuss the management of this condition.

This chapter considers the legal regulations covering drug administration by the midwife. It includes guidelines for the safe administration of medicines, including controlled drugs, and guidelines for the management of anaphylaxis. Pharmacokinetics aids the midwife's understanding of drug administration, this is discussed for both the woman and the baby.

Effective drug therapy needs the appropriately researched and manufactured medicine to enter, get around and ultimately leave the body. The action of the medicine and the effects on the person should be as expected (Jordan 2010). This all suggests that safe and effective medicine administration is a complex issue, beginning long before the midwife administers the medicine to the woman.

Some drugs in the maternal circulation do not pass through to the fetus during pregnancy and labour, as the placenta acts as a barrier. However, some drugs are able to pass through the placental barrier and can have an effect on the fetus (e.g. pethidine). Drugs may also pass from the maternal circulation to the baby via breast milk. This chapter does not consider fetal pharmacokinetics or drugs and breastfeeding, as the reader is directed towards the growing number of books that look specifically at these issues.

LEGISLATION

There are a number of Statutory Acts and Regulations that govern midwifery practice with regard to medicines management in the United Kingdom (see Alexis & Caldwell (2013) for specific details). The Nursing and Midwifery Council (NMC) provide the minimum standard of practice expected, based on the laws that govern. All midwives adhere to Standards for Medicines Management (NMC 2007) for example, or risk losing their registration to practice.

The Human Medicines Regulations 2012 categorized medicines in three ways:

- General sales list (GSL). These can be sold in a variety of places, e.g. supermarkets.
- Pharmacy only (P). Frequently known as 'over the counter' medicines. These medicines require the supervision of a registered pharmacist and therefore are sold in pharmacies only, with the pharmacist present.
- Prescription only medicines (POM) require a prescription from an appropriately qualified practitioner, e.g. registered doctor or dentist, or qualified non-medical prescriber and can only be supplied by a pharmacy or dispensing doctor.

Each of the above categories is reviewed periodically. The abbreviation 'POM' can be found on the packaging the medicine is supplied in, making it clear that it cannot be supplied without a prescription, except under certain circumstances (see Midwives Exemptions below). Sometimes medicines may be used in a different way from what they were originally licensed for, e.g. given via a different route. When a medicine is used in this way ('off label' or 'off licence'), the prescriber and dispenser take full responsibility for its use (NMC 2007), recognizing that it is a risky action to undertake. It can also mean that gaining informed consent is more difficult. Medicines should always be stored according to the guidance on the label and, in hospitals, in agreed storage facilities (in locked cupboards or fridges, with only approved staff able to carry or access the keys).

Midwives Exemptions

Under the Acts of Parliament that govern midwifery practice, midwives are given exemption to supply medicines, in the course of their professional practice, that are on the P and GSL lists, and some items that are POM. Midwives exemptions were previously called standing orders, but this term is no longer applicable. Midwives should be clear that they can only administer medication if they are familiar with its use, dosage, side effects, precautions, contraindications and method of administration (NMC 2007, Anon 2010). This administration does not need a prescription, a patient-specific direction (PSD) or a patient group direction (PGD) (see below). If, however, the medicine is not on the exemptions list then one of these will be required.

Which medicines may be given under 'Midwives Exemption'?

The full Midwives Exemptions POM list can be viewed on the NMC website (NMC 2011). Examples include diclofenac, hydrocortisone acetate, miconazole, nystatin, phytomenadione, sodium chloride 0.9%, cyclizine lactate, anti-D immunoglobulin, pethidine hydrochloride, oxytocin, and lidocaine. Student midwives were, from 2011, permitted, when under the supervision of a sign-off mentor, to administer the medications on the Midwives Exemption list, except for controlled drugs (NMC 2011). Being supervised by a sign-off mentor means in this context that the student must be physically watched administering the medicines. Student midwives may participate in the preparation and checking of controlled drugs if they are again being directly supervised by a sign-off mentor.

The administration of any medicine

Medicines, prescribed and given correctly, can make a significantly positive difference to patients. However, given incorrectly, the harm caused can have far-reaching consequences both in human and monetary terms. Matthew

(2007) suggested that up to 10,000 preventable deaths occur each year due to medication errors. In promoting safer administration of medicines, Elliott & Liu (2010) describe the nine 'rights' that should be considered with each medicine administration:

- Is the right medicine being given to the right patient in the right dose, right preparation, via the right route?
- Is it being given at the right time and is the midwife confident that the original order is right for the patient, e.g. antibiotics inappropriately for a viral infection?
- Is it being administered according to the right documentation?
- Has the midwife observed for the right response (and acted accordingly) following the administration?

It is clear that all systems need to be robust; there is the possibility for error to occur within research and development, manufacture, packaging and prescribing as well as administration. Elliott & Liu (2010) cite studies that show that the largest and most consistent errors in drug administration are human errors, 'at the bedside'. These may result from inexperience, lack of care and attention or the pressures of the daily workload. The midwife does not blindly comply with instructions but has to be knowledgeable and fully aware of what they are complicit in. For drug administration the midwife should be familiar with the drug to be administered, knowing why it is to be given, normal dosage, precautions, contraindications and side effects (NMC 2007). If this knowledge is not known, the British National Formulary (BNF)/BNF for Children (BNFc), other colleagues, the prescriber or the pharmacist could all be consulted. The electronic BNF/BNFc is updated monthly and should be the initial checking reference.

Prescriptions

Medicines that are on the POM list require a prescription. Midwives Exemptions (NMC 2011), as discussed earlier, allow midwives in the UK to administer some medicines from this list under their own autonomous practice. For all other POM, a PSD or prescription is required. This means that the prescriber (medical or approved non-medical) has reviewed the patient and assessed their need. For inpatients a PSD is often recorded on a medicine administration record; in the community, anti-forgery prescription forms are used.

Given that a PSD is specific to an individual, it should be written clearly as to identify that named client. Three identifiers constitute good practice; name and address, date of birth and NHS number are the best three. The presence of allergies should be established and documented. If appropriate, an alert identity band should be on the client's wrist when hospitalized. Any prescription should be written in black ink and should be legible. It should also contain details of:

- the name, form and strength of the drug (generic name where possible)
- dose, and unit (e.g. mg, g, or microgram) with clear wording or appropriate abbreviations and careful placing of decimal points
- route/method of administration
- frequency of administration, including maximum dose over 24 hours if appropriate
- date of prescription and if appropriate, date of completion
- prescriber's signature. This should be recognizable as that of one of the medical team overseeing the woman or the baby (GMC 2013).

E-prescribing (electronically) has been shown to reduce some of the errors; all of the above information still has to be included.

Patient group direction

A PGD is a specific written instruction covering the supply and administration of a named (prescription only) medicine or vaccine. It allows specific health care professionals to supply/administer a medicine directly to a patient with an identified clinical condition, without the need for a prescription, e.g. for labour care. The midwife is responsible in these circumstances for establishing that the client they are working with meets the criteria laid out as part of the PGD before the medicine is administered (Bussey 2011). PGDs are determined locally in consultation with medical staff, pharmacists and relevant healthcare professionals. They have a set of specific legal requirements (Griffith 2010) and can include controlled and 'off licence' medicines. A midwife must know and understand the PGD in order to practice under it; in many NHS Trusts midwives sign annually to confirm their understanding and compliance.

PROCEDURE: administration of a non-controlled drug

- Aim to be uninterrupted. Wash and dry hands.
- Obtain the signed medicine administration chart (if not covered by a PGD) and ensure it is legible and completed correctly and that the medicine has not already been given.
- Obtain the correct medicine from the correct storage facility. Ensure the label on the medicine dispensed is clearly written and unambiguous and check for any signs of possible tampering or medicine deterioration.

- Check the name, dose and expiry date of the drug (including weight related doses where relevant) and ensure the method of administration, route and timing are appropriate to the choice of drug being administered.
- Ensure the woman is not allergic to the drug and that it is compatible with breastfeeding (where appropriate).
- Prepare the medication correctly (as needed), e.g. draw up an intramuscular injection.
- Take the drug to the woman and confirm her identity (ask her to verbally state her name and date of birth) and confirm details on her identity band against the medicine administration chart.
- Explain to the woman the nature and expected action of the drug, informally gaining her consent, and ensuring that the drug is being given for something related, as she expects. For a baby, consent is given from a parent/guardian following the same discussion.
- Observe the woman taking the drug if able to administer it herself (e.g. with oral drugs or subcutaneous injections) or administer the drug for her (*per vaginam*, intramuscularly, rectally; see following chapters) with re-cleaned hands. Seeing the medication is taken ensures that it is also administered at the correct time.
- Dispose of equipment correctly. Wash and dry hands.
- Complete and sign the medicine administration chart and record the dose given, route, date and time of administration in other relevant documentation, e.g. obstetric notes, partogram.
- If any contraindications are found or a reaction develops following administration, or if the drug/route of administration is no longer suitable, contact the doctor/prescriber immediately and take appropriate action.
- Note and document the effect of the drug, e.g. good/poor response to analgesia.

Self-administration of medicines

The majority of women will be fully competent and able to self-medicate, both at home and in hospital. When in hospital it is necessary to assess the situation carefully; risk management requires that medicines are stored securely (generally at the bedside) and that clients have an assessment to ensure suitability for the task. The assessment includes:

- willing participation, leading to signed consent
- sufficient physical and mental wellbeing to cope with safe self-administration – no confusion or forgetfulness, able to read labels, and open packets and bottles, etc.

- no history of drug or substance abuse, or self-harm
- level of understanding of the medicines, their dosage, timings, effects, and possible side effects.

In the event of self-medicating, all records are kept accordingly, many medicine administration records have a coding system so that the code for self-medicating is entered by the midwife each day for that client. Regular review must take place (and be documented) to ensure that the woman remains competently able to self-medicate.

Controlled drugs (CDs)

A controlled drug refers to narcotic drugs and those that cause drug dependence. There are five controlled drug schedules:

- Schedule 1: drugs with no medicinal purpose – usually used illegally, e.g. cannabis – available only with a Home Office licence
- Schedule 2: drugs licensed as medicines that are extremely addictive, e.g. pethidine, morphine, diamorphine (heroin)
- Schedule 3: some barbiturates, analgesics and sleeping tablets, e.g. phenobarbitone, temazepam, pentazocine, tramadol
- Schedule 4: includes benzodiazepine tranquillizers, e.g. diazepam, nitrazepam
- Schedule 5: medicines containing a small amount of a controlled drug, e.g. codeine cough mixtures, analgesia.

The supply, storage, administration, surrender and destruction of controlled drugs is tightly controlled by the legislation. CDs from schedule 1 and 2 and some in schedule 3 are stored in a locked cupboard made to controlled drug cupboard specifications contained within a locked room or in a locked cupboard within a non-moveable locked cupboard. They are ordered and received in a particular way and their administration is recorded within the CD register in each ward area. There should be no alteration or crossing out in the CD register. Any errors should be bracketed, an explanation written, and the entry signed by the midwife and witness.

Supply of controlled drugs

The supply is different according to working location. Midwives who work in the community may possess diamorphine, morphine, pethidine and pentazocine for the purposes of labour care. In these situations a supply order is obtained from a Supervisor of Midwives who is satisfied that the locally agreed policy is being adhered to (NMC 2007). The Midwives Supply Order must be in writing, and provide details of the midwife's name and occupation, the drug and dose required, purpose for which it is required and total quantity to be supplied.

PROCEDURE: obtaining a supply of controlled drugs – midwives supply order

- The supply order is taken to the Supervisor of Midwives or an Appropriate Medical Officer (a doctor authorized in writing by the local supervising authority) for signing (inspection of the midwife's drug register, record of cases and remaining stock may be undertaken prior to signing).
- The signed supply order is taken to a pharmacist who has a prior agreement to supply the drug and who has a record of the midwife's signature.
- On supply of the drug, the name, amount and form of the drug supplied and name and address of supplier are recorded in the midwife's drugs book (this also contains details of the dates the drug is administered, the woman's name and amount).

The alternative, and usually preferable, option is for the general practitioner to prescribe the controlled drug directly to the pregnant woman; the woman then becomes responsible for the destruction or return of any unused ampoules.

Midwives working in NHS Trusts should follow their local policy for obtaining controlled drugs. This will vary, but in principle (NMC 2007):

- All CD stationery is stored securely with limited access to it.
- The ward and pharmacy have an agreed stock list, against which the authorized midwife on the ward can requisition further supplies.
- The midwife-in-charge carries the keys, they can be passed to other qualified midwives, but must be returned swiftly to the midwife-in-charge.
- On receipt of controlled drugs from the pharmacy, they are handed to an authorized person who signs the 'receipt' section of the order book, places the drugs in the CD cupboard and itemizes their addition into the record book, ensuring that the new tally is correct. Tamper proof seals should remain intact.

Administration of controlled drugs

Drugs should be administered in line with relevant legislation and local standard operating procedures. In addition, it is recommended that the controlled drug is checked by two people, one of whom should be a registered midwife, nurse, doctor or operating department practitioner (ODP) although this may vary according to local standard operating practices. It is recommended that the second signatory is a registered health care professional – doctor, midwife, nurse or student midwife (NMC 2007). Both people should

witness the drug being prepared and administered and the destruction of any surplus drug (e.g. part of the ampoule not administered). Where it is necessary to administer only part of a vial, both the amount given and the amount wasted should be recorded, e.g. morphine 15 mg given and 5 mg wasted.

The controlled drugs register and medicine administration chart should be completed and signed by both the person administering the drug and the witness, indicating:

- name of person receiving the drug (CD register only)
- date and time of administration
- dose administered
- CD register: any medicine from the vial not needed/wasted
- route
- both signatures.

PROCEDURE: administration of a controlled drug

- Obtain the signed medicine administration chart (if not covered by a PGD) and ensure it is completed correctly.
- Wash and dry hands.
- In the presence of the second practitioner (from now on), unlock the controlled drugs cupboard, check the stock of the drug in the cupboard with the drug register total, check that tamper proof seals are still intact
- Record the woman's name, amount of drug to be given, date of administration and amount remaining in the drug register.
- Check the name, amount and expiry date of the ampoule.
- Draw up the drug, take to the woman.
- Confirm her identity (ask her to verbally state her name and date of birth) and confirm the details on her identity band against the medicine administration chart.
- Explain to the woman the nature and expected action of the drug, informally gaining her consent, and ensuring that the drug is being given for something related, as she expects.
- Administer the drug and dispose of equipment safely. The second practitioner must witness the administration of the drug.
- Sign the drug register, recording details of the time of administration.
- Record the amount and name of the drug, route, time and date of administration in the appropriate documentation, e.g. medicine administration chart, obstetric notes, partogram. Re-clean hands. The

second practitioner can now return to their original work.
- Note and document the effect of the drug, e.g. good/poor response to analgesia.

Surrender of controlled drugs

Stocks of controlled drugs no longer required are surrendered to an authorized person (e.g. the pharmacist who supplied the drugs). A record of when and to whom the drugs were surrendered is made in the midwife's CD register.

Destruction of controlled drugs

Unwanted or expired controlled drugs can be destroyed by the midwife in the presence of an authorized person, and both should sign the midwife's controlled drug register confirming this. In the UK the authorized people most commonly used are a pharmacist or a Supervisor of Midwives (see new information from NICE in 2016 (www.nice.org.uk/)).

Unused drugs supplied to a woman on prescription should be returned to their community pharmacy.

ROLE AND RESPONSIBILITIES OF THE MIDWIFE

The midwife has a significant number of responsibilities in relation to the safe administration of medicines. Elliott & Liu (2010) describe it as a high-risk procedure. Midwives Rules and Standards (NMC 2012) are clear in Rule 5 that a midwife can only administer medicines following appropriate training in their use, dosage and methods of administration. Therefore midwives need not only to have a good working knowledge of the legal framework that applies to the administration of medicines, but also pharmacokinetics, local protocols regarding supply, storage, disposal, etc., training and updating of knowledge and skills and competent use of reporting systems. Midwives have to apply their knowledge and skills to pregnant, labouring and postnatal women, and to neonates, all of which require specialist knowledge. Record keeping is an essential part of drug administration.

Summary

- Legislation, the NMC and local policy govern the administration of drugs by the midwife; the midwife requires a good working knowledge of how these affect the safe administration, and also the supply, storage, surrender and destruction of medicines.

- Midwives may supply and administer medicines on their own autonomy from the Midwives Exemptions list (NMC 2011). Alternatively, all medications for administration should be prescribed on a prescription or PSD or permitted under PGD. Good practice requires the use of medicine administration charts for PSDs, which allows documentation to be robust and complete.
- The midwife should receive appropriate, thorough, and ongoing training in the administration of drugs, no medicine can be administered unless the midwife is familiar with its effects, possible side effects, normal dosage, precautions, contraindications, method of administration, and timing (NMC 2007).
- The correct administration of a drug should consider the nine 'rights'.
- Student midwives may administer medicines under Midwives Exemptions, except for controlled drugs and providing that they are under the direct visual supervision of a sign-off mentor.
- Controlled drugs and every aspect of obtaining, using and returning them is tightly controlled by law. The midwife should be familiar with the standard operating procedures in their area of employment.

PHARMACOKINETICS

Pharmacokinetics is an understanding of the absorption, distribution, metabolism, and excretion of drugs. As part of drug administration, an understanding of pharmacokinetics is important and may help the midwife to:
- recognize adverse reactions early
- minimize the risk of unwanted drug interactions occurring
- prevent drugs being used inadvertently during pregnancy and lactation
- educate the woman to help her make an informed choice regarding drug administration.

Adult pharmacokinetics

Absorption

Drugs administered orally are usually absorbed from the gastrointestinal (GI) tract (a small number from the stomach, e.g. alcohol, but the majority from the small intestine), entering the bloodstream (some drugs bind to plasma albumin – protein binding) via the portal vein to pass through to the liver, where metabolism begins. Capsules and tablets must disintegrate prior to absorption;

liquid or soluble drugs are sometimes absorbed quicker than capsules and tablets. Modified-release drugs are designed to release evenly over a longer time period to aid compliance and are often inappropriate if a rapid response is required. It is important not to crush drugs that are intended to be swallowed whole, as this may destroy the modified-release system, releasing a whole day's dose in a few hours at a dangerously high level or may render them ineffective. Crushed drugs are not covered by the product licence (if the woman is unable to swallow drugs, the pharmacist should be consulted).

Drug absorption via the oral route is influenced by:

- gut motility and transit time – less drug is absorbed if it passes rapidly; the reverse is also true
- presence of food in the stomach – always follow the recommendations of taking the drug before, with or after food
- acid and enzymes of the GI tract
- lipid solubility (lipid-soluble drugs are easily absorbed and distributed throughout the body water compartments)
- drug formulation
- pregnancy, due to reduced GI motility
- labour, which slows gastric emptying.

Certain drugs cannot be administered orally because the acid or enzymes of the GI tract would destroy them and so are administered parenterally (e.g. benzylpenicillin, insulin).

Drugs administered via all other routes, e.g. sublingual, rectally, *per vaginam* nasal, spinal, epidural, all enter the circulation directly and avoid the liver. Drugs administered intravenously enter the bloodstream immediately and can be distributed to the tissues quickly.

Drug plasma concentrations can be measured. The therapeutic range is the 'window' in which the drug is able to have its maximum good effect, with minimal harmful effect. Each drug differs, but ideally drug administration is timed to keep plasma levels in the therapeutic range. Antibiotics should be regularly spaced in this way, if the gap between doses is too long, the microorganisms will commence growing again. A peak in plasma concentration will occur following administration, the rate of concentration usually declines rapidly, but then slows over several hours.

Distribution

The drug is distributed around the body via the circulation until it penetrates the organs or tissues and has an effect. Drugs generally bind to plasma proteins, but this is to varying degrees. Drugs that distribute into body fluid can be affected by fluid balance (e.g. dehydration, oedema) and those that distribute into fatty tissues are influenced by the amount of fat (e.g. malnutrition, obesity). Different drug dosages may be required depending on the clinical condition of the person, pregnancy (which changes blood chemistry) and the effectiveness of cardiovascular circulation.

Metabolism

This usually occurs within the liver and may be impaired by:

- age
- liver impairment
- respiratory or cardiac disease affecting hepatic blood flow and oxygenation
- drug interaction
- genetic factors.

Liver enzymes can be accelerated or inhibited, depending on what has been ingested. From the GI tract the products of digestion are metabolized (or detoxified) by the liver enzymes and are then rendered water soluble by the liver. This action allows the kidneys to excrete waste products (Jordan 2010).

Elimination

As discussed above, the kidneys are responsible for the majority of drug excretion. The half-life of a drug is the time taken for the plasma concentration of the drug to reduce by 50%. A drug that has a short half-life is quickly removed, necessitating frequent doses, whereas a drug with a long half-life requires smaller doses as it remains in the body having an effect for longer periods. Loading doses – an initial total dose given to attain high plasma concentrations – may be needed with long half-life drugs to achieve a therapeutic plasma concentration.

Changes in pregnancy

As suggested, physiological changes occurring during pregnancy can affect pharmacokinetics. Decreased absorption in the stomach and increased absorption in the small intestine may occur due to decreased transit time. The latter may increase the time taken to attain optimal plasma concentration. The increase in plasma volume increases the volume of distribution of water-soluble drugs. The increased renal blood flow and liver activity increase drug clearance and elimination, which may necessitate higher dosages. Different doses may be required during pregnancy and their effect may be slower; thus it is important for pregnant women with pre-existing medical conditions requiring medication to have their medication requirements reviewed by their specialists/GPs on a regular basis, e.g. anti-epileptic drugs.

Neonatal pharmacokinetics

Absorption

A variety of factors may affect drug absorption via the oral route. At birth, the pH of the term baby's stomach is 7. It becomes more acidic (pH 1.5–3.0) over the first hours of life, followed by a decrease in acid production during the first 10 days of life. Preterm babies have less ability to secrete gastric acid (Jackson 1999).

Drugs remain longer in the baby's stomach as gastric emptying time is slower. The stomach surface is less absorptive than the small intestine (Jackson 1999); thus it can take longer to achieve the desired plasma concentration of the drug. Less absorption of fat-soluble drugs occurs as bile output is reduced.

Intramuscular absorption is dependent on blood flow to the muscle, muscle activity, muscle mass and amount of subcutaneous fat. Decreased blood flow to the muscle is common during the first few days of life and absorption is unreliable.

Distribution

Drugs are more able to affect the brain due to greater membrane permeability of the blood–brain barrier. The baby, particularly preterm, has a higher percentage total body water content, necessitating higher doses (mg/kg) of water-soluble drugs to achieve an effective plasma concentration. However, lower doses of lipid-soluble drugs are required as the proportion of adipose tissue is reduced for both term and preterm babies.

Protein binding is decreased in the neonate, possibly due to competing substances (e.g. bilirubin) attaching to the plasma albumin. Toxicity may occur as a result of high levels of the unbound drug (e.g. theophylline, diazepam) in the body; lower plasma concentrations are desirable. Drugs such as sulphonamides may displace bilirubin from its protein-bound site, increasing the risk of jaundice.

Metabolism and excretion

Metabolism and elimination are both reduced in the baby. Equally, the fetus eliminates the medicines taken by the mother into the amniotic fluid, which is then ingested again. Consequently some medicines such as magnesium sulphate may still have an effect on the neonate for around 48 hours after delivery.

Summary

- Pharmacokinetics is the absorption, distribution, metabolism and excretion of drugs.
- Pregnancy affects pharmacokinetics and optimal plasma concentrations may take longer to attain.

- The differences with neonatal pharmacokinetics result in the oral and intramuscular routes being unreliable.

ANAPHYLAXIS

The administration of a drug is not without risk; many drugs have known side effects and the midwife should be familiar with these. Any known allergies should be discussed and recorded at the initial booking interview, as well as on any medicine administration records and alert identity bands. Anaphylaxis is a rare but potentially fatal hypersensitivity reaction that can occur following the administration of any drug, as well as food, fluids, foreign proteins (e.g. blood transfusion, insect sting) or topical applications (e.g. plasters, latex gloves, hair dye). It can take anything from several minutes to several hours to appear, although most severe reactions occur within several minutes. Most reactions occur in people with no known risk factors, although it occurs more commonly with drugs such as antibiotics (e.g. penicillin) and whole blood transfusions. Those with atopic disorders, e.g. asthma or eczema, are considered to be more vulnerable to a hypersensitivity response. Early recognition of the signs and symptoms is essential to ensure prompt management of the condition (see below).

Mild anaphylaxis occurs more slowly, and symptoms tend to be less serious; it is managed by the administration of oral antihistamines with close observation for signs of improvement or deterioration and reassurance. Those who have experienced an itchy rash following the administration of a medicine should be considered to be sensitized and therefore at high risk of anaphylaxis should another exposure to the same medicine occur (Jordan 2010).

Severe anaphylaxis presents with cardiovascular collapse and is more urgent. The Resuscitation Council (2008) suggest anaphylaxis is likely when the following three criteria are all present:

- sudden onset and rapid advancement of symptoms
- life-threatening airway and/or breathing and/or circulation problems
- mucosal and/or skin changes, e.g. angioedema, flushing, urticaria (although these may be absent in up to 20% of cases).

Signs and symptoms

- Airway – pharyngeal/laryngeal oedema as the throat and tongue swell causing the woman to experience difficulty with swallowing and breathing and the feeling her throat is closing up; hoarseness; stridor.
- Breathing – tachypnoea (followed later by bradypnoea), shortness of breath, wheezing, hypoxia

resulting in confusion and cyanosis (late sign), fatigue, respiratory arrest.

- Circulation – shock, tachycardia, hypotension, dizziness, collapse, loss of consciousness, myocardial ischaemia and electrocardiograph (ECG) changes, cardiac arrest.
- Disability problems – the problems encountered with airway, breathing and circulation changes decrease brain perfusion and can alter the woman's neurological status causing agitation, confusion and loss of consciousness. There may also be accompanying GI symptoms of abdominal pain, vomiting, incontinence, diarrhoea.
- Mucosal and/or skin changes – erythema, urticaria, angioedema.

Management of severe anaphylaxis (Resuscitation Council 2008)

- Call for medical assistance urgently; do not leave the woman.
- If anaphylaxis is the result of a substance being administered, stop administration immediately.
- Position the woman in the left lateral position. When this is not possible and the woman is on her back, place a wedge under her right side to prevent aortocaval occlusion (if pregnant) and raise her legs.
- Follow the principles of resuscitation (Chapter 55) using ABCDE, establish an airway and resuscitate as needed while treating the anaphylaxis.
- Administer 100% oxygen therapy using a high-flow mask (>10 L/min) with an oxygen reservoir to prevent collapse of the reservoir during inspiration.
- Administer intramuscular adrenaline (epinephrine) 1 : 1000 solution (1 mg/mL); repeated at 5-minute intervals if needed (adult dose 500 micrograms, 0.5 mL; under 6 yrs 150 micrograms, 0.15 mL). If repeated doses are required, intravenous adrenaline may be administered only by a doctor who uses this in their everyday practice, e.g. anaesthetist. Continuous ECG and pulse oximetry will be required with frequent monitoring of blood pressure.
- To correct hypotension, shock, and vasodilation, administer 500–1000 mL intravenous crystalloid solution (e.g. 0.9% sodium chloride) rapidly. If hypotension persists, administer further doses.
- Anticipate the need for a chest X-ray, blood samples for urea and electrolytes, blood gases, etc., as for any emergency. If pregnant, rapid caesarean section may be required, depending upon the mother's response to resuscitation. At some point fetal monitoring should be attempted.

- As a second line of treatment, an antihistamine (chlorphenamine) 10 mg can be administered intramuscularly or by slow intravenous injection (neonatal dose 250 microgram/kg).
- Following initial resuscitation, hydrocortisone 200 mg may be administered intramuscularly or by slow intravenous injection (neonatal dose 25 mg initially).
- If bronchospasm persists, administration of a bronchodilator may be required, e.g. nebulized/intravenous salbutamol, inhaled ipratropium, intravenous aminophylline or magnesium (the latter may cause further flushes and hypotension).
- Blood should be taken to measure mast cell tryptase. This aids the diagnosis of anaphylaxis. The first specimen should be taken as soon after the reaction as is convenient, the second is taken 1–2 hours post the event and the third is taken after 24 hours.
- Document the cause and management clearly, informing the woman of this (to avoid recurrence).
- Closely observe the woman or baby's condition over the next 6 hours in a clinical area able to monitor and treat life-threatening conditions, a secondary reaction may occur. Observation is required for at least 24 hours, following a serious anaphylactic reaction.
- Following an anaphylactic reaction, referral to an allergy clinic should be made for follow-up consultation and management (NICE 2011). It may be necessary for the client to carry adrenaline for potential self-administration in the future.

Where an actual or suspected adverse drug reaction has occurred, the midwife should report this in the UK to the Medicines and Healthcare Products Regulatory Agency (MHRA) using the yellow card scheme. This can be undertaken online: www.yellowcard.mhra.gov.uk or by completing the yellow card at the back of the British National Formulary (BNF). Such monitoring exists in most countries.

ROLE AND RESPONSIBILITIES OF THE MIDWIFE

These can be summarized as:
- being familiar with pharmacokinetics and the implications for drug administration
- understanding how pregnancy affects pharmacokinetics
- understanding why pharmacokinetics is different for the baby
- asking about known allergies at the booking interview and on each admission to hospital where medication may be required
- recognizing and managing anaphylaxis correctly
- correct documentation
- informing the MHRA of a suspected or actual adverse drug reaction.

Summary

- Anaphylaxis is a rare but potentially fatal reaction that can result from (amongst other things) drug administration. It is recognized by a sudden and worsening response following administration of the trigger. The woman may experience mucosal and/or skin changes, with respiratory or cardiovascular collapse. The immediate management includes the giving of I.M. adrenaline and action as for cardiopulmonary resuscitation.

- Where an actual or suspected drug reaction has occurred, the midwife should notify the MHRA who are responsible for monitoring such events.

SELF-ASSESSMENT EXERCISES

The answers to the following questions may be found in the text:

1. From where can 'P' classified medicines be obtained?
2. What does a midwife need to know about a medicine before they can administer it?
3. Which medicines can a midwife administer autonomously under Midwives Exemptions?
4. List the nine 'rights' of medicine administration.
5. What information is needed on a correctly completed prescription?
6. List the steps taken to ensure that (a) a non-controlled drug and (b) a controlled drug are correctly administered.
7. Describe the ways in which a midwife could access pethidine for a woman labouring at home.
8. Describe how a woman can be assessed for suitability for self-medicating.
9. What are the four aspects of pharmacokinetics?
10. How does pregnancy affect pharmacokinetics?
11. How would the midwife recognize and manage anaphylaxis?
12. What is the name of the agency that monitors adverse drug reactions?

REFERENCES

Alexis, O., Caldwell, J., 2013. Administration of medicines- the nurse role in ensuring patient safety. Br. J. Nurs. 22 (1), 32–35.

Anon (Anonymous), 2010. Changes to midwives exemptions. Pract. Midwife 13 (7), 8.

Bussey, A., 2011. What is a Patient Group Direction (PGD)? Available online: <http://www.medicinesresources .nhs.uk/en/Communities/NHS/ PGDs/FAQs/What-is-a-Patient-Group -Direction-PGD/> (accessed 5 March 2015).

Elliott, M., Liu, Y., 2010. The nine rights of medication administration: an overview. Br. J. Nurs. 19 (5), 300–305.

GMC (General Medical Council), 2013. Good practice in prescribing and managing medicines and devices. GMC, London. Available online: <www.gmc-uk.org/guidance> (accessed 15 December 2015).

Griffith, R., 2010. Law, medicines and the midwife. In: Jordan, S. (Ed.), Pharmacology for Midwives, second ed. Palgrave Macmillan, Basingstoke, pp. 62–74. (Chapter 3).

Human Medicines Regulations, 2012. Available online: <http://www .legislation.gov.uk/uksi/2012/1916/ made> (accessed 26 February 2015).

Jackson, M.P., 1999. Impact of age, pregnancy, disease and food on drug action. In: Luker, K., Wolfson, D. (Eds.), Medicines Management for Clinical Nurses. Blackwell Science, Oxford. (Chapter 4).

Jordan, S., 2010. Principles of Pharmacology. In: Jordan, S. (Ed.), Pharmacology for Midwives, second ed. Palgrave Macmillan, Basingstoke. (Chapter 1).

Matthew, L., 2007. Injectable medication therapy: a patient safety challenge. Nurs. Stand. 21 (31), 45–48.

NICE (National Institute for Health and Clinical Excellence), 2011. Anaphylaxis: assessment to confirm an anaphylactic episode and the decision to refer after emergency treatment for a suspected anaphylactic episode. NICE Guideline 134. Available online: <www.nice.org.uk/> (accessed 5 March 2014).

NMC (Nursing and Midwifery Council), 2007. Standards for medicine management. NMC, London. Available online: <http://www.nmc-uk .org/Publications/Standards/> (accessed 5 March 2015).

NMC (Nursing and Midwifery Council), 2011. Changes to Midwives Exemptions. NMC Circular 07/2011. NMC, London. Available online: <www.nmc-uk.org> (accessed 5 March 2014).

NMC (Nursing and Midwifery Council), 2012. Midwives Rules and Standards. NMC, London.

Resuscitation Council UK, 2008. Emergency treatment of anaphylactic reactions. Guidelines for healthcare providers. Available online: <www.resus.org.uk> (accessed 5 March 2015).

Chapter 19

Principles of drug administration: oral administration

LEARNING OUTCOMES

Having read this chapter, the reader should be able to:

- discuss the advantages and disadvantages of the oral route, identifying what should be included in a risk assessment
- describe the different preparations available for oral use, giving an example of each
- describe the procedure for administering a drug orally to a woman and a baby
- summarize the role and responsibilities of the midwife.

This chapter considers the safe management of medication for the oral route, the preparations available and the role and responsibilities of the midwife. The procedures are described for adult and neonatal administration. It should be read in conjunction with Chapter 18.

The majority of medication taken via the mouth (orally) is absorbed by the gastrointestinal tract, often in the stomach. However, the distinction is made between medication that is swallowed and that which is held in the mouth.

- Medication to be given orally is swallowed, 'p.o.' is the agreed abbreviation.
- Buccal refers to medication that is absorbed through the vessels in the mouth; in this case the medication is lodged in the cheek. On a medicine administration record (see Chapter 18) 'buccal' is often written in full and not abbreviated.
- Sublingual preparations sit under the tongue. They are often abbreviated as 's.l.'. Both these and buccal preparations avoid the gastrointestinal tract, enter the circulation directly via the superior vena cava, and therefore have a rapid response. Jordan (2010) suggests that if there has not been a response within 5 minutes of receiving the medication, then there is not likely to be one.
- Lozenges are often sucked (systemic effect) or used for local effect, e.g. anaesthetic relief of sore throats, antifungal coating of the tongue. Some medications are chewed, this should be clear in the prescription.

Oral medication

Ansell & Dougherty (2011) suggest there are distinct advantages in using the oral route for medication. It is often an easy and convenient route without too much disruption or embarrassment, and often the medications are the least expensive. However, for some situations alternative routes or preparations may be needed:

- Compliance: is the woman/baby awake, sufficiently alert, understanding, and physically able to swallow?

- Is there gastrointestinal disturbance, e.g. vomiting, nil by mouth, that would make taking oral medication difficult or inappropriate?
- Can the woman swallow tablets? Some people find this a difficult skill.

These questions and the answers to them constitute a risk assessment. If the oral route is not safe or inappropriate at that time, an alternative route/medication should be prescribed. Oral medication is given via nasogastric or other enteral feeding tubes in particular circumstances.

Oral preparations may be affected by other constituents in the stomach, and so the manufacturer's directions should be followed (e.g. before, during or after a meal) for maximum effectiveness. In the same way, the medication should be administered in the form that it comes in; crushing, dissolving, cutting or opening a tablet/capsule when this is not indicated can cause under- or overdose and also constitutes using a medication 'off licence' – the midwife becomes fully liable for its effects (Chapter 18). Medication that is modified in its release is designed to pass through the stomach and be absorbed in the small intestine. Altering this medication in any way can cause inactivity or immediate activity, both of which can be dangerous. Some medications have an enteric coating to prevent damage to the lining of the stomach. Oral medications are:

- Tablets, caplets, capsules: these are generally swallowed whole, sitting up if possible and with a glass of water (Jordan 2010). If possible the woman should remain sat upright for a further 30 minutes. This prevents irritation to the oesophagus and other tissues. If scored, tablets/caplets may be divided in half using a tablet cutter, according to the required dosage. The cutter is washed and dried after use. Examples of tablets include analgesics, antibiotics, iron supplementation.
- Granules, powders and soluble tablets: these need to be thoroughly dissolved before administration. This is generally in water, but the manufacturer's guidelines should be followed. Examples include analgesics, e.g. paracetamol.
- Elixir: this may be supplied prepared, or require careful dilution according to the instructions. Some solutions require refrigeration. The bottle needs inverting several times to ensure thorough mixing before administration. Examples include antacids and antibiotics.
- Sprays: these should be used according to the manufacturer's instructions but are often sprayed into the cheek or under the tongue. Examples include glyceryl trinitrate, nicotine replacement therapy.
- Gels: some gels are used for their local action, e.g. pain relief for teething or antifungal treatment, others

such as dextrose (hypoglycaemia) or midazolam (epilepsy) are used when a rapid effect is needed.

Equipment

Medicine cups with gradations on the side are used; ideally they are disposable. As a clean transport medium their use allows the medication to be transferred from the packet to the mouth without it being touched. The gradations on the side allow liquids to be measured, as do medicine spoons. However, small or very accurate doses, e.g. paediatric doses, should be measured using an oral (enteric) syringe. In the UK these are purple in colour, non-luer (will not connect as an ordinary syringe would into intravenous tubing) and marked 'enteric' (NPSA 2007). They are sterile for single use only, but in some circumstances may be reused for the same client after washing. (They are then stored in a labelled plastic box). The medication is 'drawn up' using the bung that fits into the bottle neck, ideally in the presence of the woman and given straight to her.

Education

Helping the woman to understand her medication – how to take it correctly, what to expect, and what to report – is a significant part of the drug administration process. Informed consent must always be gained; it is those with legal responsibility (parents often) who give consent on behalf of children. Ideally the midwife watches the client swallowing the medication; deception is more common in some client groups and if suspected should be discussed with the woman and her multidisciplinary team.

PROCEDURE: oral administration to a woman

- Ensure the woman/baby is accessible and ready for the medication prior to dispensing it
- Undertake the thorough checking procedure as described on p. 145.
- With clean hands, select the preparation, check the expiry date, and dispense the correct dose of the drug:
  - tablets and capsules: tip the required number into the bottle cap, then into a medicine cup. If in foil packaging, check the strip, then push the tablets through the foil into the cup (avoid handling the medication). Return remaining medication to a safe place
  - elixir: invert the bottle several times, hold the bottle with the label to the rear (to avoid obscuring the label with spilt medicine), hold the medicine cup at eye level and pour the liquid into it, ensuring the fluid is accurately on the line. Alternatively, insert

an enteric syringe into the bung, invert the bottle and draw the correct number of millilitres into the syringe, also at eye level.

- Confirm the woman's identity: ask for her full name and date of birth, check her identity bracelet if necessary.
- Advise the woman on how to take the medication, providing a glass of water if necessary, encouraging her to be in an upright posture and to remain so for 30 minutes. Observe her swallowing the drug. For sublingual preparations, the medication should be placed/sprayed beneath the tongue; for buccal preparations they should be placed/sprayed into the cheek or placed next to the gum; other directions to suck, chew, etc. should be given as prescribed.
- Dispose of equipment correctly, decontaminate hands, and document the administration in the medicine administration record and any other agreed places, e.g. partogram.
- Observe for the effects of the medication and take any necessary action.

Precautions

- If the woman is unable to take the medication at the time of administration, it is recorded and the late administration checked before being given. A drug dispensed but not administered should be disposed of safely, never left in anticipation or returned to the bottle. The omission or late administration of some medications instigates an investigation in some NHS Trusts.
- Compliance is increased if the woman understands the reason for the medication, likely effects and possible side effects. Refusal to take a drug should be recorded, with the reason and the prescribing medical officer informed.
- If the woman vomits soon after administration and only if the tablet is clearly visible, a further stat. dose may be prescribed after consultation with the obstetrician.
- Controlled drugs may also be prescribed in an oral form; administration should be according to the local policy for controlled drug administration (Chapter 18). Tablets are counted; elixir should be measured very carefully using an enteric syringe.

ORAL ADMINISTRATION TO A BABY

The baby needs to be awake and able to swallow. The parents should have given consent and should be taught the procedure if they are going to need to repeat it themselves. The prescription is scrutinized as per all prescriptions (Chapter 18) and local protocols are adhered to, e.g. double independent checking by two registered practitioners. An enteric syringe is used (as above). The majority of oral medications are in the form of elixir for babies.

Patience is needed when administering medication to babies and children; it can be difficult to assess how much the baby has taken if some is seen to dribble down the chin. If this occurs, consultation with the paediatrician is necessary regarding the necessity of a further dose. For a baby that is formula-fed, Miller-Bell et al (2011) suggest mixing the medication with a small amount of formula.

PROCEDURE: oral administration to a baby

- Decontaminate hands and undertake the thorough checking process described in Chapter 18 (p. 145) independently of a second colleague.
- Confirm the identity of the baby, and reaffirm parental consent.
- Decontaminate hands and draw up the drug accurately in a sterile enteric syringe (see above), being confident that the dosage is correct.
- The baby may be more comfortable held in the parent's arms.
- Place the syringe into the baby's mouth towards the cheek, squeeze a small amount (0.5–1 mL maximum) into the mouth, and observe the baby swallowing.
- Administer the next part of the dose, observe the swallow, and continue in this way until the drug is fully administered.
- Dispose of the syringe correctly and decontaminate hands.
- Document administration.
- If appropriate, observe for the effects of the medication and take any necessary action.

ROLE AND RESPONSIBILITIES OF THE MIDWIFE

These can be summarized as:

- practising within the NMC (2007) standards for the safe and effective administration of medicines
- ensuring the drug is dispensed correctly, ideally in the woman's presence and given straight to her/her baby, after thorough identity checking
- observing the effects and side effects of the drug administered
- education of the woman to aid compliance and effectiveness, ensuring where possible that she has swallowed it
- correct record keeping.

SUMMARY

- Oral drug administration involves thorough checking in all parts of the process, as for any other drug administration (see Chapter 18 for details).
- Oral medication may come in different forms; while the majority of oral preparations are swallowed, some are for sucking, chewing, buccal, or sublingual use. Liquid preparations may be given using a medicine cup or spoon; alternatively, an enteric syringe is used.
- An assessment should be made as to whether for this woman/baby the oral route is an appropriate one for this medication at this time.

SELF-ASSESSMENT EXERCISES

The answers to the following questions may be found in the text:

1. List the advantages and disadvantages of the oral route.
2. What should the midwife consider before administering an oral medication?
3. What would the midwife do if the drug was dispensed but the woman was not available to take it?
4. Describe how a midwife would administer a sublingual drug to a woman.
5. What would the midwife do if the woman vomited her medication shortly after taking it?

REFERENCES

Ansell, L., Dougherty, L., 2011. Medicines Management. In: Doughty, L., Lister, S. (Eds.), The Royal Marsden Hospital Manual of Clinical Nursing Procedures, eighth ed. Wiley Blackwell, Chichester, pp. 956–961. (Chapter 16).

Jordan, S., 2010. Administration of medicines. In: Jordan, S. (Ed.), Pharmacology for Midwives, second ed. Palgrave Macmillan, Basingstoke, pp. 39–40. (Chapter 2).

Miller-Bell, M., Cotton, C.M., Buschbach, D., 2011. Pharmacology in neonatal care. In: Gardner, S.L., Carter, B.S., Enzman Hines, M., Hernandez, J.A. (Eds.), Merenstein & Gardner's Handbook of Neonatal Intensive Care, seventh ed. Elsevier, St. Louis. (Chapter 10).

NMC (Nursing and Midwifery Council), 2007. Standards for Medicine Management. NMC, London.

NPSA (National Patient Safety Agency), 2007. Alert No. 19, Promoting Safe Measurement and Administration of Liquid Medicines Via Oral and other Enteral routes. NPSA, London. Available online: <www.npsa.nhs.uk/> (accessed 26 February 2015).

Chapter 20

Principles of drug administration: injection technique

LEARNING OUTCOMES

Having read this chapter, the reader should be able to:

- list the situations in which a midwife is likely to administer medication by injection
- describe, with a rationale for choice, the suitable sites for I.M., S.C., and I.D. injections in the adult and I.M. in the baby
- demonstrate an injection, giving a rationale for each action
- summarize the role and responsibilities of the midwife.

Preparations are administered via an injection if they cannot be absorbed, or are absorbed too slowly, when given via other routes. In this chapter the safe administration of drugs via intramuscular (I.M.), subcutaneous (S.C.) and intradermal (I.D.) injection will be reviewed. Intravenous injection is reviewed in Chapter 23. Suitable injection sites in the adult and baby are highlighted and there is discussion about appropriate equipment to use. It is important that this chapter is read in conjunction with Chapter 18.

INDICATIONS

The midwife administers drugs by injection on a number of occasions; the following is an indicative, but not exhaustive list:

- uterotonic agent, e.g. active third stage of labour, postpartum haemorrhage
- analgesia or antidote, e.g. pethidine, morphine
- anti-D immunoglobulin
- rubella vaccine
- vitamin K (babies)

- subcutaneous heparin (thromboembolic prophylaxis)
- iron therapy
- steroids (fetal lung maturity prior to preterm birth)
- intradermal local anaesthetics.

As for all medications, the midwife should be competent to identify and manage any unforeseen emergencies, e.g. anaphylaxis or cardiac arrest. Medication given via an injectable route cannot be withdrawn.

Many people are uncomfortable with the idea of having an injection. The midwife has a responsibility to ensure that the woman is 'put at ease' and is aware of what is being administered, why and how. She also needs to be assured that the equipment chosen and technique used will promote both safety and comfort. For the client with significant needle phobia, alternative strategies may be needed and assistance from a colleague should be sought.

SAFETY CONSIDERATIONS

Giving an injection exposes midwives to potential needle-stick injury. Used needles must never be resheathed and sharps must be disposed of immediately into a sharps box at the point of care. However, in many situations a needle safety device is already fitted; these should be used on every occasion. Needle safety devices are all different in appearance but in principle work so that as soon as the needle is withdrawn from the tissue it is covered and protected. It can appear as a type of trough for the needle to sit into. Often the practitioner initiates the shield by flicking it over using the same hand as injecting with. Filter/filtered needles are used to draw solutions up into the syringe, these prevent shards of glass or shavings of rubber from entering the syringe.

Hands should be decontaminated; the World Health Organization (WHO 2010) suggest that gloves are not necessary. Skin cleansing remains an unresolved issue, Public Health England (Public Health England (PHE) 2013) suggest that none is necessary for immunizations while Ansell & Dougherty (2011) advocate its use as per the Aseptic Non Touch Technique (ANTT) (Rowley & Clare 2011) approach (see p. 89). This involves at least 30 seconds of up and down, right to left skin cleansing that creates friction, using a locally agreed alcohol-based product, then the skin dries for at least 30 seconds. ANTT themselves are in the process of producing guidelines for skin preparation prior to injection (personal communication), the reader is encouraged to be alert to this and in the meantime to practice according to locally agreed protocols. Visibly unclean skin is always cleansed prior to injection. Whether the skin is cleansed or not, the injection should be prepared and administered using ANTT.

INTRAMUSCULAR INJECTION (I.M.)

Choice of site in the adult

As suggested, intramuscular (I.M.) is injection into muscle. It can be painful and absorption can be unreliable (Jordan 2010) but the response is often seen quickly, e.g. the use of oxytocin in the third stage of labour. The choice of site is important. It may depend upon:

- the number of millilitres to be injected (although this is questionable)
- the nature of the drug
- the speed of administration. Malkin (2008) suggests that it should be 10 seconds/mL
- the mobility of the woman and accessibility of the site
- the anatomical relation of other structures (nerves, bones, blood vessels)
- the skin and general condition of the woman (presence/absence of fat and subcutaneous tissue, good muscle presence, adequate circulation, any signs of bruising, infection, swelling, inflammation, abscess, frequent or over use of the site)
- the woman's preference
- the manufacturer's guidelines.

Recommended sites (adults)

There are five recommended sites for I.M. injection (Workman 1999). However, despite Rodger & King's recommendations (based on a literature search of all available evidence) in 2000 to use the ventrogluteal site for preference (Hall 2015 agrees), it is still rarely seen in UK practice. It remains the preferred/recommended site of choice. The chosen site is often the gluteus maximus but this is the only site that has close proximity to significant vessels and nerves and so should be avoided (Malkin 2008). These are the five sites:

- Deltoid muscle of upper arm (maximum 1 mL) (Fig. 20.1A): the site is approximately 2.5 cm below the acromial process on the lateral surface of the arm, extending to the level of the axilla (an inverted triangle in shape). Often the choice of site for vaccinations, often easily accessible.
- Quadriceps muscle (vastus lateralis, maximum 5 mL): this is found on the thigh by measuring a hand's breadth down from the greater trochanter, and one up from the knee, this middle third of the lateral aspect of the thigh is the correct muscle (Fig. 20.1B). The rectus femoris is adjacent on the anterior aspect of the thigh; it is used less and is not appropriate in children (Fig. 20.1B).

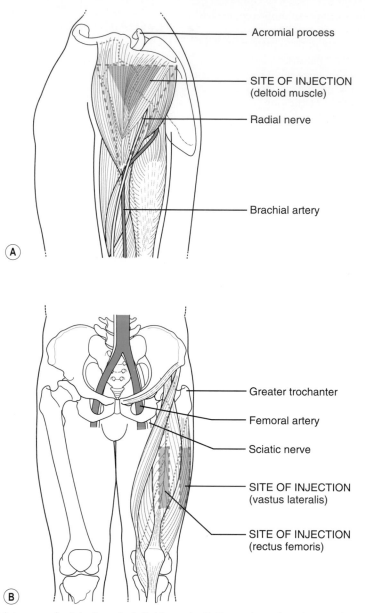

Figure 20.1 Sites for adult intramuscular injection. **A,** Deltoid muscle; **B,** Rectus femoris and vastus lateralis (vastus lateralis is the one suitable site for I.M. injection in neonates also);

- Gluteus maximus muscle (dorsogluteal) (maximum 4 mL): found on the upper outer quadrant of the buttock (Fig. 20.1C). As suggested above, this should be avoided. Ansell & Dougherty (2011) point out that without correct assessment of the muscle position and an appropriately long needle, many medications are placed into gluteal fat. Zaybak et al (2007) agree,

suggesting that the deltoid, rectus femoris or vastus lateralis should all be considered as sites of preference for an obese woman, there being less fat and subcutaneous tissue on these sites than on the buttocks.

- Ventrogluteal site (maximum 2.5 mL), the site of choice: the palm of the midwife's right hand is placed on the greater trochanter of the woman's left hip (or

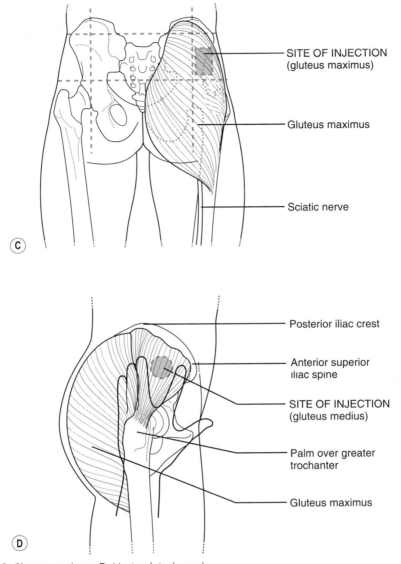

Figure 20.1, cont'd C, Gluteus maximus; **D,** Ventrogluteal muscle.
(Adapted with kind permission from Jamieson et al 1997)

vice versa). The index finger is extended to touch the anterior superior iliac crest while the middle finger stretches as far along the iliac crest as possible. The site is in the 'V' between the index and middle fingers (Fig. 20.1D).

PHE (2013) recommend the thigh or upper arm as their preferred injection sites for vaccinations, I.M. or S.C.

The volume of solution that the muscle can accommodate seems to be inconclusive (Malkin 2008), the figures suggested above are a guide. The Department of Health (PHE 2013) suggest in their immunization directives that if greater than 4 mL needs to be administered, the dose should be divided and given into different sites.

The muscle should be relaxed for minimal discomfort, the site may be supported by the non-injecting hand and some commentators recommend a slight stretching of the skin prior to needle insertion (Hunter 2008). 'Bunching up' the muscle in a thin woman may sometimes be necessary (Workman 1999).

Z-track

A Z-track technique (Fig. 20.2) ensures the solution does not leak back to the skin and so irritate the subcutaneous tissue or stain the skin. The skin and subcutaneous tissue are moved sideways or downwards 2–3 cm, the needle is inserted into the original site chosen, the solution is injected and after 10 seconds the needle is removed as the skin is released simultaneously (Workman 1999). There are advocates in the literature of Z-track being the technique of choice for all I.M. injections (Rodger & King 2000, Ogston-Tuck 2014a). The reader will need to consult their local protocol.

Choice of equipment

In an average sized woman a 21 g (green) needle is used at a 90° angle (see Fig. 20.3A), in any of the recommended sites. However, as suggested, this assessment is individualized, and the needle chosen should reach the muscle with approximately 1 cm of it still visible externally (Ansell & Dougherty 2011). This is important; I.M. injections should be into muscle tissue, so too short a length of needle would make it an S.C. injection. If the full needle is inserted and were to break, there would be no means of removing it.

The use of a filter needle for drawing up the solution means that a 'new' sharp sterile needle is used for injecting;

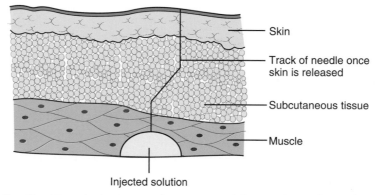

Figure 20.2 Z-track injection. The skin and subcutaneous tissue are moved downwards or sideways for 2–3 cm prior to insertion of the needle and then released as the needle is removed. The solution is prevented from back tracking to the skin.

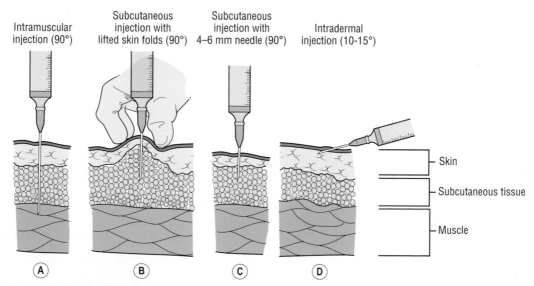

Figure 20.3 **A,** I.M. injection (90°). **B,** S.C. injection with lifted skin folds, 90°. **C,** S.C. injection using 4–6 mm needle length, 90°. **D,** I.D. injection (10–15°).

this is more comfortable. The syringe is held like a dart, this prevents the accidental injection of solution when injecting. Post-injection, a cotton wool ball or gauze swab is used to cover the puncture site and a plaster applied if necessary.

To aspirate or not?

Traditionally, after inserting the needle into the muscle, care is taken to aspirate the plunger backwards (for 10 seconds) to check that a vein has not been punctured. If it had, the medication would inappropriately be given intravenously. However, Malkin (2008) suggests that it is only the gluteus maximus muscle that is near to major arteries and that therefore if one of the other sites is being used, aspiration should not be necessary. Equally, some needle safety devices are activated when the plunger is drawn backwards, clearly this is highly inappropriate when the needle is in the muscle! Ogston-Tuck's (2014a) conclusion is that aspiration should be removed from injection technique, while Ansell & Dougherty (2011) continue to recommend the practice.

Ampoules and vials

Ampoules may be glass or, increasingly, plastic, with a top that 'snaps off'. Vials tend to be glass with a rubber bung beneath the metal top. This needs cleaning with an alcohol-impregnated wipe before use to reduce the cross-infection risk. Ampoules and vials may be completely inverted so that the substance can be drawn up without any air, and so that the scale on the syringe can be read correctly at eye level. Preparations may come as solutions or powder for reconstitution. In the event of needing to reconstitute a drug (e.g. diamorphine) a diluent e.g. sterile water, will be required according to the manufacturer's instructions.

I.M. injection for a baby

There is one main site for I.M. injection in the baby: quadriceps muscle (vastus lateralis), lateral mid-third of the thigh (Fig. 20.1B). The deltoid muscle may be used for vaccinations only.

Other sites (e.g. gluteus maximus and ventrogluteal) may be used in older babies, but Hemsworth (2000) suggests that muscular development in these sites is insufficient in neonates. The maximum dose that can be injected is 1 mL. The baby should be in a safe place (e.g. held or in a cot). A 25 g (orange) or 23 g (blue) needle is inserted at a 90° angle (Anon 2007), generally up to about half of the needle is within the tissue, but this will vary according to the baby's size.

SUBCUTANEOUS INJECTION (S.C.)

An S.C. injection places the medication into the connective tissue and fat beneath the skin. These tissues have a reduced blood supply in comparison to muscle, so drug absorption is slow and steady. Common preparations for S.C. use include insulin and low-molecular-weight heparin. As a single injection it is considered that only 1–2 mL can be accommodated, but S.C. infusions can also be established and can add up to 3 L of fluid into the circulation over 24 hours.

Subcutaneous injections can be inadvertently placed into muscle and so it is generally necessary to grasp the skin and lift the subcutaneous tissue away from the muscle before injecting (Peragallo-Dittko 1997, Workman 1999) (Fig. 20.4). Needle depth and the amount of subcutaneous tissue determine whether the needle is inserted into the skin at a 45° angle or a 90° angle. A shorter needle (that which is often in pre-prepared doses or injection pens, 6 mm) can be used at 90° generally without lifting the skin (Diggle 2014) (Fig. 20.3C); however, the technique (known as lifted skin folds) is necessary when a longer needle is used (Fig. 20.3B). To ensure the medication is deposited in the subcutaneous tissue, Hall (2015) advocates the rule that if able to grasp 5 cm (2 inches) of tissue, the needle is inserted at 90°, only 2.5 cm (1 inch) grasped means insert it at 45°. Jordan (2010) suggests that if the needle length is greater than 2.4 cm then the injecting angle should be 45°. Hall (2015) suggests that a 25 g needle is inserted at 45°, a shorter one would be inserted at 90°.

Choice of site

The preferred sites for an adult are:

- outer surface of the upper arm
- lateral upper-third of the thigh
- umbilical region of the abdomen
- on the back, beneath the scapulae, either side of the spine.

However, in assessing the evidence Ogston-Tuck (2014b) suggests that absorption changes from different sites at different rates, the fastest being the abdomen, then the arms, then thighs, and lastly hip and buttock. The arms are often the site of choice, having less blood vessels, less discomfort and being easily accessible. The site should be examined prior to injection for inflammation, infection, scarring or hardness, which may all indicate poor absorption and increase the level of pain. The question of skin cleansing prior to administration (as for I.M. injections above) remains unanswered. The reader should consult their local protocol. Aspiration (drawing back the plunger once in the

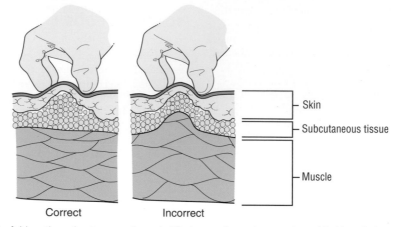

Figure 20.4 Lifted skin folds – the subcutaneous tissue is lifted away from the muscle and held until the needle has been removed.

tissue) is not considered necessary for an S.C. injection (Nicol et al 2004).

Speed of delivery

As before, all injections are more comfortable if injected slowly. Ogston-Tuck (2014b) recommends Enoxaparin should be injected over 30 seconds, the literature does not appear to cite a time scale for other S.C. injections but suggests 'slowly' (Ansell & Dougherty 2011). Slow delivery of the medication aids comfort and reduces bruising.

Specific considerations for Enoxaparin (EMC 2014)

Enoxaparin sodium (POM) is available in dose related pre-prepared syringes. In pregnancy the dose is adjusted according to body weight. It is generally administered once a day. It is administered by the midwife or the woman, with decontaminated hands, using an S.C. technique. The needle is inserted at 90° with the lifted skin folds technique (see above and Fig. 20.3B). Only when the injection is complete should the skin fold be released. It should be administered into the abdomen, for which site rotation is necessary for long-term use. That advocated by Gelder (2014) is with diabetes in mind but is eminently sensible. The site is rotated, e.g. right or left, and within that area the site moves by at least 1 cm each day. Gelder (2014) shows this as circular pattern similar to a snail shell. The woman should be lying down. The abdomen remains a safe site during pregnancy and postnatally.

The safety device fitted to the needle is activated automatically when the plunger is depressed far enough. The air bubble remains in the syringe as a mechanism of ensuring that the full dose has been delivered. Rubbing the injection site may cause bruising and so should be avoided.

In some instances the woman may be taught to self-administer medication by injection; insulin is commonly given in this way, as is low-molecular-weight heparin. Hicks (2012) suggests that many insulin-dependent diabetics have no recollection of being taught a good injection technique, and so it is noted (Hicks et al 2011) that many use an incorrect one. The midwife has a responsibility for anyone who self-medicates with subcutaneous injection both in teaching a correct technique and in assessing that this continues.

INTRADERMAL INJECTION (I.D.)

A small amount of solution (up to 0.5 mL) is injected locally into the skin using a 25 g (orange) needle at a 10–15° angle (Workman 1999) (Fig. 20.3D). The bevel of the needle is inserted upwards so that a small weal forms and is seen on the skin. The commonest sites are the scapulae or the inner forearm, but frequently midwives inject intradermally prior to cannulation (Chapter 47) and therefore inject over the site of the vein to be cannulated. Local anaesthetic is also injected intradermally when infiltrating for perineal repair (Chapter 34).

PROCEDURE: I.M. and S.C. injections in the adult

- Undertake the thorough checking procedures as for any medication administration (see Chapter 18).
- Decontaminate hands, put on non-sterile gloves and clean a plastic tray with the locally approved

alcohol wipes. Remove gloves and wash and dry hands.
- Gather equipment:
  - 1 sterile filter needle, 1 sterile needle with protection system, assessed to be the correct size for the type of injection and size of the client (see above)
  - 1 sterile syringe (an appropriate size, in date, undamaged and confirmed to be sterile)
  - portable sharps box
  - approved skin cleanser, often 70% alcohol wipe
  - cotton wool or gauze
  - ampoule (already checked thoroughly)
  - medicine administration chart.
- Open the plunger end of the syringe packaging, 'prepare' the syringe ensuring that the plunger moves within the barrel. Connect the filter needle firmly, using a non-touch technique (Key-Parts are the syringe tip and needle hub). Place connected syringe and needle onto the tray. Drop the other needle from its packaging onto the tray also (with protection system if separate).
- For a glass ampoule ensure all of the solution is in the ampoule (not retained in the top), snap off the top (protect fingers). For a plastic ampoule, snap off the top.
- Unsheath the needle and draw up the required amount of solution using a non touch technique (Key-Parts are the solution and the needle), remove the ampoule.
- Invert the syringe and examine it for air. If necessary tap it gently to encourage the air up to the top of the syringe; push the plunger to exclude the air from the syringe, ensuring none of the solution is lost and the dosage in the syringe is correct.
- Remove the needle, discard it into the sharps box, replace with the protected needle using a non touch technique, place onto the tray. Take the medicine administration chart, sharps box and tray to the woman, include the skin cleanser if required, cotton wool or gauze.
- Confirm her identity by asking her to state her name and date of birth, ensure privacy and expose the injection site, positioning the woman accordingly, (often left lateral for I.M. right ventrogluteal muscle).
- Decontaminate hands, if local policy suggests: clean the injection site (Key-Site) for 30 seconds, up and down, side to side, creating friction. Leave to dry for at least 30 seconds.
- For S.C. injection: identify the site, lift the skin folds (away from the muscle, Fig. 20.4) with the non-injecting hand, decisively inject at a 90° angle, continuing to hold the folds. Inject slowly until the injection is complete. Wait for 10 seconds then

remove the needle and release the skin folds. Apply gentle pressure with cotton wool or gauze, activate the needle defence system, put the used sharps straight into the sharps box
- For I.M. injection: using the landmarks for the chosen injection site (ventrogluteal recommended), identify the specific site for puncture. Remove hands (to prevent needle stick injury) but retain the site of entry in the 'mind's eye'. Using the non-dominant hand gently stretch the skin/subcutaneous tissue 2–3 cm sideways or downwards, then decisively inject at a 90° angle, holding the syringe like a dart and inserting the needle with approximately 1 cm of it still visible. Push on the plunger smoothly at a rate of 10 seconds/mL to inject the solution. Wait 10 seconds, remove the needle and release the skin at the same time. Press gently on the puncture site with the gauze or cotton wool; avoid massage which may cause irritation. Activate the needle defence system and place the used sharps straight into the sharps bin
- Assist the woman to a comfortable position, decontaminate hands.
- Dispose of remaining equipment correctly.
- Document administration and act accordingly; examine the site 2 hours later for any possible reactions.

ROLE AND RESPONSIBILITIES OF THE MIDWIFE

These can be summarized as:
- correct use of equipment and choice of site to facilitate a safe and comfortable injection technique
- knowledge and application of evidence based best practice
- education and support of the woman, particularly if anxious
- correct disposal of sharps
- correct contemporaneous record keeping.

SUMMARY

- Injections require the midwife to choose an appropriate length of needle and correct angle of insertion to ensure that the medication is placed into the correct tissue.
- A number of factors determine which site is chosen, the ventrogluteal site is the one of choice for I.M. injections.
- Whether the skin is cleansed or not prior to injection remains an unanswered question.

- Aspiration is not necessary for S.C. injections, Malkin (2008) suggest that it is not necessary for I.M. either unless using the gluteus maximus site.

- Care is taken to avoid needlestick injury by using needle defence systems and sharps boxes at the point of care, and not resheathing needles.

SELF-ASSESSMENT EXERCISES

The answers to the following questions may be found in the text:

1. Cite examples of when injections may be necessary for a childbearing woman.
2. List the sites suitable for I.M. injection for both the woman and the baby.
3. List the considerations necessary for the safe administration of S.C. Enoxaparin.
4. Demonstrate an I.M. injection for a baby.
5. Compare and contrast the similarities and differences between an I.M. and a S.C. injection in the adult, in relation to the equipment, technique and site.
6. Describe how a Z-track injection is completed.
7. Summarize the role and responsibilities of the midwife when administering an injection.

REFERENCES

Anon., 2007. Intramuscular injection technique. Paediatr. Nurs. 19 (2), 37.

Ansell, L., Dougherty, L., 2011. Medicines management. In: Doughty, L., Lister, S. (Eds.), The Royal Marsden Hospital Manual of Clinical Nursing Procedures, eighth ed. Wiley Blackwell, Chichester, pp. 956–961. (Chapter 16).

Diggle, J., 2014. How to help patients achieve correct self-injection technique. Pract. Nurs. 25 (9), 451–454.

EMC (electronic medicines compendium), 2014. Clexane. Available online: <www.medicines.org.uk/emc/medicine/24345/SPC/Clexane+pre-filled+syringes/> (accessed 29 January 2015).

Gelder, C., 2014. Best practice injection technique for children and young people with diabetes. Nurs. Child. Young People 26 (7), 32–36.

Hall, A., 2015. Administering medications. In: Potter, P.A., Perry, A.G., Stockert, P.A., Hall, A. (Eds.), Essentials for Nursing Practice, eighth ed. Elsevier, St. Louis, pp. 377–462. (Chapter 17).

Hemsworth, S., 2000. Intramuscular injection technique. Paediatr. Nurs. 12 (9), 17–20.

Hicks, D., 2012. Diabetes focus: teaching injection technique will improve quality of life. Nurs. Times 108 (10), 16.

Hicks, D., Kirkland, F., Pledger, J., et al., 2011. Helping people with diabetes to manage their injectable therapies. Primary Health Care 21 (1), 28–31.

Hunter, J., 2008. Intramuscular injection techniques. Nurs. Stand. 22 (24), 35–40.

Jamieson, E.M., McCall, J.M., Blythe, R., et al., 1997. Clinical Nursing Practices, third ed. Churchill Livingstone, Edinburgh.

Jordan, S., 2010. Administration of medicines. In: Jordan, S. (Ed.), Pharmacology for Midwives, second ed. Palgrave Macmillan, Basingstoke, pp. 42–44. (Chapter 2).

Malkin, B., 2008. Intramuscular injection technique: an evidence-based approach. Nurs. Times 104 (50/51), 48–51.

Nicol, M., Bavin, C., Bedford-Turner, S., et al., 2004. Essential Nursing Skills, second ed. Mosby, Edinburgh, p. 130.

Ogston-Tuck, S., 2014a. Intramuscular injection technique: an evidence based approach. Nurs. Stand. 29 (4), 52–59.

Ogston-Tuck, S., 2014b. Subcutaneous injection technique: an evidence based approach. Nurs. Stand. 29 (3), 53–58.

Peragallo-Dittko, V., 1997. Rethinking subcutaneous injection technique. Am. J. Nurs. 97 (5), 71–72.

PHE (Public Health England), 2013. Immunisation procedures: the green book, Chapter 4. In: Part of Immunisation Against Infectious Disease. PHE, London. Available online: <www.gov.uk> (accessed 29 January 2015).

Rodger, M., King, L., 2000. Drawing up and administering intramuscular injections: a review of the literature. J. Adv. Nurs. 31 (3), 574–582.

Rowley, S., Clare, S., 2011. ANTT: a standard approach to aseptic technique. Nurs. Times 107 (36), 12–14.

WHO (World Health Organisation), 2010. WHO Best Practices for Injections and Related Procedures Toolkit. WHO, Geneva, p. 6.

Workman, B., 1999. Safe injection techniques. Nurs. Stand. 13 (39), 47–53.

Zaybak, A., Yapucu, U., Tamsel, S., et al., 2007. Does obesity prevent the needle from reaching muscle in intramuscular injections? J. Adv. Nurs. 58 (6), 552–556.

Chapter | 21 |

Principles of drug administration: administration of medicines *per vaginam*

LEARNING OUTCOMES

Having read this chapter, the reader should be able to:

- discuss the advantages and disadvantages of the vaginal route for the administration of medicines
- describe how a drug is administered P.V.
- discuss the role and responsibilities of the midwife before, during and after drug administration
- list the factors that are pertinent to the administration of prostaglandin P.V.

The midwife is actively involved in the administration of medicines *per vaginam* (P.V.), largely with prostaglandin for the induction of labour. There are a range of preparations that can be administered vaginally (tablet, creams, pessaries, foams, etc.), often used for the treatment of localized infections, contraceptive use or systemic use, e.g. prostaglandins. This chapter considers the midwife's role and responsibilities and the procedure for administration P.V., focusing largely on the administration of prostaglandin E$_2$ (PGE$_2$). This chapter should be read in conjunction with Chapters 18, 29, and 30.

ADVANTAGES AND DISADVANTAGES OF THE VAGINAL ROUTE

The vagina has a large surface area with a good blood supply. Medication is circulated via the internal iliac veins and therefore bypasses the liver. There are likely to be fewer peaks and troughs in plasma levels, the medication being absorbed over a given (often) slow and sustained time span. Despite these advantages, some of the disadvantages make it a less favourable route. These include:

- Embarrassment (survivors of sexual abuse will also find this a traumatic route for medication). If appropriate, can the medication be self-administered?
- Variable absorption – only certain molecules can be absorbed this way, absorption can vary with age and stage of the menstrual cycle and with the changes in pH. Some prostaglandins can be retrieved (like a tampon) if there is an adverse effect.
- Loss of medication through leakage.
- Potential for incorrect placing, e.g. prostaglandin should be placed into the posterior vaginal fornix, never into the cervix.
- Potential irritation to the vaginal wall.
- Potential to introduce infection. Personal protective equipment (PPE) should be used (Chapter 8) and asepsis maintained.

Using prostaglandin

Naturally produced prostaglandins increase towards term and appear to both ripen the cervix and contribute towards uterine contractions (Jordan 2010). Manufactured forms of the drug can be administered for the induction of labour, *per vaginam* is the route of choice. Lower doses are often as effective as higher ones and little benefit is gained by repeated doses. Vaginal gel is better absorbed than vaginal tablets or pessary. It is an unstable compound chemically and so attention should be paid to correct storage (refrigerated generally) and accurate prescribing. Dosages for the different compounds, e.g. gel, tablets, or pessary, are all different, unless otherwise prescribed, they are always placed into the posterior vaginal fornix.

It is recognized that most body systems can be affected by prostaglandins. Gastrointestinal effects, e.g. diarrhoea or nausea, are common, as are flushing, hypo- and hypertension, headache and pyrexia. Some of these effects are seen within 30 minutes of administration. Serious effects such as fetal compromise, bronchospasm, uterine hypertonus, amniotic fluid embolism and uterine rupture have all been noted and care should include specific observations for these risks. Prostaglandin should be used in extreme care with grand multiparous women.

The drug begins working within 10 minutes of administration (gel is faster than pessary) but the woman is asked to retain a semi-recumbent position for 20–30 minutes to improve absorption. She should not be left alone at this time. If a retrieval device is being used, the midwife should remove the prostaglandin if any serious adverse reactions are seen, e.g. significant fetal compromise. Many women need to exercise patience when being induced, they also need to understand the range of analgesics available, prostaglandin-induced contractions often being more painful (NICE 2014).

The NICE (2008) Induction of Labour (IOL) guideline was unchanged following its review in 2014. It suggests:

- Women with uncomplicated pregnancies can be offered induction of labour between 41 and 42 weeks to avoid the risks of prolonged pregnancy. There are fewer perinatal deaths, fewer meconium aspirations, and fewer caesarean sections with its use (Gulmezoglu et al 2012). Care should be woman-centred with the woman able to make a fully informed decision, being particularly aware of the risk of serious complications (NICE 2014). A plan should also be made in the event of a failed induction.
- Bishop's scoring (see Glossary) is undertaken prior to prescription and administration. With consent, membrane sweeping may be undertaken also (see Chapter 29). Depending on which of the preparations is prescribed, Bishop scoring may be repeated later and a second dose may be prescribed. If using a retrieval pessary, it should be removed when the cervix is ripened or after 24 hours, or 30 minutes before an oxytocin infusion (BNF 2014).
- Electronic continuous monitoring of the fetal heart rate should be confirmed as normal prior to PGE_2 administration and repeated when contractions begin. Intermittent auscultation can be used if the contraction pattern is within the sphere of normal.
- Women often prefer to begin the process in the morning, although there is no evidence to suggest that this is more effective. The venue and timing of the administration should permit electronic fetal heart rate assessment. Women who have the administration of prostaglandin as an outpatient should be given clear advice regarding when to consult/return to the maternity unit (NICE 2014).

Considerations for the midwife when administering PGE_2

These can be summarized as:

- Assessment prior to administration: the midwife must be familiar with the local protocols for the administration of PGE_2, most of which are discussed above. Does the woman meet the inclusion criteria, e.g. gestation, parity, previous history?
- Assessing the nine 'rights' of drug administration as for any prescription (p. 145), including specific information for PGE_2: the lubricant used with vaginal drugs should be appropriate, e.g. water-based lubricant, and sterile for single use. Interaction can occur with some preparations, e.g. obstetric cream and PGE_2.
- Understanding the action and side effects of the drug, and therefore education and support of the woman to prepare her for the effect. Antifungal preparations may be self-administered, for which the midwife can have a significant role in educating the woman in infection prevention and drug administration.
- Maintenance of dignity and privacy during an embarrassing procedure.
- Observations made while undertaking the drug administration: e.g. repeated Bishop's scoring, angle of pubic arch, nature of presenting part, other factors that may affect care.
- Correct administration technique, placing the medication in the correct place. The midwife must be competent in the skill of vaginal examination before administering PGE_2 P.V.
- Conscientious care following administration: observations are made both for the expected action and to exclude deviations from the norm. These include assessment of the contractions – strength,

length and frequency; assessment of fetal wellbeing; blood pressure; temperature, pulse and respiration; and assessment for levels of pain.

- Adherence to national and local protocols with regard to infection control, personal protection, the administration of medicines and care in labour.
- Contemporaneous record keeping of the care given before, during and after the administration.

PROCEDURE: administration of medicines P.V.

- Gain informed consent, confirm the prescription, ensure privacy and establish fetal wellbeing.
- Wash and dry hands, put on apron.
- Gather equipment:
  - sterile gloves and handrub
  - sterile vaginal examination pack (according to local protocol)
  - disposable sheet
  - sterile single-use water-based lubricant
  - disposable wipes
  - the drug.
- Confirm the woman's identity. Ask the woman to adopt an almost recumbent position (use a wedge to avoid aortocaval occlusion if necessary), with her knees bent, ankles together and knees parted, placing a disposable sheet beneath her buttocks.
- Remove any sanitary towels or underwear, keeping the genital area covered.
- Open the gloves, open the drug, place it and a blob of the lubricant onto the sterile side of the paper (or use the vaginal examination pack).
- Apply handrub and then gloves.
- Ask the woman to lift the covers exposing the genital area.
- For PGE$_2$ administration, part the labia with the thumb and forefinger of the non-examining hand:
  - lubricate the two fingers of the examining hand and gently insert into the vagina, in a downwards and backwards direction along the posterior vaginal wall to locate the cervix, ensuring the thumb does not come into contact with the woman's clitoris or anus. Slide the gel applicator between the vaginal wall and the examining hand, until it has been guided into the posterior vaginal fornix by the examining hand. The plunger is then depressed by the other hand and the gel administered. Lubricant may be applied to the tip to aid insertion
  - for the application of a tablet or pessary, either insert the examining hand with the pessary secured

between the fingers, guiding it into the fornix as above, or insert the examining hand into the vagina, slide the pessary in using the non-examining hand, and guide it into place using the examining hand. Lubricant may be applied to the pessary to aid insertion.

- Remove fingers, wipe the vulva with the wipes. Ensure that the retrieval string is accessible (if used); maintain the woman's dignity.
- Remove gloves, use handrub, auscultate the fetal heart and then assist the woman to resume a comfortable semi-recumbent position.
- Dispose of equipment correctly and wash and dry hands.
- Document administration and findings and act accordingly.

Other preparations

The procedure is the same for any administration of a medication P.V. except that a vaginal examination is generally not needed when positioning of the medication is not crucial. Under these circumstances the medication often has its own applicator. This is slid along the posterior vaginal wall until the medication is high in the vagina. It is removed after the medication has been ejected.

ROLE AND RESPONSIBILITIES OF THE MIDWIFE

These can be summarized as:

- practising within evidence-based protocols
- education and support of the woman
- observation of normality for mother and fetus, referral if necessary
- contemporaneous documentation.

SUMMARY

- There are both advantages and disadvantages to using the vaginal route for medication.
- For the induction of labour prostaglandin works locally to ripen the cervix. It should be used with caution, serious as well as less serious side effects are possible.
- The midwife has a number of responsibilities including all those associated with the administration of medicines and with safe and effective woman-centred care.

SELF-ASSESSMENT EXERCISES

The answers to the following questions may be found in the text:

1. Describe how the midwife prepares the woman for administration of a P.V. medication.
2. List the possible side effects of PGE$_2$.
3. Describe how PGE$_2$ is administered P.V.
4. Discuss the role and responsibilities of the midwife after the administration of PGE$_2$ P.V.

REFERENCES

BNF (British National Formulary), 2014. BNF66. BMJ Group & Pharmaceutical Press, London.

Gulmezoglu, A.M., Crowther, C.A., Middleton, P., Heatley, E., 2012. Induction of labour for improving birth outcomes for women at or beyond term. Cochrane Database Syst. Rev. (6), Art. No.: CD004945, doi:10.1002/14651858.CD004945.pub3.

Jordan, S., 2010. Drugs increasing uterine contractility: uterotonics (Oxytocics). In: Jordan, S. (Ed.), Pharmacology for Midwives, second ed. Palgrave Macmillan, Basingstoke. (Chapter 6).

NICE (National Institute for Health and Clinical Excellence), 2008. Induction of Labour. NICE, London. Available online: <www.nice.org.uk> (accessed 5 March 2015).

NICE (National Institute for Health and Care Excellence), 2014. NICE Quality Standards (QS60) Induction of Labour April 2014. NICE, London. Available online: <www.nice.org.uk> (accessed 5 March 2015).

Chapter 22

Principles of drug administration: administration of medicines per rectum

LEARNING OUTCOMES

Having read this chapter, the reader should be able to:

- describe the safe administration of suppositories and enemas, making differentiations accordingly
- discuss the issues highlighted in the literature regarding suppository use, identifying that which is researched evidence and that which is not
- discuss the role and responsibilities of the midwife in relation to per rectum (P.R.) administration.

Medicines inserted into the rectum have two predominant actions:

- for laxative purposes
- systemic treatment, e.g. analgesia (paracetamol, diclofenac), uterotonics (misoprostol), anti-emetics (systemic suppositories are sometimes called retention suppositories).

The rectum can be a useful route for the administration of some medicines if the woman is nil by mouth, unconscious, or vomiting. This chapter reviews the correct procedure and discusses the role and responsibilities of the midwife.

The rectal route

This is a commonly used route for the administration of some medicines, but it is not always the most popular route for patients. The superior rectal vein drains the upper part of the rectum, while the inferior rectal veins drain the lower part. The lining of the rectum is delicate. Medicines can be well absorbed but there are potential dangers: rupturing the mucosa, infection and haemorrhage. The nearness of some of the branches of the vagus nerve in the rectum means that a bradycardia can be induced; extreme care is taken with any women needing a suppository who have an existing cardiac condition. There may also be inconsistencies in the amount of drug absorbed via the rectal route: the inferior rectal veins enter the circulation directly (lower rectum), facilitating faster drug absorption. From the upper rectum the superior rectal vein transports medication via the liver; the absorption systemically is slower. The presence of faeces in the rectum can also reduce drug absorption. The midwife should observe the woman for any signs of under- or overdose following P.R. drug administration (Jordan 2010).

Bradshaw et al (2009) suggest that any administration of suppositories or enema should be preceded by a digital rectal examination. This includes a risk assessment: particularly in understanding the client's medical history, examining the perianal area, assessing anal sphincter tone, and noting the presence/absence of faeces in the rectum. A digital rectal examination should be carried out by an appropriately trained and competent practitioner. The author would suggest that the majority of maternity clients are unlikely to need this level of ongoing intervention, those that do should be cared for jointly by obstetric and gastroenterology teams. However, an appreciation of the client's history, and of any perianal anomalies, e.g. perineal trauma, anal sphincter damage, haemorrhoids, genital warts, helminthic infection, are clearly significant factors that impact on the suitability of administering medication P.R.

SUPPOSITORIES

The medication is contained within the pellet that dissolves at body temperature in the rectum. Sometimes ongoing use of suppositories can irritate the bowel; this often relates to whichever melting substance is used. Lubricating the suppository makes its insertion easier and improves the comfort for the woman. The instructions should be checked, some need lubricating with water alone, e.g. glycerin suppositories (BNF 2014).

Which way are they inserted?

The shaping of suppositories has traditionally suggested to practitioners that they should be inserted tapered end first. There is, however, a debate about this. Abd-el-Maeboud et al (1991) considered the anatomy and physiology of the rectum and believed that inserting a suppository blunt end first would facilitate its retention better than if inserted tapered end first. This caused a change in practice (Moppett 2000), but Kyle (2009) has questioned this change. Kyle (2009) considers that Abd-el-Maeboud's trial had a dubious methodology and that changes to practice that are based on an isolated study should be made cautiously. Abd-el-Maeboud et al (1991) suggest that if the suppository is inserted blunt end first the anatomy of the rectum 'sucks' the suppository in as the sphincter closes, whilst inserting a suppository tapered end first prevents the anal sphincter from closing properly. The manufacturers continue to suggest that tapered end first is correct in line with their product licence (Bradshaw & Price 2007). Johnson & Taylor (2010) supported the idea that suppositories for systemic use should be inserted blunt end first while laxative ones should be inserted tapered end first. As Kyle (2009) suggests, if this issue is of considerable significance then further rigorous research is needed promptly. The reader should be aware of the devolving argument, any future studies and their locally agreed protocol.

Where should they be placed?

The rectum is the last 10–12 cm of the large colon, it is straight, but then curves to follow the line of the sacrum. Its latter part is the anal canal, this includes strong muscular sphincters, internally and externally. The anatomy

suggested by Abd-el-Maeboud et al (1991) implies that the suppository is retained, even if only inserted a small way into the rectum. It is generally accepted, however, that for laxative purposes suppositories should be inserted 2–4 cm in, beyond the anal canal into the rectum. While the differences in blood supply to different parts of the rectum were noted earlier, trying to place the suppository correctly in relation to this is almost impossible.

Laxative suppositories should be placed between the faeces and the rectal wall. Suppositories for systemic use work better if the rectum is empty; they too should be in contact with the rectal wall.

ENEMAS

Enemas for systemic use are often small (microenemas) while laxative ones generally contain more fluid. Both have a nozzle that extends into the rectum (beyond the anal canal), often about 10 cm in length but only intended to be inserted 2–4 cm as for suppositories. Addison et al (2000) suggest that lengthy tubing is to aid self-administration, rather than high rectal insertion. If a large fluid enema is to be used, it should be warmed to body temperature to prevent shock occurring. The tubing is lubricated, as for suppositories, and the air is excluded before insertion.

INFORMED CONSENT

Obtaining consent for the giving of medication via the P.R. route includes (among other things) an appreciation of the type and effect of the drug. Sometimes an association is made with suppositories and the laxative effect without realizing that systemic medications are given this way also. An unconscious woman (e.g. after general anaesthetic) would need to give consent prior to the surgery commencing. All clients need to understand what administration P.R. involves in order to give informed consent.

POSITIONING OF THE WOMAN

Traditionally it is considered easier to insert laxative suppositories and all types of enemas if the woman adopts a left lateral position with one or both of her knees flexed (Fig. 22.1). In this position insertion then follows the natural anatomy of the colon, flexed knees reduce the discomfort of the anus as the suppository is passed through the sphincter. This requires the midwife to use their right hand, even if left handed. However, because of the action of only pushing it through the sphincter, the insertion of a

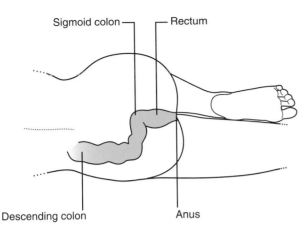

Sigmoid colon — — Rectum

Descending colon — Anus

Figure 22.1 Suggested positioning for insertion of P.R. medication. *(Adapted with kind permission from Jamieson et al 2002)*

blunt end first systemic suppository can be administered in any position, e.g. while the woman is still in lithotomy after procedures such as perineal repair. The midwife can use the hand that suits them.

PROCEDURE: administration of medicines per rectum

- The prescription is scrutinized and dispensed according to the nine 'rights' (see p. 145).
- Gain informed consent and ensure privacy. Wash and dry hands. (If the medication is for systemic use, the woman should be encouraged to open her bowels before its administration.)
- Gather equipment:
  - suppository(ies) or (warmed) enema
  - non-sterile gloves and alcohol handrub
  - disposable sheet
  - compatible lubricant, usually water-based
  - gauze swabs
  - plastic apron
  - a trolley or tray from which to work.
- After removing underwear, the woman is asked to lie in a left lateral position with one or both of her knees flexed. Place the disposable sheet beneath her buttocks and cover her with a bed sheet.
- Put on plastic apron, apply handrub, and put on gloves. Ask the woman to lift the sheet.
- Place lubricant on the gauze, lubricate the tapered end of the suppository (if laxative), the blunt end (if systemic), or the tubing tip (if an enema). Expel the air from the enema tubing by pushing the solution through to the tip.
- Ask the woman to take a deep breath (this relaxes the anal sphincter).

- Lift the woman's right buttock using the left hand:
  - laxative suppository: insert the suppository tapered end first, 2–4 cm into the rectum using the right index or middle finger. Place it between the faeces and rectal wall. Insert a second suppository in the same way if required
  - systemic suppository: gently push the blunt end first through the anal sphincter. The finger does not need to enter the rectum
  - Insert the enema tubing, advancing it slowly 2–4 cm. The fluid runs in by gravity (Addison et al 2000). Withdraw the tubing carefully once completed, maintaining pressure on the pack to prevent the fluid flowing back into it.
- Wipe the perineum with the gauze, re-cover the woman. Remove gloves and apron, apply handrub, and assist her into a comfortable position.
- Encourage her to retain the medication for as long as possible. Aim for laxatives to be retained for at least 10–20 minutes.
- Assist later, if needed, to the toilet.
- Dispose of equipment correctly and wash and dry hands.
- Document administration and effect and act accordingly.

ROLE AND RESPONSIBILITIES OF THE MIDWIFE

These can be summarized as:

- appropriate checking and dispensing of the drug (as for any prescription)
- understanding the action and possible side effects of the drug: the effect/side effect should always be reported and recorded. If given for laxative purposes, the quantity, colour and consistency of the stool should be recorded according to the Bristol stool classifications (p. 141)
- education and support of the woman: gaining informed consent so that she has realistic expectations of the procedure and outcome
- maintenance of dignity and privacy during an embarrassing procedure
- correct administration technique, placing the medication in the correct place, upholding the infection control and personal protective equipment protocols. Avoidance of potential complications
- appropriate care following administration: e.g. toilet facilities with assistance to reach them, if necessary (laxatives), assessment of pain levels or incidence of vomiting (systemic medication)
- contemporaneous record keeping of the care given before, during and after the administration.

SUMMARY

- Administration of medicines P.R. may be for laxative or systemic purposes. The debate continues as to which end of the suppository should be inserted first.
- The midwife should be familiar with the effect of the drug and how to administer it correctly.

SELF-ASSESSMENT EXERCISES

The answers to the following questions may be found in the text:

1. Discuss the advantages and disadvantages of using the rectal route for medicine administration.
2. List the information the midwife should be familiar with before administering a laxative suppository.
3. Discuss the evidence that determines which end of a suppository should be inserted first.
4. Describe how a laxative enema is administered.
5. Summarize the role and responsibilities of the midwife when administering a medicine P.R.

REFERENCES

Abd-el-Maeboud, K.H., El-Naggar, T., El-Hawi, E., et al., 1991. Rectal suppository: commonsense and the mode of insertion. Lancet. 338 (8770), 798–800.

Addison, R., Ness, W., Swift, I., 2000. How to administer enemas and suppositories. Nurs. Times NT Plus 96 (6), 3–4.

BNF (British National Formulary), 2014. BNF 66. British Medical Association, Royal Pharmaceutical Society, London.

Bradshaw, A., Price, L., 2007. Rectal suppository insertion: the reliability of the evidence as a basis for nursing practice. J. Clin. Nurs. 16 (1), 98–103.

Bradshaw, E., Collins, B., Williams, J., 2009. Administering rectal suppositories: preparation, assessment and insertion. Gastrointest. Nurs. 7 (9), 24–28.

Jamieson, E.M., McCall, J., Whyte, L., 2002. Clinical Nursing Practices, fourth ed. Churchill Livingstone, Edinburgh.

Johnson, R., Taylor, W., 2010. Skills for Midwifery Practice, third ed. Elsevier, Edinburgh, p. 161.

Jordan, S., 2010. Administration of medicines. In: Jordan, S. (Ed.), Pharmacology for Midwives, second ed. Palgrave Macmillan, Basingstoke, pp. 39–61. (Chapter 2).

Kyle, G., 2009. Practice questions. Nurs. Times 105 (2), 16.

Moppett, S., 2000. Which way is up for a suppository? Nurs. Times 96 (19), 12–13. NT Plus Supplement.

Chapter 23

Principles of drug administration: intravenous drug administration

Midwives are required to administer intravenous (I.V.) drugs to women, and sometimes babies, and should be trained and assessed as competent in this procedure, with regular updating to maintain this competency (NMC 2012). Intravenous drugs can be given as a small 'bolus' or 'push', as a large-volume infusion, or via a volume-controlled or patient-controlled infusion device. While antibiotics are the most common I.V. drugs administered, opioids, paracetamol, and uterotonics are examples of other drugs that may be given. This chapter considers the administration of I.V. medication for women as a 'bolus/push' or an intermittent infusion and concludes with a discussion on the use of continuous I.V. administration using a syringe-driver and patient-controlled analgesia. Administration of I.V. drugs to the neonate is not discussed. This chapter should be read in conjunction with Chapters 10, 18, 47 and 48.

LEARNING OUTCOMES

Having read this chapter, the reader should be able to:

- list the indications for using the intravenous route
- discuss the possible disadvantages of using the intravenous route
- describe each of the different ways that drugs can be administered intravenously
- demonstrate giving an intravenous drug as a bolus and by intermittent infusion
- discuss the role and responsibilities of the midwife when undertaking intravenous drug administration.

INDICATIONS FOR I.V. USE

- When rapid absorption and effect is required.
- When constant therapeutic blood levels of a drug are required.
- When drugs are contraindicated by other routes, e.g. oral, intramuscular (I.M.).
- Where peripheral perfusion is poor, reducing the effect of drugs administered by injection.

DISADVANTAGES OF THE I.V. ROUTE

- It requires a patent peripheral I.V. cannula which may cause pain in the short-term.
- It is an invasive procedure increasing the risk of infection.

- The rapid absorption of the drug increases the risk for a reaction to the drug to occur.
- There is increased potential for medication errors, e.g. drug and physiochemical incompatibility, particularly if multiple drug infusions are required at the same time and the drugs are able to mix (Bertsche et al 2008, Nemec et al 2008).
- There is increased potential for bacterial or particulate contamination if drugs are being diluted or added to other fluids (Bertsche et al 2008).

SAFETY CONCERNS

Aceves et al (2013) caution that despite all the improvements in I.V. medication administrations, particularly with advancing technology, there still remains a high-risk for error compared with other forms of drug administration. Shane (2009) suggests that 61% of serious and life-threatening drug errors are related to the administration of I.V. drugs with 73% of I.V. boluses being given too quickly. Cousins et al (2005) found this centred around four areas:

1. Unlabelled prepared drugs that were left for short periods were being administered to the wrong patient.
2. The wrong diluent was used resulting in the powder not dissolving or being inactivated.
3. The drug being given too quickly when administered as a bolus, which can cause phlebitis but may also result in an adverse event for the patient.
4. Loss of patency of the cannula and, more concerning, not adhering to the principles of an Aseptic Non Touch Technique (see Chapter 10 and discussed below).

The Institute for Safe Medication Practice (ISMP) (2015) advise discarding any unattended unlabelled syringes containing any type of solution and recommend that the syringe is always labelled once the drug is drawn up, unless this is done by the patient's bedside and administered immediately. They also recommend using, wherever possible, medication in a ready-to-administer form (ISMP 2015). However, this is often not possible and it is important to follow the manufacturer's instructions on which diluent to use (usually water or normal saline 0.9%). Powder must be diluted. If the powder is not dissolving it should be discarded and another dose of the drug and diluent mixed.

To promote safe medication management, the 'nine rights' should be checked in relation to the drug, the diluent, and the flush (see p. 145) by two midwives, one of whom must be the administrator of the drug (NMC 2008). Both midwives should ensure they independently check the medical infusion device is set to the correct programme for delivery of the medication (if used).

The cannulation site should be assessed before the drug is drawn up, with signs of infiltration and extravasation looked for (see Chapter 47). The cannula should be confirmed as being patent before administering the bolus as Hall (2015) cautions that accidental injection of drugs into the tissues rather than the vein can result in pain, sloughing of the tissues and abscess formation. If there is any doubt, the cannula should be flushed and if not patent, the cannula should be removed and a new one sited elsewhere if there is still a need for I.V. medication.

Flush

The site should be flushed with 2–5 mL of normal saline before and after the administration of drugs; if more than one drug is given, the cannula should be flushed between drugs to avoid drug incompatibilities (Ansell & Dougherty 2011).

Aseptic Non Touch Technique (ANTT)

It is important to use an ANTT approach to reduce the very real risk of infection occurring (see Chapter 10). An ANTT should be used when reconstituting the drug and when handling the syringe and cannula/needleless port (Key-Parts). The use of gloves will also protect the midwife's hands from contact with the drug constituents whilst the drug is being drawn up.

BOLUS/PUSH ADMINISTRATION (DIRECT INTERMITTENT INJECTION)

An I.V. bolus introduces a concentrated dose of a drug through a needless port (often via an extension set) directly into the circulation, usually with a small amount of fluid (Hall 2015). This is useful when there is concern about fluid overload, but the high concentration can also cause a chemical phlebitis, particularly if administered quickly (Scales 2008). The bolus is administered as a 'push' as the midwife will physically push the drug through the woman's cannula. Hall (2015) considers this to be the most dangerous way to administer drugs as they will be absorbed quickly with no time to correct errors. It is important the midwife is aware of the manufacturer's recommendations for the speed of administration or where these are not available, the local approved guideline should be followed. deWit & O'Neill (2014) caution that no intravenous drug should be administered in less than 60 seconds and

Ansell & Dougherty (2011) suggest most drugs would be administered between 3 and 10 minutes but if there are no recommendations regarding the rate of administration, they suggest proceeding slowly over 5–10 minutes. Further advice can be sought from the hospital pharmacist if any doubt exists. It is particularly helpful to give the drug slowly if there is a possibility of an anaphylactic reaction occurring, as this usually happens quickly and it enables the midwife to stop administering the drug (see Chapter 18).

PROCEDURE: 'push' administration

- Check that the cannula is patent and has an injection port, preferably a needleless one, attached (and an extension set if used).
- Undertake the thorough checking procedures, as for any medication administration (see Chapter 18).
- Decontaminate hands, clean a plastic tray with the locally approved cleanser to establish a General Aseptic Field, wash and dry hands.
- Gather equipment:
  - the medicine administration chart
  - the drug, including correct solution if it is to be diluted
  - appropriately sized sterile syringes, sterile syringe caps/covers and filter needles
  - non-sterile gloves (ensure the woman does not have a latex allergy)
  - pre-prepared 10-mL sodium chloride 0.9% flush or 10-mL sodium chloride 0.9% ampoule/vial with 10-mL syringe for flushing (or locally approved flushing solution)
  - cleaned plastic tray
  - approved skin cleanser, often 70% alcohol/2% chlorhexidine wipe
  - portable sharps box.
- Wash and dry hands and put on non-sterile gloves.
- Open the plunger end of the syringe packaging, 'prepare' the syringe by ensuring that the plunger moves within the barrel. Connect the filter needle firmly, using an ANTT (Key-Parts are the syringe tip and needle hub). Place the connected syringe and sheathed needle onto the tray.
- If a diluent is used:
  - open the diluent by snapping off the top
  - unsheath the needle and insert into the diluent, keeping the end of the needle within the solution to reduce the aspiration of air bubbles
  - draw up the required amount of diluent (Key-Parts are the diluent and needle) by either keeping the ampoule/vial upright on a flat surface or inverting the ampoule/vial and keeping the needle central (McKenna & Lim 2014)

- place on tray
- open the drug by snapping off the top, having first ensured all the powder/liquid is at the bottom of the ampoule/vial and insert the needle into the ampoule/vial (Key-Parts are the needle and the ampoule/vial top)
- gently mix the drug and diluent to ensure the drug dissolves
- withdraw the volume required (Key-Part is the needle).
- If there is no diluent:
  - open the drug by snapping off the top, having first ensured all the liquid is at the bottom of the ampoule/vial. If a vial is used with a rubber bung, the bung should be cleaned with the approved cleanser for 20 seconds, up and down, side to side, creating friction then left to dry for at least 30 seconds
  - unsheath the needle and insert into the ampoule/vial to withdraw the required amount of drug (Key-Parts are the needle and drug). If the ampoule has a rubber bung McKenna & Lim (2014) recommend air is drawn into the syringe equal to the volume of the drug required, the needle is inserted centrally, and the air injected taking care not to inject into the solution. Keep the needle in the solution to prevent air from being aspirated into the syringe.
- When the required volume of drug is drawn up, invert the syringe and examine it for air. If necessary tap the syringe gently to encourage the air up to the top of the syringe; push the plunger to exclude the air from the syringe, ensuring none of the solution is lost and the dosage in the syringe is correct.
- Remove the needle from the syringe without touching the end of the syringe and place in the sharps box.
- Cover the end of the syringe with a sterile cap/cover without touching the Key-Parts and place on the plastic tray.
- Label the syringe.
- Draw up a flush if required, using the ANTT described above, label and place on the plastic tray.
- Remove gloves and wash and dry hands.
- Take the medicine administration chart, sharps box, approved skin cleanser and tray to the woman.
- With both checkers present, confirm her identity by asking her to state her name and date of birth and checking her identity label with the medication administration chart.
- Decontaminate hands and apply non-sterile gloves.

- Scrub the tip of the I.V. port (Key-Site) with the approved cleanser for 20 seconds, up and down, side to side, creating friction and using different parts of the wipe. Then clean away from the tip using a non touch technique. Leave to dry for at least 30 seconds.
- If present, check the infusion for its smooth running then stop it.
- If using a flush, remove the cap/cover from the syringe containing the flush.
- Attach the syringe to the needleless port and inject half of the flush observing around the cannula site for swelling, then disconnect the syringe, recover with a sterile cap/cover using a non touch technique, and replace onto the tray.
- Remove the cap/cover from the syringe containing the drug.
- Attach the syringe and inject the first 1 mL of the drug according to the manufacturer's recommendations, observing the woman's condition throughout (Hayes & Williamson 1998).
  - if an infusion is present, it can be restarted and if no problems are noticed, stop the infusion, and continue to administer the rest of the drug at the correct rate
  - if the infusion fluid is incompatible with the medication, Ansell & Dougherty (2011) recommend stopping the infusion and flushing the line before and after the medication administration and then restarting the infusion
  - if no infusion is present continue to inject the drug according to the manufacturer's instructions.
- If an adverse reaction develops while administering the drug, stop the administration, call the doctor, and manage accordingly.
- Repeat the flushing with the remaining normal saline, using pulsation and positive pressure, as described on page 354. If present recommence the infusion at the appropriate rate.
- Dispose of equipment correctly.
- Remove gloves.
- Wash and dry hands.
- Document administration and effects and act accordingly.

INTERMITTENT INFUSION (LARGER VOLUME)

The medication can be added to a larger volume (25–250 mL) of compatible fluid and administered as an infusion over 15 minutes to 2 hours (Ansell & Dougherty 2011). This should be in line with the manufacturer's instructions or follow the locally approved guideline. The infusion should preferably be administered through a medical infusion device to ensure it runs over the correct time period (see Chapter 48). The intermittent infusion is achieved by:

- adding drugs to a burette giving set of an existing infusion, with the existing infusion being stopped until the drugs have been administered, or
- attaching a prepared infusion containing the drug to a giving set and connecting this to the cannula if there is not an existing infusion, or
- connecting the prepared infusion of the drug (and giving set) to a needless port (ideally the one closest to the cannula) (ISMP 2015) when there is an existing infusion, with the existing infusion being stopped until the drugs have been administered to prevent back-tracking of fluid (MHRA 2010).

If there is not a current infusion running, the cannula will require flushing before and after administration, as described above. The administration set may be retained for the next dose provided sterility is maintained, but should be renewed after 24 hours. Hand decontamination is essential at each stage of the procedure and it is important that care is taken not to introduce microorganisms into the closed system and using an ANTT.

If drugs are added to a bag of fluid, it is important that:

- an ANTT is used when drawing up and adding medication to the fluid, the fluid to the burette or giving set and the needleless port (all Key-Parts)
- the fluid and drug are compatible
- care is taken not to puncture the bag with the needle
- an additive label is applied with the drug, dose, name, and number of the woman, and date and time the drug was added and signed by the two midwives involved in the checking procedure
- the drug and fluid are thoroughly mixed (by inverting the bag gently)
- the checking procedures are the same as for bolus administration
- the flow rate is correct.

Documentation in the woman's notes should include the amount of the drug and diluent used (if any), time and duration of administration and whether by a bolus or intermittent infusion. The response of the woman should be noted and documented. If the cannula has been flushed, documentation should also include what was used, the amount and whether it was before, after or both. The medication chart should also be signed.

ADMINISTRATION USING A SYRINGE DRIVER

A syringe driver (or pump) is a small powered (mains and battery) infusion pump that gradually administers small amounts of a drug or fluid contained within a syringe by driving the plunger of the syringe at an accurately controlled rate thereby maintaining constant blood levels of the drug. Tubing connects the syringe to the needleless port of the cannula and this is primed as for any other I.V. tubing prior to use. The syringe contains a drug that is usually prediluted to a specific strength and this should not be diluted further, although the initial dilution can be made up in the clinical area. A 60-mL syringe is usually the largest size syringe that can be accommodated with these devices and most pumps can use smaller syringes.

Errors in the use of syringe drivers occur in a number of areas – incorrect drug calculation, drug incompatibility and instability, equipment failure, incorrect infusion rate, inadequate user training, inadequate documentation and poor servicing of equipment (Kain et al 2006). Thus it is vital the midwife has received training in how to use the equipment (particularly how to correctly insert the syringe), can use a second checker to confirm the infusion rate and that the device has been serviced according to manufacturer's instructions.

The majority of new syringe drivers use mL/hr to calculate the administration rate. Many pumps are programmable and each NHS Trust will have a number of regimes programmed so that all the midwife needs to do is find the appropriate programme.

However, older ambulatory syringe drivers may use millimetres to calculate the administration rate which is not intuitive. Their use is not common in the Western world. The length of fluid to be administered must be known and the drug is diluted so that the total length is divisible by 12. Instruction booklets will be provided with each driver, but the general rule is:

$$\{\text{Length of fluid (mm)/Delivery time (hours)}\} = \text{rate setting (mm/hour)}$$

For example, if 36 mm of fluid is to be infused over 12 hours then the rate would be 3 mm/hour.

The setting up of the pump relies on several standard principles:

- use of an ANTT
- calculation of the amount of drug required over the given period of time with appropriate solution for dilution
- use of a sterile syringe, correctly sized to fit the driver and inserted so that the plunger is secure
- sterile preparation and dilution of the drug (may be supplied pre-prepared)
- use of sterile tubing that will fit the needleless port; the tubing must be primed and attached, after measurement and calculation of the rate or accessing the correct programme
- the syringe must be labelled correctly with the name, dose and volume of the drug and expiry date
- the driver should be maintained and in full working order; alarms for 'occlusion' and 'infusion complete' must be working and the midwife must make regular observations of the pump to ensure it is running to time.

PATIENT-CONTROLLED ANALGESIA

Patient-controlled analgesia (PCA) is primarily used for postoperative analgesia particularly with I.V. opioid use but may also be used during labour with some epidurals. The syringe driver has a button the woman presses to administer a pre-set dose of the drug giving the woman the control of when and how much of the drug to have. A lockout interval can be programmed to prevent doses being administered too quickly resulting in overdose and providing time for the initial dose to take effect (usually 5–10 minutes). The pump can also be programmed to deliver a given dose over a set period of time usually 1–4 hours. Each device has an inbuilt tamper-proof mechanism to prevent the woman, visitors or others changing the dose and or frequency of the bolus.

McKenna & Lim (2014) suggest that when a PCA is used, there is a tendency to use less medication as women are able to self-administer before the pain becomes very difficult to manage and deWit & O'Neill (2014) report greatly reduced anxiety levels in regard to pain because the woman is in control. Ismail et al (2012) also found there was improved pain control, less need for rescue analgesia for breakthrough pain, lower incidence of nausea and vomiting, and greater patient satisfaction when PCA pethidine was used for post–caesarean section analgesia. Demirel et al (2014) found similar results when tramadol was administered via a PCA rather than as a continuous intravenous infusion. Another advantage of PCAs is that they can maintain a fairly constant concentration of the drug within the blood.

Side effects of the PCA are related to the drug being administered and for opioid use include nausea, vomiting, pruritus, respiratory depression, sedation, confusion and urinary retention (Momeni et al 2006).

The midwife setting up the infusion must set:

- the lockout interval
- a 1- or a 4-hour dose limit
- limit of the drug that the woman can receive with each boost.

ROLE AND RESPONSIBILITIES OF THE MIDWIFE

These can be summarized as:

- adherence to local regimes for training and updating of skills
- using an ANTT for all procedures
- correct administration procedure, as per the NMC (2008) and local regimes
- observation of the woman for any unexpected or adverse responses
- contemporaneous record keeping.

SUMMARY

- I.V. drugs have a swift effect which, while advantageous, can also be problematic if an adverse drug reaction occurs.
- An ANTT should be used throughout the setting up and administration of an I.V. drug.
- I.V. drugs may be given in the following ways:
  - intermittent direct bolus or 'push' injection
  - intermittent infusion
  - additives to an infusion
  - syringe driver 12- or 24-hour infusion
  - syringe driver with patient control.
- The midwife needs to be competent in the administration of medication I.V. and the correct use of all devices used in her clinical area of practice and maintain this competency.
- When given as a 'bolus' injection, it is important to administer the drug slowly to reduce the risk of phlebitis and adverse reactions.

SELF-ASSESSMENT EXERCISES

The answers to the following questions may be found in the text:

1. What are the advantages and disadvantages of administering drugs via the I.V. route?
2. Discuss the ways in which I.V. drugs can be administered.
3. Describe how you would administer a bolus dose of I.V. antibiotics.
4. How do the principles of ANTT apply to I.V. drug administration?
5. Discuss the advantages of patient-controlled analgesia.
6. Summarize the role and responsibilities of the midwife when administering drugs intravenously.

REFERENCES

Aceves, C.M., Oladimeji, P., Thimbleby, H., Lee, P., 2013. Pre prescribed infusions running as intended? Quantitative analysis of log files from infusion pumps used in a large acute NHS hospital. Br. J. Nurs. Carefusion Suppl: 22 (14), 15–21.

Ansell, L., Dougherty, L., 2011. Medicines management. In: Dougherty, L., Lister, S. (Eds.), The Royal Marsden Manual of Clinical Nursing Procedures, eighth ed. Wiley-Blackwell, Chichester.

Bertsche, T., Mayer, Y., Stahl, R., et al., 2008. Prevention of intravenous drug incompatibilities in an intensive care unit. Am. J. Health Syst. Pharm. 65 (19), 1834–1840.

Cousins, D.H., Sabatier, B., Begue, D., et al., 2005. Medication errors in intravenous drug preparation and administration: a multicentre audit in the UK, Germany and France. Qual. Saf. Health Care 14 (3), 190–195.

Demirel, I., Ozer, A.B., Atilgan, R., et al., 2014. Comparison of patient-controlled analgesia versus continuous infusion of tramadol in post-cesarean section pain management. J. Obstet. Gynaecol. Res. 40 (2), 392–398.

deWit, S.C., O'Neill, P., 2014. Fundamental Concepts and Skills for Nursing, fourth ed. Elsevier, St. Louis, pp. 720–726.

Hall, A., 2015. Administering medications. In: Potter, P.A., Perry, A.G., Stockert, P.A., Hall, A. (Eds.), Essentials for Nursing Practice, eighth ed. Elsevier, St. Louis, pp. 423–458.

Hayes, C., Williamson, E., 1998. Injection technique: intravenous 2. Nurs. Times 94 (46), 40.

Ismail, S., Afshan, G., Monem, A., Ahmed, A., 2012. Postoperative analgesia following caesarean section: intravenous patient controlled analgesia versus conventional continuous infusion. Open J. Anesthesiol. 2, 120–126.

ISMP (Institute for Safe Medication Practice), 2015. ISMP's National Summit on safe practices associated with intravenous push medication administrations for adults: Draft Consensus Statement. Available online: <www.ismp.org/Tools/guidelines/IVSummitPush/statements.aspx> (accessed 8 February 2015).

Kain, V.J., Yates, P.M., Barrett, L., et al., 2006. Developing guidelines for syringe driver management. Int. J. Palliat. Nurs. 12 (2), 60–67.

McKenna, L., Lim, A.G., 2014. Medications. In: Dempsey, J., Hillege, S., Hill, R. (Eds.), Fundamentals of Nursing and Midwifery second Australian and New Zealand Edn. Lippincott

Williams & Wilkins, Sydney, pp. 768–773.

MHRA (Medicines and Healthcare products Regulatory Agency), 2010. Medical safety alert Intravenous (IV) extension sets with multiple ports – risk of backtracking. Available online: <https://www.gov.uk/drug-device -alerts/medical-device-alert -intravenous-iv-extension-sets-with -multiple-ports-risk-of-backtracking> (accessed 8 February 2015).

Momeni, M., Crucitti, M., De Kock, M., 2006. Patient-controlled analgesia in the management of postoperative pain. Drugs 66 (18), 2321–2337.

Nemec, K., Kopelent-Frank, H., Greif, R., 2008. Standardization of infusion solutions to reduce the risk of incompatibility. Am. J. Health Syst. Pharm. 65 (17), 1648–1654.

NMC (Nursing and Midwifery Council), 2008. Standards for Medicine Management. NMC, London. Available online: <http://www .nmc-uk.org/Publications/Standards/> (accessed 3 March 2015).

NMC (Nursing and Midwifery Council), 2012. Midwives Rules and Standards. NMC, London. Available online: <http://www.nmc-uk.org/ Publications/standards/> (accessed 3 March 2015).

Scales, K., 2008. Intravenous therapy: a guide to good practice. Br. J. Nurs. 17 (19), S4–S12.

Shane, R., 2009. Identifying the risk points: Back to the basics. Available online: <http://www.ashpadvantage .com/3CPE/p3-handout.pdf> (accessed 8 February 2015).

Chapter 24

Principles of drug administration: inhalational analgesia: Entonox

LEARNING OUTCOMES

Having read this chapter, the reader should be able to:

- describe the safe and effective use of oxygen and nitrous oxide (50/50)
- identify the signs and symptoms that accompany adverse reactions and discuss appropriate management should any occur
- detail the role and responsibilities of the midwife when administering it.

Midwives will be familiar with the use of medication to inhale for the purposes of general anaesthesia, and with the administration of oxygen by inhalation, but the primary inhalational medication used by midwives is Entonox.

Entonox (one of its trade names) is a 50%-each mixture of oxygen and nitrous oxide. In this concentration it acts as an effective analgesic when inhaled. Its use in UK maternity settings is, potentially, for all stages of labour, where the analgesic effect is achieved with only minimal side effects for the mother and fetus. Entonox is used increasingly across other areas of medical care including paediatrics and trauma care. This chapter reviews its safe use and the role and responsibilities of the midwife.

UNDERSTANDING ENTONOX

Entonox is a colourless gas, supplied piped or in cylinders. If piped, the tubing is a blue and white stripe, if supplied in a cylinder, the cylinder shoulders are blue and white. Newer cylinders have the name written on the side. For the purposes of analgesia, Entonox is self-administered by the woman, under the supervision of an appropriately trained midwife. In the UK Entonox is on the P (Pharmacy) list of medicines (see Chapter 18) and so may be administered by midwives in the course of their professional practice. As for any medication, the midwife must be satisfied that its use is indicated and that they have been trained accordingly. The woman uses a mouthpiece or mask to which a demand/expiratory valve is attached. The mask is held over the nose and mouth with an airtight seal, or the mouthpiece is placed in the mouth. As the woman breathes in, the Entonox is heard to be released; the apparatus should remain in place during expiration. Self-administration allows the woman to regulate the amount taken according to need and to avoid overdosing. The apparatus also includes a microbiological filter to prevent any cross-infection. It has a slightly sweet smell and taste (Nagele et al 2014) but often not enough for women to notice or comment.

Analgesia can be achieved within a few breaths (25–35 seconds), the maximum peak occurring after only 2–3 minutes of breathing it. For the most effective use of Entonox, the contractions are palpated so that the gas is taken immediately when the contraction commences, and before the perception of pain. Just as the effects are seen rapidly, the gas is also excreted from the lungs rapidly. This means that the effects are present for approximately 60 seconds after breathing it has ceased, with no effects after that, until breathing it recommences. Consequently the woman can stop inhaling the gas at the peak of the contraction, knowing that the analgesic effect is still in place. This is also one way to avoid an excessive intake of Entonox (see below).

It is a suitable analgesic for labour, often giving sufficient pain relief while allowing the woman to retain control within her labour. Her ability to experience contractions remains, as does her level of consciousness, rationality and mobility. NICE (2014) suggest that it should be available in all birth settings, although it is acknowledged that its effectiveness is not proven. Green (1993) indicates that women have good levels of satisfaction with Entonox use in labour. From their observations in practice many midwives will agree that one of the benefits of inhalational analgesia is that the woman focuses on breathing regularly, has something to hold on to and therefore has a certain level of distraction that may help her through each contraction.

In the second stage of labour breathing the analgesia may help the woman in the interim if waiting for the presenting part to descend before actively pushing. It can be used effectively for examining the perineum and for suturing at the end of the third stage of labour. Without uterine contractions the woman is able to breathe the Entonox for a minute or more before any part of the procedure is undertaken.

It is noted that Entonox crosses the placenta, but it has no known negative effects on the fetus (BOC 2011). The neonate also excretes it via their lungs at birth, this effective form of excretion avoids the less mature liver and kidneys (Jordan 2010).

POTENTIAL COMPLICATIONS

- Hypoxia. There are two possible causes for potential hypoxia when using Entonox. Firstly, it is noted that at the end of an anaesthetic procedure when nitrous oxide is stopped abruptly (and room air breathed), oxygen tension can fall as nitrous oxide floods the alveoli. This is known as 'diffusion hypoxia', and is generally a transient situation. Oxygen should be available to administer to the woman or neonate, should this occur. Care should also be taken to ensure that Entonox is not used for longer than 24 hours. For some labours this means commencing it when labour is established, rather than using it in the latent phase.

- Secondly, Entonox needs to be stored in such a way that the two gases do not separate out. At $-6°C$ for cylinders, or piped at $-30°C$, the gas separation means pure oxygen would be administered first, followed by pure nitrous oxide. Both of these are life-threatening situations. Entonox cylinders should be stored horizontally and at room temperature (at least $>10°C$) to prevent this separation. Community midwives should be particularly alert to this in the winter months if the cylinder is left in the car.

- Hyper- and hypoventilation. The self-administration of Entonox means that often women hyperventilate during a contraction in order to achieve maximum pain relief. This is often followed by hypoventilation between contractions. Excessive breathing (hyperventilation) results in a reduction of carbon dioxide, this commences a cascade of effects that can include dizziness, fetal hypoxia and tetany. Tetany may result in spasm of the larynx and airway obstruction, early signs include involuntary spasms in the muscles of the extremities. Jordan (2010) recommends that the breaths taken when using Entonox should be slow and with reasonable depth. Dizziness, tingling, or twitching in the hands are all suggestive signs of hyperventilation.

- Depth of anaesthesia. Nitrous oxide, as for all anaesthetic gases, depresses the nervous system. Women can become drowsy, self-administration determines that were this to happen, the mask or mouthpiece would fall away and the gas would be excreted from the lungs in the next few breaths. Sedation greater than this, or an obvious detachment from the situation (often with hallucinations) would suggest that a deeper stage of anaesthesia has been reached than is desired. (In deeper anaesthesia the woman is unable to respond to verbal commands). The Entonox should be stopped and medical assessment organized. Nausea is a common side effect; vomiting, if the woman is sedated in this way, is potentially life threatening. Entonox is often used alongside other analgesics; level of sedation, respiration rate and respiration depth should be monitored, particularly if opioids have been administered as well. BOC (2008) specifically caution against the use of Entonox with high dose of fentanyl, the two can cause a reduced heart rate and cardiac output.

- Existing pathology. The effectiveness of Entonox as an analgesic will potentially be impaired for some groups of women. This includes any compromise to the cardiovascular system, e.g. pre-eclampsia; nervous system damage, e.g. muscular sclerosis; and haematology changes, e.g. sickle cell anaemia. It is also noted that nitrous oxide can expand any existing pockets of gas within the body (BOC 2011). Anyone with known sinus or ear problems should use nitrous oxide with caution.

- Fire risk. As for all combustible gases care should be taken to avoid sources of fire and any grease. This is pertinent in the home as well as medical establishments.
- Staff exposure. Robertson (2006) reiterates the need for occupational awareness of health and safety. Maternity units should have effective ventilation and scavenger systems, staff should also consider wearing personal exposure monitors, particularly if working consistently on labour wards. Care should be taken to avoid standing in front of women when Entonox is being breathed out. Vitamin B_{12} can be inhibited with exposure to nitrous oxide and fertility may be affected. Robertson (2006) urges midwives who are planning to become pregnant to consider working in non-nitrous oxide environments.

PROCEDURE: using Entonox in labour

- Ensure that the equipment is correct and working, that the midwife is trained in its use, and that the woman does not have any allergies or contraindications.
- Ensure also that the woman understands how Entonox is safely used and that she agrees to this administration.
- Allow the woman to place the mouthpiece or mask in place.
- With a hand on the uterine fundus, palpate for the presence of a contraction.
- As the contraction begins, encourage the woman to breathe in the gas taking slow breaths with reasonable depth.
- At the peak of the contraction encourage the woman to remove the mask/mouthpiece and to breathe normally in air (aim to stand at the side as she breathes out, rather than in front of her). Continue to assist the woman through that contraction in a way that helps her.
- Observe and question the woman as to the effects of the gas, and any side effects, particularly as time passes.
- Monitor all vital sign observations as for care in labour, ensuring that respiration rate and depth are noted. Consider the use of pulse oximetry if any observations are outside of normal parameters.

- Understand and observe for the possible effects/side effects of multiple pharmacology, e.g. use of opioid analgesics concurrently.
- Ensure that all records are contemporaneously kept including the duration of use, effects and possible side effects.
- Ensure that all apparatus is cleaned/serviced and ready to use again on completion.

ROLE AND RESPONSIBILITIES OF THE MIDWIFE

These can be summarized as:
- if appropriately trained in its use, the midwife may administer Entonox to labouring women – all stages of labour are permitted
- as a self-administered medication, the midwife has a significant role in ensuring that the woman uses it correctly, and in helping her to gain the maximum benefit
- as well as monitoring the woman's vital signs as part of labour care, the midwife must monitor her respiration rate and depth, encouraging her to breathe slowly but with reasonable depth. Action should be taken should there be any signs or symptoms of overdose, hyperventilation or hypoxia
- full and contemporaneous records are kept
- the midwife should be fully aware of how to use, store and clean the apparatus (particularly if using a portable cylinder), and of how to ensure that potential faults are corrected
- Health and Safety at Work Regulations should be upheld with regard to nitrous oxide use. Midwives should consider their own safety.

SUMMARY

- Due to the nature of its administration (i.e. the need to breathe early in each contraction) its effect as a labour analgesic can be variable, but it is appreciated by many women. The side effects for the women are transitory and there are no documented negative effects (at this time) for the fetus.
- The midwife has responsibilities to ensure that it is stored, serviced and used correctly. The midwife should be alert to any signs of adverse reactions with its use.
- Working in environments of extensive nitrous oxide use may pose health threats to employees. Health and Safety Regulations should be upheld.

SELF-ASSESSMENT EXERCISES

The answers to the following questions may be found in the text:

1. Describe how a midwife should support a woman to use Entonox effectively in the first and second stages of labour.
2. Discuss the advantages and disadvantages of Entonox as a labour analgesic.
3. Summarize the role and responsibilities of the midwife when caring for a woman using Entonox in labour.
4. a) Which vital sign observations should be undertaken regularly when a woman is using Entonox? b) Why?

REFERENCES

BOC, 2008. New Zealand Data Sheet: Entonox. BOC, Australia. Available online: <http://www.medsafe.govt.nz/profs/datasheet/e/entonoxgas.pdf> (accessed 1 March 2015).

BOC, 2011. Entonox: Essential Safety Information. BOC, Manchester. Available online: <http://www.bochealthcare.co.uk/en/Products-and-services/Products-and-services-by-category/Medical-gases/ENTONOX/ENTONOX.html> (accessed 1 March 2015); (safety data sheet).

Green, J., 1993. Expectations and experiences of pain in labour: findings from a large prospective study. Birth 20 (2), 65–72.

Jordan, S., 2010. Pain relief. In: Jordan, S. (Ed.), Pharmacology for Midwives, second ed. Palgrave Macmillan, Basingstoke. (Chapter 4).

Nagele, P., Duma, A., Kopec, M., et al., 2014. Nitrous Oxide for treatment-resistant major depression: A proof-of-concept trial. Biol. Psychiatry Journal. Available online: <http://www.biologicalpsychiatryjournal.com/article/S0006-3223(14)00910-X/fulltext> (accessed 3 January 2015).

NICE (National Institute for Health and Care Excellence), 2014. Intrapartum Care: Care of Healthy Women and their Babies during Childbirth. NICE, London. Available online: <www.nice.org.uk> (accessed 5 March 2015).

Robertson, A., 2006. Nitrous oxide – no laughing matter. MIDIRS Midwifery Digest. 16 (1), 123–128.

Chapter | 25 |

Principles of drug administration: epidural analgesia

LEARNING OUTCOMES

Having read this chapter, the reader should be able to:

- discuss the differences between epidural, spinal and combined spinal epidural analgesia
- list the indications and contraindications for epidural analgesia

- discuss the side effects and how these are recognized and managed
- discuss the complications and how these are recognized and managed
- describe how an epidural is sited and a bolus administered
- describe how to remove an epidural catheter safely.
- discuss the role and responsibilities of the midwife throughout and following the procedure

Epidural analgesia generally appears to be an effective way of reducing pain during labour (Simmons et al 2012); it involves the administration of drugs into the epidural space which generally cause loss of pain and loss of sensation. A 24-hour epidural service is offered in most consultant delivery units using skilled obstetric anaesthetists and midwives who have been trained and are considered to be competent in epidural management with annual recertification to ensure their knowledge and skills are maintained (OAA/AAGBI 2013). The epidural rate in the UK is around 22% (Kemp et al 2013), although Odibo (2007) suggests the demand is closer to 70–90%; rates in the US are much higher than the UK at 58% (Simmons et al 2012). It is a useful analgesia in situations where operative surgery may be required as an effective epidural should be topped up and used as the intraoperative anaesthesia (McClure et al 2011). Halpern et al (2009) recommend that the incidence of a general anaesthetic being required as anaesthesia for caesarean section when the woman already has an epidural *in situ* should not be more than 3%.

This chapter clarifies the terminology and details the procedures for epidural insertion, intermittent bolus administration and removal. The indications, contraindications, side effects, complications – recognition and management – and midwife's role and responsibilities are discussed. The reader is encouraged to be aware that the debates surrounding epidural use and normal birth are greater than this text can examine.

THE EPIDURAL SPACE

The spinal cord is protected by three meninges (membranes) made of connective tissue with spaces between them – the tough outer dura mater, the arachnoid mater (the main physiological barrier for drugs passing between the epidural space and the spinal cord), and the inner, more delicate, pia mater. Between the pia and arachnoid mater is the subarachnoid space (also referred to as the intrathecal space) containing the cerebrospinal fluid (CSF); the subdural space is between the dura and the arachnoid mater. The meninges are surrounded by a layer of fat and connective tissue contained within the epidural space which is situated between the wall of the vertebrae and ligamentum flavum and the dura mater (Fig. 25.1). The epidural space is a potential space, 5–6 mm thick in the lumbar region, containing blood and lymphatic vessels. According to Sharma et al (2011), the mean distance from the skin to the epidural space is 5.4 mm, whereas two decades ago it was 4.8 mm, reflecting increasing obesity levels. The spinal nerves also pass through the epidural space and intervertebral spaces; the area of skin relating to where each nerve emerges is a dermatome.

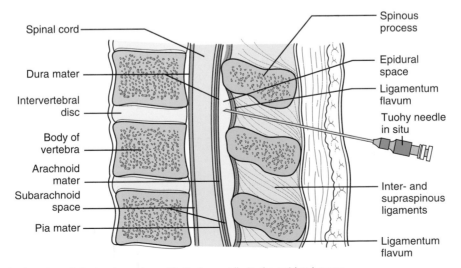

Figure 25.1 Sagittal section of the lumbar spine with Tuohy needle in the epidural space.

EPIDURAL ANALGESIA

This involves the introduction of a local anaesthetic, often combined with an opioid, into the epidural space through a small catheter either as a continuous epidural infusion (CEI) or an intermittent epidural bolus (IEB). Some of the drug can enter into the systemic circulation or attach to the epidural fat content (with no analgesic effect). The remainder of the drugs cross the dura and arachnoid mater into the intrathecal space and the CSF (Bowrey & Thompson 2008).

Successful placement of the epidural catheter is essential if effective analgesia is to be achieved. The anaesthetist has to estimate the distance from the woman's skin to her epidural space, as this varies between women. Sharma et al (2011) suggest that ethnicity and body mass index are two main factors affecting distance suggesting Asian (including Chinese) women, who have smaller spinous and transverse processes but larger vertebral bodies compared with Caucasian women, have a shorter skin-to-epidural space distance. They also found that the distance was further in Black/British Black and Chinese labouring women who had a body mass index (BMI) >40. The risk of a dural puncture occurring is increased if the distance to insert the epidural needle is overestimated. Ultrasound imaging is being used more frequently for measuring the skin to epidural space distance where there is concern (Loubert et al 2011).

LOW-DOSE 'MOBILE' EPIDURAL

Some hospitals use low-dose epidurals which provide good analgesia without loss of motor function. While this is referred to as a 'mobile' epidural women are usually restricted in how they can mobilize – moving between the bed and a chair. As full motor strength is not guaranteed, women should be cautioned not to walk around. The observations recorded are the same as for a normal-dose epidural with the addition of assessing the woman's ability to ambulate 20–30 minutes after each bolus. This is assessed by asking the woman to raise each leg straight off the bed and hold its position for at least 5 seconds – if this is achieved weight bearing is likely to be satisfactory.

SPINAL ANALGESIA

Spinal analgesia is achieved by injecting a single bolus of the drug/s through the epidural space, dura and arachnoid membranes, into the intrathecal (subarachnoid) space.

Lower doses of the drug(s) can be used as it is placed directly into the CSF where the opioid can bind to the opioid receptor sites in the dorsal horn of the spinal cord. Onset of analgesia is rapid but not as long lasting as an epidural and therefore is rarely used for labour on its own (Simmons et al 2012). It is often the analgesia/anaesthesia of choice for emergency caesarean section where rapid anaesthesia is required or for an elective caesarean section. Spinal anaesthesia may be used for emergency caesarean section if the epidural block is insufficient, although Vaida et al (2009) advise caution if a bolus has just been administered. They suggest the CSF may be compressed so when the drugs are injected in the intrathecal space, they may be displaced upwards which can lead to an unpredictable high block. This is not an issue with a continuous infusion.

COMBINED SPINAL EPIDURAL ANALGESIA

Combined spinal epidural (CSE) analgesia involves a spinal injection of a small amount of local anaesthetic and/or a lipophilic opioid, e.g. fentanyl, into the intrathecal space immediately before or after the placement of the epidural catheter. This can be achieved by using the epidural needle to locate the epidural space at the level of L3 then passing a smaller-diameter longer spinal needle through the epidural needle lumen to pierce the dura and arachnoid membranes. The drug is injected into the CSF and the spinal needle removed to allow the epidural catheter to be inserted into the epidural space for maintenance of analgesia (Loubert et al 2011, Simmons et al 2012). Anim-Somuah et al (2011) suggest CSE combines the advantages of the faster onset and more reliable analgesia achieved with the spinal with the continuing pain relief of the epidural while allowing the woman to remain alert; however, there is a greater incidence of pruritus than with epidural analgesia alone (Loubert et al 2011). Simmons et al (2012) suggest there is no advantage in offering CSE over epidural for labour analgesia.

DRUGS

Local anaesthetics (e.g. bupivacaine, ropivacaine) cross the dura and arachnoid membranes, where they are in contact with the nerve roots and spinal cord. Once there, they plug the sodium channels and dampen down the excitation of the nerve cell, preventing it from passing the impulse to another nerve cell. This prevents transmission of the pain impulses to the higher centres and can take effect within 10–20 minutes of administration.

The combination of a local anaesthetic and a strong opioid in low doses infused into the epidural space is synergistic with the potential to produce analgesia without increasing the incidence of side effects seen when the drugs are administered separately at higher doses (Bowrey & Thompson 2008).

Opioids bind to opioid receptors, primarily mu opioid receptors, in the dorsal horn. They inhibit the release of neurotransmitters such as substance P and glutamate, further reducing the transmission of the pain impulses as well as producing an analgesic effect. Fentanyl is 75–125 times more potent than morphine because it is lipophilic (fat-soluble) (Bowrey & Thompson 2008) but has a shorter duration and half-life.

CONTINUOUS VERSUS INTERMITTENT DRUG ADMINISTRATION

CEI provides a constant flow of a small amount of the drug(s) into the epidural space via an epidural infusion pump, whereas IEB is in the form of manually administered boluses given either on a regular basis or as needed. Boluses can also be provided as an adjunct to continuous administration via the pump. George et al (2013) suggest that small, regularly spaced boluses provide a more extensive spread of local anaesthetic within the epidural space which may result in improved analgesia. Skrablin et al (2011), however, propose that CEI provides a more consistent analgesia without excessive fluctuations in anaesthetic level than IEB but is also associated with insufficient or excessive analgesia and blockade.

INDICATIONS FOR EPIDURAL ANALGESIA

- Pain relief/maternal request
- Where there is likelihood of instrumental or operative delivery, e.g. malposition, malpresentation, multiple pregnancy, prolonged labour
- Hypertension
- Preterm labour, where there may be an early desire to push
- Postoperative analgesia opioid administration.

CONTRAINDICATIONS

Some of the contraindications for epidural analgesia are absolute while others are relative:

Absolute

- patient refusal
- coagulation defects
- localized or general sepsis
- haemorrhage and cardiovascular instability
- hypovolaemia
- known allergy to drugs used
- raised intracranial pressure
- unavailability of appropriately trained staff in setting up and ongoing care of epidurals
- insufficient midwifery staff to provide one-to-one care for the duration of epidural.

Relative

- spinal deformity
- some neurological disorders, e.g. multiple sclerosis.

Although an increased BMI is not a contraindication, there is a higher failure rate when the woman's BMI is >30, often requiring the epidural to be resited (Dresner et al 2006).

SIDE EFFECTS OF EPIDURAL ANALGESIA

The side effects associated with epidural analgesia usually result from the effects of the drugs used:

Opioid side effects:

- respiration depression
- sedation
- nausea and vomiting
- pruritus (itching)
- urinary retention.

Local anaesthetic side effects vary depending on the drug and dosage used:

- peripheral vasodilatation and resulting hypotension (if severe, will also cause loss of consciousness)
- leg weakness
- urinary retention
- drug toxicity: restlessness, dizziness, tinnitus, metallic taste, drowsiness
- anaphylactic drug reaction (see Chapter 18).

Women with an epidural are also more likely to develop a fever during labour than women who do not have an epidural (Segal 2010) although the aetiology for this is not clear. It is possibly multifactorial, a combination of an imbalance between heat production and heat-dissipating mechanisms, a side effect of opioids, particularly fentanyl, and maternal inflammation; the latter is now the dominant view (Segal 2010).

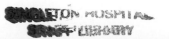

MANAGEMENT OF SIDE EFFECTS

Respiration depression

Although this can occur early, within the first 2 hours of drug administration, it may also be a late and unreliable sign of opioid overdose (6–24 hours). It occurs as a result of the opioid being absorbed from the epidural space into the systemic circulation and the intrathecal space. It is likely that there is a rostral/cephalad spread of the opioids which means it spreads towards the head with the brain stem and respiratory centre being reached early in the spread. The effect is more profound with morphine and diamorphine (as they are water-soluble) than fentanyl.

Bowrey & Thompson (2008) define respiratory depression as a respiratory rate <8 and an increased sedation score on two occasions after the administration of spinal opioids. An increasing sedation score may be noted before the decrease in the respiratory rate. Monitoring the sedation level and respiration rate is important for anyone who has received opioids so that respiratory depression is detected and treated early. The woman should be kept upright, given oxygen (titrated to maintain oxygen saturation levels ≥95%), help called and naloxone administered. As the effect of naloxone wears off after approximately 1 hour, further doses may be required.

Sedation

Opioids can cause sedation, which for some women is very welcome and allows them to rest, even sleep, throughout labour. The woman's sedation level should be monitored with the vital signs as an increasing sedation level may herald the onset of respiratory depression.

Nausea and vomiting

Low doses of opioids activate the mu opioid receptors in the chemoreceptor trigger zone (CTZ), which can result in nausea and vomiting although the effects are not as evident as when opioids are administered intravenously. Not all women will experience nausea and vomiting, as higher doses of opioids can suppress vomiting by acting at receptor sites deeper in the medulla. Where it does arise, it is usually managed easily with the administration of an intravenous anti-emetic.

Pruritus (itching)

This occurs more commonly over the face, chest, and abdomen. It may be a result of the opioids causing histamine release or a side effect from the activation of the mu opioid receptors. Treatment is administration of an antihistamine with or without a decrease in the infusion rate if a CEI is used or if severe, administration of a small dose of naloxone – however this will decrease the analgesic effect of the opioid.

Urinary retention

If the woman is unable to pass urine (usually encouraged by sitting on a bedpan) then insertion of an indwelling urinary catheter may be required (see Chapter 14).

Hypotension

Hypotension can occur due to the action of the local anaesthetic on the sympathetic nerves by relaxing the smooth muscle of the blood vessel walls and reducing the tone, which results in vasodilation. Hawkins (2010) suggests it affects up to 80% of women undergoing an epidural. It is important to establish the woman's baseline blood pressure before the epidural commences. Hypotension is usually easily treated by fluid replacement; thus it is important the woman has a peripheral intravenous cannula *in situ*. If this is ineffective, a vasopressor such as phenylephrine or metaraminol may be required either as a bolus or by infusion. The midwife should also consider turning the woman to a left lateral position until the hypotension is corrected. Correcting hypotension is important as the drugs cause a decrease in vascular resistance and with a normal blood pressure there is a significant improvement in uteroplacental blood flow (Hawkins 2010).

Leg weakness

The woman is advised not to mobilize following birth until she has full leg strength and is able to weight bear. The midwife should be with the woman when this is first attempted. With reduced mobility the woman is at increased risk of a pressure injury, particularly around the heels (Loorham-Battersby & McGuiness 2010), and the midwife should take appropriate precaution to minimize this risk (see Chapter 53). Increasing leg weakness noted in labour or after delivery may be associated with an infusion rate that is too high, epidural haematoma or abscess, particularly if the effects of the epidural on the motor block have been decreasing. If there is any concern about a haematoma forming during labour the epidural infusion should be turned off and no further boluses given and leg strength assessed every 30 minutes – an increase in leg strength should be seen and the infusion/bolus administration can recommence. The same applies if the woman is receiving epidural analgesia postnatally.

Drug toxicity

It is important to note that local anaesthetic toxicity does not always occur at the time of the initial injection. Severe toxicity will present as a sudden alteration in the woman's mental status accompanied by severe agitation and/or loss of consciousness with or without tonic-clonic convulsions and a metallic taste. Cardiovascular collapse can occur with bradycardia (AAGBI 2010).

Should this occur while the injection is being given, the anaesthetist will stop the injection. Help should be called and assistance given to maintain the airway. If the anaesthetist is not present he should be summoned urgently as intubation may be indicated. The woman will require oxygen administration to maintain oxygen saturation levels ≥95% and intravenous cannulation (see Chapter 47). Observation of vital signs should be undertaken and fluids administered to reverse the effects of hypotension. If seizures continue, medication may be required. If circulatory arrest occurs, cardiopulmonary resuscitation should commence using a left tilt (see Chapter 55) and boluses of intravenous lipid emulsion given. Lipids are an effective remedy for the cardiotoxic effects of lipid-soluble local anaesthetics such as bupivacaine and ropivacaine (Hawkins 2010).

COMPLICATIONS

These are associated with siting or removing the epidural catheter or problems that arise throughout epidural use. The associated signs and symptoms may occur immediately or be delayed for several days after removal of the epidural catheter. As some of these complications are extremely serious, it is important that the midwife is vigilant so early referral and treatment can be provided. There appears to be no consensus as to the incidence of complications occurring in practice, which Middle & Wee (2009) suggest is due to the available studies being too small to be reliable. Fortunately the majority of complications are rare. Risks for intrathecal injection are 1 : 2900, intravascular injection 1 : 5008 and high/total spinal block 1 : 16 200 according to Jenkins (2005).

The risks determined by the Obstetric Anaesthetists Association for Great Britain and Ireland, which should be given to the woman are:

- epidural not working effectively and requiring additional pain relief 1 : 8
- epidural not working effectively at caesarean section necessitating a general anaesthetic 1 : 20
- significant drop in blood pressure 1 : 50
- severe headache with epidural 1 : 100
- absolute failure rate 1 : 1000

- nerve damage (numb patch on leg or foot, weakness) 1 : 1000 (temporary), lasting beyond 6 months 1 : 13 000
- abscess formation 1 : 50 000
- meningitis 1 : 100 000
- accidental unconsciousness 1 : 100 000
- haematoma 1 : 170 000
- severe injury including paralysis 1 : 250 000 (OAA 2008).

Partial block ('breakthrough' pain)

This occurs when contractions are still felt over one area of the abdomen due to the non-uniform spread of local anaesthetic (Anim-Somuah et al 2011). Hawkins (2010) suggests one cause is the presence of fibrous bands within the epidural space preventing an even spread of the infusate – this can be difficult to treat. The catheter should be checked to ensure it has not moved from its insertion point. If pain is felt in the upper part of the abdomen, the basal rate of the infusion can be increased as per the anaesthetist's instructions or a bolus given. If there is a missed segment, a bolus can be given with the woman lying on the side where the pain is felt. If this does not help, the anaesthetist should review the woman and may want to consider pulling the catheter back slightly (the midwife should NOT attempt this), giving a bolus of a different drug or resiting the epidural catheter. If the pain is unilateral it may be due to the tip of the catheter being lodged on one side of the epidural space during its insertion resulting in the drugs preferentially bathing the nerve roots on that side. Withdrawing the catheter slightly (undertaken by the anaesthetist) may correct this.

Dural puncture

This occurs when the epidural needle or catheter accidentally punctures the dura mater resulting in leakage of the CSF and reduced intracranial pressure. This causes traction on the innervated tissues around the brain and can result in a severe headache occurring usually in the following few days. Leakage of CSF may be noted at the time of insertion of the Tuohy needle or epidural catheter – the fluid can be tested for the presence of glucose and protein using a urinary reagent strip to distinguish it from normal saline that may have been used during the procedure. If drugs are given immediately following an inadvertent dural puncture, they will be administered into the intrathecal rather than the epidural space, resulting in a total spinal block. If the dural puncture is noticed before the epidural catheter is inserted, the anaesthetist is likely to resite the epidural or insert an intrathecal catheter. If there is no headache, labour continues, and the woman can push during the second stage.

Postdural puncture headache (PDPH)

Hawkins (2010) agrees with the OAA (2008) that the risk of a dural puncture is 1% and suggests that 70% of these women will develop a PDPH. PDPH classically presents with a moderate to severe postural headache felt like a tight band in the frontal region which may radiate to both temples, be felt behind the eyes or in the occipital region. It is usually alleviated by lying down and increases in severity on standing or sitting. Associated symptoms include neck stiffness, photophobia, nausea, vomiting, diplopia, hyperacusia, hearing loss, and tinnitus (Darvish et al 2011). The headache usually begins around 24–48 hours post-puncture (although rarely it may happen immediately following the dural puncture) and can resolve spontaneously within 5–10 days (but may take up to 3 weeks); however, the symptoms can be very debilitating necessitating treatment of an epidural blood patch (EBP). Darvish et al (2011) suggest that a subdural haematoma may form if the PDPH is not treated.

PDPH is classified according to its severity and effects on the woman:

- Mild PDPH causes a slight restriction in daily activities and the woman is not bedridden. There are usually no other associated symptoms and the pain responds well to non-opiate analgesia.
- Moderate PDPH results in significant restriction of daily activities with the woman needing to spend most of her time lying down. Associated symptoms may be present and pain management involves the use of opiates.
- Severe PDPH causes complete restriction of daily activities as the woman is unable to do anything other than lie down without severe pain. Associated symptoms are present and conservative management is ineffective.

Diagnosis is usually made based on the symptoms alone, but if there is any doubt, magnetic resonance imaging (MRI) can be performed, which may also show other causes of the headache. Discussion with the consultant anaesthetist is warranted as soon as PDPH is suspected, who will then review the woman on a daily basis and consider whether conservative management of adopting whatever posture is most comfortable, maintaining hydration and simple analgesia is sufficient. Caffeine may also be prescribed, as it will help to dilate the constricted intracranial veins.

Where conservative management does not work, an EBP can be used. It is not advisable to use this form of treatment if the woman is pyrexial or within the first 24–48 hours due to its lower success rate and higher risk of bacteraemia. EBP is usually undertaken in the operating theatre or a delivery suite room under aseptic conditions. If the woman is receiving an anticoagulant, at least 12 hours should have passed since the last dose was given. The woman is usually positioned in the left lateral position which is more comfortable but also decreases the risk of further CSF leakage. Twenty millilitres of blood is taken from the woman and, after a Tuohy needle has been inserted into the epidural space below or at the site of the dural puncture, the blood is slowly injected into the epidural space. The woman may feel some relief immediately as the blood exerts a mass effect within the epidural space which increases the CSF pressure. A clot forms and blocks the puncture site stopping further leakage of CSF allowing the CSF to regenerate and return to a normal volume. Following the procedure the woman should lie flat for 2 hours and then begin to mobilize slowly. Over the next 48 hours the woman should avoid heavy lifting, excessive bending or straining when defaecating. If the headache recurs, the EBP can be repeated although OAA (2014) state that 60–70% of headaches are resolved within a few minutes to a few hours.

Catheter migration

This is an extremely rare complication where the catheter migrates into the CSF causing a total spinal block from an intrathecal injection or a blood vessel resulting in an intravascular injection. Intravascular administration of the epidural drugs can result in sedation from excess opioids or local anaesthetic toxicity noticed by tingling, numbness, twitching, convulsions, apnoea and loss of consciousness. Occasionally the catheter falls out causing an increase in pain and a feeling of wetness from leakage of the infusate.

Abscess formation

A rare but serious complication is the formation of an abscess within the epidural space. It usually occurs after the epidural catheter has been removed. The abscess can compress the spinal cord leading to nerve damage and paralysis in addition to being the cause of sepsis. It manifests as back pain, tenderness and erythema around, and purulent discharge from, the insertion site; there may also be swelling around the insertion site. If the woman is pyrexial, a sample of the discharge should be sent for culture and sensitivity analysis. If this is noted before the epidural catheter is removed, the tip of the catheter should also be sent for analysis once it is removed.

Haematoma

This is fortunately a very rare but also very serious complication. A haematoma forms as a result of trauma to the epidural blood vessels during catheter insertion or more likely, on removal. It is usually self-limiting and may be of no consequence. However, if the woman is receiving an anticoagulant, it can quickly become more serious. It presents as back pain and tenderness accompanied by sensory and/or motor weakness – particularly increasing leg weakness and bladder and/or bowel dysfunction. Untreated an epidural haematoma can compress the spinal cord leading to permanent nerve damage and paralysis within 6–8 hours. Diagnosis should be made early with an MRI or computed tomography (CT) scan. The haematoma should be evacuated before permanent damage occurs.

High regional/total spinal anaesthesia

This is an excessively high block, above T4, requiring tracheal intubation and may arise due to inadvertent placement of the epidural catheter into the intrathecal rather than the epidural space. This results in rapid onset of analgesia accompanied by a dense motor block of the legs, symptomatic hypotension, dyspnoea, slurred speech and hoarseness, arm weakness/tingling, sedation/anxiety, high level of insensitivity to cold and touch, and unconsciousness. Help should be called immediately, particularly the anaesthetist, as the woman will require intubation and ventilatory support and oxygen administered to maintain oxygen saturation levels ≥95%. If there is an epidural infusion running, it should be turned off. Hypotension should be corrected with intravenous fluids and vasoconstrictors, e.g. ephedrine, phenylephrine, metaraminol, adrenaline, to maintain blood pressure and reduce the risk of cardiac arrest. The woman should not be laid flat until the anaesthetist requests this, as it will result in the block becoming higher. Observations of pulse, blood pressure, respirations and oxygen saturation should be undertaken. The consultant obstetrician should be informed, as urgent delivery of the baby may be required once the woman's condition has stabilized; vaginal delivery may still be possible.

Meningitis

Fortunately, meningitis – an infection within the meninges and CSF – is an extremely rare complication of epidural. The woman may develop fever, headache, neck stiffness, photophobia, and nausea and vomiting and should be referred for urgent medical treatment to reduce the risk of complications.

EFFECT ON LABOUR

Traditionally, epidural use during labour was associated with an increased risk of instrumental delivery, caesarean section, oxytocin augmentation and lower Apgar scores. This may have been due to the high dose of local anaesthetic drugs that were used when epidural use was first introduced. Odibo (2007) suggests these drugs affect the pelvic autonomic and parasympathetic nerves inhibiting oxytocin release and reducing the strength and frequency of contractions. During the second stage, the expulsive nature of contractions may be affected as the urge to push is lost due to the sensory blockade and pelvic floor muscle tone is reduced, which can affect rotation of the presenting part. Different drugs and dosages have been used over time to reduce the adverse effects on labour but epidural analgesia may still impact on labour. Women are more likely to have a longer second stage, reduced mobility, hypotension, urinary retention, fever and an increased need for oxytocin augmentation and instrumental delivery; however, Anim-Somuah et al (2011) found no significant adverse impact on maternal satisfaction, long-term backache, Apgar scores or the risk of caesarean section.

Changes in practice are also helping to overcome the risks (e.g. delayed pushing; see Chapter 31). Torvaldsen et al (2004) reviewed the evidence concerning the practice of discontinuing the epidural analgesia late in labour to decrease the risk of instrumental deliveries and conclude that there is insufficient evidence to support or refute the practice. The timing of when the epidural is commenced does not appear to adversely affect the type of delivery. Sng et al (2014) found there was no increase in the risk of caesarean section or instrumental delivery for women who had an early epidural (cervical dilatation ≤3 cm in comparison with those who had an epidural when the cervix was dilated to 4 cm or more) and suggest it should be initiated when the woman requests it.

Cheng et al (2014) agree that the second stage is longer with epidural use and propose the definition of prolonged second stage should be reviewed for epidural use. Many intrapartum policies now provide for a longer second stage with delayed pushing. Cheng et al (2014) suggest that the length of the second stage for nulliparous women with an epidural should be 4 hours and 3 hours for multiparous women. In support of a longer 'normal' second stage timeframe, Gillesby et al (2010) found that by delaying active pushing for up to 2 hours, the amount of time nulliparous women pushed for reduced by 27% (68 minutes compared to 94 minutes). The women in the delayed pushing group rested for up to 2 hours but the length of the second stage was only 59 minutes longer than the group who did not delay pushing. Additionally the 1-minute Apgar score was higher in the delayed pushing group, although scores at 5 minutes were similar.

The woman should be encouraged to adopt whatever position is comfortable for her during the second stage as there is currently insufficient evidence on which position to adopt (Kemp et al 2013).

When comparing CEI and IEB drug administration George et al (2013) found the two methods were comparable in terms of labour duration but the length of the second stage was significantly shorter (up to 22 minutes) and maternal satisfaction higher when IEB was used. They did not find any difference in the mode of delivery. However, Skrablin et al (2011) found women using CEI were more likely to have a caesarean section than those receiving IEB but agree there was no difference in labour duration.

PROCEDURE: siting an epidural catheter and analgesia

If a woman is requesting or requires an epidural, the anaesthetist should be informed and should attend within 30 minutes if the hospital offers a 24-hour epidural service, unless there are exceptional circumstances (these must be documented) (OAA/AAGBI 2013). Staffing levels and skill mix on the delivery suite should be considered as there must be an epidural-competent midwife and enough staff for her to undertake the ongoing one-to-one care of the woman and the epidural (OAA/AAGBI 2013). Although the midwife may have discussed the advantages, disadvantages and risks of epidural with the woman while she was considering whether to have an epidural, the anaesthetist is ultimately responsible for obtaining informed consent prior to siting one, which includes a discussion of the risks involved (Middle & Wee 2009). Written information can be provided by the midwife prior to the anaesthetist's arrival to assist with this (a two-sided epidural information card is available by download from the Obstetric Anaesthetists Association of Great Britain and Ireland website (OAA 2008)).

The midwife is responsible for organizing the anaesthetist and the equipment required, assisting as needed and supporting the woman. Her partner, e.g. boyfriend, husband, may be able to provide support although Orbach-Zinger et al (2012) found that the woman's anxiety levels increased during epidural insertion when the partner was present.

- Inform the anaesthetist and gather the equipment (this is often contained together on a trolley ready for use):
  - equipment for peripheral intravenous cannulation (see Chapter 47) and intravenous infusion (usually crystalloid fluid) (see Chapter 48)
  - cardiotocograph (CTG) monitor (see Chapter 1)
  - trolley top or area for a sterile field to be set up
  - sterile gown and gloves
  - sterile dressing pack, with fenestrated drape and gauze
  - antiseptic lotion, e.g. chlorhexidine in 70% isopropyl alcohol
  - epidural pack, usually containing a Tuohy needle with stylet, syringe, epidural catheter and antibacterial filter
  - local anaesthetics for the skin and epidural, e.g. lidocaine (lignocaine) and bupivacaine
  - opiate analgesia, if required (administered according to controlled drug administration; see Chapter 18) – this is usually combined with the local anaesthetic
  - sterile syringes and needles
  - tape/plastic skin dressing
  - appropriate documentation (including MEOWS chart if not already in use), often specific epidural chart and coloured stickers to differentiate epidural and intravenous lines (if using CEI).
- Encourage the woman to empty her bladder.
- Cannulate and commence an intravenous infusion: the use of crystalloids to increase blood volume is often used as it can reduce the risk of hypotension (Hofmeyr et al 2004).
- Record baseline observations of blood pressure, pulse, respiration, pain and sedation score and commence CTG monitoring.
- Position the woman according to her comfort and the anaesthetist's wishes (usually one of two ways), to promote curvature of the spine so that access can be gained between the vertebrae:
  - in left lateral with knees flexed and pulled up towards her chest with her head flexed forwards 'chin on chest' – this encourages anterior flexion of the vertebral column. The woman's back should be very close to the edge of the bed and a pillow placed under her head and another between her knees
  - sitting on the edge of the bed with feet supported on a chair/stool, shoulders hunched forwards with arms resting upon a bed table or hugging a pillow and head resting on her arms to encourage anterior flexion of the spine.
- Assist the anaesthetist to 'gown and glove' and to establish a Critical Aseptic Field pour the lotion, open the needles and syringes, hold ampoules of drugs for drawing up, etc. (see Chapter 10).
- Support the woman with remaining still and keep her informed of what is happening while the epidural is sited by the anaesthetist:
  - the woman's back is cleansed, the drapes put in place, and the local anaesthetic inserted into the skin
  - while the woman is between contractions and very still, the Tuohy needle is inserted between the lumbar vertebrae to the ligamentum flavum where resistance is noted
  - as the ligamentum flavum is punctured there will a sudden loss of resistance to pressure noted on the

syringe plunger and the anaesthetist may feel a slight clicking sensation as the needle enters into the epidural space

- the stylet will be removed and normal saline injected to assess the resistance and ensure that the Tuohy needle is in the correct place
- when the anaesthetist is confident the needle tip is correctly placed the epidural catheter is threaded through the needle 4–6 cm into the epidural space and the Tuohy needle removed over the catheter.

- If used, spray plastic skin around the puncture site and/or secure the catheter with tape; the filter will be connected by the anaesthetist and this should be positioned for ease of access.
- A small test dose is given and if satisfactory the first complete dose is given or a syringe driver/infusion pump attached for a CEI.
- Assist the woman into the position advised by the anaesthetist for the initial 20 minutes after administration (often semi-recumbent).
- Record the woman's blood pressure, respiration and pulse every 5 minutes for the next 20 minutes and then every 30 minutes.
- The woman's condition should also be observed including her level of pain/block, respiratory rate, her warmth, safety, intravenous infusion, colour, sedation level and signs of nausea.
- The anaesthetist completes their contemporaneous records including the controlled drug register if appropriate.
- Refer to the anaesthetist if any observations give cause for concern (hypotension may be corrected by increasing the rate of the intravenous infusion, but the anaesthetist should always be informed).
- Ensure the anaesthetist has disposed of the equipment correctly, including sharps.
- Continue to monitor the fetal heart rate and uterine activity, recording the epidural and times of boluses on the CTG tracing.
- If all observations are within normal limits after 20 minutes and the level of analgesia has been achieved, the woman can be assisted to change her position to one of her choice (avoiding aortocaval compression).
- Normal labour care continues including care of the bladder, (catheterization may be necessary as urinary retention is a common problem, see Chapter 14), pressure-area care (see Chapter 53), and the maintenance of contemporaneous records (NMC 2008).
- If a CEI is not used, the midwife should observe for signs of recurring sensation usually after 2–8 hours and administer a bolus before the woman becomes uncomfortable.

- Administration of patient-controlled analgesia (PCA) (see Chapter 23) allows the woman to administer her own intermittent boluses with or without a low-dose background CEI but will still require assessment of her vital signs and condition as described above following each bolus.

CHECKING THE LEVEL OF THE BLOCK

While the epidural block level is initially assessed by the anaesthetist after 20 minutes, the midwife will undertake subsequent assessments – at least once an hour to ensure it is at the correct level (this will have been previously determined by the anaesthetist). The level is checked using temperature change with either an ice cube (wrapped in gauze or tissue to protect the midwife's fingers) or a cold solution (e.g. ethyl chloride spray). Touch alone is unreliable and use of a pinprick is traumatic (Ousley et al 2012). Either gently rub the ice cube or spray the cold solution at the top of the woman's chest, moving downwards one side at a time. The woman will be able to feel the coldness of the ice cube/spray in areas where the block is not present but when placed against an area where the block is effective, will not feel it as cold – this area is compared against a dermatome chart (Fig. 25.2) and the level recorded. Normally the level is kept below T4; if it rises above this, the anaesthetist should be informed and the infusion stopped if it is continuous, as there is a risk of respiratory arrest. When the level is too low, the woman is likely to be feeling pain and require a bolus or an increase in the basal infusion rate. If the woman is receiving a continuous infusion and the block is too low to be beneficial, the midwife should check that the catheter is still *in situ* and connected to the bacterial filter with no leaks in the tubing and consider increasing the basal rate before calling the anaesthetist, who may need to resite the catheter.

INTERMITTENT EPIDURAL BOLUS ADMINISTRATION

Boluses are used when CEI is not used or if there is break-through pain with a CEI. This should only be undertaken by a midwife who has been trained and assessed as competent with this procedure and who is familiar with local protocol. The anaesthetist prescribes the concentration and volume of the dose and the frequency with which a bolus can be administered. They may also state a preference for the position the woman should adopt. It is advisable to administer the dose in two halves with 5 minutes between them in case the catheter has migrated into the CSF. The

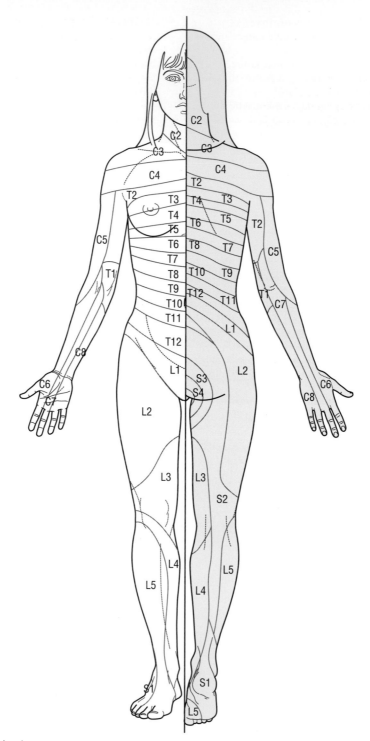

Figure 25.2 Dermatome levels.
(Adapted with kind permission from Walsh 1997)

observations recorded following a bolus also apply to a bolus administered via a PCA pump by the woman and the midwife should remain with the woman for 20 minutes, or longer if her vital signs are unstable or any signs of sepsis develop.

PROCEDURE: manual intermittent epidural bolus administration

- Establish the need for the bolus, check the intravenous infusion is running correctly, and gather equipment:
  - the prescribed drug(s)
  - the medicine administration chart and epidural chart
  - non-sterile gloves
  - sterile needle and syringe
  - locally approved cleanser, usually 70% alcohol/2% chlorhexidine wipe.
- Assist the woman into the position requested by the anaesthetist, either lateral or sitting.
- Wash and dry hands, apply gloves, check the drugs with another midwife and draw up the correct dose using an Aseptic Non Touch Technique (ANTT).
- Confirm the woman's identity on the medicine administration chart both verbally with the woman and against her identity band.
- Following a contraction, remove the filter cap, scrub the tip of the port with the approved wipe using and up-and-down and side-to-side movements for at least 20 seconds using different parts of the wipe, then scrub the sides and allow to dry for at least 30 seconds.
- Inject half of the medication at a rate of 5 mL per 30 seconds using an ANTT (if local protocol is to administer all the medication, do so).
- Observe the woman throughout for adverse reactions such as tinnitus, drowsiness and slurred speech.
- Reapply the cap.
- Repeat the procedure in 5 minutes if administered in two halves.
- Observations of the maternal pulse, respiration, blood pressure and general condition are recorded as before: every 5 minutes for at least 20 minutes, every 30 minutes thereafter, and with continuous monitoring of the fetal heart.
- If required, assist the woman into a comfortable position.
- Dispose of equipment correctly.
- Wash and dry hands.
- Document the administration in all the relevant places and the effect of the drug(s), act accordingly.
- Continue to observe for the effects, side effects and complications of the block; summon the anaesthetist if required.

PROCEDURE: removing an epidural catheter

The catheter is removed once the epidural is no longer required, usually once labour is over. If the woman is on anticoagulants, the midwife should wait at least 12 hours after the last dose and 4–6 hours before the next dose before removing the catheter to decrease the risk of bleeding around the site. If there is any concern about the coagulation status of the woman, coagulation studies should be undertaken and the catheter removed only when agreed by the anaesthetist. It is preferable to remove the catheter during the day so that the woman can be monitored more easily for signs of haematoma formation. The epidural catheter may be attached to a clot which can dislodge as the catheter is removed, resulting in bleeding. It is often easier to remove the catheter if the woman adopts the position she used when the catheter was inserted.

- Discuss the procedure with the woman and gain informed consent.
- Assist the woman into a suitable position and expose her back ensuring privacy throughout.
- Wash and dry hands.
- Remove the tape and carefully pull the catheter out swiftly in one movement.
- Clean around the site with skin cleansing agent, e.g. chlorhexidine in 70% alcohol/2% chlorhexidine for 30 seconds (Key-Site) using an up-and-down and side-to-side movement and allow to dry for 30 seconds.
- Apply an occlusive dressing for 24 hours.
- Examine the tubing for completeness by assessing the gradations and the rounded appearance of the blue catheter tip; checking with a second person may be required.
- Document removal and act accordingly.
- Observe the woman for signs of haematoma formation.

POSTNATAL CARE

Until the effects of the epidural wear off, there will be a degree of numbness affecting the legs; thus mobilization will be delayed. During this time the woman may require assistance to care for her baby and with breastfeeding. She will also need observing for signs of urinary retention and headache, two of the most common short-term side effects. Observations for backache may be needed in the longer term and women should be given written information regarding when and how to seek help should complications arise, particularly for women who have an early discharge from hospital (OAA/AAGBI 2013). Once the woman feels ready to mobilize the midwife should ensure the woman is able to weight bear before mobilization occurs.

Further observations, particularly of respiration, may be required where the woman has had neuraxial analgesia (e.g. epidural, spinal) that includes opioids because of the risk of delayed respiratory depression (OAA/AAGBI 2013).

ROLE AND RESPONSIBILITIES OF THE MIDWIFE

These can be summarized as:

- completing the training and maintaining competence for the provision of boluses and/or care of a continuous infusion
- giving consideration to the delivery suite workload and whether the woman can be given the 'one-to-one' care required
- education and preparation of the woman
- assisting the anaesthetist during preparation and siting
- assisting with the correct positioning and support of the woman during and following the siting of the epidural
- providing the ongoing care including appropriate observations of the woman and fetus
- recognizing complications as they arise and responding appropriately
- being able to remove the epidural catheter correctly
- providing appropriate postnatal care
- maintaining contemporaneous, thorough documentation.

SUMMARY

- Epidural analgesia can be a very effective form of labour analgesia but it is not without potential complications.

- A local anaesthetic and an opioid are usually given together either as a continuous infusion or as intermittent boluses.
- The side effects of epidural generally relate to the side effects of the drugs administered.
- The midwife has a responsible role at the time of siting the epidural, with the ongoing care and with the management of the infusion or intermittent bolus administration, both during labour and postnatally.
- Complications can be very serious and the midwife should be able to recognize these and respond accordingly.

SELF-ASSESSMENT EXERCISES

The answers to the following questions may be found in the text:

1. What are the differences between epidural and spinal analgesia?
2. List the indications and contraindications for epidural analgesia.
3. Identify three complications of epidural analgesia and discuss how these are recognized and managed.
4. Describe the midwife's role while the epidural is being sited.
5. What observations should be undertaken on a woman who has an epidural *in situ*?
6. How can a midwife assess the level of the block?
7. Describe how an intermittent epidural bolus is administered safely by a midwife.
8. Describe how an epidural catheter is removed correctly.

REFERENCES

AAGBI (Association of Anaesthetists of Great Britain and Ireland), 2010. AAGBI Safety Guideline Management of Severe Local Anaesthetic Toxicity. Available online: <http://www.aagbi.org/publications/publications-guidelines/M/R> (accessed 3 March 2015).

AAGBI (Association of Anaesthetists of Great Britain and Ireland), OAA (Obstetric Anaesthetists' Association), 2013. OAA/AAGBI, 2013. Guidelines

for Obstetric Anaesthetic Services 2013. Available online: <http://www.oaa-anaes.ac.uk/ui/content/content.aspx?id=152> (accessed 3 March 2015).

Anim-Somuah, M., Smyth, R.M.D., Jones, L., 2011. Epidural versus non-epidural or no analgesia in labour. Cochrane Database Syst. Rev. (12), CD000331, doi:10.1002/14651858.CD000331.pub2.

Bowrey, S., Thompson, J., 2008. Spinal opioids in postoperative pain relief 2:

adverse effects. Nurs. Times 104 (31), 28–69.

Cheng, Y.W., Shaffer, B.L., Nicholson, J.M., Caughey, A.B., 2014. Second Stage of Labor and Epidural Use. Obstet. Gynecol. 123 (3), 527–535.

Darvish, B., Gupta, A., Alahuhta, S., et al., 2011. Management of accidental dural puncture and post-dural puncture headache after labour: a Nordic survey. Acta Anaesthesiol. Scand. 55, 46–53.

Dresner, M., Brocklesby, J., Bamber, J., 2006. Audit of the influence of body mass index on the performance of epidural analgesia in labour and the subsequent mode of delivery. Br. J. Obstet. Gynaecol. 113 (10), 1178–1181.

George, R.B., Allen, T.K., Habib, A.S., 2013. Intermittent epidural bolus compared with continuous epidural infusions for labor analgesia: a systematic review and meta-analysis. Anesth. Analg. 116 (1), 133–144.

Gillesby, E., Burns, S., Dempsey, A., et al., 2010. Comparison of delayed versus immediate pushing during second stage of labor for nulliparous women with epidural anaesthesia. J. Obstet. Gynecol. Neonatal Nurs. 39, 635–644.

Halpern, S.H., Soliman, A., Yee, J., et al., 2009. Conversion of epidural labour analgesia to anaesthesia for Caesarean section: a prospective study of the incidence and determinants of failure. Br. J. Anaesth. 102 (2), 240–243.

Hawkins, J.L., 2010. Epidural analgesia for labor and delivery. NEJM 362, 1503–1510.

Hofmeyr, G.J., Cyna, A.M., Middleton, P., 2004. Prophylactic intravenous preloading for regional anaesthesia in labour. Cochrane Database Syst. Rev. (4), CD000175, doi:10.1002/14651858.CD000175.pub2.

Jenkins, J., 2005. Some immediate serious complications of obstetric epidural analgesia and anaesthesia: a prospective study of 145000 epidurals. Int. J. Obstet. Anesth. 14, 37–42.

Kemp, E., Kingswood, C.J., Kibuka, M., Thornton, J.G., 2013. Positions in the second stage of labour for women with epidural anaesthesia. Cochrane Database Syst. Rev. (1), CD008070, doi:10.1002/14651858.CD008070.pub2.

Loubert, C., Hinova, A., Fernando, R., 2011. Update on modern neuraxial analgesia in labour: a review of the literature of the last 5 years. Anaesthesia 66, 191–212.

Loorham-Battersby, C.M., McGuiness, W., 2010. Heel damage and epidural analgesia: is there a connection? J. Wound Care 20 (1), 28–34.

McClure, J.H., Cooper, G.M., Clutton-Brock, T.H., on behalf of the Centre for Maternal and Child Enquiries, 2011. Saving Mothers' Lives: reviewing maternal deaths to make motherhood safer: 2006-8: a review. Br. J. Anaesth. 107 (2), 127–132.

Middle, J., Wee, M., 2009. Informed consent for epidural analgesia in labour: a survey of UK practice. Anaesthesia 64 (2), 161–164.

NMC (Nursing and Midwifery Council), 2008. The Code: Standards of Conduct, Performance and Ethics for Nurses and Midwives. NMC, London.

OAA (Obstetric Anaesthetists' Association), 2008. Epidural information card. Available online: <http://www.labourpains.com/ui/content/content.aspx?id=45> (accessed 3 March 2015).

OAA (Obstetric Anaesthetists' Association), 2014. Headache after epidural or spinal injection – what you need to know. Available online: <http://www.labourpains.com/ui/content/content.aspx?ID=316> (accessed 3 March 2015).

Odibo, L., 2007. Does epidural analgesia affect the second stage of labour? Br. J. Midwifery 15 (7), 429–435.

Orbach-Zinger, S., Ginosar, Y., Sverdlik, J., et al., 2012. Partner's presence during initiation of epidural labor analgesia does not decrease maternal stress: a prospective randomized controlled trial. Anesth. Analg. 114 (3), 654–660.

Ousley, R., Egan, C., Dowling, K., Cyna, A.M., 2012. Assessment of block height for satisfactory spinal anaesthesia for caesarean section. Anaesthesia. 67, 1356–1363.

Segal, S., 2010. Labor epidural analgesia and maternal fever. Anesth. Analg. 111 (6), 1467–1475.

Sharma, V., Swinson, A.K., Hughes, C., et al., 2011. Effect of ethnicity and body mass index on the distance from skin to lumbar epidural space in parturients. Anaesthesia 66, 907–912.

Simmons, S.W., Taghizadeh, N., Dennis, A.T., et al., 2012. Combined spinal-epidural versus epidural analgesia in labour. Cochrane Database Syst. Rev. (10), CD003401, doi:10.1002/14651858.CD003401.pub3.

Skrablin, S., Grgic, O., Mihaljevic, S., Blajic, J., 2011. Comparison of intermittent and continuous epidural analgesia on delivery and progression of labour. J. Obstet. Gynaecol. 31 (2), 134–138.

Sng, B.L., Leong, W.L., Zeng, Y., et al., 2014. Early versus late initiation of epidural analgesia for labour. Cochrane Database Syst. Rev. (10), CD007238, doi:10.1002/14651858.CD007238.pub2.

Torvaldsen, S., Roberts, C., Bell, J., Raynes-Greenow, C., 2004. Discontinuation of epidural analgesia late in labour for reducing the adverse delivery outcomes associated with epidural analgesia. Cochrane Database Syst. Rev. (4), CD004457, doi:10.1002/14651858.CD004457.pub2.

Vaida, S., Dalal, P., Mets, B., 2009. Spinal anesthesia for Cesarean delivery following pre-existing epidural labour analgesia. Can. J. Anaesth. 56, 988.

Walsh, D., 1997. TENS: Clinical Applications and Related Theory. Churchill Livingstone, Edinburgh.

Chapter | 26 |

Principles of drug administration: transcutaneous electrical nerve stimulation

LEARNING OUTCOMES

Having read this chapter, the reader should be able to:
- discuss the principles by which TENS is considered to be effective when in labour
- describe how it is applied and used
- summarize the role and responsibilities of the midwife.

This chapter considers the midwife's role in the application and use of transcutaneous electrical nerve stimulation (TENS) for the purposes of pain relief in labour. TENS is not a pharmaceutical drug, but it is widely used for analgesia in labour.

HOW DOES TENS WORK?

The 'gate control' theory of pain suggests that stimulation of larger peripheral (sensory) nerve fibres inhibits pain signals entering the central pain pathway, reducing the perception of pain; TENS provides this stimulation (Francis 2014). Additionally, it is believed that the electrical stimulation also activates the release of the body's own endorphins (Bedwell 2011).

TENS is available as a handheld battery-operated unit. Four electrodes (sticky) are placed onto the skin over specific spinal nerves. The electrical output is adjusted according to the frequency (the number per second), duration and amplitude of the pulse (strength of the current), determining how often, how strong and how long the pulses are. Francis (2014) suggests that the conventional use of TENS for labour should have a high rate of pulses with a strong but painless tingling sensation. He is also clear that as the pain of a contraction increases, the TENS intensity should be increased, too, reducing it when uterine muscles relax. Many TENS machines for labour have the facility to boost the intensity in this way.

There are contraindications for the use of TENS. It should be avoided:

- when immersed in water
- in the presence of a cardiac pacemaker
- over damaged or sore skin
- in the first trimester (Poole 2007a)
- on the abdomen at any stage of pregnancy
- if less than 37 weeks' gestation (Bedwell 2011).

It should also be used with caution for women who have epilepsy.

SUITABILITY AS A LABOUR ANALGESIC

Studies conflict when considering the effectiveness of TENS, so much so that NICE (2014) state that TENS should not be offered to women in established labour. However, levels of consumer satisfaction are good (Carroll et al 1997) and Francis (2014) suggests that it is the inadequacy and poor quality of the research that causes professionals to doubt TENS, rather than TENS itself. As a non-pharmacological analgesic, it has no known ill effects for the mother (so long as it is used according to the manufacturer's instructions) or fetus. It allows the woman to mobilize, to utilize other analgesics as well and to have some control – aiding both her physiological and psychological equilibrium. It also offers some distraction. Francis (2014) believes it to be an easy to use, safe and inexpensive non-pharmacological pain reducer. Poole (2007b) suggests that it may take 20–30 minutes for the effects of TENS to be felt.

POSITIONING OF TENS

Hawkins (1994) suggests that correct positioning of the electrodes is essential. Jackson et al (2014) and Coates (1998) both indicate (when labouring) the need to place the electrodes over the spinal nerves that supply the uterus and pelvic floor: T10–L1 and S2–S4. Francis (2014), however, challenges this approach by suggesting that the electrodes should be placed either side of the lower spine or at the lowest part of the spine and that the woman should be encouraged to move them to find the optimal position for her. In his example, one pair of electrodes is placed on the bottom left of the back, the other pair on the bottom right.

If using conventional placing, Coates (1998) suggests that if the woman's arms are relaxed and hanging loosely by her sides, then the lower tip of her scapula is at T7. Three spinal vertebrae can then be counted down to locate T10. The top of the upper pad is placed level with T10. S2 is located by identifying the iliac crests and placing the top of the lower electrode one vertebra below this. The pads should be placed centrally either side of the spinal column, with 3 cm between them (Fig. 26.1).

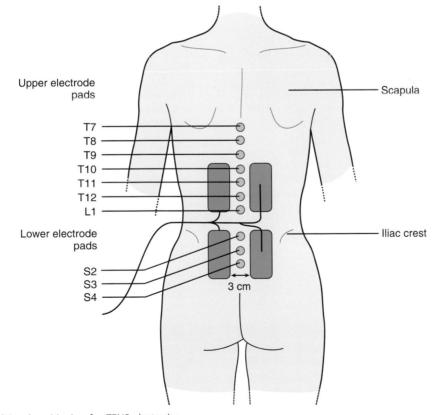

Figure 26.1 Traditional positioning for TENS electrodes.
(Adapted from Jackson et al (2014) with permission of Elsevier)

PROCEDURE: applying a TENS unit for a labouring woman

- Clarify that this is the woman's choice of analgesia; discuss what to expect and establish that none of the contraindications listed above exists.
- Decontaminate hands. Position the woman so that access can be gained to her back.
- Ensure the unit is switched off, but fully charged with the electrodes connected and all the controls on the lowest possible setting.
- Identify suitable positions for the electrodes (see Fig. 26.1 for the traditional locations) and apply them to the skin.
- Switch the unit on so that the woman can feel a strong tingling sensation, demonstrate the boost and how to increase and decrease the intensities according to need.
- Ensure that the woman is comfortable.
- Replace clothing, securing the unit in a pocket if appropriate, leaving the boost button accessible. Decontaminate hands.
- Continue to monitor the woman, aiding her to gain maximum effectiveness from TENS throughout her labour.
- Document application and effect, ensure that there is no electrical interference with any other items being used.
- Discontinue the use of TENS at the end of labour or according to the woman's wishes (switch the unit off, remove electrodes, clean reusable electrodes, service and maintain the unit according to the manufacturer's instructions).

ROLE AND RESPONSIBILITIES OF THE MIDWIFE

These can be summarized as:
- education and empowerment of the woman in her choice of analgesia, but cautiously and with informed consent given that NICE (2014) suggest not to recommend it
- appropriate training, updating, and application of TENS
- care and maintenance of the TENS unit
- observation of the effectiveness
- contemporaneous record keeping.

SUMMARY

- TENS works on the 'gate control' theory of pain: electrical impulses stimulate the sensory nerves to 'close the gate'. It is also believed to encourage the body to release endorphins.
- Many women view TENS as being a good non-pharmacological analgesic for labour; research questions its validity, but some academics question the validity of the research (Francis 2014, Bedwell et al 2011).
- It has minimal side effects and allows both mobility and control.
- The midwife has a role in ensuring that it is applied, used, and maintained correctly.

SELF-ASSESSMENT EXERCISES

The answers to the following questions may be found in the text:
1. How are the effects of TENS achieved?
2. How does a midwife decide where to place the electrodes?
3. Which signs indicate to the woman and the midwife that the TENS unit is working effectively?
4. When should TENS not be used?
5. Summarize the role and responsibilities of the midwife in relation to the use of TENS in labour.

REFERENCES

Bedwell, C., 2011. Why do women use TENS equipment and how effective is it? Br. J. Midwifery 19 (6), 348–351.

Bedwell, C., Dowswell, T., Neilson, J., Lavender, T., 2011. The use of transcutaneous electrical nerve stimulation (TENS) for pain relief in labour: a review of the evidence. Midwifery 27, e141–e148.

Carroll, D., Tramer, M., McQuay, H., et al., 1997. Transcutaneous electrical nerve stimulation in labour pain: a systematic review. Br. J. Obstet. Gynaecol. 104 (2), 169–175.

Coates, T., 1998. Transcutaneous electrical nerve stimulation: TENS. Pract. Midwife 1 (11), 12–14.

Francis, R., 2014. TENS (Transcutaneous electrical nerve stimulation) for labour pain. Pract. Midwife 15 (5), 20–23.

Hawkins, J., 1994. The use of TENS for pain relief in labour. Br. J. Midwifery 2 (10), 487–490.

Jackson, K., Marshall, J., Brydon, S., 2014. Physiology and care during the first stage of labour. In: Marshall, J., Raynor, M. (Eds.), Myles Textbook for Midwives, seventeenth ed. Elsevier, Edinburgh, p. 353.

NICE (National Institute for Health and Care Excellence), 2014. Intrapartum Care: Care of Healthy Women and Their Babies during Childbirth.

Clinical Guideline 190. NICE, London. Available online: <www.nice.org.uk/> (accessed 5 March 2015).

Poole, D., 2007a. Use of TENS in pain management Part One: how TENS works. Nurs. Times 103 (7), 28–29.

Poole, D., 2007b. Use of TENS in pain management Part Two: how to use TENS. Nurs. Times 103 (8), 28–29.

Chapter | 27 |

Facilitation of skills related to childbearing: optimal fetal positioning

LEARNING OUTCOMES

Having read this chapter, the reader should be able to:

- discuss the different positions and postures a woman can use during pregnancy to encourage the fetal occiput to rotate from a posterior to an anterior position and the evidence relating to this
- discuss the different methods that may change the presentation from breech to cephalic and the supporting evidence

- identify some of the hazards associated with malpositions and malpresentations for the woman and baby.

It has long been recognized that both malposition and malpresentation are associated with an increased risk of intervention during labour, including instrumental and operative delivery and increased morbidity for both the woman and the baby. Where it is possible to reduce the incidence of malposition and malpresentation before labour commences, the associated risks will also be reduced. This chapter considers the how the incidence of malposition and malpresentation can be reduced by encouraging the fetus into an optimal fetal position. It will consider the use of maternal positioning and alternative therapies. It does not discuss manual rotation of an occipitoposterior position during labour.

MALPOSITION OF THE OCCIPUT: OCCIPITOPOSTERIOR POSITION

A malposition is any position than is not occipitoanterior (OA) when the vertex is presenting.

The RCM (2012) suggest that between 15–32% of fetuses commence labour in an occipitoposterior (OP) or occipitolateral position, and it is more common in nulliparous women. Carseldine et al (2013) propose the rate of OP positions in the first stage of labour is 25%; many of these will rotate to an OA position during labour so that 5% of births are in a persistent OP position. Phipps et al (2014) suggest that about 70% of babies in an OP position in the early second stage will be born by caesarean section or instrumental delivery.

OP labour and deliveries have an increased risk of adverse effects for the mother and baby, including:

- higher presenting part with wider diameters that will take longer to negotiate the pelvis
- early rupture of membranes, increasing the risk of ascending infection
- back pain
- cord prolapse
- uncoordinated uterine action leading to prolonged labour
- premature urge to push
- prolonged first and second stages
- urinary retention
- trauma to the vagina and pelvic floor including third and fourth degree tears
- instrumental and/or operative delivery, which may be associated with an increased blood loss and neonatal trauma from the forceps or ventouse cup
- abnormal moulding which may result in an unsettled baby and increase the risk of intracranial haemorrhage
- Apgar scores <7 at 5 minutes
- increased perinatal mortality and morbidity.

(Adapted from Carseldine et al 2013, Coates 2013, Simkin 2010)

Sutton & Scott (1996) strongly advocate the use of different positions and postures from 34 weeks' gestation to encourage the fetus to rotate to a lateral or anterior position and so facilitate engagement. They do advise women to discuss this with the health professional overseeing their pregnancy to ensure there are no contraindications to this.

The rationale for these positions is to provide the fetus with room to rotate within the uterus and adopt a position that is more comfortable and better for delivery. The fetus will be able to adopt a more flexed position if in a lateral or anterior position; as the head flexes, the engaging diameters will reduce and hence engagement is likely to occur earlier rather than later. Their advice centres on the regular use of upright and forward leaning postures, particularly during Braxton Hicks contractions, as this is believed to assist the fetus to manoeuvre into the optimum position.

Favourable positions to adopt

- Upright and forward leaning postures, as they create more space for the fetus to turn.
- When reading, sitting on a dining chair with elbows resting on the table and leaning slightly forwards, keeping the knees apart.
- Sitting on a dining chair facing the back, stretching and resting arms over the back of the chair.

- When sitting generally, the knees should be lower than the hips and the back kept straight by placing a small cushion over the small of the back for support.
- While watching television, kneeling on the floor leaning over a large bean bag or cushion
- When driving, place a wedge cushion under the buttocks.
- When swimming, keep the abdomen forwards; breast stroke is better than back stroke.
- When lying on one side, place a pillow between the legs with the top knee resting on the bed.

Positions that increase the likelihood of an OP position

- Relaxing in semi-reclining positions with knees higher than the hips.
- Sitting for long periods in a bucket seat when driving – encourage regular stops to change position and use of a wedge cushion under the buttocks.
- Sitting with crossed legs or legs up.
- Deep squatting in late pregnancy as the head may be forced into the pelvis in the OP position.

The work by Sutton & Scott (1996) is not research-based; rather, their claims are supported by strong anecdotal evidence. This is an under-researched area and at present these positions do not appear to have any disadvantages for suitable women.

The use of an 'all-fours' position using knees and hands for support in conjunction with pelvic rocking has been used since the 1950s with little research as to its effectiveness. Hunter et al (2007) undertook a systematic review of the literature evaluating this intervention and concluded that while adopting this position for 10 minutes twice daily resulted in a positional change at the time, it had no effect on the fetal position at term. Even though there were no adverse effects, they do not recommend the hands–knees position as an intervention; however, they did find this position reduced the incidence of backache during labour. Kariminia et al's (2004) small study compared this intervention (for 10 minutes twice daily) with a control group who had to undertake walking each day from 37 weeks. They concluded that although the hands–knees posture combined with pelvic rocking exercises is commonly used to encourage rotation from the posterior to the anterior position, their results did not support this practice and recommended that in the absence of any beneficial effects, the practice should be discontinued. However Simkin (2010) questions whether the intervention was too slight to fairly assess the potential value of pelvic rocking. Encouraging rotation of the occiput from a posterior to an anterior position remains an area for further research.

MALPRESENTATION: BREECH PRESENTATION

The usual presentation in labour is vertex. A malpresentation refers to any presentation that is not vertex, e.g. breech, face, brow. Breech presentation occurs in approximately 3–4% of pregnancies at term; this figure is higher earlier in pregnancy. As Jackson et al (2013) suggest approximately one-third of breech presentations are not diagnosed until labour, midwives need to maintain their skills in undertaking a vaginal breech delivery through simulation.

Breech labour and delivery is associated with a number of complications:

- early rupture of membranes, with increased risk of ascending infection and cord prolapse
- uncoordinated contractions leading to prolonged labour
- increased risk of cord compression during first and second stage
- foot, leg, and arm prolapse
- early urge to push
- increased risk of operative delivery
- no moulding; head undergoes compression and decompression increasing the risk of intracranial haemorrhage during vaginal birth
- increased risk of trauma to vagina and pelvic floor
- increased risk of birth asphyxia
- increased perinatal morbidity and mortality.

There are a number of techniques that can be used to encourage the fetus to turn from the breech to a cephalic presentation, including external cephalic version, postural management and acupuncture, including moxibustion.

External cephalic version

External cephalic version (ECV) can be undertaken on women with a breech presentation and an uncomplicated pregnancy after 37 weeks to reduce the incidence of term breech presentation (Hofmeyr & Kulier 2012a, Hutton & Hofmeyr 2006). The RCOG (2010) suggest nulliparous women be offered ECV from 36 weeks and multiparous women from 37 weeks' gestation. NICE (2008) agree that all women with breech presentation should be offered ECV at 37 weeks and if this is not possible, it should be at 36 weeks. However, Hutton & Hofmeyr (2006) suggest there is insufficient evidence regarding ECV between 34–36 weeks and state there is no difference to the presentation at term or the caesarean section (CS) rate if it is undertaken earlier, between 32–34 weeks.

ECV is undertaken by experienced personnel, usually obstetricians. The RCOG (2010) suggest success rates of ECV at term are 30–80% with less than 5% spontaneous reversion to breech presentation after a successful ECV. Steen & Kingdon (2008) suggest that ECV has a 50% success rate and consider it an important intervention in reducing the CS rate when performed routinely for breech presentation.

Although Cluver et al (2015) found the use of beta-stimulant tocolytics, e.g. terbutaline, salbutamol, ritodrine, to facilitate ECV increased the number of cephalic presentations in labour and reduced the number of CSs, they caution there is insufficient data on possible adverse effects for the mother or the baby. While increasing the amount of amniotic fluid has been suggested to improve the success of ECV, Burgos et al (2014) found it made no difference.

The RCOG (2010) advise there are absolute and relative contraindications to ECV.

- Absolute:
  - where delivery by CS is required
  - ruptured membranes
  - multiple pregnancy (unless for delivery of the second twin)
  - antepartum haemorrhage within the previous 7 days
  - abnormal cardiotocography
  - major uterine abnormality.
- Relative:
  - small-for-gestational fetus with abnormal Doppler parameters
  - oligohydramnios
  - severe congenital abnormality, e.g. hydrocephalus
  - proteinuric pre-eclampsia
  - scarred uterus (however, Burgos et al (2013) did not find any contraindications for ECV for women who have had a previous CS)
  - unstable lie.

Complications

Hofmeyr & Kulier (2012a) suggest the rates of complications associated with ECV are low with the most frequently reported complication being a transient abnormal fetal heart rate (FHR) pattern. Rarer complications include persistent pathological FHR pattern, vaginal bleeding, placental abruption, emergency CS, and perinatal mortality. They also recommend administration of anti-D prophylactically for non-sensitized rhesus-negative women.

For safety reasons the ECV should be undertaken during daylight hours in a unit where emergency facilities are available. Very occasionally, the fetus becomes compromised during the procedure requiring immediate delivery as a result of placental abruption or knotting of the umbilical cord.

It is important to ensure the following points are adhered to and the midwife can undertake many of these:

- determine the location of the placenta by ultrasonography
- perform an abdominal palpation before the procedure to ensure there has been no spontaneous version and that the breech has not engaged
- cardiotocography should be undertaken before and after the procedure and should be normal
- the woman's bladder should be empty
- the uterus should not be contracting
- the procedure should be stopped if pain is felt
- rhesus negative women should receive anti-D immunoglobulin within 72 hours of the procedure
- cord prolapse should be excluded if the membranes rupture during the procedure
- the procedure is abandoned if the fetus does not turn easily (it can be re-attempted after several days).

ECV encourages the fetus to rotate 180° by moving the breech away from the pelvic brim and then with one hand over each fetal pole, the fetal head is turned downwards while the breech is rotated upwards. The fetus is usually rotated face downwards to maintain flexion. However, if this is unsuccessful, an attempt can be made to turn the fetus backwards but it is important to maintain flexion of the head.

Posture

While the majority of the literature discussing postural techniques discuss the knee–chest position, Sàrries Zgonc (2011) discusses other positions used by Shiatsu therapists to disengage the breech and rocking the baby to show him/her where the exit is. These do not have a large evidence base and would benefit from good-quality research into their effectiveness.

Disengaging the breech (Sàrries Zgonc 2011)

This involves the woman adopting an inverted posture by lying with her head on the floor, her legs upright with her heels high up against a wall and her body and legs supported with pillows and blankets to maintain a straight but relaxed position from shoulders to feet. The woman is encouraged to remain in this position for 5 minutes to encourage the breech to disengage from the pelvis. The shiatsu therapist then regulates the energy flow from the upper to the lower abdomen to increase the flow towards the symphysis pubis which in turn is thought to encourage the fetal head to move down. The woman then takes two to three deep sighs and is helped to roll slowly onto her side and rest. The woman is then taught some exercises to do each day.

Rocking the baby and showing him/her where the exit is (Sàrries Zgonc 2011)

The woman lies on the floor with her knees bent and feet flat on the floor with arms outstretched. The woman identifies which hip feels the loosest and straightens the opposite leg. She then lifts up the looser hip towards the opposite side by moving her bent leg out and away from the other leg but keeping the knee bent and pointing at the ceiling. Her lumbar spine should not be arched and her upper body should remain still. The hip then returns to the floor and the exercise slowly repeated four times. The woman is finally encouraged to place one hand on her pubic bone and the other on her sacrum with her fingertips pointing downwards. She then talks to her baby to show him the way out of the pelvis between her hands. This is all then repeated using the opposite hip.

Knees–chest position

Traditionally, women have been encouraged to adopt a knees–chest posture. There is no clear regimen for how long they should remain in this position and how often it should be done. For example, Hofmeyr & Kulier (2012b) describe the Elkins regime whereby a knee–chest position is adopted for 15 minutes every 2 hours when awake for 5 days; a modified Elkins regime whereby the women assume the position three times a day for 7 days but also with a full bladder; and an Indian version where the woman adopts a supine, head-down position with the pelvis supported by a wedge for 10–15 minutes once or twice a day. Hofmeyr & Kulier (2012b) conclude from their meta-analysis that there is insufficient evidence to support or refute the routine use of postural management.

Acupuncture

Acupuncture is a form of traditional Chinese and Japanese medicine that uses energy (meridian) lines and acupuncture points that are believed to run throughout the body. If there is a difficulty within one of the energy lines it will disrupt the body–mind–spirit relationship; thus correcting and rebalancing the energy levels is at the centre of this treatment. Acupuncture should only be administered by a trained acupuncturist who may use conventional acupuncture (insertion of needles into the skin at acupuncture sites), electroacupuncture (passing a small electric current through the needles inserted into the skin at acupuncture points) and moxibustion. Several studies report on the efficacy of acupuncture, although the study numbers are generally small. One small study of 67 women demonstrated a highly significant effect of acupuncture in altering the presentation (78.7% of the intervention group versus 21.2% of the control group, $p < 0.001$) when undertaken twice a week from 34 to 37 weeks (Habek et al 2003).

MOXIBUSTION

Moxibustion for turning the breech involves the burning of the herb *Artemisia vulgaris* on or over the skin at the acupuncture point BL67 using moxa sticks or cones (Coyle et al 2012) between 28 and 37 weeks of pregnancy. This point is located at the lateral corner of the fifth toenail bed. The sticks are lit and allowed to smoke which applies heat to the acupuncture points. The duration and frequency of treatment can vary immensely, e.g. for 15 minutes up to 10 times each day for a set number of days to twice weekly treatments. Grabowska (2006) recommends using moxibustion twice a day for 15–20 minutes until the presentation changes to cephalic and Neri et al's (2007) small study found only three treatments were needed to change the presentation. Moxibustion is thought to stimulate placental oestrogen and prostaglandin production, encouraging fetal activity through contraction of the uterine lining (Coyle et al 2012).

Moxibustion has received favourable reports that it encourages the fetus to move from a breech to a vertex presentation (Steen & Kingdon 2008). Coyle et al (2012) found that moxibustion, with or without acupuncture or postural techniques, can reduce the number of breech presentations at birth, it also helps to reduce the number of operative deliveries and reduced use of oxytocin during labour. However, Coulon et al (2014) did not show any advantage with using moxibustion once every 48 hours for 20 minutes. Their control group received a 20 minute treatment using an inactivated laser at the same acupoint. They did find, however, that women undergoing moxibustion had a higher success rate when ECV was undertaken. The RCOG (2010) agree that moxibustion appears to be safe and has some success; however, they conclude there is insufficient evidence to support its use. Guttier et al (2009) found no beneficial effect of moxibustion in changing the presentation but found the women who used it had very positive opinions about its use and over 95% would recommend it to a friend with a breech presentation. Furthermore, the control group had been asked not to undertake any form of intervention to attempt to change the presentation, yet one-third attempted at least one intervention which included moxibustion, which may have influenced the outcome.

This is an area of growing interest and the reader is advised to keep abreast of the developments within acupuncture.

ROLE AND RESPONSIBILITIES OF THE MIDWIFE

These can be summarized as:
- keeping up-to-date with current opinion and advice in optimal fetal positioning to provide good evidence-based advice and care
- education and support of the woman
- assisting at ECV.

SUMMARY

- The evidence around postural management for rotating the occiput from a posterior to an anterior position is mainly anecdotal, with little support for undertaking the hands–knees position during pregnancy although there do not appear to be any adverse side effects.
- Postural management for breech appears to bring no benefit but is not considered harmful.
- In uncomplicated pregnancies, ECV has a high success rate, although complications can arise during the procedure.
- Acupuncture, particularly moxibustion, increases fetal activity to encourage the breech to change to a cephalic presentation.
- Further research into postural intervention is required to evaluate its efficacy.

SELF-ASSESSMENT EXERCISES

The answers to the following questions may be found in the text:
1. List the hazards associated with malposition and malpresentation for the woman and the baby.
2. A woman who has a baby in an occipital posterior position asks for advice on postures and positioning to attempt to encourage the fetal occiput to rotate. What advice will you give?
3. Discuss the procedures that can be used to change the presentation from breech to cephalic.
4. What are the role and responsibilities of the midwife in relation to optimal fetal positioning?

REFERENCES

Burgos, J., Cobos, P., Rodriguez, L., et al., 2013. Is external cephalic version at term contraindicated in previous caesarean section? A prospective comparative cohort study. BJOG 121, 230–235.

Burgos, J., Quinta, E., Cobos, P., et al., 2014. Effect of maternal intravenous fluid therapy on external cephalic version at term: a prospective cohort study. Am. J. Obst. Gynecol. 211 (665), e1–e7.

Carseldine, W.J., Phipps, H., Zawada, S.F., et al., 2013. Does occipit posterior position in the second stage of labour increase the operative delivery rate? Aust. N. Z. J. Obstet. Gynaecol. 53, 265–270.

Cluver, C., Gyte, G.M.L., Sinclair, M., et al., 2015. Interventions for helping to turn term breech babies to head first presentation when using external cephalic version. Cochrane Database Syst. Rev. (1), CD000184, doi:10.1002/14651858.CD000184.pub4.

Coates, T., 2013. Malpositions of the occiput and malpresentations. In: Marshall, J., Raynor, M. (Eds.), Myles Textbook for Midwives, sixteenth ed. Elsevier, Edinburgh, pp. 435–453.

Coulon, C., Poleszczuk, M., Paty-Montaigne, M.-H., et al., 2014. Version of breech fetuses by moxibustion with acupuncture. Obstet. Gynaecol. 124 (1), 32–39.

Coyle, M.E., Smith, C.A., Peat, B., 2012. Cephalic version by moxibustion for breech presentation. Cochrane Database Syst. Rev. (5), CD003928, doi:10.1002/14651858.CD003928.pub3.

Grabowska, C., 2006. Turning the breech using moxibustion. Midwives 9 (12), 484–485.

Guttier, M.-J., Pichon, M., Dong, H., et al., 2009. Moxibustion for breech version. Obstet. Gynecol. 114 (5), 1034–1040.

Habek, D., Habek, J.C., Jagust, M., 2003. Acupuncture conversion of fetal breech presentation. Fetal Diagn. Ther. 18 (6), 418–421.

Hofmeyr, G.J., Kulier, R., 2012a. External cephalic version for breech presentation at term. Cochrane Database Syst. Rev. (10), CD000083, doi:10.1002/14651858.CD000083.pub2.

Hofmeyr, G.J., Kulier, R., 2012b. Cephalic version by postural management for breech presentation. Cochrane Database Syst. Rev. (5), CD000051, doi:10.1002/14651858.CD000051.pub2.

Hunter, S., Hofmeyr, G.J., Kulier, R., 2007. Hands and knees posture in late pregnancy or labour for fetal malposition (lateral or posterior). Cochrane Database Syst. Rev. (4), CD001063, doi:10.1002/14651858.CD001063.pub3.

Hutton, E.K., Hofmeyr, G.J., 2006. External cephalic version for breech presentation before term. Cochrane Database Syst. Rev. (1), CD000084, doi:10.1002/14651858.CD000084.pub2.

Jackson, K., Marshall, J.E., Brydon, S., 2013. Physiology and care during the first stage of labour. In: Marshall, J., Raynor, M. (Eds.), Myles Textbook for Midwives, sixteenth ed. Elsevier, Edinburgh, pp. 327–366.

Kariminia, A., Chamberlain, M.E., Keogh, J., Shea, A., 2004. Randomised controlled trial of effect of hands and knees posturing on incidence of occiput posterior position at birth. Br. Med. J. 328 (7438), 490.

Neri, I., De Pace, V., Venturini, P., Facchinetti, F., 2007. Effects of three different stimulations (acupuncture, moxibustion, acupuncture plus moxibustion) of BL.67 acupoint at small toe on fetal behavior of breech presentation. Am. J. Chin. Med. 35 (1), 27–33.

NICE (National Institute for Health and Care Excellence), 2008. Antenatal care: routine care for the healthy pregnant woman. NICE, London. Available online: <www.nice.org.uk> (accessed 3 March 2015).

Phipps, H., de Vries, B., Jagadish, U., Hyett, J., 2014. Management of occiput posterior position in the second stage of labor: a survey of midwifery practice in Australia. Birth 41 (1), 64–69.

RCM (Royal College of Midwives), 2012. Evidence Based Guidelines for Midwifery-Led Care in Labour. Persistent Lateral and Posterior Fetal Positions at the Onset of Labour. Available online: <https://www.rcm.org.uk/content/evidence-based-guidelines> (accessed 4 February 2015).

RCOG (Royal College of Obstetricians and Gynaecologists), 2010. External cephalic version and reducing the incidence of breech presentation Green Top Guideline 20a. Available online: <http://www.rcog.org.uk/womens-health/clinical-guidance/external-cephalic-version-and-reducing-incidence-breech-presentation> (accessed 3 March 2015).

Sàrries Zgonc, I., 2011. The breech: from experience to knowledge. MIDIRS Midwifery Dig. 21 (1), 37–40.

Simkin, P., 2010. The fetal occiput posterior position: state of the science and a new perspective. Birth 37 (1), 61–71.

Steen, M., Kingdon, C., 2008. Breech birth: reviewing the evidence for external cephalic version and moxibustion. Evid. Based Midwifery 6 (4), 126–129.

Sutton, J., Scott, P., 1996. Understanding and Teaching Optimal Fetal Positioning, second ed. Bay Print, Tauranga, New Zealand.

Chapter | 28 |

Facilitation of skills related to childbearing: Cusco speculum use

LEARNING OUTCOMES

Having read this chapter, the reader should be able to:

- discuss the indications for using a Cusco speculum
- describe how to insert and remove the speculum
- discuss what to do if the cervix cannot be visualized
- discuss the role and responsibilities of the midwife in relation to speculum use.

A Cusco speculum is a medical instrument that is inserted into the vagina for access to the top of the vagina and cervix. For the woman this may be an uncomfortable and embarrassing procedure; thus it is important that the midwife undertakes this sensitively and correctly.

INDICATIONS

The midwife may need to use a Cusco speculum:

- to assess cervical dilatation during suspected preterm labour
- to examine the top of the vagina and cervix for the presence of amniotic fluid when prelabour rupture of membranes is suspected
- to assess for the source of bleeding following bleeding *per vaginam*
- to obtain a high vaginal swab.

CUSCO SPECULUM

The Cusco speculum is made of metal (reusable) or plastic (single use, disposable) and usually comes in three sizes – small, medium, and large. It has two short hinged blades that are curved across their width to give a duckbill shape (Fig. 28.1). The blades are close together when the speculum is closed, but when open they separate and press against the vaginal walls. At one end there is a circular opening through which the vagina and cervix can be visualized and swabs inserted when required. Attached to this are the handles that open and close the speculum using a screw mechanism. When the handles are apart the blades are closer together and as the handles are brought closer together the blades open. It is worth practising the opening and closing of the blades a few times before inserting it to ensure familiarity with how it works.

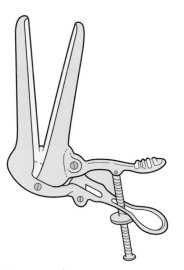

Figure 28.1 Cusco speculum.
(Adapted with kind permission from Chilman & Thomas 1987)

INSERTION OF THE SPECULUM

The insertion of a speculum, whilst usually not painful, can be uncomfortable, particularly if there is a vaginal infection or lacerations, and using a cold speculum can make this discomfort worse. It can also be an embarrassing procedure for some women, which can be a source of anxiety. In their study with non-pregnant women, Wright et al (2005) found both discomfort and anxiety were reduced when women were offered the opportunity for self-insertion of the speculum. There do not appear to have been any studies looking at the effects of self-insertion of speculums during pregnancy.

When inserting the speculum, it is advisable to apply a thin coating of lubricating gel over the outer aspects of the blades to reduce friction between the blades and the vaginal wall. Hill and Lamvu (2012) found the use of 0.3 mL lubricating gel, compared with water for lubrication, reduced the degree of pain experienced during insertion. Use of aqueous gel for lubrication does not appear to affect the detection of infection from any swabs taken (Harmanli & Jones 2010). The blades should be inserted either obliquely or in the anteroposterior diameter while gently applying a 45° downward pressure. The speculum is rotated during insertion so that the handles are facing the clitoris or anus.

The speculum should be inserted far enough to facilitate visualization of the cervix and, if required, swab taking (Hardy 2007). If the cervix is not visualized, it is possible the speculum is not inserted far enough, in which case the blades should be closed slightly and the speculum inserted deeper or a larger speculum with longer blades be used. The tip of the speculum may have slipped into the anterior fornix which is more likely to occur if a downward pressure is not used during insertion. If this has occurred, the speculum should be withdrawn slightly and the hand holding the end of the speculum raised slightly to depress the speculum tip into the same axis as the cervix.

If the lateral walls of the vagina bulge inwards on opening the blades, visualization of the cervix will also be difficult. This is more likely to occur with obese women or where the woman has a vaginal prolapse. To overcome this, a condom with a small cut at the tip can be placed over the speculum prior to insertion or a larger speculum can be used (although the latter may increase the discomfort for the woman).

Once in position the blades are opened and the cervix and upper part of the vagina can be visualized. This is facilitated by using a good light source and many speculums use a light source that is clipped to the speculum. The light should be positioned so that the midwife is looking just over the top of it. When undertaking the procedure to assess for ruptured membranes, it is important that the woman has been lying down for at least 30 minutes to allow the amniotic fluid to pool in the vagina.

When removing the speculum, care should be taken to ensure the blades are not shut quickly while still in the vagina as they can pinch the walls of the vagina. It is better to close the blades completely once the speculum has been removed. The speculum can be rotated so that it is removed using the same position as it was inserted in.

ASEPSIS

Insertion of a speculum during pregnancy should be with a sterile speculum and follow the principles of asepsis to reduce the risk of ascending infection which can lead to uterine and neonatal sepsis. Tattersall (2006) advocates the use of single-use disposable speculums; these should never be reused (Wilkinson 2006). In the presence of ruptured membranes, sterile gloves should be worn but non-sterile gloves are acceptable for obtaining a swab when the membranes are intact. A sterile vaginal examination (VE) pack and warm water should be used to clean the vulva if required.

PROCEDURE: using a speculum

- Discuss the procedure with the woman and gain informed consent.

- Encourage the woman to empty her bladder.
- If suspected ruptured membranes, the woman should lie down for 30+ minutes.
- Gather equipment:
  - sterile or non-sterile gloves (depending on the reason for speculum use)
  - speculum and lubricating gel, e.g. KY Jelly
  - disposable sheet
  - sterile VE pack containing swabs and a bowl (if indicated)
  - warm water (if indicated)
  - swab stick and medium (if indicated)
  - light source.
- Ensure privacy.
- Place the disposable sheet so that it will be under the woman's buttocks and thighs.
- Ask the woman to remove her underwear and any sanitary towels, lay down (if not already doing so) in an almost recumbent position (using a wedge to avoid aortocaval occlusion if necessary), and cover her lower abdomen and upper thighs.
- The woman should be asked to flex her legs at the knees with her ankles together and knees parted.
- Wash and dry hands and apply gloves.
- Remove the cover to expose the genital area – the woman can be asked to do this if sterile gloves are used.
- If being used, open the VE pack and ask the assistant to put warm water into the bowl.
- Lubricate the outer aspect of the blades of the speculum with a water-soluble lubricant, keeping the blades closed.
- If indicated, clean the genital area by swabbing the perineum from front to back using cotton-wool balls or gauze soaked with the warm water, passing the swabs from the examining (clean) hand to the non-examining (dirty) hand; use each swab once and dispose of it (see p. 225).
- Using the non-dominant hand, part the labia and insert the speculum into the vagina in a downwards direction with the dominant hand.
- During insertion, rotate the speculum to position the handles towards the clitoris or anus.
- Open the blades by unscrewing the handles and bringing them closer together, informing the woman that she may feel pressure as the blades stretch the vagina.
- Inspect the vagina and cervix using a good light source and, if indicated, obtain the high vaginal swab (see Chapter 11).

- Remove the speculum by closing the blades slightly, taking care not to trap any maternal tissue, and rotating the speculum back to its insertion position then withdraw the speculum.
- Remove the disposable sheet and assist the woman to replace her sanitary towel and knickers.
- Remove and dispose of gloves and equipment.
- Assist the woman into a comfortable position.
- Wash and dry hands.
- Document findings and act accordingly.

ROLE AND RESPONSIBILITIES OF THE MIDWIFE

These can be summarized as:
- recognizing the need for using a Cusco speculum
- ensuring the procedure is undertaken correctly, with minimal discomfort
- recognizing what to do if the cervix is not visualized initially
- correct documentation.

SUMMARY

- The woman may find this an embarrassing and uncomfortable procedure.
- It is important to undertake the procedure correctly and use lubrication to reduce the discomfort.
- Asepsis is important to reduce the risk of uterine and neonatal infection.

SELF-ASSESSMENT EXERCISES

The answers to the following questions may be found in the text:
1. When might a midwife need to use a Cusco speculum?
2. How may discomfort and embarrassment be reduced for the woman during this procedure?
3. Describe how the speculum should be inserted and removed.
4. What can the midwife do if the cervix is not visualized initially?

REFERENCES

Chilman, A., Thomas, M., 1987. Understanding Nursing Care, third ed. Churchill Livingstone, Edinburgh.

Hardy, J., 2007. How to take a sample for cervical screening. Nurs. Stand. 21 (50), 40–44.

Harmanli, O., Jones, K.A., 2010. Using lubricant for speculum insertion. Obstet. Gynecol. 116 (2), 415–417.

Hill, D.A., Lamvu, G., 2012. Effect of lubricating gel on patient comfort during vaginal speculum examination. Obstet. Gynecol. 119 (2), 227–231.

Tattersall, S., 2006. The use of vaginal specula in improving infection control. Nurs. Times 102 (9), 53–55.

Wilkinson, E., 2006. The implications of reusing single-use medical devices. Nurs. Times 102 (45), 23.

Wright, D., Fenwick, J., Stephenson, P., Monterosso, L., 2005. Speculum 'self-insertion': a pilot study. J. Clin. Nurs. 14 (9), 1098–1111.

Chapter | 29 |

Facilitation of skills related to childbearing: membrane sweep

LEARNING OUTCOMES

Having read this chapter, the reader should be able to:

• discuss the indications for membrane sweeping

• discuss the current evidence available

• describe how the procedure is performed

• discuss what the midwife can do if the cervix is closed

• summarize the role and responsibilities of the midwife.

NICE (2008) recommend that while the majority of women will go into spontaneous labour by 42 weeks, the midwife should discuss the risks associated with prolonged pregnancy (>42 weeks) with women at the 38-week antenatal appointment. This discussion should include membrane sweeping, also referred to as a 'stretch and sweep'. This chapter considers the skill of sweeping or 'stripping' the membranes.

MEMBRANE SWEEPING

Yildirim et al (2010) define membrane sweeping as 'the digital separation of the chorioamniotic membranes from the lower uterine segment'. It involves a vaginal examination (VE) (p. 224), so the midwife can use her fingers to gently dilate (stretch) the cervical os, and then separate the membranes from the lower segment (sweep). This is performed on a cervix that is beginning to dilate, as it requires entry of the fingers through the cervix. If the cervix is not dilated, cervical massage can be undertaken (NICE 2008). This causes an increase in the local production of prostaglandin and increases prostaglandin metabolites within the maternal circulation (Boulvain et al 2005, Yildirim et al 2010) with labour following over the next few days.

de Miranda et al (2006) undertook membrane sweeping every 48 hours, performing three 360° sweeps on each occasion until labour commenced or the pregnancy reached 42 weeks' gestation. Yildirim et al (2010) used the same technique but only performed it once. NICE (2008) do not specify how to undertake a membrane sweep but recommend nulliparous women be offered the procedure at the 40- and 41-week antenatal visits, while parous women should be offered it at the 41-week visit. Additionally they suggest membrane sweeping should be offered whenever a VE is undertaken to assess the cervix or additional membrane sweeping offered if labour does not commence spontaneously. The frequency at which membrane sweeping should be undertaken is still subject to debate.

Cervical massage can be achieved on a closed cervix by using the fore- and middle fingers to make circular pushing and massaging movements on the surface of the cervix for 15–30 seconds' duration (de Miranda et al 2006, Yildirim et al 2010). Gibbon (2012) recommends massaging the cervix around the vaginal fornices.

BENEFITS AND RISKS

Membrane sweeping does appear to reduce the time to spontaneous onset of labour and the need for formal methods of induction, e.g. prostaglandin (PGE$_2$) (de Miranda et al 2006, Mozurkewich et al 2011, NICE 2008). Yildirim et al (2010) found an increase in spontaneous labour within 7 days. de Miranda et al (2006) concluded membrane sweeping significantly reduced the time to delivery by 1 day when undertaken at 41 weeks' gestation. Their study reduced the number of women with post-term pregnancies from 41 to 23% and found the effects were more evident for cervical sweeping than massage with significant effects for both primi- and multigravid women. However, Hamdan et al (2009) in their study looking at serial membrane sweeping at 36^{+6}–40^{+6} weeks for women planning a vaginal birth after caesarean delivery found no significant effect on the spontaneous onset of labour. Hill et al (2008) undertook weekly sweeps from 38 weeks and found no difference in the number of post-term pregnancies or inductions of labour.

There are no differences in adverse maternal and neonatal outcomes for women who had membrane sweeping or massage compared with those who did not, e.g. prelabour rupture of membranes, maternal and neonatal infection requiring antibiotic treatment, meconium-stained liquor, vaginal bleeding, instrumental and operative delivery, neonatal morbidity (Boulvain et al 2005, de Miranda et al 2006, Hamdan et al 2009, Yildirim et al 2010).

Membrane sweeping is associated with increased maternal discomfort and vaginal bleeding with and following the procedure (Boulvain et al 2005, de Miranda et al 2006, Mozurkewich et al 2011) and it is important the woman is aware of this before she consents to the procedure. Yildirim et al (2010) found that 19.5% of women found membrane sweeping resulted in discomfort.

Sweeping the membranes appears to be a safe procedure which may reduce the incidence of prolonged pregnancy. Provided there are no complications, e.g. placenta praevia, contraindication to labour or vaginal birth, it can be offered to women over 40 weeks' gestation. Local protocols should be followed but generally this procedure can be undertaken in an outpatient setting such as the woman's home or antenatal clinic. Asepsis should be maintained and the midwife should be trained in this aspect of care prior to undertaking the procedure.

The midwife should maintain contemporaneous records and should document the discussion with the woman, that consent is obtained, when and how the procedure was undertaken, and the findings from the VE.

PROCEDURE: stretch and sweep of the membranes

- Discuss the procedure including the benefits and risks with the woman and gain informed consent.
- Prepare for and undertake the examination *per vaginam* (as detailed on p. 225 as far as 'Locate the cervix …') expecting to find a posterior, largely uneffaced, almost closed cervix.
- Undertake a Bishop's scoring (or similar) assessment (see Glossary) of the cervix.
- Insert one or two fingers into the cervix to gently dilate the os, moving the finger(s) between the lower uterine segment and fetal membranes.
- Using some inward pressure, move the finger(s) with a sweeping circular action through 360° (Fig. 29.1). This should be undertaken fairly decisively as the woman will be uncomfortable, which will increase if the procedure is unnecessarily prolonged.
- If the cervix is closed, perform cervical massage for 15–30 seconds using the fore- and middle fingers to make circular pushing and massaging movements on the cervix.

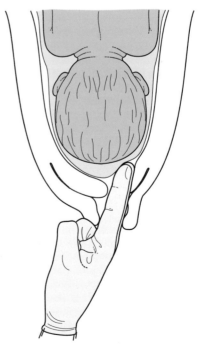

Figure 29.1 Sweeping the membranes.

- Remove the examining hand gently, remove gloves.
- Auscultate the fetal heart.
- Assist the woman to dress and resume a comfortable position; discuss the findings.
- Dispose of equipment appropriately and wash and dry hands.
- Document the findings and act accordingly.

- Cervical massage can be undertaken on a closed cervix.
- Membrane sweeping reduces the risk of prolonged pregnancy but is associated with maternal discomfort and vaginal bleeding.
- It appears to be a safe procedure with no serious adverse effects for the woman or the baby.

ROLE AND RESPONSIBILITIES OF THE MIDWIFE

These can be summarized as:

- discussing the procedure with the woman at 38 weeks providing information on the benefits and risks
- undertaking the procedure correctly having gained informed consent
- thorough contemporaneous documentation.

SELF-ASSESSMENT EXERCISES

The answers to the following questions may be found in the text:

1. When should membrane sweeping be offered and undertaken?
2. On which women should this procedure not be undertaken?
3. What information would the midwife discuss with the woman to help her make an informed decision about whether or not to undergo membrane sweeping?
4. Discuss how membrane sweeping and cervical massage can be undertaken.
5. Summarize the role and responsibilities of the midwife in relation to this procedure.

SUMMARY

- Sweeping the membranes involves gently dilating the cervical os and digitally separating the membranes from the lower uterine segment.

REFERENCES

Boulvain, M., Stan, C.M., Irion, O., 2005. Membrane sweeping for induction of labour. Cochrane Database Syst. Rev. (1), Art No.: CD000451, doi:10.1002/14651858.CD000451; pub2.

de Miranda, E., van der Bom, J.G., Bonsel, G.J., et al., 2006. Membrane sweeping and prevention of post-term pregnancy in low-risk pregnancies: a randomised controlled trial. Br. J. Obstet. Gynaecol. 113 (4), 402–408.

Gibbon, K., 2012. How to … perform a stretch and sweep. Midwives. Available online: <https://www.rcm.org.uk/news-views-and-analysis/how-to%E2%80%A6-perform-a-stretch-and-sweep> (accessed 3 March 2015.).

Hamdan, M.L., Sidhu, K., Sabir, N., et al., 2009. Serial membrane sweeping at term in planned vaginal birth after cesarean: a randomized controlled trial. Obstet. Gynecol. 114 (4), 745–751.

Hill, M.J., McWilliams, G.D., Garcia-Sur, D., et al., 2008. The effect of membrane sweeping on prelabour rupture of membranes. Obstet. Gynecol. 111 (6), 1313–1319.

Mozurkewich, E.L., Chilimigras, J.L., Berman, D.R., et al., 2011. Methods of induction of labour: a systematic review. BMC Pregnancy Childbirth 11, 84. <http://www.ncbi.nlm.nih.gov/pmc/articles/PMC3224350> (accessed 27 October 2015).

NICE (National Institute for Health and Clinical Excellence), 2008. Induction of Labour. NICE, London. Available online: <www.nice.org.uk> (accessed 3 March 2015).

Yildirim, G., Güngördük, K., Karadağ, Ö.İ., et al., 2010. Membrane sweeping to induce labor in low-risk patients at term pregnancy: a randomized controlled trial. J. Matern. Fetal Neonatal Med. 23 (7), 681–687.

Chapter 30

Principles of intrapartum skills: first-stage issues

LEARNING OUTCOMES

Having read this chapter, the reader should be able to:

- discuss what is meant by the latent and established phase of the first stage of labour and how this affects subsequent assessment of progress
- discuss the different positions that a woman may adopt during the first stage of labour and when each of these may be recommended
- list the indications for undertaking a vaginal examination (VE) during labour
- discuss the information that may be obtained from a VE and how this assesses progress
- describe the procedures for VE, amniotomy, and the application of a fetal scalp electrode.

The National Institute for Health and Care Excellence (NICE 2014) advise that the first stage of labour has two phases – latent and established (active). NICE (2014) suggest that the latent phase is from the onset of painful contractions (although they may be irregular) and a time during which there are cervical changes including effacement and dilatation up to 4 cm. Thus an established first stage of labour is from when the cervix is 4 cm dilated and there are regular painful contractions. This chapter focuses on a selection of the skills used by the midwife when caring for a woman during the first stage of labour (some of which may also be used at other times, e.g. second stage of labour). The chapter begins with a discussion of the definition of latent and active phases as progress is assessed on the basis of how these are defined. The use of different positions the woman can adopt follows and concludes with some of the skills used during the first stage of labour. The skills reviewed are examination *per vaginam*, often referred to as a vaginal examination (VE), amniotomy (artificial rupture of membranes, ARM), and application of a fetal scalp electrode (FSE) which may occur during a VE. It is recognized that the midwife uses other important skills during labour, in particular communication with and observation of the woman, as much information can be gleaned from this. However, this is not discussed within this text.

THE LATENT AND ESTABLISHED PHASES OF THE FIRST STAGE OF LABOUR AND PROGRESS OF LABOUR

While the first stage of labour is classified as having latent and established phases, there is no universal agreement as to when one phase ends and the other begins, which makes assessing progress difficult. Women who present to hospital in the latent phase are often encouraged to go home and wait for labour to establish. NICE (2014) provide a very clear definition based around whether painful contractions are regular and whether the cervix is dilated from and beyond 4 cm. However, some multiparous women are assessed as being in the latent phase when they have painful contractions every 15 minutes and their cervix is 4 cm dilated as this may be considered a 'multips os'. However, the woman herself may consider she is in labour and not wish to go home. Equally, some women will never have regular contractions yet still manage to birth their baby – are they in the established phase at any point? A medicalized definition of when the different phases of labour begin and end may be very different to the woman's perception of her labour (RCM 2012a).

McDonald (2010) questions whether the latent phase actually exists or whether it is 'pre-labour' with the body undergoing the physical changes needed in preparation for birth, or is the latent phase the end of 'pre-labour'. The RCM (2012a) suggest the latent phase and its duration and impact on labour is poorly understood. However, if the latent phase is taken into account when considering the overall length of the first stage, it can make the first stage appear longer and progress slower, leading to increased intervention (particularly if a partogram is used with alert and action lines).

NICE (2014) suggest the average length of time for the duration of labour for first labours is around 8 hours, and it is unusual for it to last longer than 18 hours, whereas for second and subsequent labours, the duration is around 5 hours and is unlikely to last over 12 hours. Thus they expect the duration of labour to vary between first and subsequent labours. However, they also state that delay in the established first stage is suspected when there is cervical dilatation of <2 cm in 4 hours for first and subsequent labours or there is slowing in the progress of labour for second and subsequent labours (NICE 2014). They also consider the amount of descent and rotation of the presenting part and any changes in the strength, duration, and frequency of uterine contractions should be considered (NICE 2014). However, a reduction in the frequency of contractions and slowing of cervical dilatation may be experienced as part of normal labour. Schmid & Downe (2010) suggest the woman will undergo a number of transition phases during labour which include a period when the cervix is dilated to 5–6 cm and again around 8–9 cm. During these transition periods, for some women, contractions slow and labour can slow down, perhaps even stop. Schmid & Downe (2010) suggest this is a time when the woman is able to restore her physical energy and as such should not be considered abnormal otherwise unnecessary intervention will occur. Zhang et al (2010) found it can take >6 hours for the cervix to dilate from 4 to 5 cm, and over 3 hours to move from 5–6 cm and suggest that with both first and subsequent labours the progress of cervical dilatation is the same up to 6 cm, after which the multiparous labour often progresses quicker than the first labour. They argue that, particularly for nulliparous women, labour does not progress in a consistent manner (Zhang et al 2010) yet women can birth their babies vaginally without adverse outcomes to mother or baby, a view supported by Incerti et al (2011). They also suggest that the established phase of labour should not be considered to begin until cervical dilatation is ≥6 cm, as before that no change in cervical dilatation is often normal (Zhang et al 2010).

Grasek et al (2014) studied the descent of the fetal head during term labour and calculated the median station for each centimetre of cervical dilatation for nulliparous and multiparous women. Nulliparous women had a median station of −3 at 0–1 cm, −2 at 2–3 cm, −1 at 4–5 cm, 0 at 6–8 cm, +1 at 9 cm, and +2 at 10 cm whereas multiparous had a slower descent of −3 at 0–3 cm, −2 at 4–5 cm, −1 at 6 cm, 0 at 7–9 cm, and +2 at 10 cm (Grasek et al 2014). Descent time between each of the stations was significantly quicker in multiparous women except for descent between +2 and +3.

When assessing progress, the midwife should take into account more than cervical dilatation but should also consider whether the position of the cervix has moved, whether it has ripened (softened), become effaced and whether the presenting part has rotated, flexed and descended (RCM 2012b). She should also consider where the woman is in her labour, what is happening with the contractions, whether the woman has entered a transition phase (as may be noted by her changing behaviours), and what definition of latent and established labour and 'progress' is being used. One advantage of assessing progress is that it allows time to transfer the woman to a facility with a higher level of care if delay is suspected (Downe et al 2013).

MATERNAL POSITIONING

Women should be encouraged to adopt whichever positions they find comfortable during the first stage of labour (NICE 2014). Lawrence et al (2013) suggest that, given the freedom to do so, women will change position throughout labour and a change in positions should be encouraged to avoid the occurrence of pressure ulcer formation (see Chapter 53). For some women, changing position is more difficult due to constraints such as epidural anaesthesia or continuous fetal heart rate monitoring; however, the midwife can still enable the woman to make some positional changes, e.g. side-lying. The RCM (2012c) acknowledge that midwives should be proactive in demonstrating and encouraging different positions in labour, particularly for women with challenges such as continuous fetal heart rate monitoring and intravenous tubing. The environment is often the key to freedom of movement – one without a variety of furniture and props that encourage positional changes are more likely to have women who remain semi-reclined on the bed (Cutler 2012, RCM 2012c). When the bed is the dominant feature in the room women are likely to adopt this position; it is also a convenient position for the midwife when certain procedures are required (e.g. abdominal palpation, examination *per vaginam*). Lawrence et al (2013) suggest many women will be upright throughout labour but within the Western world, there is a preference for lying down when the cervix is around 5–6 cm. This would tie in with the transitional phase that occurs around this time in labour and the woman is in need of recharging her energy. Once this has happened the woman should be encouraged to be upright again. Cutler (2012) cautions midwives not to guide the woman onto the bed for their own convenience. Equally, after procedures such as abdominal palpation and VE undertaken with the woman on the bed, the midwife should encourage her to adopt her previous position.

Positions adopted can vary from upright (including walking, sitting, kneeling, squatting, all-fours) to recumbent (including supine, semi-recumbent, lateral, or side-lying); Chapman (2009) suggests that upright positions are more comfortable than sitting positions, with which the RCM (2012c) agrees. Upright positions encourage the fetus to descend into the pelvis (Lawrence et al 2013) and may also result in a shorter first stage, less severe pain, and less narcotic and epidural use (RCM 2012c). The National Childbirth Trust (NCT 2011) encourage women to keep moving in labour and also advocate rocking against the wall or holding on to an open door, swaying, walking around and up and down stairs, and the use of a birthing ball to remain upright. Simkin & Ancheta (2005) support the use of upright positions, suggesting moving around during labour can help the pelvic bones accommodate the fetus during its travels through the pelvis. Baker (2010) agrees, suggesting upright positions optimize the changes that occur within the pelvic joints during the end of pregnancy and labour (increasing pelvic diameters and causing slight changes in pelvic shape). Midwives advocate the use of stair walking or lifting one leg onto a surface so that the knee is higher than the other where labour appears to be slowing or asynclitism is present. The NCT (2011) suggest that if a woman has been mobilizing but is getting tired she could try kneeling or if she wants to sit, to ensure her feet are lower than her pelvis.

Squatting makes use of gravity and the pelvic changes (Sanderson 2012) but Cutler (2012) cautions that women in the Western world find it hard to maintain a squatting position as a result of shortening of the Achilles tendon from the use of chair sitting, wearing heeled shoes, and not using squatting for defaecation. For a woman to use squatting during labour, it is worth discussing this during pregnancy and encouraging her to practice, particularly if her partner is going to support her in the squat.

All-fours

Hunter et al (2007) found that women who were labouring with fetuses in an occipitoposterior position experienced less backache when adopting an all-fours position. This may also be achieved by leaning over a birthing ball to relieve pressure on the woman's arms. It may be more comfortable for the woman if she has support/cushioning under her knees (e.g. pillow, padded mat). Hanson (2009) suggests an open knee–chest position (the buttocks are high, with the thighs at right angles to lower legs) can help to reduce the premature urge to push while a closed knee–chest position (the buttocks are lower to the ground, with knees and hips flexed and abducted beneath the abdomen) is useful if the cervix is oedematous.

Lateral (side-lying)

Ridley (2007) recommends women with an occipitoposterior position should lie on their side, ensuring it is the same side as the position of the fetal spine, to encourage fetal rotation to an occipitoanterior position (e.g. lie on right side for right occipitoposterior position), as this was found to increase the incidence of spontaneous vaginal delivery, decrease the length of labour, and reduce the risk of caesarean section compared with lying on the opposite side or any other position. This may be a way of alternating the position of a woman with restricted mobility, e.g. with epidural use, and relieving pressure from the buttocks, sacral area, and heels.

Supine

Women should be discouraged from lying supine. When the woman lies flat, the weight of the pregnant uterus can compress the major blood vessels (aortocaval compression) which can compromise maternal cardiac function and uterine blood flow. This reduces fetal oxygenation and causes alterations in the fetal acid–base status. If a woman wishes to lie supine, it is advisable to place a wedge under her right side to relieve the pressure off the major vessels. Contractions can appear to be less strong in the supine position compared to upright or lateral positions but if the woman becomes upright again, the contractions should return to their previous state (Lawrence et al 2013).

Semi-recumbent

Kerrigan (2006) suggests there is little evidence to support use of this position; however, some women may need to rest and adopt this position periodically during labour.

EXAMINATION *PER VAGINAM*

A VE is an intimate, invasive procedure with the potential to cause distress and pain to the woman; thus it should only be undertaken when there is a clear clinical indication. Hassan et al (2012) remind us that for women, VE is a living experience that they may feel empowers them by increasing their self-confidence and belief in their childbearing ability or, equally, increase their feeling of vulnerability. While it is often undertaken to assess progress, it is imprecise when performed by different clinicians (RCM 2012b). There is also a risk of ascending infection with multiple examinations, particularly once the membranes have ruptured, although Cahill et al (2012) suggest the risk of maternal fever is not significantly increased by the number of VEs. While Lewin et al (2005) found women experience an average of three VEs during labour some women will have far more than this. Shepherd & Cheyne (2013) found the number of VEs undertaken increased as

the length of time in labour in hospital increased, with 52% of women undergoing ≥3 VEs during labour with the most common rationale given by midwives was to assess labour progress.

Dixon & Foureur (2010) suggest that it is an intervention which disrupts the woman's concentration and interferes with the labour rhythm, particularly as the woman may be required to change her position. There is no research-based information on which to make a recommendation for the timing and frequency of VEs during labour (RCM 2012b). Hassan et al (2012) caution that a VE should be done only when necessary and consideration should be given to the woman's feelings and experiences during a VE. However, NICE (2014) recommend it should be undertaken 4-hourly, if there is concern about progress or in response to the woman's wishes. An abdominal palpation should be undertaken prior to the VE so that the results of each can be correlated.

Indications

A VE may be undertaken prior to labour as part of an induction of labour procedure to insert a prostaglandin pessary or gel (Chapter 21) or to perform a membrane sweep (Chapter 29).

During labour, the midwife may undertake a VE to:

- confirm the onset of labour
- identify the presentation and position
- assess progress during labour
- perform an artificial rupture of membranes
- apply a fetal scalp electrode
- exclude cord prolapse following spontaneous rupture of the membranes where there is an ill-fitting or high presenting part
- confirm the onset of the second stage of labour, especially with a breech presentation and multiple pregnancy.

Contraindications

The midwife should not undertake a VE when there is:

- no consent from the woman
- active bleeding
- placenta praevia
- suspected preterm labour
- pre-labour rupture of the membranes.

This can be a very distressing procedure for some women and it is important the procedure is discussed with the woman before the VE is undertaken. Her informed consent should be obtained and the VE is not undertaken if the woman does not agree. The discussion should include the rationale for the procedure, what will happen, what is required of the woman, and confirmation that the VE will be stopped at any point if requested by the woman. The ideal time for much of this discussion is before the onset of labour but it should be repeated each time a VE is indicated. The discussion should also occur in a manner that allows the woman to ask questions and refuse the examination. Verbal and non-verbal communication should be continued during the procedure not only to provide the woman with information about what is happening but also so the midwife can recognize when the woman is experiencing discomfort/pain and requires the VE to end (Stewart 2005). Lewin et al (2005) found only 70% of women recalled a discussion of VE occurring prior the procedure, although 95% considered they were well informed of the findings. Only 40% felt they could refuse the examination and sadly, 22.2% felt their permission was not sought!

INFORMATION GAINED FROM UNDERTAKING AN EXAMINATION *PER VAGINAM*

External genitalia

Prior to performing the VE the external genitalia should be observed for abnormalities such as varicosities, oedema, warts, signs of infection, and scarring, particularly if indicative of previous perineal or labial trauma or female genital mutilation. NICE (2014) advise that a VE may be very difficult in the presence of infibulated genital mutilation as may catheterization and applying a fetal scalp electrode. They further advise that if this is noted, a discussion should occur with the woman to inform her of the risks around delay in the second stage of labour and spontaneous 'perineal' trauma and the need for an anterior episiotomy and possibly defibulation in labour (NICE 2014), although this discussion should ideally take place during pregnancy.

If there is any discharge or bleeding from the vagina, the colour, consistency, amount and odour should be recorded. If the membranes have ruptured, amniotic fluid may be seen and the colour and odour should be noted. Clear liquor with a non-offensive odour is normal.

Vagina

The vagina should feel warm and moist, with soft distensible walls. A hot, dry vagina could be indicative of dehydration, infection or obstructed labour and a vagina that feels 'tense' may be associated with fear or previous scarring. The presence of varicosities, a cystocele, or a rectocele should be noted. A full rectum may be felt through the posterior vaginal wall which may lead the midwife to suggest the use of suppositories or an enema.

Cervix

The cervix is assessed for position, consistency, effacement, dilatation, and application to the presenting part. The cervix is usually in a central or posterior position, firm, non-effaced with the os closed (unripe) during pregnancy. However during the latter weeks of pregnancy and early labour, the structure and position of the cervix alters as the cervix 'ripens', causing the cervix to feel less rigid and adopt an anterior position. A soft and stretchy 'ripe' cervix is often associated with good dilatation of the os uteri, whereas a tight unyielding unripe cervix at term is more likely to be associated with prolonged labour. An unripe cervix requires three to four times more uterine effort than a ripe cervix (Burnhill et al 1962).

With the primigravid woman, effacement usually precedes dilatation but they can appear to occur simultaneously with the multigravid woman. Effacement is assessed by the length of the cervix and the degree to which it protrudes into the vagina. A non-effaced cervix feels long and tubular, with the os closed or partly dilated. The cervix thins out and becomes shorter with effacement, as the lower uterine segment 'takes it up' (Fig. 30.1). A fully effaced cervix feels continuous with the lower uterine segment and does not protrude into the vagina.

In the primigravid woman, the os uteri is usually closed until labour begins, but with a multigravid woman the os may allow one or two fingers through before labour, commonly referred to as a 'multips os'. With a breech presentation the fetal anus should not be mistaken for a closed cervix as the anus will be traumatized if fingers are inserted through it (Warwick et al 2013).

Dilatation of the os uteri, measured in centimetres, is assessed by inserting one or both fingers through the external os and parting the fingers to assess the diameter. In early labour, when the cervix is less than 2 cm dilated, usually only one finger can be inserted. It may be easier to feel around the remaining rim of cervix towards the end of the first stage to estimate dilatation; for example, a rim of 1 cm equates to a dilatation of 8 cm, as there is 2 cm of cervix remaining. When feeling a rim that is stretchy, it is important to assess dilatation without stretching it, this may be easier to achieve by using fingertips on the edge of the cervix. Full dilatation occurs when the cervix can no longer be felt and is equal to 10 cm. This is the point at which the fetal head can pass through the cervix; although for the preterm fetus this may happen before full dilatation. If the presentation is breech, the foot and leg can protrude through the cervix before it is fully dilated (footling breech). Dilatation of the os uteri should occur progressively throughout the first stage of labour and is one factor in determining progress.

A cervix that is well applied to the presenting part is associated with good uterine activity (Blackburn 2013). The

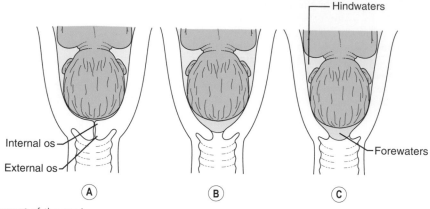

Figure 30.1 Effacement of the cervix.

reverse may also be true, that a poorly applied cervix is associated with less efficient uterine activity and slower progress. For example, when the fetus is in an occipitoposterior position, the head is not pushed directly onto the cervix; rather, it is directed downwards and forwards against the back of the symphysis pubis, leading to a decrease in the effectiveness of uterine contractility, slower cervical dilatation and prolonged labour (Chamberlain 1993). The application of the cervix to the presenting part can be assessed by feeling between them.

The membranes

The membranes should be felt to determine if they are intact or ruptured. Intact membranes can be felt as a shiny surface over the presenting part but may be difficult to feel especially in early labour or when the forewaters are shallow with the membranes tightly pressed against the presenting part. In this situation they may be mistaken for ruptured membranes. Bulging forewaters may be felt when the cervix is poorly applied to the presenting part as amniotic fluid is positioned between the membranes and the presenting part. During a contraction the pressure within the forewaters increases, causing the membranes to feel tense with a predisposition to rupturing spontaneously. This is more likely to occur if the presenting part is poorly applied, e.g. high or ill-fitting presenting part, malposition or malpresentation. Occasionally the membranes are intact but amniotic fluid is leaking – this is most likely caused by a hindwater leak. Care should be taken not to rupture the membranes (unless there is an indication to do so and consent obtained), particularly if a pulsation is felt beneath the membranes as this could be due to either a cord presentation or vasa praevia. Referral should be sought as an emergency caesarean section may be indicated to prevent cord prolapse or fetal haemorrhage from ruptured vasa praevia.

Presentation

The information gained from the abdominal examination is used in conjunction with the landmarks identified on the presenting part to confirm the presentation:

- A cephalic presentation will feel smooth, round and firm, and sutures or fontanelles may be felt which can help confirm the position and the degree of flexion. Moulding can be assessed by the degree of overlapping of the bones of the vault. No moulding is when there is normal separation of the bones with open sutures. 1+ occurs when the bones are touching each other, and if they overlap but can be separated with gentle digital pressure 2+. Severe moulding (3+) occurs when the bones are overlapping and cannot be separated with gentle digital pressure. Caput succedaneum may also be felt as a soft or firm mass on the presenting part, which can make the identification of sutures and fontanelles more difficult.
- Both the breech and face presentation feel soft and irregular. With the breech presentation the sacrum may be palpable as a hard bone, with the anus close by and the landmarks of the ischial tuberosities and sacrum are located in a straight line. A finger inadvertently inserted into the anus will be gripped and no gum margins will be felt. Fresh meconium is also likely to be present.
- With a face presentation, the orbital ridges may be felt, a finger inserted into the mouth may be sucked and gum margins felt, the landmarks of the malar bones and mouth are located in a triangular position and an ear may be felt. If a face presentation is suspected or confirmed, care should be taken to avoid damaging the eyes; application of a fetal scalp electrode is not recommended and obstetric cream

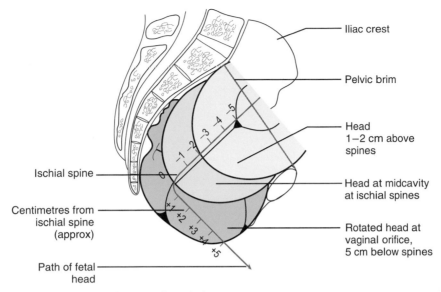

Figure 30.2 Level of presenting part in relation to the ischial spines.

should not be used, as it could initiate a chemical conjunctivitis.

- When the cord presents, the pulsations may be palpated through the membranes – the membranes should not be ruptured due to the danger of cord prolapse. If a cord is felt without membranes the emergency procedure for managing cord prolapse should be instigated while the examining midwife keeps her fingers in the vagina and attempts to push the presenting part off the cord.

Level of the presenting part

The level of the presenting part is determined by assessing the distance between the presenting part and the ischial spines in centimetres (Fig. 30.2). The ischial spines are referred to as zero station, with the presenting part being above (−cm) or below (+cm) this. The ischial spines may be difficult to palpate; thus this becomes a subjective measurement. The midwife should ensure it is the level of the presenting part being assessed and not caput succedaneum. Descent of the presenting part is one indicator of progress during labour and the assessment should correlate with the findings from the degree of engagement assessed during the abdominal examination.

Position

With a cephalic presentation, identification of sutures and fontanelles will confirm the position and attitude. The

sagittal suture is easily identified as a long straight suture; its position is taken in relation to the maternal pelvis, moving from back to front.

- If it is in the anteroposterior diameter, it is indicative of a direct occipitoanterior or occipitoposterior position.
- A sagittal suture in the right oblique (felt moving from the posterior right quadrant of the maternal pelvis obliquely forwards to the left anterior quadrant) (Fig. 30.3) is indicative of left occipitoanterior or right occipitoposterior position. If in the left oblique diameter, it is indicative of a right occipitoanterior or a left occipitoposterior position.
- Where the sagittal suture is in the transverse diameter, it is indicative of a right or left occipitolateral/ transverse position.
- A sagittal suture that does not run centrally through the pelvis but is located more to one side than the other may be indicative of asynclitism.

The posterior fontanelle is felt as a small triangular area, with three sutures running from it and is indicative of a well-flexed cephalic presentation, usually occipitoanterior position if felt in the upper quadrant of the pelvis. As labour progresses the posterior fontanelle may close due to moulding and it may not be possible to feel three sutures if a caput succedaneum is present.

The anterior fontanelle is felt as a larger, diamond-shaped area, with four sutures running from it. However if a caput succedaneum is present, it may not be possible to feel all four sutures. Palpation of the anterior fontanelle is

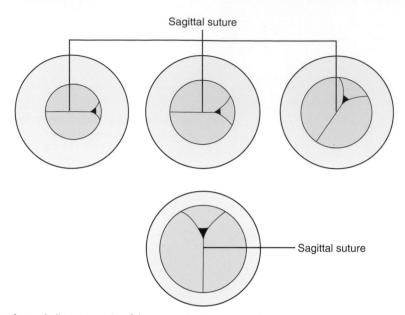

Figure 30.3 Rotation of a cephalic presentation felt on examination *per vaginam*.

usually associated with a deflexed head, often with an occipitoposterior position (where it will be felt in the upper quadrant of the pelvis). If felt centrally, it could be indicative of a brow presentation.

Progress is indicated where there is progressive flexion (or extension with a face presentation), descent and rotation. Comparing the position of the landmarks from all previous VEs should demonstrate this. Some midwives will draw what they felt and this will also reflect the changing attitude and rotation.

Pelvic outlet

The adequacy of the pelvis for the size of the baby can be assessed as part of the VE. However this is a subjective assessment and the pelvis is a dynamic structure with measurements that can vary according to the position of the woman. The assessment of the size of the fetus may also be considered a 'best estimate'; even the use of ultrasound scans to assess weight gives a weight range. For the midwife undertaking the VE, usually two assessments of pelvic adequacy are undertaken which give an indication of whether the pelvic outlet is narrowed. The first is to assess the distance between the ischial spines. Ischial spines are difficult to palpate – if they are prominent and easily felt, the transverse diameter of the outlet is reduced, which could affect progress, particularly in the second stage of labour. The second assessment is of the subpubic angle and is assessed by moving the top part of the two examining

fingers towards the pubic arch. Two fingers should fit snugly under the pubic arch, indicating an angle of 90° or greater. A reduced subpubic angle is often found with prominent ischial spines and may be associated with an android pelvis. This can result in more pressure being placed on the perineum and perineal trauma, as well as delay in the second stage. Care should be taken when assessing the subpubic angle to avoid pressing on the clitoris which can be painful.

PROCEDURE: examination *per vaginam* (VE)

A VE should be carried out using an Aseptic Non Touch Technique with the wearing of sterile gloves providing the non touch component. Although sterile VE packs and lotions to wash the genital area are used in many labour wards, McCormick (2001) has demonstrated that the infection rate is unaffected by their use and recommends stringent hand decontamination and using sterile gloves (avoiding their contamination) to reduce the risk of infection. It is also more cost effective than using VE packs and lotions. NICE (2014) advise that tap water is sufficient for perineal cleansing where it is required, in support of this Ohlsson et al (2014) and Lumbiganon et al (2014) found the use of chlorhexidine did not reduce the incidence of maternal and neonatal infection; the midwife should refer to the hospital policy for local requirements on perineal cleansing. The procedure for perineal cleansing follows this procedure. If an assistant is present, she can open packs and equipment for the midwife.

- Confirm the woman's identity if she is not known to the midwife.
- Discuss the procedure fully with the woman and gain informed consent.
- Ensure privacy.
- Gather equipment:
  - apron
  - sterile gloves
  - lubricant, e.g. water-soluble lubricant, obstetric cream (the latter should not be used with a face presentation)
  - disposable sheet
  - alcohol handrub
  - other equipment as necessary, e.g. amnihook, fetal scalp electrode
  - Pinard stethoscope or sonicaid.
- Encourage the woman to empty her bladder if she is not catheterized.
- Wash and dry hands.
- Perform an abdominal palpation to determine the lie, presentation, position and degree of engagement, and auscultate the fetal heart.
- Ask the woman to adopt an almost recumbent position (use a wedge to avoid aortocaval occlusion if necessary), with her knees flexed and parted, and ankles together (be aware of the difficulty experienced by women with pelvic girdle pain when opening their legs).
- Place the disposable sheet beneath her buttocks.
- Ask the woman to remove any sanitary towels or underwear, keeping the genital area covered.
- Wash and dry hands, apply apron.
- Open the equipment to be used including the lubricating gel.
- Apply handrub, allow to dry, then put on gloves.
- Ask the woman to lift up the cover to allow access to the genital area.
- Lubricate the first two fingers of the dominant hand with lubricant/antiseptic cream.
- Advise the woman that she will feel her labia being touched and with the thumb and forefinger of the non-examining hand, part the labia, observing the condition of the vulva.
- Inform the woman of what is about to happen, then, if no contraction present, gently insert the first two fingers of the examining hand into the vagina, in a downwards and backwards direction along the anterior vaginal wall, ensuring the thumb does not come into contact with the woman's clitoris or anus.
- Locate the cervix and determine the position, tone, consistency, degree of effacement and dilatation, and

application to the presenting part (if the cervix is not located, ask the woman to make a couple of fists and place them under her buttocks, tilting her pelvis upwards).
- Gently move the fingers through the cervical os to ascertain the presence/absence of the forewaters, the presentation, position, degree of flexion and level of the presenting part, the presence of caput succedaneum and the degree of moulding.
- If necessary and consent has been gained prior to the examination, rupture the membranes (p. 227) and/or apply a fetal scalp electrode (p. 227).
- Withdraw the fingers gently, assessing the pelvic outlet.
- Auscultate the fetal heart.
- Assist the woman into a comfortable position, reapply sanitary pad if required, and discuss the findings.
- Dispose of equipment appropriately, removing the gloves then apron.
- Wash and dry hands.
- Document the findings in the notes (also the partogram and or cardiotocograph [CTG] if being used) and act accordingly.

PROCEDURE: perineal cleansing

A VE pack and warm water for cleansing will be required. The midwife should follow the procedure for examination *per vaginam* up to 'Ask the woman to lift up the cover …'. The midwife is then required to:

- Swab the vulva and perineum from front to back using cotton-wool balls or gauze soaked with warm water, passing the swabs from the examining hand to the non-examining hand and taking care not to touch the examining hand with the non-examining hand; use each swab once and dispose of it.
- The procedure then continues as described above in the procedure on examination per vaginam from the point 'Lubricate the first two fingers of the dominant hand …'.

AMNIOTOMY (ARTIFICIAL RUPTURE OF MEMBRANES)

Intact membranes provide a cushion for the presenting part, providing protection from compression and infection. They also apply an even pressure on the cervix to assist with effacement of the cervix. Vincent (2005) suggests bulging membranes at the introitus help to prestretch the perineum prior to crowning.

Over two-thirds of women can reach full dilatation prior to the membranes rupturing spontaneously (Romano 2008); however, for many women this is not achieved, as the membranes have been ruptured artificially (ARM). While many midwives would not rupture the membranes without a clear clinical indication, ARM remains one of the most commonly performed procedures in both obstetric and midwifery practice (Smyth et al 2013).

A disposable, sterile amnihook should be used for the procedure; this is a crochet-like long-handled hook with a very sharp tip that is pressed against the chorion with the intention of tearing a hole in the membranes. The amniotic fluid can leak out through the hole increasing the size of it or the membranes can be torn apart digitally.

ARM should not be undertaken with a labour that is progressing normally, as removing the cushion of the intact membranes means the presenting part will press directly onto the cervix. The RCM (2012d) argue that an ARM can have a negative impact on the woman by altering her ability to cope and recommend that benign measures, e.g. positional changes, are used to increase the strength of contractions if progress is considered 'slow'. An ARM, 'breaking the waters', is not part of physiological labour and can disrupt the normal process of labour, often leading to other interventions (Andrees & Rankin 2007, Svardby et al 2007) such as continuous electronic fetal monitoring (CEFM). However, NICE (2014) are clear that ARM alone for suspected delay in labour is not an indication for CEFM. Prostaglandin PGE_2 is released by the amnion and cervix while the chorion produces prostaglandin dehydrogenase (PDHG), an enzyme that prevents the cervix from ripening (Smyth et al 2013). It has been proposed that the part of the chorion in contact with the cervical os at term releases less PDHG, thus allowing PGE_2 to exert its effect. However, if an amniotomy is performed early in labour (<3 cm) this effect is lost and labour may slow down (Smyth et al 2013). Olsen et al (2010) caution that the risk of endometritis increases approximately 1.7-fold within 1 hour following amniotomy; thus it is important to monitor the woman for signs of this if an ARM is undertaken.

Amniotomy is often undertaken to 'speed up' labour by increasing the frequency of contractions possibly by releasing prostaglandins and oxytocin, NICE (2014) concur, advising an ARM shortens labour length by 1 hour but the strength of contractions will increase, increasing the degree of pain felt. However, Smyth et al (2013) found no evidence that this was a significant outcome from performing an ARM.

The RCM (2012d) caution that fetal heart rate abnormalities can be seen after ARM, which can result in intervention with an increased risk of caesarean delivery. Dilbaz et al (2006) suggest there is an increase in variable decelerations with early amniotomy. These changes may be a result of fetal haemodynamic changes. Fok et al (2005) found there was a significant reduction in the impedance of the fetal middle cerebral artery (MCA) and renal artery, which they attribute to being a response to fetal stress and release of vasoactive substances following ARM. Amniotic fluid embolism (anaphylactoid syndrome of pregnancy) is a rare side effect associated with ARM (Mato 2008).

Indications

- Induction of labour
- Augmentation of labour
- Application of fetal scalp electrode and/or assessment of liquor colour
- Maternal request
- Often prior to birth of second twin.

Contraindications

- No maternal consent
- High presenting part (risk of cord prolapse)
- Preterm labour
- Known vaginal infection
- Maternal HIV-positive status
- Caution is taken with polyhydramnios or any malposition or malpresentation
- Placenta praevia
- Vasa praevia.

If the presenting part is high and ballotable, it is unwise to perform an ARM. However, the obstetrician may choose to perform a controlled ARM and the midwife may be asked to apply light pressure to the fundus to encourage the presenting part to engage in the pelvis as the membranes rupture. The obstetrician ensures the fluid has drained and no cord has prolapsed before removing the hand. Cord prolapse does occur following ARM; Dilbaz et al (2006) suggest this is more likely to occur if there is a malpresentation, multiparity, low birth weight, prematurity or polyhydramnios, but it may still be unexpected. Thus it is important the midwife feels for the presence of cord following the ARM and takes appropriate steps if it is found.

Standard precautions should be followed and the sharpness of the amnihook means that the midwife must take care to avoid personal injury and dispose of the hook into a sharps box. It is also important to confirm the membranes are intact, as trauma to the fetal scalp or anus (if a breech presentation) (Warwick et al 2013) can occur if the membranes have already ruptured and the amnihook is scraping the fetal skin. This can be difficult to ascertain when the membranes are tight across the presenting part and no liquor is draining. It may be easier to rupture the membranes when a contraction is present and the membranes are bulging under the pressure; however, this is not an absolute necessity.

PROCEDURE: artificial rupture of the membranes

- Discuss the indication with the woman and gain her informed consent.
- Gather equipment:
  - equipment as for vaginal examination
  - amnihook.
- Undertake a vaginal examination as detailed on p. 225, maintaining sterility of the amnihook.
- With the examining hand, locate the cervix and ensure conditions are favourable for an ARM to be performed, e.g. descent of presenting part, no pulsation felt beneath the examining fingers.
- Holding the amnihook with the non-examining hand, slide the amnihook carefully between the examining hand and anterior vaginal wall with the point of the hook pointing downwards.
- Use the examining hand to guide the amnihook into position with the hook pressed against the membranes.
- Use the non-examining hand to twist the amnihook slightly to tear the membranes.
- Withdraw the amnihook gently while retaining the fingers in the cervix as the amniotic fluid drains out (ensuring the amniotic fluid does not come into contact with the midwife's clothing).
- The examining fingers can then locate the tear and digitally increase the size of the opening.
- Reassess the cervix, fetal descent and position, and feel for the presence of the umbilical cord.
- If indicated, a fetal scalp electrode can be applied at this point (see below).
- Withdraw the hand, auscultate the fetal heart.
- Assist the woman with regard to hygiene, comfort and position.
- Discuss the findings with the woman.
- Dispose of equipment correctly, wash and dry hands.
- Document the indications for ARM with the findings and act accordingly.

APPLICATION OF A FETAL SCALP ELECTRODE

A fetal scalp electrode (FSE) can be used when continuous CTG monitoring is indicated to ensure continuity of contact. Fetal cardiac electrical activity is detected through the fetal scalp electrode to a transducer usually located on the woman's thigh. This is then attached to the electrocardiograph (ECG) port on the monitor. The sound of the fetal heart is continuous regardless of maternal or fetal position and movement, and is not accompanied or confused by sounds of fetal movement or uterine blood flow. Harper et al (2013) found a decrease in caesarean section delivery with FSE use which they attribute to an improved ability to monitor fetal heart tones compared with external monitoring. However, it is an invasive procedure for both the woman and the fetus; the electrode is secured under the fetal scalp, with either a clip or spiral connection. It is assumed that the fetus experiences some pain from its application and the transfer of viruses such as HIV and herpes simplex from mother to child is more likely (Baker 2007) (both are contraindications to FSE use). Skin infection or long-term scarring on the baby's scalp can also occur. Harper et al (2013) did not find an increase in maternal infection with FSE use.

Needs et al (1992) found clip electrodes performed better than other types with regard to attachment. The clip is applied by rotating the end of the electrode: anticlockwise rotation causes the clip to recede into the electrode head while clockwise rotation causes it to emerge from the electrode head and be caught on the scalp. It is usually spring loaded and therefore rarely requires an active rotation clockwise to apply the clip. The Copeland FSE is commonly used and is considered to reduce the risk of needlestick injury as it has a protecting penetrating needle; this also controls the depth of penetration reducing the risk of fetal injury to the skull (Cutlan 2006). If using a spiral electrode, it is rotated in the direction of the spiral, usually clockwise, until caught under the scalp.

Accuracy of scalp electrodes depends upon their correct application. If membrane is between the electrode and the scalp the tracing is likely to be unreliable, sometimes known as 'artefact' and interpretation of the trace is impossible. The electrode should not be placed near or through a fontanelle or suture line, the cervix or vagina – it should be positioned on the skin folds of the scalp. It can be used on the buttocks of a breech presentation, but causes obvious scarring. It should not be used with a face presentation.

PROCEDURE: application of a fetal scalp electrode

- Discuss the indication with the woman and gain her consent.
- Ensure that the monitor has an ECG facility and the correct leads and attachments.

- Gather equipment:
  - equipment as for vaginal examination with amnihook if membranes are intact
  - sterile fetal scalp electrode.
- Perform a vaginal examination as detailed on p. 225.
- Undertake an ARM (p. 227) if membranes intact.
- With the examining hand, locate the fetal scalp; ensure that sutures and fontanelles are avoided.
- Slide the FSE (using the non-examining hand) between the examining hand and vaginal wall.
- Use the examining hand to guide the electrode into place and support the head of the electrode against the scalp.
- With the non-examining hand, turn the end of the electrode anticlockwise, then release to attach to the scalp, maintaining support of the electrode against the scalp.
- The electrode should be attached to the scalp; a gentle pull will confirm whether it is attached.
- An assistant may attach the leads to the transducer and the transducer to the monitor while the examining hand remains in place; if the electrode is not working, reapplication may be attempted.
- Before withdrawing the examining hand, check the electrode is securely placed over an appropriate area of the scalp.
- Apply conductive gel to the transducer or the appropriate fastening and attach around the woman's thigh using a small belt or attach to the monitor on the woman's abdomen if appropriate (e.g. EZIplug 3 attaches to either the leg or the abdomen, Cutlan 2006); ensure that monitoring is occurring satisfactorily.
- Assist the woman with regard to hygiene, comfort, and position.
- Explain the differences in the fetal heart sounds heard.
- Dispose of equipment correctly, wash and dry hands.
- Document the indications for FSE with other aspects of the examination and act accordingly.

Removal of the fetal scalp electrode

It is important that the FSE is removed from the baby's scalp at or just before birth. This is particularly important to remember if the woman has an emergency caesarean section to avoid trauma to the fetal scalp as the baby is removed from the uterine cavity while the FSE is attached to the external monitor. It is imperative that the FSE is also removed from the woman's vagina to avoid it being retained within her body (Valenzuela 2006).

To remove the clip-style FSE, the electrode head is held against the scalp while the end is rotated anticlockwise. Whilst an anticlockwise rotation can remove the spiral electrode, it is quicker to take hold of the two wires hanging from it and pull them apart – this will cause the clip to rotate and come loose from the scalp as the wires unravel. Care should be taken not to create any trauma while removing it. Any obvious puncture marks should be noted on the initial birth examination. The electrode should be disposed of in the sharps box.

ROLE AND RESPONSIBILITIES OF THE MIDWIFE

These can be summarized as:
- encouraging and supporting the woman in the use of appropriate positions to enhance her comfort and labour progress
- undertaking a competent examination *per vaginam* in which all of the information is gained without causing distress to the woman
- undertaking an amniotomy correctly, when indicated
- appropriate application of a fetal scalp electrode, when indicated
- recognizing deviations from normal and instigating referral
- education, explanations and support of the woman
- appropriate record keeping.

SUMMARY

- Progress in labour is very individual and can be assessed using a variety of indicators.
- Women should be encouraged and supported to change position during the first stage of labour and use those which are most comfortable while avoiding the supine position.
- There is a need for more high-quality evidence regarding the advantages and disadvantages of the different positions used.
- An examination *per vaginam* is an invasive procedure but one that can yield valuable information in relation to the assessment of progress in labour.
- Amniotomy should not be undertaken routinely in a labour that is progressing normally.
- Fetal scalp electrodes offer continuity of contact if continuous fetal monitoring is indicated.
- The risk of ascending infection is high; an Aseptic Non Touch Technique should be used throughout.

SELF-ASSESSMENT EXERCISES

The answers to the following questions may be found in the text:

1. How is progress assessed during the first stage of labour?
2. What advice can the midwife give to a woman regarding positioning during the first stage of labour?
3. For what reasons would the midwife undertake an examination *per vaginam* during labour?
4. What should be discussed with the woman to gain her informed consent regarding an examination *per vaginam*?
5. How would you perform an examination *per vaginam*?
6. How could the midwife identify a flexed cephalic presentation?
7. What information can be gained from an examination *per vaginam* and what is the significance of it?
8. Describe how to perform an amniotomy and apply a fetal scalp electrode.
9. What are the role and responsibilities of the midwife in relation to an examination *per vaginam*, artificial rupture of the membranes, and application of a fetal scalp electrode?

REFERENCES

Andrees, M., Rankin, J., 2007. Amniotomy in spontaneous, uncomplicated labour at term. Br. J. Midwifery 15 (10), 612–616.

Baker, D., 2007. Consequences of herpes simplex virus in pregnancy and their prevention. Curr. Opin. Infect. Dis. 20 (1), 73–76.

Baker, K., 2010. Midwives should support women to mobilise during labour. Br. J. Midwifery 18 (8), 492–497.

Blackburn, S.T., 2013. Maternal, Fetal and Neonatal Physiology: A Clinical Perspective, fourth ed. Saunders, St. Louis, pp. 119–130.

Burnhill, M.S., Donezis, J., Cohen, J., 1962. Uterine contractility during labour studied by intra-amniotic fluid pressure recordings. Am. J. Obstet. & Gynecol. 83, 561–571.

Cahill, A.G., Duffy, C.R., Odibo, A.O., et al., 2012. Number of cervical examinations and risk of intrapartum maternal fever. Obstet. Gynecol. 119 (6), 1096–1101.

Chamberlain, G.V.P., 1993. Obstetrics by Ten Teachers, sixteenth ed. Arnold, London.

Chapman, V., 2009. Slow progress and malpresentations/malpositions in labour. In: Chapman, V., Charles, C. (Eds.), The Midwife's Labour and Birth Handbook, second ed. Wiley-Blackwell, Chichester, pp. 106–134.

Cutlan, C., 2006. Electronic fetal monitoring and infection control. Br. J. Midwifery 14 (10), 584–585.

Cutler, L., 2012. A consideration of the positions women adopt for labour. Br. J. Midwifery 20 (5), 346–350.

Dilbaz, B., Ozturkoglu, E., Dilbaz, S., et al., 2006. Risk factors and perinatal outcomes associated with umbilical cord prolapse. Arch. Gynecol. Obstet. 274, 104–107.

Dixon, L., Foureur, M., 2010. The vaginal examination during labour: is it benefit or harm? NZCOM J. 42 (May), 21–26.

Downe, S., Gyte, G.M.L., Dahlen, H.G., Singata, M., 2013. Routine vaginal examinations for assessing progress of labour to improve outcomes for women and babies at term. Cochrane Database Syst. Rev. (7), Art. No.: CD010088. doi:10.1002/14651858 .CD010088.pub2.

Fok, W.Y., Leung, T.Y., Tsui, M.H., et al., 2005. Fetal hemodynamic changes after amniotomy. Acta Obstet. Gynecol. Scand. 84, 166–169.

Grasek, A., Tuuli, M., Roehl, K., et al., 2014. Fetal descent in labor. Am. Coll. Obstet. Gynecol. 123 (3), 521–526.

Hanson, L., 2009. Second stage labor: challenges in spontaneous bearing down. J. Perinatol. Neonatal. Nurs. 23 (1), 31–39.

Harper, L.M., Shanks, A.J., Tuuli, M.G., et al., 2013. The risks and benefits of internal monitors in laboring patients. Am. J. Obstet. Gynecol. 209 (38), e1–e6.

Hassan, S.J., Sundby, J., Husseini, A., Bjertness, E., 2012. The paradox of vaginal examination practice during normal childbirth: Palestinian women's feelings, opinions, knowledge and experiences. Reprod. Health 9, 16.

Hunter, S., Hofmeyr, G.J., Kulier, R., 2007. Hands and knees in late pregnancy or labour for fetal malposition (lateral or posterior). Cochrane Database Syst. Rev. (4), Art. No.: CD001063. doi:10.1002/14651858.CD001063.pub3.

Incerti, M., Locatelli, A., Ghidini, A., et al., 2011. Variability in rate of cervical dilation in nulliparous women at term. Birth 38 (1), 30–35.

Kerrigan, A., 2006. The mother-midwife partnership: a critical analysis of intrapartum care. Br. J. Midwifery 14 (6), 346–350.

Lawrence, A., Lewis, L., Hofmeyr, G.J., Styles, C., 2013. Maternal positions and mobility during the first stage of labour. Cochrane Database Syst. Rev. (10), Art. No.: CD003934. doi:10.1002/14651858.CD003934. pub4.

Lewin, D., Fearon, B., Hemmings, V., Johnson, G., 2005. Informing women during vaginal examination. Br. J. Midwifery 13 (1), 26–29.

Lumbiganon, P., Thinkhamrop, J., Thinkhamrop, B., Tolosa, J.E., 2014. Vaginal chlorhexidine during labour for preventing maternal and neonatal infections (excluding Group B streptococcal and HIV). Cochrane Database Syst. Rev. (9), Art. No.: CD004070 doi:10.1002/14651858. CD004070.pub3.

Mato, J., 2008. Suspected fluid embolism following amniotomy: a case report. AANA J. 76 (1), 53–59.

McCormick, C., 2001. Vulval preparations in labour: use of lotions or tap water. Br. J. Midwifery 9 (7), 453–455.

McDonald, G., 2010. Diagnosing the latent phase of labour: use of the partogram. Br. J. Midwifery 18 (10), 630–637.

NCT (National Childbirth Trust), 2011. Positions for labour and birth. Available online: <http://www.nct.org.uk/sites/default/files/related_documents/NCT%20Positions%20for%20labour%20birth.pdf> (accessed 8 February 2015).

Needs, L., Grant, A., Sleep, J., et al., 1992. A randomised controlled trial to compare three types of fetal scalp electrode. Br. J. Obstet. Gynaecol. 99 (4), 302–306.

NICE (National Institute for Health and Care Excellence), 2014. Intrapartum care. Care of healthy women and their babies during childbirth. NICE, London. Available online: <www.nice.org.uk> (accessed 3 March 2015).

Ohlsson, A., Shah, V.S., Stade, B.C. 2014 Vaginal chlorhexidine during labour to prevent early-onset neonatal group B streptococcal infection. Cochrane Database Syst. Rev. (12), Art. No.: CD003520. doi:10.1002/14651858. CD003520.pub3.

Olsen, M.A., Butler, A.M., Willers, D.M., et al., 2010. Risk factors for endometritis after low transverse cesarean delivery. Infect. Control Hosp. Epidemiol. 31 (1), 69–77.

RCM (Royal College of Midwives), 2012a. Evidence Based Guidelines for Midwifery-Led Care in Labour. Latent Phase. RCM, London.

RCM (Royal College of Midwives), 2012b. Evidence Based Guidelines for Midwifery-Led Care in Labour. Assessing Progress in Labour. RCM, London.

RCM (Royal College of Midwives), 2012c. Evidence Based Guidelines for Midwifery-Led Care in Labour. Positions for Labour and Birth. RCM, London.

RCM (Royal College of Midwives), 2012d. Evidence Based Guidelines for Midwifery-Led Care in Labour. Rupturing Membranes. RCM, London.

Ridley, R.T., 2007. Diagnosis and intervention for occiput posterior malposition. J. Obstet. Gynecol. Neonat. Nurs. 36 (2), 135–143.

Romano, A.M., 2008. Research summaries for normal birth. J. Perinat. Educ. 17 (1), 48–52.

Sanderson, T.A., 2012. The movement of the maternal pelvis: a review. MIDIRS Midwifery Dig. 22 (3), 319–326.

Schmid, V., Downe, S., 2010. Midwifery skills for normalizing unusual labours. In: Walsh, D., Downe, S.

(Eds.), Essential Midwifery Practice Intrapartum Care. Wiley-Blackwell, Chichester, pp. 159–190.

Shepherd, A., Cheyne, H., 2013. The frequency and reasons for vaginal examination in labour. Women Birth 26 (1), 49–54.

Simkin, P., Ancheta, R., 2005. The Labor Progress Handbook: Early Interventions to Prevent and Treat Dystocia, second ed. Blackwell, Oxford.

Smyth, R.M.D., Markham, C., Dowsell, T., 2013. Amniotomy for shortening spontaneous labour. Cochrane Database Syst. Rev. (6), Art. No.: CD006167. doi:10.1002/14651858. CD006167.pub4.

Stewart, M., 2005. 'I'm just going to wash you down': sanitizing the vaginal examination. J. Adv. Nurs. 51 (6), 587–594.

Svardby, K., Nordstrom, L., Sellstroni, E., 2007. Primiparas with or without oxytocin augmentation: a prospective descriptive study. J. Clin. Nurs. 16 (1), 179–184.

Valenzuela, P., 2006. Removal of a fetal scalp electrode lodged in the vagina of a patient for 23 years. J. Obstet. Gynecol. 26 (7), 704–705.

Vincent, M., 2005. Amniotomy: to do or not to do? Midwifery 8 (5), 228.

Warwick, A., Strachan, B., McNally, J., 2013. The bottom line: Iatrogenic fetal anal trauma in undiagnosed breech presentation. Br. J. Midwifery 21 (7), 481–483.

Zhang, J., Landy, H.J., Branch, D.W., et al., 2010. Contemporary patterns of spontaneous labor with normal neonatal outcomes. Obstet. Gynecol. 116 (6), 1281–1287.

Chapter | 31 |

Principles of intrapartum skills: second-stage issues

LEARNING OUTCOMES

Having read this chapter, the reader should be able to:

- discuss the evidence and opinions surrounding the definition, recognition, and duration of the second stage, directed and spontaneous pushing, positions used, as well as nuchal cord and perineal management
- discuss the preparation for, and conduct of, a normal delivery
- describe how to infiltrate the perineum and perform an episiotomy
- discuss the role and responsibilities of the midwife during the second stage of labour.

During the second stage of labour the baby descends and rotates through the pelvis, the symphysis pubis width increases (Rustamova et al 2009), contractions become expulsive, the perineum stretches and thins out, and the baby is born. This chapter will review the current evidence and clinical skills utilized during care in the second stage of labour and will include a discussion on the definition and duration of the second stage, the effects of directed and spontaneous pushing, different maternal positions and the management of a nuchal cord. The chapter concludes with a discussion on the 'management' of the perineum, including when and how to undertake an episiotomy.

Definition

Traditionally the second stage of labour has been defined by a very clinical description: from full dilatation of the os uteri to the complete birth of the baby. It is now recognized that this stage of labour has both a passive and an active phase (NICE 2014). Lai et al (2009) acknowledge there is more to the second stage than cervical dilatation, with descent of the presenting part and maternal feelings also being important considerations. Recognition of the passive phase is important so that the woman is discouraged from pushing as soon as the cervix is fully dilated, as this can have adverse outcomes.

The passive phase describes the time from when the cervix is fully dilated but there is no strong urge to push and the presenting part may still be high but is beginning to descend and rotate through the pelvis. It has been referred to as 'rest and be thankful', 'rest and descent' and the 'pause for rotation' (Brancato et al 2008, Long 2006). The woman may feel drowsy and relaxed (Long 2006) and the contractions may appear less frequent and strong, giving the woman the opportunity to recharge, ready for the active phase. Ideally the woman should be discouraged from pushing, allowing descent to occur passively to avoid maternal exhaustion. Yildirim & Beji (2008) claim women cannot push effectively when the urge to push is absent. Lai et al (2009) argue that the fetus will descend more rapidly once it is approximately 1 cm past the ischial spines and has rotated to an occipitoanterior position.

NICE (2014) state the active phase is when the woman experiences expulsive contractions, with a strong urge to push, the cervix is fully dilated, and the presenting part is visible. The urge to push begins with the initiation of the Ferguson's reflex as the fetus descends past the ischial spines onto the pelvic floor stimulating the stretch receptors in the posterior vaginal wall. This causes the posterior lobe of the pituitary gland to secrete more oxytocin and a positive feedback mechanism is created. Lai et al (2009) suggest the reflexive need to push hard in the active phase is three-four times higher when there has been descent of the presenting part. If the woman is pushing when the cervix is fully dilated but expulsive contractions are absent, NICE (2014) suggest this should also be considered the active phase.

There are many advantages in delaying pushing until the active phase has been reached, including decreased maternal exhaustion; less perineal, bladder, and pelvic trauma; reduced incidence of instrumental delivery; increased self-belief and confidence in the woman's ability to birth; fewer fetal heart abnormalities; higher Apgar scores at 1 and 5 minutes and higher umbilical cord arterial pH levels (Albers & Borders 2007, Brancato et al 2008, Lai et al 2009, Nicholl & Cattell 2006, Roberts & Hanson 2007, Schaffer et al 2005, Yildirim & Beji 2008).

RECOGNITION

As women transition from the first to the second stage, a number of signs may be seen. The woman may become quiet and withdrawn or particularly vocal and feel that she 'can't go on', 'doesn't want to do this anymore'. Equally she may feel renewed with energy. The Royal College of Midwives (RCM 2012a) suggest there may be changes in

facial expression and the woman will begin to breathe harder. A heavy blood-stained show may be noted as the operculum descends and a change in the nature of contractions is felt with an overwhelming urge to push. There will be occasions when the urge to push does not signal the advent of the second stage, so if in doubt, undertake a vaginal examination (VE). The contractions may slow initially but then return stronger and are more expulsive in nature. As the presenting part descends, pouting of the vulva and anus may be seen and the presenting part will become visible at the introitus. Other physical signs include a purple line extending up the anal cleft (Hobbs 1998), changes in abdominal shape (Burvill 2002) or the sacral curve (rhombus of Michaelis; Sutton 2003). Equally, in the absence of visible signs and expulsive contractions, the passive phase of the second stage may be diagnosed following a VE when the cervix is noted to be fully dilated. This is essential when the breech is presenting to avoid head entrapment where the body is delivered through a partially dilated cervix that the head cannot pass through. A VE may also reveal the presence of a caput succedaneum that is giving the appearance of a descending presenting part.

DURATION

While the RCM (2012a) advise there is no good evidence to justify arbitrary time limits on the length of the second stage of labour, NICE (2014) suggest the baby should be born within 3 hours (nulliparous women) or 2 hours (multiparous women) from the beginning of the active phase for most women. They advise referral may be required an hour before the end of these time limits. The importance of recognizing progress is also emphasized by NICE (2014); rotation and descent of the presenting part should be assessed if there is inadequate progress by 1 hour of active pushing for nulliparous women or 30 minutes for multiparous women, as a VE and amniotomy (Chapter 30) may be required.

Downe (2011) considers the second stage to be extremely variable and may be extremely quick, particularly for the multiparous woman. The length of the second stage will be affected by factors such as maternal position and epidural anaesthesia and the midwife should continue to observe for signs of normality and progress while recognizing and managing any deviations from normal. The American College of Obstetricians and Gynecologists suggest the second stage is prolonged if delivery has not occurred within 3 hours for nulliparous women with an epidural or 2 hours without and for multiparous women, within 2 hours with an epidural and 1 hour without (Laughon et al 2014). However, Gillesby et al (2010) found outcomes were better when women with an epidural delayed active pushing for 2 hours.

Cheng et al (2007) found a second stage lasting longer than 3 hours for multiparous women was associated with increased risk of operative delivery, increased maternal morbidity and lower Apgar scores. Allen et al (2009) found the risks of adverse outcomes for mother and baby increased when the duration of labour was longer than 2 hours for the multiparous woman and 3 hours in the nulliparous woman. A prolonged second stage is also associated with an increased incidence of postpartum haemorrhage (Lu et al 2009), chorioamnionitis, and third- and fourth-degree tears (Laughon et al 2014).

PUSHING: SPONTANEOUS OR DIRECTED

The RCM (2012a) remind us there is no good evidence for directed pushing using the Valsalva manoeuvre or that women need to be instructed on how and when to push. Women should be encouraged to follow what their bodies are telling them to do and push when they have the urge (NICE 2014). The verbal communication used during the second stage is vital so the woman is empowered and able to take control of the birth. Borders et al (2013) suggest this is achieved when the midwife uses affirmation, information sharing, direction (e.g. with changing position) and baby talk (talking to and about the baby). Delaying active pushing and waiting for the urge to push with descent of the fetus has been referred to as 'labouring down' (Borders et al 2013). During the active phase of the second stage, women develop a strong urge to push and will do so without instruction often once the contraction has built up rather than at the beginning of it (Hanson 2009). This form of physiological spontaneous pushing uses a resting respiratory volume, not a deep breath, and short pushes lasting 3–6 or 5–7 seconds, three to five times during a contraction (Borders et al 2013, Di Franco et al 2007, Perez-Botella & Downe 2006). Spontaneous pushing is not thought to significantly increase the duration of the second stage (Sampselle et al 2005); indeed it may even shorten it (Jahdi et al 2011, Yildirim & Beji 2008). Naranjo et al (2011) found the second stage was longer overall with spontaneous pushing; however, the amount of time spent physically pushing was less, resulting in fewer adverse outcomes than women who experienced directed pushing. Gillesby et al (2010) had similar results when women with an epidural delayed pushing. With less time spent pushing, Lai et al (2009) found women who pushed spontaneously experienced less fatigue at 1 and 24 hours post-delivery.

Directed pushing generally involves taking a deep breath and holding it, taking breaths quickly between pushes and 3–4 sustained pushes from when the contraction begins to when it ends. This is the Valsalva manoeuvre that was originally used to clear pus from the middle ear. It causes the glottis to close and increases intrathoracic pressure which decreases venous return to the heart resulting in reduced cardiac output and blood pressure. This can result in reduced uterine blood flow and placental perfusion increasing the likelihood of the fetus becoming hypoxic and acidotic (Perez-Botella & Downe 2006, Prins et al 2011, Roberts & Hanson 2007). This may also be a factor involved with perineal trauma and stress incontinence due to the increased downward stress on the anterior vaginal wall and bladder supports (Prins et al 2011, Roberts & Hanson 2007, Schaffer et al 2005). The woman may feel dizzy from holding her breath which may cause her to gasp, allowing a sudden increase in the amount of blood returning to the heart and increasing blood pressure (Dempsey et al 2014, Perez-Botella & Downe 2006). Using the Valsalva manoeuvre can also result in a temporary reduction in vision and subconjunctival haemorrhage, which can occur as a result of transient subclinical retinal oedema (Connor 2010). Women may experience more fatigue up to 24 hours post-delivery, which can indirectly affect the physical and mental health of the new mother (Lai et al 2009).

In situations where the woman does not experience the urge to push (e.g. epidural anaesthesia) she may need some instruction on when and how to push (Osborne & Hanson 2012). The principles of spontaneous pushing should be followed, for example, no breath holding, short bursts allowing the contraction to build up first.

POSITION

The position adopted by women during the second stage of labour is influenced by many factors, including cultural and societal norms. Meyvis et al (2011) suggest the two major positions are horizontal and vertical (upright). Within many of the Western countries a semi-recumbent position with legs on a support has been commonplace which Meyvis et al (2011) and Gupta et al (2012) suggest is to allow a good view of the perineum and facilitate manoeuvres such as assisted delivery. De Jonge et al (2007) consider routine use of the supine position as an intervention when used in normal labour. In traditional cultures the vertical position is often the position of choice (Gupta et al 2012). While there may be advantages and disadvantages with each of the different positions Gupta et al (2012) and Kemp et al (2013) consider women should be able to deliver in whichever position is comfortable for them (even with an epidural *in situ*) and given the choice, women do opt to use a variety of positions during the second stage

(De Jonge et al 2007, Kemp et al 2013). Women should also be aware of the positive and negative effects of upright and horizontal positions to enable them to make an informed choice. Women who are able to choose and change positions appear to have a greater sense of control and less need for analgesia (Lawrence et al 2013). NICE (2014) agree women should be encouraged to use which-ever position they choose but advise they should be dis-couraged from lying supine or semi-supine. The midwife has an important role in encouraging women to use differ-ent positions and supporting women in their choice. This is particularly important if a VE is performed during the second stage as De Jonge & Lagro-Janssen (2004) found women were more likely to remain supine following the VE. A positive and supportive environment can promote a sense of competence and personal achievement (Gupta et al 2012). Cotton (2010) argues that a comfortable posi-tion will facilitate beta-endorphin production, thus enhanc-ing analgesia at this time.

Sanderson (2012) suggests the pelvis should be viewed as a dynamic structure during birth and recommends a 'sacrum-free' position for delivery to make use of the increased pelvic diameters. In 1969, Russell demonstrated an increase in both the transverse and anteroposterior diameters when the woman is in a squatting position (Russell 1969) and, according to Sutton (2003), pelvic diameters also increase when the woman adopts a lateral position. These suggest horizontal positions should be avoided where possible.

Horizontal positions include lithotomy, semi-recumbent (sitting, semi-sitting) and left lateral (although it could be argued lateral positions are similar to vertical as there is no pressure on the sacrum). When the woman is sat on her pelvis and the sacrum is unable to move, the pelvic diam-eters of the outlet are reduced. The woman may attempt to lift her buttocks off the bed, push her pelvis forwards and throw her arms back to rectify this (Downe 2011), although this practice is often discouraged unnecessarily. Downe (2011) suggests this is the opposite of the commonly encouraged semi-recumbent position with the woman holding onto her thighs to pull her legs towards her and suggests it is more logical to allow the woman to follow her instincts. Bayes & White (2011) found lithotomy was used more when an instrumental delivery was anticipated and argue this should be the only reason for its use as it is associated with an increased risk of third- and fourth-degree tears (Gottvall et al 2007). The lithotomy position is less likely to empower the woman and may be embar-rassing for her as it can feel as if her genitals are on display with everyone looking down at her (De Jonge & Lagro-Janssen 2004). When a semi-recumbent position is used, Downe (2011) recommends the woman is well-supported by pillows and or a wedge to prevent her sliding into a dorsal position.

Vertical or upright positions include standing, squatting, also kneeling and all-fours. Upright positions are thought to encourage descent of the presenting part, strong, efficient contractions, enhanced alignment of the fetus and assist the fetal ejection reflex (Cotton 2010). Pearson (2012) also claims the second stage is shorter, with fewer instrumental deliveries and fetal heart abnormalities when an upright position is adopted.

Perineal damage includes spontaneous first- to fourth-degree tears and episiotomy, but does the position adopted affect the likelihood of this occurring? Meyvis et al (2011) compared lithotomy with the left lateral position and found perineal damage increased with the use of the lithot-omy position. This appears to be due to more episiotomies, but women in the left lateral group had significantly more first- and second-degree perineal tears. Gupta et al (2012) suggest an upright position or use of the birthing stool is associated with fewer episiotomies but an increased risk of second-degree tears occurring. However, Albers & Borders (2007) found upright and lateral delivery positions were associated with fewer perineal tears. When using a semi-sitting position during the expulsive phase, Da Silva et al (2012) found an increased risk of second-degree tears and episiotomy compared to women who adopted a lateral, squatting or all-fours position. Soong & Barnes (2005) found a significant increase in perineal trauma in women adopting the semi-recumbent position compared with the all-fours position. These effects were more noticeable with women undergoing their first vaginal birth and where the birth weight was in excess of 3500 g. Women with epidural anaesthesia are more likely to adopt a horizontal position; for these women, Soong & Barnes (2005) found suturing was more likely to be required in a semi-recumbent rather than a lateral position. Nicholl & Cattell (2006) agree, sug-gesting if a horizontal position is used for delivery, a lateral position is preferable, as it results in more intact perineums and less risk of fourth-degree tears. De Jonge et al (2010) compared sitting, semi-sitting, and recumbent positions and found similar rates of intact perineums but more peri-neal tears with the sitting group and more labial tears with the semi-sitting group. Gottvall et al (2007) found there was a greater risk of third- and fourth-degree tears when women were in lithotomy (regardless of mode of delivery) or squatting.

Blood loss may increase in the presence of perineal tears or episiotomy but there is little evidence to suggest blood loss increases with one or more particular positions. Gupta et al (2012) did find a greater blood loss >500 mL associ-ated with an upright birthing position but also noted the blood loss was collected in a receptacle; thus it could be measured rather than inaccurately estimated, and there were no differences in the rate of blood transfusions required.

Di Franco et al (2007) consider upright positions make use of gravity and increase the pelvic diameters but acknowledge they are more tiring than semi-recumbent positions. To counteract this, they recommend using a supported squat, supporting the woman under her arms. This results in less weight on her legs and feet, and lengthening of her trunk, which provides more space for the fetus to move through the pelvis.

When comparing the use of kneeling and sitting upright, Ragnar et al (2006) concluded the outcomes do not differ significantly, although kneeling was associated with more favourable maternal experiences and reduced pain. Kneeling also allowed women the freedom to modify their position more easily, allowing them to feel more in control.

When adopting a supine, semi-recumbent or prolonged squatting position, it is important to avoid excessive and prolonged thigh-holding, as this can cause compressive peroneal neuropathy (functional and/or pathological changes to the peroneal nerve which supplies the calf and foot). This presents with knee tenderness, foot drop, and decreased sensation over the dorsum of the foot (Sahai-Srivastava & Amezcua 2007).

Midwives should therefore:

- inform and advise women about the advantages and disadvantages of the various positions that can be used in the second stage of labour
- encourage and support women to adopt the positions of their choice in which they are most comfortable, while remembering the advantages of an upright position (or lateral where an epidural anaesthesia is present)
- show women and their birthing partners how to utilize upright positions together
- utilize available equipment such as beanbags, birthing balls/chairs/stools, etc.
- have confidence in their ability to facilitate safe deliveries in different positions.

ASEPSIS

While it is often considered the delivery should be an aseptic procedure to reduce the incidence of postnatal infection for mother and baby, this is not always possible when the midwife is delivering without assistance. In this situation the midwife should consider how she can reduce the risk of infection. Equipment used should be sterile at the onset of the delivery and a sterile field established on the working surface and, with horizontal positions, the area of the woman's perineum. It is important to keep sterile and non-sterile equipment separate. Adaptations are necessary according to the environment and the position that the woman has adopted. Hand hygiene (Chapter 9) and use of personal protective equipment (Chapter 8) are

essential. Once the sterile gloves have been applied for delivery, they should be kept sterile or changed as needed. An anal pad may be used to cover or remove any faeces that may escape from the anus in horizontal positions.

MANAGEMENT OF THE PERINEUM

Effective management of the perineum is a priority for midwives according to Albers et al (2005) because of the short- and long-term effects perineal trauma has for the woman. Pain is not only unpleasant for the woman but affects her ability to function normally and care for her baby (Albers & Borders 2007, Way 2012). Sufficient time is helpful for the perineum to distend and stretch slowly. Moore & Moorhead (2013) suggest routine infiltration of the perineum is not evidence-based and may cause harm by increasing volume within the perineum, which can alter the elasticity of the perineal tissue, increasing the risk of spontaneous trauma.

PERINEAL MASSAGE

The literature regarding the value of perineal massage is conflicting and many of the studies are small. While Beckmann & Stock (2013) suggest women who perform antenatal perineal massage have a lower risk of perineal trauma primarily through a reduced risk of episiotomy, Seehusen & Raleigh (2014) suggest this is only for women who had not had a vaginal birth previously. Aasheim et al (2011) suggest perineal massage may reduce the risk of third- and fourth-degree tears, although Karaçam et al (2012) found perineal massage during the second stage had no effect on the amount or degree of perineal trauma, pain and wound healing. However, Geranmayeh et al (2012) suggest the use of Vaseline for perineal massage significantly reduces the amount and type of perineal trauma experienced. At present there is not conclusive evidence for or against perineal massage antenatally or during labour and the reader should be vigilant for new evidence in this matter.

WARM COMPRESSES

Moore & Moorhead (2013) suggest women may find it beneficial to have their perineum soaked with warm or cool water during the second stage. Aasheim et al (2011) recommend the use of warm compresses to reduce perineal trauma, suggesting it is acceptable to both the women and the midwives.

HANDS ON OR HANDS OFF?

The RCM (2012b) suggest there is no evidence to support either technique and recommend either be used. Aasheim et al (2011) found that the definition of hands-off varies in the literature from no hand on the perineum or baby's head with or without the shoulders delivering with assistance, to not touching the baby's head until it crowns. The hands-on approach generally encompasses placing a hand on the baby's head in an attempt to control the speed of delivery of the head, placing the other hand next to the perineum to support it (often with a swab held against the perineum) and using traction to assist the shoulders to birth with anterior shoulder first. McCandlish et al (1998) found the hands-on approach resulted in less perineal pain at 10 days but little or no difference in other outcomes. It may be possible to achieve control of the speed of delivery with verbal guidance, but equally the woman may wish to deliver the baby herself onto her abdomen; both of these methods are modifications of the hands-on technique. NICE (2014) advise either technique can be used. The RCOG (2015) recommend a hands-on approach to reduce the incidence of anal sphincter injury.

THE NUCHAL UMBILICAL CORD

Checking for a nuchal cord around the baby's neck at delivery has its origins in the medical textbooks of the late seventeenth century (Jefford et al 2009) and is still recommended in midwifery textbooks today (Downe & Marshall 2014). Reed et al (2009) suggest a nuchal cord occurs in 10–37% of deliveries and is thought to be commoner in males due to their tendency to have longer cords with tight cords being rare (Jefford et al 2009). There is no high-level evidence to support the practice of feeling around the baby's neck for the presence of the umbilical cord and Jefford et al (2009) are concerned this will involve a vaginal examination for which the woman has usually not consented to and which is invasive and possibly painful.

If the nuchal cord is felt for, the next question is what to do with it – looping a loose cord over the baby's head, delivering the baby through the cord or clamping and cutting a tight cord? There is little evidence supporting these practices and the literature does not always distinguish between loose and tight cords (Reed et al 2009). The option of slipping a loose cord over the baby's head is favoured by midwives but does involve handling the cord while the woman stops pushing. Clamping and cutting the cord severs the oxygen supply completely for the baby which will be detrimental should shoulder dystocia occur and Reed et al (2009)

suggest this could be the reason why babies have lower Apgar scores and pH levels in the studies reviewing the management of nuchal cords. It would appear to be preferable to leave the cord intact and deliver the baby with the nuchal cord in place as placental blood flow can resume once the baby is born; thus there is no spasm of the umbilical vessels from handling the cord and the baby has the advantage of the additional blood volume from delayed cord clamping. Sadan et al (2007) agree; they found leaving the nuchal cord intact or cutting it once the anterior shoulder has delivered had no adverse effects on perinatal outcomes.

To deliver the baby through the nuchal cord, Reed et al (2009) recommend using the Somersault technique – both shoulders are delivered slowly without handling the cord and as the shoulders deliver, the baby's head is flexed to push his face close to his mother's thigh (Fig. 31.1). Then, keeping the head next to the perineum, assist the baby to somersault out of the vagina and unwrap the cord.

Management of the nuchal cord at delivery remains a contentious issue with little evidence to support a particular management option. However, with the risk of shoulder dystocia and the advantages of delayed cord clamping it would appear prudent not to clamp and cut the cord unless the delivery is prevented by a tight short cord. Therefore it may be unnecessary to feel for a nuchal cord unless there is a clear clinical indication.

PREPARATION OF THE ENVIRONMENT

The support, communication, physical care, observations and record keeping that have extended through the first stage of labour should continue throughout the second stage. NICE (2014) recommend hourly blood pressure, 4-hourly temperature, half-hourly recording of the frequency of the contractions, intermittent auscultation of the fetal heart for 1 minute immediately following a contraction every 5 minutes and palpation of maternal pulse every 15 minutes to differentiate between the two heart rates. Additionally, NICE (2014) suggest the frequency with which urine is passed should be recorded, and a VE offered hourly in the active phase or according to the woman's wishes, but stress this should only occur after an abdominal palpation and assessment of vaginal loss has been undertaken.

The environment of the second stage should:

- have a midwife present throughout, with an assistant for delivery (depending on local protocol, but ideally a second midwife)
- be calm and relaxed
- be warm and ready to receive the baby
- contain all that is required for the birth

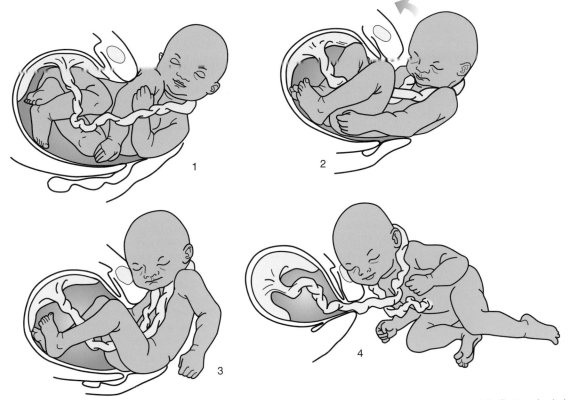

Figure 31.1 The Somersault manoeuvre. Both shoulders are delivered slowly without handling the cord, while flexing the baby's head to push his face close to his mother's thigh. Keeping the head next to the perineum, assist the baby to somersault out of the vagina. *(From Mercer et al. 2005. Reproduced with kind permission of Elsevier.)*

- have a recognized system for calling emergency assistance
- be equipped to begin emergency management for mother or baby; all equipment should be checked and the midwife must be competent in its use.

Swabs and sharps

All swabs and sharps opened should be counted and recorded and the count repeated after the delivery with an entry in the woman's notes to record they are both correct. Double counting, out loud, with a colleague is best practice and swabs should be separated during the counting. Lamont et al (2010) report that there were 99 incidents, e.g. swabs retained within the woman, reported in England and Wales between April 2007 and March 2009. The swabs should be woven gauze with a radiopaque thread throughout so they are detectable on X-ray. When soaked in blood, swabs can be difficult to identify and may occasionally be left inside the vagina by mistake leading to fever, infection, pain, secondary postpartum haemorrhage and psychological harm (Lamont et al 2010).

PROCEDURE: normal delivery

Adaptations are made according to the birth environment and position of the woman. Note should be taken of the discussions above. Undertake a VE to confirm second stage if there is a clear clinical indication, e.g. with breech presentation.

- Prepare the environment and gather equipment:
  - delivery trolley or clean surface to work from
  - sterile delivery pack, including warm towels to dry/ wrap the baby
  - sterile gloves
  - Personal protective equipment (PPE) – apron, eye protection
  - disposable sheets, non-sterile gloves and sanitary towels

- extras: urinary catheter, amnihook, lidocaine, needles and syringes, uterotonic agent
- an infectious waste refuse bag should be available, usually a floor bin
- Resuscitaire should be switched on and checked it is working.

- Ensure that the room temperature is warm (21–24°C) and draughts excluded.
- Continue to provide ongoing reassurance and explanations to the woman, supporting her with spontaneous pushing, choice of position and analgesia and maintaining maternal and fetal observations.
- Position the disposable sheets strategically in the area of the perineum, while wearing non-sterile gloves.
- When the delivery is imminent, put on apron and eye protection, wash and dry hands, and open the outer covering of the delivery pack.
- Place all other sterile items onto the delivery pack using an Aseptic Non Touch Technique (ANTT) (if there is an assistant present, they can do this).
- Apply handrub, allow to dry, and then put on the sterile gloves.
- Count the swabs and sharps, and check the instruments in the delivery pack preferably with the assistant as a second checker.
- Organize the delivery trolley/surface in a way that suits, having cord clamps and a receiver for the placenta close by.
- Keep observing the advancing presenting part while carrying out these procedures as some women experience short second stages!
- Position any sterile drapes appropriately to provide a sterile field.
- If being used, place a warm compress on the perineum.
- If being used, place the anal pad in position.
- Have a warm towel close by to dry the baby.
- The perineum will stretch as the fetus reaches the perineum, this may sting and feel sore so continue to encourage and support the woman.
- As the head crowns, apply gentle pressure to it with one hand to slow the delivery and 'guard' the perineum with the other hand if adopting a hands-on approach otherwise remain hands-off.
- Encourage the woman to breathe slowly and give gentle pushes as the head extends and emerges, note the time. Do not feel around the neck for a nuchal cord.
- Restitution will be seen followed by external rotation of the head as the shoulders rotate internally.
- The next contraction usually occurs within 1–3 minutes and the woman will have the urge to push again. Apply traction to the anterior shoulder (in a direction away from the symphysis pubis) to deliver it, followed by traction in the opposite direction to deliver the posterior shoulder if hands-on, otherwise allow the shoulders to deliver spontaneously if hands-off.
- The body and limbs of the baby are delivered by lateral flexion, following the curve of the birth canal, in an upward direction towards the woman's abdomen. The woman or her partner may assist with this.
- Note the time of delivery.
- Ideally the baby is placed skin-to-skin with his mother and dried completely with the wet towel replaced with a dry warm one; parents or midwife will check the gender.
- Drying acts as stimulation, during which time the baby will take its first breath and cry; assess the Apgar score (see Chapter 37) at 1 minute. Act swiftly (before 1 minute) if resuscitation is required (see Chapter 56).
- Clamping and cutting of the cord will be undertaken according to the parents' wishes and chosen management of the third stage of labour (Chapter 32). Breastfeeding may be facilitated (Chapter 41).
- Share in the joy of the moment, but stay alert to the clinical situation.
- Care moves into management of the third stage of labour; this may have included the administration of an intramuscular or intravenous uterotonic following the birth of the baby.

EPISIOTOMY

Episiotomy is the surgical incision into the perineum to widen the vulval outlet, usually undertaken with scissors. Rates of episiotomy vary across the world from 9.7% (Sweden) to 100% (Taiwan) with reported rates of 30% in Europe (Carroli & Mignini 2009). Frankman et al (2009) report the episiotomy rate in the US has reduced from 60.9% to 24.5% between 1979 and 2004, which has been accompanied by a reduction in anal sphincter tears and conclude that not performing an episiotomy is an important step in reducing rates of third- and fourth-degree tears. Aasheim et al (2011) found a 'hands-off' approach to the perineum resulted in fewer episiotomies being performed.

Episiotomy should not be undertaken routinely but only when there is an indication because of concerns about maternal and or fetal wellbeing or with instrumental delivery (Sleep et al 1984); restricted use of episiotomy is associated with less posterior perineal trauma (posterior vaginal wall, perineal muscles and anal sphincter), less suturing and fewer complications than routine use. There is an increased risk of anterior perineal trauma (labia, anterior vagina, urethra, clitoris) with little associated morbidity

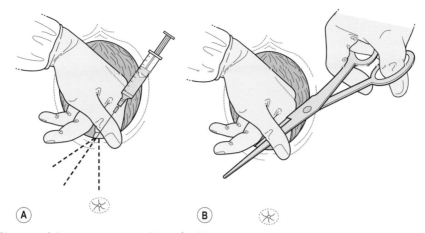

Figure 31.2 A, Infiltration of the perineum; **B,** Incision of episiotomy.

(Carroli & Mignini 2009, RCOG 2015). Chapman (2009) suggests it is harder for left-handed midwives to perform an episiotomy because the design of the scissors is for right-handed use and also the angle of the cut. Chapman (2009) ponders this and wonders if left-handed midwives undertake fewer episiotomies than right-handed midwives or whether they swap the scissors into their right hand. It is not appropriate to undertake the episiotomy to the woman's left.

If an episiotomy is indicated, the midwife may perform this with the woman's consent and if properly trained. The timing of gaining informed consent is a more difficult issue; parenthood education during the antenatal period may assist the woman to understand what it is and why it may be necessary; her birth plan may include her wishes. However, the urgency of the need to undertake an episiotomy at the time limits detailed explanations, but consent is still required and debriefing following birth is recommended.

The midwife should only perform a right mediolateral episiotomy, not midline. A midline episiotomy is more likely to extend to a third- or fourth-degree tear and increases the risk of anal incontinence (Eogan et al 2006, Lappen & Gossett 2010). The incision should begin at the posterior fourchette, at an angle of 45–60° (Fig. 31.2) (Eogan et al 2006, NICE 2014); however, Thomas & Cameron (2007) found that the angle of incision varied between 29–80° from the midline. The risk of anal sphincter injury increases with a small episiotomy angle (Eogan et al 2006).

Unless the woman has a good epidural *in situ*, infiltration of the perineum with an anaesthetic is necessary prior to the incision. Lidocaine is the drug of choice, as this can be administered using the Midwives Exemption List. The timing of the episiotomy is important as the presenting part needs to have descended sufficiently onto the perineum to displace the levator ani (deep muscles) as the incision is then likely to involve only the skin, posterior vaginal wall and superficial pelvic floor muscles (see Fig. 31.2). If the incision is performed too early, the deep pelvic floor muscles may be incised, resulting in increased bleeding from the wound. The presenting part can deliver once the episiotomy is complete; thus the midwife is required – almost simultaneously – to remove the scissors from the vulva, control the delivery of the head, and support the perineum so that the episiotomy does not extend. The procedure and repair (see Chapter 34) are both aseptic events.

PROCEDURE: infiltration of the perineum and episiotomy

- Gain informed consent.
- Between contractions, draw up the correct dose of anaesthetic agent, e.g. lidocaine, using a sterile needle (21-g green) and syringe and an ANTT and avoiding touching the Key-Parts (connecting ends of the syringe and needle and the solution).
- Insert two fingers into the vagina behind the perineum to protect the presenting part.
- Insert the full depth of the needle centrally at the introitus, draw back on the plunger to ascertain if the needle is in a blood vessel, noted by the presence of blood in the syringe. If this is seen the needle, syringe, and anaesthetic agent should be replaced and the procedure repeated. If no blood is seen, inject one-third of the anaesthetic while withdrawing the needle. Do not take the needle completely out of the tissue, but as the

introitus is reached, reposition the needle and reinsert it in a mediolateral direction. Inject the anaesthetic as described and then repeat for a third time (Fig. 31.2A) to infiltrate a fan-shaped area of the perineum.

- Allow the agent time to work, two or three contractions if possible.
- Re-insert two fingers to protect the presenting part again. Using the straight scissors supplied in the delivery pack, make one decisive right mediolateral incision of approximately 4–5 cm long, beginning at the posterior fourchette and at an angle of 45–60° from the midline, at the height of the contraction at which the delivery is anticipated (Fig. 31.2B).
- Immediately apply control to the fetal head, removing the scissors onto the trolley; guard the perineum if able and facilitate the slow delivery of the head.
- Continue with the delivery as described above.
- Ensure that after examination of the genital tract (see Chapter 32), blood loss is assessed and the episiotomy is repaired appropriately (see Chapter 34).
- Records should specifically include details of the indication, infiltration and incision.

ROLE AND RESPONSIBILITIES OF THE MIDWIFE

These can be summarized as:

- providing safe, evidence-based care for the woman and baby
- supporting and encouraging the woman to adopt a safe, comfortable position
- recognizing when an episiotomy is required and performing this safely and effectively
- recognizing and managing deviations from normal; referring as necessary
- contemporaneous record keeping.

SUMMARY

- The second stage has a passive and an active phase; the passive phase may be a time to rest while pushing occurs in the active phase.
- Restricting the length of the second stage is inappropriate providing there is progress and maternal and fetal wellbeing.
- Spontaneous pushing is safer than directed pushing and should be encouraged.
- The woman should be encouraged and supported to adopt a comfortable, preferably upright, position.
- Delivery of the baby may be 'hands-on' or 'hands-off' although controlling the speed of delivery of the head, support of the perineum and lateral flexion to the shoulders may result in less perineal pain in the short term.
- Episiotomy should not be performed routinely and should be undertaken at an angle of 45–60°.

SELF-ASSESSMENT EXERCISES

The answers to the following questions may be found in the text:

1. What might lead you to suspect the woman has reached the second stage of labour?
2. Discuss how you would encourage the woman to push and why.
3. Compare and contrast the various positions used during the second stage; which would you encourage the woman to use?
4. Demonstrate how a normal birth is conducted, including management of the equipment and positioning of the hands.
5. Describe how to infiltrate the perineum and perform an episiotomy.
6. Summarize the role and responsibilities of the midwife when providing complete care during the second stage of labour.

REFERENCES

Aasheim, V., Nilsen, A.B.V., Lukasse, M., Reinar, L.M., 2011. Perineal techniques during the second stage of labour for reducing perineal trauma. Cochrane Database Syst. Rev. (2), Art. No.:CD006672, doi:10.1002/14651858.CD006672.pub2.

Albers, L.L., Borders, N., 2007. Minimizing genital tract trauma and related pain following spontaneous vaginal birth. J. Midwifery Womens Health 52 (3), 246–255.

Albers, L.L., Sedler, K.D., Bedrick, E.J., et al., 2005. Midwifery care measures in the second stage of labor and reduction of genital tract trauma at birth: a randomized trial. J. Midwifery Womens Health 50 (5), 365–372.

Allen, V.M., Baskett, T.F., O'Connell, C.M., et al., 2009. Maternal and perinatal outcomes with increasing duration of the second stage of labor. Obstet. Gynecol. 113 (6), 1248–1258.

Bayes, S., White, C., 2011. Use of the lithotomy position for low-risk women in Perth, Australia. Br. J. Midwifery 19 (5), 285–289.

Beckmann, M.M., Stock, O.M., 2013. Antenatal perineal massage for reducing perineal trauma. Cochrane Database Syst. Rev. (4), Art. No.: CD005123, doi:10.1002/14651858. CD005123.pub3.

Borders, N., Wendland, C., Haozous, E., et al., 2013. Midwives' verbal support of nulliparous women in second-stage labor. J. Obstet. Gynecol. Neonatal Nurs. 42, 311–320.

Brancato, R.M., Church, S., Stone, P.W., 2008. A meta-analysis of passive descent versus immediate pushing in nulliparous women with epidural analgesia in the second stage of labor. J. Obstet. Gynecol. Neonatal Nurs. 37 (1), 4–12.

Burvill, S., 2002. Midwifery diagnosis of labour onset. Br. J. Midwifery 10 (10), 600–605.

Carroli, G., Mignini, L., 2009. Episiotomy for vaginal birth. Cochrane Database Syst. Rev. (1), Art. No.: CD000081, doi:10.1002/14651858.CD000081.pub2.

Chapman, V., 2009. Clinical skills: issues affecting the left-handed midwife. Br. J. Midwifery 17 (8), 588–592.

Cheng, Y.W., Hopkins, L.M., Laros, R.K. Jr., Caughey, A.B., 2007. Duration of the second stage of labor in multiparous women: maternal and neonatal outcomes. Am. J. Obstet. Gynecol. Neonatal Nurs. 196 (6), 585.e1–585.e6.

Connor, A., 2010. Valsalva-related retinal venous dilation caused by defaecation. Acta Ophthalmogica 88 (4), e149. doi:10.1111/j.1755-3768.2009.01624.x.

Cotton, J., 2010. Considering the evidence for upright positions in labour. MIDIRS 20 (4), 459–463.

Da Silva, F.M.B., de Oliveira, S.M.J.V., Bick, D., et al., 2012. Risk factors for birth-related perineal trauma: a cross-sectional study in a birth centre. J. Clin. Nurs. 21, 2209–2218.

De Jonge, A., Lagro-Janssen, A.L., 2004. Birthing positions: a qualitative study into the views of women about various birthing positions. J. Psychosom. Obstet. Gynecol. 25 (1), 47–55.

De Jonge, A., Teunissen, D.A.M., van Diem, M.T., et al., 2007. Women's positions during the second stage of labour: views of primary care midwives. J. Adv. Nurs. 63 (4), 347–356.

De Jonge, A., van Diem, MT, Scheepers, P.L.H., et al., 2010. Risk of perineal damage is not a reason to discourage a sitting position: a secondary analysis. Int. J. Clin. Pract. 64 (5), 611–618.

Dempsey, J., Hillege, S., Hill, R., 2014. Fundamentals of Nursing and Midwifery a Person-Centred Approach to Care, second ed. Australian and New Zealand Edition. Lippincott, Williams & Wilkins, Sydney, pp. 1132–1168.

Di Franco, J.Y., Romano, A.M., Keen, R., 2007. Care practice #5: spontaneous pushing in upright or gravity-neutral positions. J. Perinat. Educ. 16 (3), 35–38.

Downe, S., 2011. Care in the second stage of labour. In: McDonald, S., Magill-Cuerden, J. (Eds.), Mayes' Midwifery, fourteenth ed. Baillière Tindall, London, pp. 510–514.

Downe, S., Marshall, J.E., 2014. Physiology and care during the transition and second stage phases of labour. In: Marshall, J.E., Raynor, M.D. (Eds.), Myles Textbook for Midwives, sixteenth ed. Elsevier, Edinburgh, pp. 367–393.

Eogan, M., Daly, L., O'Connell, P., O'Herlihy, C., 2006. Does the angle of episiotomy affect the incidence of anal sphincter injury? Br. J. Obstet. Gynaecol. 113, 190–194.

Frankman, E.A., Wang, L., Bunker, C.H., Lowder, J.L., 2009. Episiotomy in the United States: has anything changed? Am. J. Obstet. Gynecol. 200 (573), e1–e7.

Geranmayeh, M., Habibabadi, Z.R., Fallahkish, B., et al., 2012. Reducing perineal trauma through perineal massage with Vaseline in the second stage of labor. Arch. Gynecol. Obstet. 285 (1), 77–81.

Gillesby, E., Burns, S., Dempsey, A., et al., 2010. Comparison of delayed versus immediate pushing during second stage of labor for nulliparous women with epidural anesthesia. J. Obstet. Gynecol. Neonatal Nurs. 39, 635–644.

Gottvall, K., Allebeck, P., Ekeus, C., 2007. Risk factors for anal sphincter tears: the importance of maternal position at birth. Br. J. Obstet. Gynaecol. 114, 1266–1272.

Gupta, J.K., Hofmeyr, G.J., Shehmar, M., 2012. Position in the second stage of labour for women without epidural anaesthesia. Cochrane Database Syst. Rev. (5), Art No.: CD002006, doi:10.1002/14651858.CD002006.pub3.

Hanson, L., 2009. Second stage labor care: challenges in spontaneous bearing down. J. Perinatol. Neonatal Nurs. 23 (1), 31–39.

Hobbs, L., 1998. Assessing cervical dilatation without VEs – watching the purple line. Pract. Midwife 1 (11), 34–35.

Jahdi, F., Shahnazari, M., Kashanian, M., et al., 2011. A randomized controlled trial comparing the physiological and directed pushing on the duration of the second stage of labor, the mode of delivery and Apgar score. Int. J. Nurs. Midwifery 31 (5), 55–59.

Jefford, E., Fahy, K., Sundin, D., 2009. Routine vaginal examination to check for a nuchal cord. Br. J. Midwifery 17 (4), 246–249.

Karaçam, Z., Ekmen, H., Çalişer, H., 2012. The use of perineal massage in the second stage of labor and follow-up of postpartum perineal outcomes. Health Care Women Int. 33 (8), 697–718.

Kemp, E., Kingswood, C.J., Kibuka, M., Thornton, J.G., 2013. Positions in the second stage of labour for women with epidural anaesthesia. Cochrane Database Syst. Rev. (1), Art. No.: CD008070, doi:10.1002/14651858.CD008070.pub2.

Lai, M.-L., Lin, K.-C., Li, H.Y., et al., 2009. Effects of delayed pushing during the second stage of labor on postpartum fatigue and birth outcomes in nulliparous women. J. Nurs. Res. 17 (1), 62–71.

Lamont, T., Dougall, A., Johnson, S., et al., 2010. Reducing the risk of retained swabs after vaginal birth: summary of a safety report from the National Patient Safety Agency. Br. Med. J. 341, c3679.

Lappen, J.R., Gossett, D.R., 2010. Changes in episiotomy practice: evidence-based medicine in action. Expert Rev. Obstet. Gynecol. 5 (3), 301a.

Laughon, S.K., Berghella, V., Reddy, U.M., et al., 2014. Neonatal and maternal outcomes with prolonged second stage. Obstet. Gynecol. 124 (1), 57–67.

Lawrence, A., Lewis, L., Hofmeyr, G.J., Styles, C., 2013. Maternal positions and mobility during first stage labour. Cochrane Database Syst. Rev. (10), Art. No.: CD003934, doi:10.1002/14651858.CD003934.pub4.

Long, L., 2006. Redefining the second stage of labour could help to promote normal birth. Br. J. Midwifery 14 (2), 104–107.

Lu, M.C., Muthengi, E., Wakeel, F., et al., 2009. Prolonged second stage of labor and postpartum hemorrhage. J. Matern. Fetal Neonatal Med. 22 (3), 227–232.

McCandlish, R., Bowler, U., van Asten, H., et al., 1998. A randomised controlled trial of care of the perineum during second stage of normal labour. Br. J. Obstet. Gynaecol. 105 (12), 1262–1272.

Mercer, J.S., Skovgaard, R.L., Peareara-Eaves, J., Bowman, T.A., 2005. Nuchal cord management and nurse-midwifery practice. J. Midwifery Womens Health 50 (5), 373–379.

Meyvis, I., van Rompaey, B., Goormans, K., et al., 2011. Maternal position and other variables: effect on perineal outcomes in 557 births. Birth 39 (2), 115–120.

Moore, E., Moorhead, C., 2013. Promoting normality in the management of the puerperium during the second stage of labour. Br. J. Midwifery 21 (9), 616–620.

Naranjo, C.M., Puertas, E.C., Lopez, E.L., 2011. Obstetrical perinatal and maternal implications of spontaneous pushing and directed pushing. Metas. Enferm. 14 (5), 8–11.

NICE (National Institute for Health and Care Excellence), 2014. CG190

Intrapartum Care: Care of Healthy Mothers and Their Babies During Childbirth. NICE, London. Available online: <www.nice.org.uk> (accessed 3 March 2015).

Nicholl, M.C., Cattell, M.A., 2006. Getting evidence into obstetric and midwifery practice: reducing perineal trauma. Aust. Health Rev. 30 (4), 462–467.

Osborne, K., Hanson, L., 2012. Directive versus supportive approaches used by midwives when providing care during the second stage of labor. Birth 20, 142–147.

Pearson, S., 2012. Warwick midwives are delivering women in upright positions. Br. J. Midwifery 20 (7), 522–523.

Perez-Botella, M., Downe, S., 2006. Stories as evidence: why do midwives still use directed pushing? Br. J. Midwifery 14 (10), 596–599.

Prins, M., Boxem, J., Lucas, C., Huttone, E., 2011. Effect of spontaneous pushing versus Valsalva pushing in the second stage of labour on mother and fetus: a systematic review of randomised trials. Br. J. Obstet. Gynaecol. 118, 662–670.

Ragnar, I., Altman, D., Tyden, T., Olssen, S.-E., 2006. Comparison of the maternal experience and duration of labour in two upright delivery positions – a randomised controlled trial. Br. J. Obstet. Gynaecol. 113 (2), 165–170.

RCM (Royal College of Midwives), 2012a. Evidence Based Guidelines for Midwifery-Led Care in Labour Second Stage of Labour. Royal College of Midwives, London.

RCM (Royal College of Midwives), 2012b. Evidence Based Guidelines for Midwifery-Led Care in Labour Care of the Perineum. Royal College of Midwives, London.

RCOG (Royal College of Obstetrics & Gynaecologists), 2015. The Management of Third or Fourth Degree Perineal Tears. RCOG Green-top Guidelines No 29. RCOG, London. Available online: <www.rcog.org.uk> (accessed 29 August 2015).

Reed, R., Barnes, M., Allan, J., 2009. Nuchal cords: sharing the evidence

with parents. Br. J. Midwifery 17 (2), 106–109.

Roberts, J., Hanson, L., 2007. Best practices in second stage labor care: maternal bearing down and positioning. J. Midwifery Womens Health 52 (3), 238–247.

Russell, J.G.B., 1969. Moulding of the pelvic outlet. J. Obstet. Gynaecol. 76, 817–820.

Rustamova, S., Predanic, M., Sumersille, M., Cohen, W.R., 2009. Changes in symphysis pubis width during labor. J. Perinat. Med. 37, 370–373.

Sadan, O., Fleischfarb, Z., Everon, S., et al., 2007. Cord around the neck: should it be severed at delivery? A randomized controlled study. Am. J. Perinatol. 24 (1), 61–64.

Sahai-Srivastava, S., Amezcua, L., 2007. Compressive neuropathies complicating normal childbirth: case report and literature review. Birth 34 (2), 173–175.

Sampselle, C.M., Miller, J.M., Luecha, Y., et al., 2005. Provider support of spontaneous pushing during the second stage of labor. J. Obstet. Gynecol. Neonatal Nurs. 34 (6), 695–702.

Sanderson, T.A., 2012. The movements of the maternal pelvis: a review. MIDIRS Midwifery Dig. 22 (3), 319–326.

Schaffer, J.I., Bloom, S.L., Casey, B.M., 2005. A randomized trial of the effects of coached versus uncoached maternal pushing during the second stage of labor on postpartum pelvic floor structure and function. Am. J. Obstet. Gynecol. 192 (5), 1692–1696.

Seehusen, S., Raleigh, M., 2014. Antenatal perineal massage to prevent birth trauma. Am. Fam. Physician 89 (5), 335–356.

Sleep, J.M., Grant, A., Garcia, J., et al., 1984. West Berkshire perineal management trial. Br. Med. J. 289, 587–590.

Soong, B., Barnes, M., 2005. Maternal position at midwife-attended birth and perineal trauma: is there an association? Birth 32 (3), 164–169.

Sutton, J., 2003. Birth without active pushing. In: Wickham, S. (Ed.),

Midwifery Best Practice. Elsevier Science, Edinburgh, pp. 90–92.

Thomas, E., Cameron, H., 2007. Midwives' management of episiotomy at a district general hospital. Br. J. Midwifery 15 (11), 680–683.

Way, S., 2012. A qualitative study exploring women's personal experiences of their perineum after childbirth: expectations, reality and returning to normality. Midwifery 28 (5), e712–e719.

Yildirim, G., Beji, N.K., 2008. Effects of pushing techniques in birth on mother and fetus: a randomized study. Birth 35 (1), 25–30.

Chapter | 32 |

Principles of intrapartum skills: third-stage issues

LEARNING OUTCOMES

Having read this chapter, the reader should be able to:

- recognize the importance of the third stage of labour for the health and wellbeing of the mother and baby
- describe the physiology of the third stage of labour
- discuss the effects of delayed cord clamping and umbilical cord milking on the baby
- discuss the different methods of managing the third stage
- list the uterotonics used for third stage management, identifying when they should be used and how they work
- discuss how blood loss is estimated
- describe how the genital tract is examined following delivery.

For the majority of women the third stage of labour occurs with no adverse outcomes but it has the potential to be a hazardous time for the woman, as primary postpartum haemorrhage (PPH) remains a direct cause of maternal mortality. While in the UK the risk of death from haemorrhage is very small (11 women died from PPH during 2010–2012) (Knight et al 2014), worldwide, particularly in developing countries, the death rate can be much higher, accounting for 30% of maternal deaths in Africa and Asia (Fawole et al 2012). The midwife has a responsibility to ensure the placenta and membranes are delivered safely and competently following the delivery of the baby. This chapter focuses on the principles of the management of the third stage of labour, discussing both expectant and active management, examination of the genital tract following delivery of the placenta and estimation of blood loss; relevant anatomy and physiology are included.

PHYSIOLOGY OF THE THIRD STAGE OF LABOUR

The third stage is from the birth of the baby to the complete expulsion of the placenta and membranes, involving the separation, descent, and expulsion of the placenta and membranes; the control of haemorrhage from the placental site; and examination of the genital tract following delivery. Perineal repair is occasionally undertaken while awaiting the birth of the placenta.

The physiology of placental separation has been revised in recent years following ultrasound visualization of placental separation (Herman 2000, Herman et al 2002, Krapp et al 2000) with three phases identified: latent, contraction/detachment, and expulsion. The intrauterine volume reduces drastically (from 4 L prelabour to 0.5 L) as the uterus becomes smaller following the delivery of the baby. Pressure within the uterus increases from 100 mmHg in the second stage to 140 mmHg in the third stage.

Phase 1: latent phase

The myometrium continues to contract and retract as with the first and second stages of labour resulting in extensive thickening of most of the myometrium; the area of myometrium beneath the placental site does not thicken to the same degree. This takes 101 ± 87 seconds.

Phase 2: contraction/detachment phase

The myometrium under the lower pole of the placenta begins to contract with a reduction in the surface area. Consequently, the shearing forces cause the placenta to separate from the spongy layer of the decidua. With the onset of placental detachment, the wave of separation passes upwards and the remaining placenta detaches, with the uppermost part of the placenta detaching last, leaving the maternal sinuses within the decidua exposed. The oblique muscle fibres surrounding the blood vessels contract to seal the torn ends of the maternal vessels to prevent haemorrhage. This phase lasts 56 ± 45 seconds.

Phase 3: expulsion phase

As the placenta descends into the lower uterine segment, the membranes (which had begun to detach from the uterine wall as the internal cervical os dilated) peel away from the walls of the uterus. With further contractions the placenta descends into the vagina, assisted by gravity, with the membranes following. This takes 77 ± 63 seconds.

Maternal effort will birth the placenta and membranes with the fetal surface appearing at the vulva, with the membranes behind containing any blood loss within them; this is often referred to as the 'Schultze' method of expulsion (Fig. 32.1A). Sometimes the lower edge of the placenta will descend first with the maternal surface appearing at the vulva and sliding out lengthways with the membranes (Fig. 32.1B). This is a slower process, with increased blood loss as the mechanisms to control haemorrhage are less effective when the placenta is still partially attached. This has been referred to as the 'Matthews Duncan' method of expulsion.

Radiological studies have demonstrated that the placenta usually separates within 3 minutes of the birth of the baby (Brandt 1933). Herman (2000) suggests the duration of the third stage varies according to the length of the latent phase; however, the time taken for the descent and birth of the placenta and membranes can also vary individually, influenced by factors such as posture and whether the third stage is managed actively or expectantly. Harris (2011) suggests the placenta begins to separate with the birth of the baby and is completed within one to two contractions.

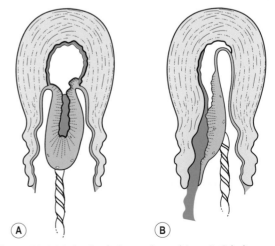

Figure 32.1 Methods of placental expulsion. **A,** Schultze. **B,** Matthews Duncan.

Signs of separation and descent

These are not absolute and may occur for other reasons:

- Bleeding: a trickle of 30–60 mL of blood from the vagina; this could also be from a laceration or a partially separated placenta (although bleeding is often heavier).
- Cord lengthening: this may occur as the placenta descends or from a coiled cord that is straightening out.
- A change in the shape and position of the uterus: the uterus becomes globular, hard, high, mobile and ballottable. Before placental separation and descent into the lower uterine segment, the fundus is broad and palpable, usually below the umbilicus. With separation and descent, the fundus narrows and fundal height increases, usually above the umbilicus (Fig. 32.2). This can be assessed by gently palpating the fundus (it may provoke irregular contractions which can interfere with placental separation and cause a partially separated placenta, resulting in excessive bleeding). The placenta may also appear as a bulge just above the symphysis pubis.
- The woman feels pressure or an urge to push as the placenta enters the vagina.

Control of haemorrhage

The placental circulation is approximately 500–800 mL/min at term; thus bleeding from the placental site can be profuse and rapid and it is vital that haemorrhage is controlled. This is achieved in three ways:

1. The middle oblique fibres of the uterus contract, constricting and kinking the blood vessels passing through them. Blood flow slows down and stops, allowing time for clot formation at the placental site.
2. The uterine walls become in apposition to each other, exerting pressure on the placental site.
3. The coagulation process begins to work at the placental site, within the sinuses and torn vessels. The damaged tissues release thrombokinase which converts prothrombin to thrombin. Thrombin combines with fibrinogen to form fibrin, which forms a clot by combining with platelets. Vitamin K, calcium and the other clotting factors are required for this process to happen efficiently.

CORD CLAMPING

With the introduction of active management, the practice of immediate cord clamping following birth (within 30 seconds) became widespread. However, placental separation is reliant on the ability of the uterus to continue to contract and retract. Clamping the cord can set up a counter-resistance in the placenta preventing the transfer of blood to the baby. This can prevent the placenta from reducing in size with the potential to inhibit contraction

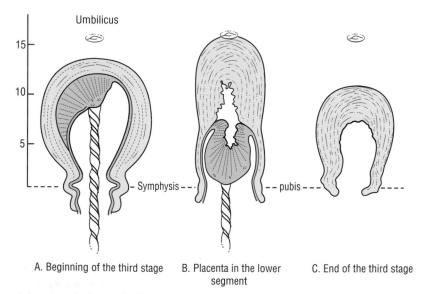

A. Beginning of the third stage   B. Placenta in the lower segment   C. End of the third stage

Figure 32.2 Position of the uterus before and after placental separation.

and retraction of the uterus resulting in a slower separation process. This has two effects:

1. Delay in complete separation causes the torn maternal vessels to seal off more slowly, producing a retroplacental clot and increasing the risk of haemorrhage.

2. A retained placenta may occur if the cervix retracts before it is expelled, often necessitating a manual removal of the placenta and membranes under epidural, spinal, or general anaesthetic.

When the cord is not clamped immediately, the process of placental separation is unaffected and the baby receives the extra blood contained within the placenta. Scheans (2013) suggests that blood flow via the umbilical arteries from baby to placenta stops after 20–25 seconds following birth, whereas the blood flow from the placenta to the baby via the umbilical vein continues for up to 3 minutes. McAdams (2014) refers to the importance for the baby of receiving this additional iron-rich blood, suggesting the first minute before cord clamping is the 'iron minute'.

When it is time to clamp the cord, the clamp should be applied 3–4 cm from the abdominal wall. If the baby is preterm the cord should be longer, as catheterization of the umbilical vessels may be required; this is more successful with a longer cord. A clamp is usually applied to the maternal end of the cord and the section of cord between the two clamps cut. This may be something that the woman's partner or family member will want to do and the midwife should direct them where to cut.

Delayed cord clamping (DCC)

Short-term benefits

DCC has many short-term benefits. The most obvious benefit is the increased blood volume (ACOG 2012, Meyer & Mildenhall 2012, Scheans 2013). Mercer et al (2010) suggest the very low birthweight baby receives 10–15 mL/kg of extra blood with even a brief delay in cord clamping while Raju (2013) advises the amount increases with time, suggesting 16 mL/kg by 60 seconds and 23 mL/kg by 180 seconds for the term baby. Airey et al (2008) propose DCC increases placental transfusion to the baby by 20%, providing an extra 20–40 mg/kg of iron for the term baby whereas Blouin et al (2013) advise the extra 15–40 mL/kg of blood received increases blood volume by 30–50% and provides an additional 30–75 mg of iron with 3 minutes of DCC. McDonald et al (2013) suggest blood volume increases by 30% and the baby receives 60% more red blood cells. This can significantly increase the haemoglobin for both the preterm (Aziz et al 2012, Ghavam et al 2014) and the term (Raju 2013) baby and increases circulating ferritin levels (Raju 2013) and iron stores at 2–4 months (Raju

2013), decreasing the risk of iron-deficiency anaemia between 4–6 months (Scheans 2013) and the need for blood transfusions (ACOG 2012, Ghavam et al 2014, Rabe et al 2012, Raju 2013, Scheans 2013). The extra blood volume also assists with facilitating the pulmonary adaptation required at and following birth and Baenziger et al (2007) suggest this is why there is less need for medical interventions such as mechanical ventilation in the preterm baby following DCC.

The increased blood volume improves blood flow in the superior vena cava and may decrease vascular resistance, improving the preterm baby's ability to autoregulate cerebral blood flow in early life (Meyer & Mildenhall 2012). Blood pressure is increased for the preterm baby (within normal limits) (Ghavam et al 2014, Rabe et al 2012, Raju 2013) possibly reducing the risk (up to 50%) of intraventricular haemorrhage for the preterm baby who has DCC (ACOG 2012, Ghavam et al 2014, Rabe et al 2012, Raju 2013, Scheans 2013). There is improved cerebral perfusion and oxygenation (Baenziger et al 2007, Raju 2013) which potentially improves perfusion generally, reducing the risk of organ injury occurring from decreased perfusion. Overall there is also a decreased incidence of intracranial haemorrhage (ACOG 2012, Raju 2013, Scheans 2013).

Tolosa et al (2010) refer to the transfusion of placental blood as 'nature's first stem cell transplant'. The stem cells within the blood have anti-inflammatory, neurotrophic, and neuroprotective effects (Raju 2013, Tarnow-Mordi et al 2014). Ghavam et al (2014), Rabe et al (2012) and Scheans (2013) found DCC helps reduce the incidence of late-onset sepsis and necrotizing enterocolitis for preterm babies.

Other benefits include increased duration of early breastfeeding for preterm babies <32 weeks (Mercer et al 2006), significantly less hypothermia (Aziz et al 2012), and increased urinary output in the first 48 hours (Raju 2013).

From the maternal perspective, McDonald et al (2013) found no significant difference in the incidence of severe PPH or haemorrhage of 500 mL and no significant difference in mean blood loss at delivery or postnatal maternal haemoglobin levels when DCC was undertaken for term babies.

Long-term benefits

There is little evidence currently for or against longer-term benefits. Blouin et al (2013) reviewed the effect of DCC on babies whose mothers were anaemic compared to non-anaemic mothers. They found at 8 months there was significantly less iron deficiency in babies who had DCC and whose mothers were anaemic. Mercer et al (2010) suggest that DCC seems to be a protective factor against motor disability at 7 months corrected age for very low birthweight infants (they studied babies at 24–31[+6] weeks' gestation); however, Ghavam et al (2014) found no difference in disability between babies who had early or late delayed cord clamping or cord milking. Andersson et al (2013a) agree, they found no difference at 4 months on neurodevelopment of symptoms of infection.

Risks of delayed cord clamping

Tarnow-Mordi et al (2014) are concerned about an increase in the incidence and severity of jaundice, a view supported by Raju (2013) who suggests there is an increased need for phototherapy. However, Scheans (2013) and Cernadas et al (2006) found asymptomatic polycythaemia, (haematocrit >65%) was more common in babies who had DCC but this was not associated with a significant difference in serum bilirubin levels or the need for phototherapy in the first 1–3 days.

In certain situations DCC may not be advisable, e.g. where there are maternal antibodies circulating and are destroying fetal cells, as the baby receives not only extra red blood cells during the placental transfusion of blood but also everything else in the blood. These cases are less common in the developed world and are considered on an individual basis.

Duration of DCC

If the third stage is expectant, clamping and cutting the cord would not occur until after the cord has stopped pulsating. For the baby having a lotus birth (see Chapter 33), there would be no clamping or cutting of the cord. But if the third stage is to be actively managed, how long should the cord pulsate and transfer blood before it is clamped and cut?

The consensus appears to be that DCC should take somewhere between ≥30 seconds and up to or longer than 3 minutes (ACOG 2012, McAdams 2014, Raju 2013, Scheans 2013, WHO 2014) for a term baby. The longer the cord pulsates, the greater the placental transfusion of blood to the baby. ACOG (2012) suggest the ideal duration for the preterm baby has not been established and the need for resuscitation overrides DCC; Rabe et al (2012) and WHO (2014) suggest it should be for 30–120 seconds.

Position of the baby

Early studies recommended positioning the baby 40 cm below the introitus for 30 seconds for maximal transfer of blood (Palethorpe et al 2010). More recent studies of DCC position the baby at the level of the introitus for a vaginal birth (McAdams 2014, Meyer & Mildenhall 2012) or below the introitus (Andersson et al 2013b, Mercer et al 2010) and above the level of the uterus, usually on the maternal legs, following a caesarean birth (McAdams 2014, Meyer &

Mildenhall 2012). Blouin et al (2013), however, positioned the baby on the mother's abdomen, which is more realistic of what happens following the vaginal birth of the baby, a position supported by Cook (2007). Palethorpe et al (2010) found no reliable research to demonstrate whether the position of the baby during DCC makes a difference to the health of the baby or the mother. It would make sense to continue placing the baby skin-to-skin with his mother during DCC, with its known benefits (Moore et al 2012) until good evidence suggests otherwise.

Milking the cord

Tarnow-Mordi et al (2014) suggest that milking the umbilical cord disrupts the fetoplacental circulation and the transition of the cardiopulmonary and cerebral circulation. However, in situations where there is no time for DCC, e.g. resuscitation, milking the cord may offer some advantages (Raju 2013). But how much of the cord should be milked, how quickly, and how many times? And does it vary according to gestational age? Much of the research around milking the cord involves preterm babies who are likely to experience early cord clamping due to resuscitation needs but who would benefit from delayed cord clamping – 24–28 weeks (March et al 2013), 32 weeks (Backes et al 2010).

March et al (2013) held babies at or below the level of the placenta following a vaginal birth and at the same level following an operative birth; 20 cm of cord was milked three times. Patel et al (2014) held babies 10 cm below the placenta, pinching the cord as close to the placenta as possible and milking it towards the baby for 2–3 seconds, then released the cord for 2–3 seconds and repeated twice more but for <30 seconds in total. Upadhyay et al (2013) undertook cord milking on babies who were placed on a resuscitaire by leaving the cord 25 cm long. The cord was then milked three times at 10 cm/sec after which it was clamped. Takami et al (2012) used a 20 cm segment of cord two to three times at 20 cm/sec.

Advantages of cord milking include reduced rates of mortality (Backes et al 2010), intraventricular haemorrhage (IVH) (Backes et al 2010, March et al 2013), transfusion (IVH) (Backes et al 2010, March et al 2013), higher haemoglobin (Hb) and serum ferritin at 6 weeks (Upadhyay et al 2013), and relatively higher blood pressure (within the normal range) during the first 48 hours of life (Upadhyay et al 2013). Higher initial Hb, mean arterial blood pressure, and urine output levels within the first 24 hours decreased the need for volume expanders (Patel et al 2014, Takami et al 2012). Takami et al (2012) conclude that cord milking improves cerebral perfusion. Additionally there is no increased risk of hyperbilirubinaemia and phototherapy (March et al 2013).

Backes et al (2010) advise caution though, as the effects of milking on the fragile germinal matrix vessels in the preterm baby are unknown and suggest this warrants further consideration in future studies.

MANAGEMENT OF THE THIRD STAGE

There are considerable variations between and within countries in policies for the management of the third stage of labour and the pharmacological agents used (Winter et al 2007). Midwives should be competent with both expectant (physiological, passive) and active management (RCM 2012).

EXPECTANT MANAGEMENT OF THE THIRD STAGE OF LABOUR (EMTSL)

Women who have experienced a physiological labour and birth can be offered a physiological third stage for birthing their placenta (NZCOM 2013, RCM 2012); the physiological process of placental separation and delivery are dependent on a finely tuned balance of hormonal, physiological, psychological and neurological interactions, which if any of these have been disturbed, can compromise safety at this time (Fry 2007). With EMTSL the placenta is delivered by maternal effort assisted by gravity and the baby suckling at the breast. There should be no intervention – no drugs, no cord clamping (unless it has stopped pulsating), no palpation of the abdomen. Signs of separation and descent are usually seen.

A calm, warm, relaxed environment with skin-to-skin contact with the baby (NZCOM 2013, RCM 2012) should be maintained so that fear, anxiety, and tension are dissipated. If not, adrenaline levels increase which can inhibit oxytocin release and interfere with the physiological process of uterine contraction and retraction, and thus placental separation and descent (Blackburn 2008, Buckley 2004, Page 2007). Indeed, Kanikasamy (2007) advises oxytocin release is enhanced when the midwife is calm and confident and able to instill confidence. Blackburn (2008) agrees, suggesting the woman should be undisturbed to lower catecholamine levels and encourage oxytocin and prolactin release.

EMTSL can be undertaken with preterm labour; however, it is acknowledged that this may not be possible if the baby requires active resuscitation as the cord may require early clamping. However, the maternal end of the cord can be left unclamped (place the cord in a sterile receiver) to facilitate a limited amount of blood to drain from the placenta, helping to reduce its overall size. According to Lucas (2006), this helps minimize retroplacental bleeding and decreases the risk of partial separation and isoimmunization. The other principles of EMTSL are the same, but this is not as effective and may inhibit the physiological process. In the presence of haemorrhage, a uterotonic drug is required and a move to actively managing the third stage. The blood drained from the placenta should not be included in the total estimate of blood loss following delivery, being placental and not maternal blood.

Blood loss is higher with EMTSL (Begley et al 2015); however, if the woman is not compromised and the loss not severe, it may be a physiological loss which the body can cope with. Wickham (1999) suggests blood loss in the early postnatal period will be less when the third stage is managed expectantly compared with active management. However, it is important to discuss this with the woman, ideally during the antenatal period or early labour, as the midwife should change to active management if the woman begins to haemorrhage. As such, the woman should be aware of the risk of haemorrhage and consent to the change from expectant to active management in the presence of haemorrhage.

The duration of the third stage is often longer with EMTSL. Dixon et al (2009) suggest that in the absence of bleeding, it can last more than an hour without an increased risk of PPH. While the woman's condition remains stable, with no excessive bleeding, there is no cause for concern; breastfeeding can be initiated, with the added benefit of increased oxytocin release to promote uterine contraction. The RCM (2012) recommend the woman should be encouraged to adopt an upright position to shorten the duration of the third stage. NICE (2014) suggest the placenta should be delivered within 1 hour and if this does not happen, management should change to active. At this point the midwife should assess whether the placenta has separated by positioning the woman on her back and, using only fingertips, gently pressing her abdominal wall just above the pubic bone and observing the cord. If the cord does not move, Odent (1998) advises the placenta has separated.

Principles of expectant management

- The principles of standard precautions (Chapter 8) and an Aseptic Non Touch Technique (ANTT) (Chapter 10) are followed to reduce the risk of infection.
- Note the time of delivery of the baby.
- Keep the baby covered on the woman's abdomen, skin-to-skin.
- Maintain a safe, warm, private environment, taking steps to reduce any anxiety in the woman.
- The midwife can continue to wear the apron and gloves worn for delivery of the baby but the gloves should be changed prior to examining the genital tract.
- Ensure the woman's bladder is empty.

- Encourage the woman to adopt an upright position.
- Observe the general condition of the woman throughout, particularly blood loss *per vaginam*, colour, respirations (NICE 2014).
- Do not touch the cord, allowing it to stop pulsating naturally.
- Encourage and assist the woman to breastfeed when the baby is ready.
- Do not palpate the uterus unless blood loss becomes excessive.
- Place a bedpan or suitable receptacle under or next to the woman when she is ready to push the placenta out.
- When she has the urge to push, encourage the woman to deliver the placenta by her own efforts, bearing down to expel the placenta.
- Note the time the placenta and membranes are expelled.
- The cord can be clamped and cut when it has stopped pulsating, unless the woman has requested a lotus birth (Chapter 33).
- Assess the condition of the woman, noting the condition of the uterus (should be firm and central), amount of blood loss, pulse and blood pressure following completion of the third stage; the condition of the genital tract should also be determined, suturing can be undertaken when appropriate.
- Assist the woman into a comfortable position, removing any soiled linen; if all her observations are within the expected parameters, leave the woman and baby together (with her partner or labour supporter), ensuring the call bell is close at hand.
- Examine the placenta (Chapter 33) and record total blood loss.
- Dispose of the placenta and equipment correctly (if the woman is taking the placenta home, it should be double wrapped and placed in a suitable container).
- Document findings and act accordingly.

ACTIVE MANAGEMENT OF THE THIRD STAGE OF LABOUR (AMTSL)

Traditionally this involves the administration of an uterotonic drug, early cord clamping, and delivery of the placenta using controlled cord traction (CCT) (NICE 2014, RCM 2012, Westhoff et al 2013). Begley et al (2015) advise that AMTSL reduces the incidence of severe PPH (≥1000 mL), blood transfusion and additional uterotonics being required and results in a haemoglobin level that is higher by 0.5 g/dL. However, they further caution that for every 66 women who have AMTSL, the severe PPH rate reduces by one, diastolic blood pressure >90 mmHg will increase for 1:52 women, 1:65 will return to hospital with bleeding (Begley et al 2015), and one less woman out of every 28 will have a haemoglobin <9 g/dL. Sloan et al (2010) found AMTSL significantly reduced the risk of PPH but only marginally for those at the lower end of severity when compared with expectant management. When delivery of the placenta is prolonged >18 minutes, the risk of PPH is significant (Magann et al 2005); this increases further by 30 minutes with a risk six times higher than it was before 30 minutes. It is important women are advised of the risks and benefits of both active and expectant third stage management, preferably during the antenatal period so they can make an informed choice (Begley et al 2015).

Uterine massage

Uterine massage involves placing a hand on the lower abdomen to stimulate uterine contraction through the use of repetitive massaging or squeezing movements. Hofmeyr et al (2013) do not support the routine use of uterine massage following delivery of the placenta, suggesting that if a uterotonic has been administered the potential for further benefit is limited. WHO (2012) also do not recommend the use of uterine massage when oxytocin has been administered and advise there is insufficient evidence to support its use as part of routine PPH prevention when no uterotonic, or a uterotonic other than oxytocin, has been administered. However, Chen et al (2013) suggest it is often part of routine management of the third stage in under-resourced countries such as Uganda. Hofmeyr et al (2013) advise that the evidence as to whether uterine massage should be undertaken routinely where there is an increased risk of PPH and no uterotonics available is inconclusive. Furthermore, Chen et al (2013) found that while uterine massage did not reduce the amount of blood lost during the first 2 hours following the birth, it did increase the number of therapeutic uterotonics administered.

Controlled cord traction

While this is a traditional component of AMTSL, there is increasing interest into what it contributes to the process. Deneux-Tharaux et al (2013) found that across Europe the guidelines for AMTSL recommend CCT but the implementation of this is highly variable – from 12% in Hungary up to 95% in Ireland; France's guidelines do not recommend CCT, suggesting that pulling on the cord in the absence of signs of placental separation is poor practice. Their study compared undertaking CCT immediately after delivery with a contraction and awaiting signs of spontaneous separation and descent assisted by maternal effort (this was sometimes helped by fundal pressure or soft tension on the cord if needed). They found that not undertaking CCT had no significant effect on the incidence of PPH, duration of the third stage, or the need for manual removal of placenta, with women experiencing less pain, discomfort, anxiety and fatigue; it was also compatible with DCC. Consequently, Deneux-Tharaux et al (2013) suggest there is no evidence to recommend CCT as part of AMTSL to reduce the incidence of PPH. Gülmezoglu et al (2012) concur, suggesting the omission of CCT results in only a very small increased risk of severe haemorrhage. They found that for every 581 women not having CCT, only one additional woman experienced blood loss ≥1000 mL; thus, as not using CCT is safe, they propose it should not be used; rather, the focus is on the uterotonic component of AMTSL. NZCOM (2013) agree, advising CCT to be optional unless syntometrine or ergometrine has been administered. Hofmeyr et al (2015) found that while the use of CCT may reduce the risk of manual removal of placenta in certain circumstances, it had little effect on the incidence and severity of PPH. Thus they suggest it can be offered routinely only if the birth attendant is competent in its use, but they do not consider the cost of implementing training in CCT for birth attendants with little or no formal training to be worthwhile; rather, they should omit CCT from their active management package (Hofmeyr et al 2015). In further support of not undertaking CCT, Begley et al (2015) suggest that CCT can cause shreds of membrane of placenta to be retained in utero, increasing the incidence of women returning to hospital with bleeding.

If undertaking CCT, an area of debate is whether signs of separation should be seen before commencing CCT. Rogers et al (2012) suggest there is a lack of consensus within the literature regarding this. Their survey found that 72% awaited signs of placental separation – generally cord lengthening or a gush of blood; 17% did CCT immediately when the uterus was contracted and none looked for changes in the uterus (firm, rounder, higher in abdomen) (Rogers et al 2012). While traditionally AMTSL does not require signs of separation to be seen, Pena-Marti & Comunian-Carrasco (2007) recommend using CCT only after signs of separation are seen and a uterotonic drug administered. NZCOM (2013) agree signs of separation should be seen before use of CCT.

Risk factors for PPH

Active management is recommended for women with risk factors. The four Ts are commonly cited as the underlying reason for PPH occurring. The list of risk factors below (adapted from the RCOG 2009) have been grouped according to which 'T' they fit into:

Tone

- Known placenta praevia
- Multiple pregnancy

- Previous PPH
- Asian ethnicity
- Obesity (body mass index [BMI] >35)
- Prolonged labour (>12 hours)
- Age (>40 years, nulliparous)
- Large-for-gestational age baby.

Trauma

- Elective or emergency caesarean section
- Episiotomy
- Operative vaginal delivery
- Large-for-gestational age baby.

Tissue

- Retained placenta or membranes.

Thrombin

- Suspected or proven placental abruption
- Pre-eclampsia/gestational hypertension
- Pyrexia in labour.

Unclassified

- Anaemia (<9 g/dL)
- Induction of labour.

Uterotonic drugs

Uterotonic are used prophylactically for women at increased risk for PPH and during PPH to stimulate the uterus to contract. They primarily consist of oxytocin in the synthetic form of syntocinon, ergometrine, or a combination of the two (syntometrine).

Oxytocin

Oxytocin is a cyclic 9-aminoacid peptide secreted by the posterior lobe of the pituitary gland (Oladapo et al 2012). It is released into the systemic circulation during labour and suckling. Syntocinon is the synthetic form of oxytocin and is identical to it. Oxytocin binds with oxytocin receptors within the uterus, triggering calcium release from intracellular stores which leads to rhythmic contraction of smooth muscle, primarily of the upper segment of uterus, mimicking the body's own actions. Oxytocin also has a weak antidiuretic activity and water intoxication can occur with repeated administration in large volumes of electrolyte-free solutions (Oladapo et al 2012).

The usual dose of syntocinon is 5 or 10 IU. When administered intravenously (I.V.), oxytocin takes effect within 60 seconds; with intramuscular (I.M.) use, it takes around 2–4 minutes to take effect with the response lasting 30–60 minutes (Medsafe 2014a, Oladapo et al 2012). It is recommended that it is diluted in a physiological electrolyte solution if given by I.V. infusion and administered as a drip infusion or, preferably, by means of a variable-speed infusion pump over 5 minutes (Medsafe 2014a). Oxytocin has a direct relaxing effect on vascular smooth muscle, Medsafe (2014a) and Oladapo et al (2012) caution that a rapid I.V. bolus injection of oxytocin can cause acute short-lasting hypotension accompanied with flushing, reflex tachycardia, and electrocardiograph changes. These rapid haemodynamic changes may result in myocardial ischaemia, particularly in women with pre-existing cardiovascular disease. Oladapo et al (2012) suggest oxytocin should not be used if the woman has an unstable cardiovascular condition, e.g. shock, hypovolaemia, and cardiac disease. Common side effects include headache, tachycardia, bradycardia, nausea, and vomiting (Medsafe 2014a). Plasma half-life of oxytocin ranges from 3–20 minutes. Mori et al (2012) found no evidence to support the practice of injecting oxytocin diluted in normal saline directly into the umbilical vein for third stage management.

Syntocinon is usually stored at temperatures of 2–8°C. However, where this is not possible it can be stored at 30°C for three months (Medsafe 2014a), although Oladapo et al (2012) recommend the temperature should be no more than 25°C, after which time it should be discarded.

Ergometrine

Ergometrine is an amine ergot alkaloid that stimulates contraction of uterine and vascular smooth muscle as well as the cervix. Ergometrine causes sustained tonic uterine contractions of both the upper and lower uterine segments via agonist or partial agonist effects at myometrial 5-HT2 receptors and alpha-adrenergic receptors. With doses around 200 mcg, the uterine contraction is intense and usually followed by periods of relaxation; however, with larger doses, the contraction is sustained and forceful with little or no period of relaxations (Medsafe 2014b). As the amplitude and frequency of uterine contraction and tone are increased by ergometrine, uterine blood flow reduces, promoting haemostasis. Constriction of vascular smooth muscle can result in an increase in both venous and arterial blood pressure and thus should not be routinely administered to women with hypertension.

When given I.V., ergometrine takes effect almost immediately and certainly within 1 minute, with the effects lasting for 45 minutes. Medsafe (2014b) recommend use of I.V. ergometrine only in situations where there is severe uterine bleeding or other life-threatening emergency and advise it should be administered slowly, at least over 1 minute and preferably diluted to 5 mL with sodium chloride 0.9% to reduce the risk of serious adverse effects occurring. I.M. administration is also quick, with effects seen within 2–5 minutes and lasting 3 or more hours and does not need diluting.

Ergometrine should be stored at temperatures of 2–8°C and protected from light. The usual dose is 250–500 mcg. Side effects are mainly related to the effects of smooth muscle contraction and include tinnitus, headache, transient chest pain and palpitations, cramp-like pains in the back and legs, nausea and vomiting, a sharp rise in blood pressure and a decreased prolactin level (if multiple doses given).

Liabsuetrakul et al (2007) suggest ergometrine significantly reduces the mean blood loss, PPH incidence, and the need for additional uterotonics but increases blood pressure and the need for analgesia.

Syntometrine

This is composed of ergometrine 500 mcg and oxytocin 5 IU in 1 mL. It combines the effects of the two drugs; unfortunately it also combines the side effects of the two drugs. Syntometrine begins to work after 2.5 minutes and its effect lasts for several hours, so it has the advantage of working more quickly than ergometrine alone and lasts longer than oxytocin alone. It is particularly useful when I.V. administration of a uterotonic is not possible. Compared with syntocinon alone, it achieves a small but significant reduction in bleeding when the blood loss is 500–1000 mL but there is no difference between syntometrine and syntocinon when the blood loss is >1000 mL (McDonald et al 2004). There is a significant increase in the incidence of diastolic hypertension, vomiting and nausea when syntometrine is used compared with syntocinon and McDonald et al (2004) suggest the advantages of reducing the risk of a blood loss of 500–1000 mL should be measured against the risk of side effects occurring when deciding whether to use syntocinon or syntometrine.

Following the change in practice from using syntometrine to syntocinon for AMTSL, Rogers et al (2011) suggest there has been a significant increase in estimated blood loss >1000 mL at delivery which they propose may be due to improved estimation of blood loss or a lack of proficiency in the use of syntocinon. They stipulate that CCT should only be used when a contraction is present and given the cyclic nature of syntocinon as opposed to the continuous ergometrine-induced contraction, it is possible that CCT is undertaken continuously even when the uterus is not contracted which, according to Rogers et al (2011), may interfere with the control of bleeding.

Westhoff et al (2013) found syntocinon at either 5 or 10 IU was superior to ergometrine for preventing PPH >500 mL with less side effects such as nausea and vomiting and did not find any improvement when they were added together.

Route and dose

Oladapo et al (2012) found no evidence to recommend the use of I.M. over I.V. syntocinon and vice versa for a vaginal birth in relation to the benefits, risks and side effects. WHO (2012) advise using 10 IU I.V. or I.M., whereas NICE (2014) suggest 10 IU I.M. Both the RCM (2012) and NZCOM (2013) recommend the use of a uterotonic when undertaking AMTSL but do not specify the amount or the route, whereas the RCOG (2009) advise 5 or 10 IU I.M.; I.M. administration is usually quicker than a slow I.V. injection and requires less skill; thus it is preferable for birth attendants with limited clinical skills (Oladapo et al 2012).

Timing of administration

Traditionally the uterotonic had been administered initially as the head crowned and then with the delivery of the anterior shoulder. However, if the drug is administered at this time, it has serious implications for DCC and it means that a second person who is qualified to administer an injection has to be present (Soltani et al 2011). Within the American literature the uterotonic is administered following the birth of the placenta to decrease the risk of retained placenta. Soltani et al (2011) found administering oxytocin (mainly I.V.) at the delivery of the anterior shoulder or after the placental birth did not significantly influence the major clinical outcomes such as PPH or the duration of the third stage. NICE (2014) recommend the uterotonic is administered as the anterior shoulder delivers or immediately after the birth of the baby but before the cord is clamped (before 5 minutes). The RCM (2012) advise that a uterotonic is given as part of active management but do not indicate when this should be, whereas the NZCOM (2013) recommend the uterotonic should be given after the cord has been clamped and cut.

Principles of active management

- The principles of standard precautions (Chapter 8) and an ANTT (Chapter 10) are followed to reduce the risk of infection.
- Following the birth of the baby, an I.V. or I.M. uterotonic drug is administered.
- Clamp and cut the cord within 5 minutes unless contraindicated, ensuring both ends are secure and placing the maternal end in a sterile receiver, positioned close to the vulva.
- Place a sterile towel over the woman's abdomen and place the non-dominant hand over the fundus and await a contraction, keeping the hand still, during which time signs of placental separation and descent may be seen.
- To deliver the placenta:
  - either encourage the woman to birth the placenta through her own effort OR
  - when the uterus is contracted and signs of separation and descent are noted, place the non-dominant hand above the symphysis pubis, with the thumb and fingers stretched across the abdomen and palm facing inwards (Fig. 32.3) to push the uterus upwards (there is no evidence this reduces the risk of uterine inversion but it may act as a counter pressure and the movement of the placenta may be felt)

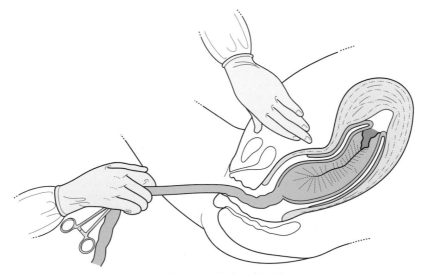

Figure 32.3 Position of hand to 'guard' the uterus during controlled cord traction.

- using the dominant hand, grasp the cord and apply steady downward traction
- controlled cord traction is accomplished more easily by keeping the hand applying traction close to the vulva. The grip should be secure by holding the artery forceps on the cord close to the vulva; as the cord lengthens, the clamp should be moved up to remain near to the vulva. Alternatively, wrap the cord around the fingers of the dominant hand, moving them nearer the vulva as necessary
- if the uterus relaxes or resistance is felt, stop, relieve the pressure from the dominant then the non-dominant hand and wait for 1 minute before attempting again, ensuring the uterus is contracted
- when the placenta appears at the vulva, traction should be applied in an upward direction to follow the curve of the birth canal
- the non-dominant hand is moved down to help ease the placenta into the receiver, allowing the membranes to be expelled slowly.

- If there is difficulty delivering the membranes, they should be 'teased out' either by moving them gently up and down (artery forceps can be positioned on the membranes to help with this) or by twisting the placenta round to make the membranes into a rope-like structure, either way encouraging the membranes to separate and be expelled.
- Observe the condition of the woman throughout, particularly any blood loss *per vaginam*.
- Note the time the placenta and membranes are expelled (often within 5–10 minutes).
- Assess the condition of the woman, noting the condition of the uterus, amount of blood loss, pulse and blood pressure following completion of the third stage; the condition of the genital tract should also be determined, suturing can be undertaken when appropriate.
- Assist the woman into a comfortable position, removing soiled sheets; if all her observations are within the expected parameters, leave the woman and her baby (skin-to-skin) together (with her partner or labour supporter), ensuring the call bell is close at hand.
- Examine the placenta (see Chapter 33) and record total blood loss.
- Dispose of the placenta and equipment correctly (if the placenta is being taken home by the woman, it should be double wrapped and placed in a suitable container).
- All swabs should be double counted and should correspond with the initial double count.
- Document findings and act accordingly.

Documentation includes completing the delivery records in detail, including the birth notification. The new family are given time together, vital sign observations are checked, as is the woman's uterus and lochial loss. Refreshments are given and baby care attended to; infant feeding should begin.

ESTIMATION OF BLOOD LOSS

Begley et al (2015) suggest many women can tolerate a blood loss of 600–750 mL, which is equivalent to a routine blood donation but acknowledge the effect of blood loss will vary considerably depending on the woman's general health state, current haemoglobin value, coagulation status and the speed of loss. Estimating blood loss is notoriously inaccurate, with estimates usually lower than the actual amount of blood lost. Underestimating blood loss will artificially 'lower' PPH rates and estimates of measures taken to prevent PPH (Sloan et al 2010). Carroli et al (2008) found the prevalence of PPH was higher in studies that measured blood loss than those that estimated it. Sloan et al (2010) suggest the recommendation for using oxytocin as the uterotonic of choice for preventing PPH has been made from the body of studies that do not distinguish between visual and measured blood loss.

Gabel & Weeber (2012) suggest measuring haematocrit as haemoglobin levels immediately after severe haemorrhage is inaccurate and women are affected differently by blood loss. Many women who are in good health with good predelivery haemoglobin levels can tolerate a 750-mL loss with little or no effect (Begley et al 2015). McDonald et al (2013) agree, suggesting healthy women are able to tolerate a blood loss up to 1000 mL without being compromised.

As early as 1967, Brant demonstrated that although blood loss up to 300 mL was accurately assessed, blood loss in excess of this was generally underestimated. Generally, as the amount of blood loss increases, the underestimation increases (Al Kadri et al 2011, Bose et al 2006, Yoong et al 2010). Al Kadri et al (2011) and Toledo et al (2007) found underestimation of blood loss was not influenced by the background or level of seniority. Bose et al (2006) assessed obstetricians', anaesthetists', midwives', nurses' and healthcare assistants' ability to assess blood loss using sanitary pads, gauze swabs, kidney dishes, inco-pads, floor spills, and a bed soaked with different amounts of blood. Anaesthetists were most accurate in their assessment but tended to overestimate blood loss, whereas all the other categories of healthcare professional seriously underestimated blood loss. In particular, Bose et al (2006) found there was significant underestimation for large floor spillages, large gauze swabs and where blood loss was over the bed and onto the floor. They developed guidelines to assist with the visual estimation of blood loss, which include looking at saturated gauze swabs (small 10 × 10 cm = 60 mL, medium 30 × 30 cm = 140 mL, large 45 × 45 cm = 350 mL), saturated sanitary pad (100 mL), floor spillages (50 cm diameter = 500 mL, 75 cm = 1000 mL, 100 cm = 1500 mL) and whether the bleeding with a PPH is restricted to the bed (unlikely to exceed 1000 mL) or spills over the bed and onto the floor (likely to exceed 1000 mL) (Bose et al 2006). Yoong et al (2010) found a tendency to overestimate small volumes of blood loss. Their participants were more accurate at 150–200 mL compared to 25 and 50 mL, suggesting that when women have frequent small losses of blood following birth, the overall accuracy of blood loss estimation will be reduced (Yoong et al 2010).

Accurate estimation of blood loss is important as it forewarns of impending haemorrhagic state (Bose et al 2006). This includes blood loss on disposable sheets and linen and collected within receivers during and after the third stage. It is important to retrieve as much blood from the sheets as possible into a container for measurement. Obvious blood loss can be measured in a jug, but when the blood has seeped onto the sheets, it becomes harder to estimate blood loss; thus these should be weighed for greater accuracy. Toledo et al (2007) found the use of drapes with calibrated markings placed under the woman to 'catch' the blood increased the accuracy of estimated loss – a 2-L blood loss was underestimated by 41% when non-calibrated drapes were used compared to 9–11% with calibrated drapes.

The measured/estimated amount of blood loss should be documented appropriately and referral should be made if this is excessive or the woman is compromised.

EXAMINATION OF THE GENITAL TRACT FOLLOWING DELIVERY

Trauma to the cervix, vagina, labia and perineum can increase blood loss; cause increased pain for the woman; and result in infection. The midwife should examine the woman's genital tract following birth to ascertain the degree of trauma and whether suturing is indicated. Stevenson (2010) recommends undertaking a digital ano-rectal examination after every vaginal birth to increase the detection of third-degree tears which may occur even when the perineum is intact. The midwife will insert her index finger into the anus and ask the woman to squeeze; the separated ends will be seen to retract backwards towards the ischiorectal fossa and a distinct gap felt anteriorly if the external anal sphincter is torn (Stevenson 2010). If the woman has an epidural she may not be able to squeeze, so Stevenson (2010) recommends inserting the index finger into the anus

and thumb into the vagina to palpate the sphincter using a 'pill-rolling' motion. She also advises the rate of detection increases if perineal trauma is examined for twice – either by two separate midwives/doctors if no suturing is required or prior to suturing (Stevenson 2010). Bruising and oedema may be evident, which can affect the examination. The area is likely to be extremely tender and the examination should be undertaken sensitively; the woman should be offered inhalational analgesia (NICE 2014). It is important there is a good light source to visualize the genital tract clearly. In many NHS Trusts, it is mandatory for two midwives or a midwife and a doctor to independently assess the genital tract.

PROCEDURE: examination of the genital tract

- The principles of standard precautions (Chapter 8) and an ANTT (Chapter 10) are followed to reduce the risk of infection.
- Explain the procedure to the woman and gain informed consent.
- The midwife continues to wear the gloves that have been used for the delivery of the placenta and membranes if they are not contaminated, otherwise a new pair of sterile gloves should be worn.
- Ask the woman to adopt an almost recumbent position, with her knees bent, ankles together and knees parted.
- Wash down the external genitalia gently with a sterile swab and warm tap water, wiping from front to back to remove any blood or debris.
- Examine the vulva, noting any trauma, particularly to the labia.
- Wrap a sterile swab around the first two fingers of the examining hand, fingers slightly parted.
- Separate the labia gently with the fingers of the non-examining hand and insert the swabbed fingers carefully into the vagina, directing the fingers in a downwards and backwards direction.
- Gently press down to examine the anterior and side walls of the vagina and cervix for trauma, replacing the gauze as necessary (if the cervix cannot be seen, the woman may need to lie flat).
- Slowly begin to remove the swabbed fingers from the vagina, examining the posterior vaginal wall.
- When the fingers have been removed, examine the perineum for trauma.
- Visually examine the anus – absence of puckering around the anterior aspect of the anus may be indicative of anal sphincter trauma.
- Undertake a rectal examination to exclude trauma to the ano-rectal mucosa and anal sphincter.

- Assist the woman into a comfortable position, remove gloves then apron, wash and dry hands, and discuss the findings.
- Suturing may be undertaken when appropriate (Chapter 34).
- Dispose of equipment appropriately.
- Document findings and act accordingly.

ROLE AND RESPONSIBILITIES OF THE MIDWIFE

These can be summarized as:
- undertaking the procedures correctly and following evidence-based and or best practice guidelines
- maintaining competency with both active and expectant management of labour
- recognizing deviations from normal, taking actions and instigating referral
- taking appropriate action to prevent and reduce the complications arising from PPH
- appropriate record keeping.

SUMMARY

- The third stage of labour is concerned with the delivery of the placenta and membranes and the control of haemorrhage.
- During this stage, the woman is at increased risk of morbidity and mortality from haemorrhage.
- The placenta and membranes may be delivered expectantly (by the woman) or actively (by the midwife).
- DCC confers many benefits for the baby and does not appear to compromise the woman.

- Active management decreases the length of the third stage and the blood loss, but is associated with increased side effects from the uterotonic drugs and retained placenta.
- Cord clamping is optional with active management but the cord should be cut within 5 minutes.
- Estimation of blood loss is often inaccurate and under-assessed; as the blood loss increases, inaccuracy also increases.
- The genital tract should be examined following delivery of the placenta and membranes for signs of trauma, including a digital rectal examination.
- All swabs used should be double counted at the end of labour care, to ensure none is retained within the woman, and documented.

SELF-ASSESSMENT EXERCISES

The answers to the following questions may be found in the text:
1. Describe how the placenta separates and descends.
2. What are the advantages for the baby of DCC?
3. What is the midwife's role when the third stage is to be expectant?
4. Identify the drugs commonly used with active management of labour and discuss their side effects.
5. How and when is CCT used?
6. How is blood loss estimated and how can accuracy be improved?
7. How does the midwife assess the genital tract for trauma following delivery of the placenta and membranes?
8. Why is it important to double count the number of swabs at the end of labour care?

REFERENCES

ACOG (American College of Obstetricians and Gynecologists), 2012. Timing of Umbilical Cord Clamping after Birth. Committee Opinion No. 543. Available online: <http://www.acog.org/Search?Keyword=delayed+cord+clamping> (accessed 3 March 2015).

Airey, R., Farrar, D., Duley, L., 2008. Timing of umbilical cord clamping: midwives views and practices. Br. J. Midwifery 16 (4), 236–239.

Al Kadri, H.M.F., Al Anazi, B.K., Tamim, H.M., 2011. Visual estimation versus gravimetric measurement of postpartum blood loss: a prospective cohort study. Arch. Gynecol. Obstet. 283, 1207–1213.

Andersson, O., Domellöf, M., Andersson, D., Hellström-Westas, L., 2013a. Effects of delayed cord clamping on neurodevelopment and infection at four months of age: a randomized trial. Acta Paediatr. 102, 525–531.

Andersson, O., Hellström-Westas, L., Andersson, D., Clausen, J., 2013b. Effects of delayed compared with early umbilical cord clamping on maternal postpartum haemorrhage and cord blood gas sampling: a randomized trial. Acta Obstet. Gynecol. Scand. 92, 567–574.

Aziz, K., Chinnery, J., Lacaze-Masmonteil, T., 2012. A single-center experience of implanting delayed cord clamping in babies born at less than 33 weeks gestational age. Adv. Neonatal Care 12 (6), 371–376.

Backes, C.H., Rivera, B.K., Haque, U., et al., 2010. Placental transfusion strategies in very preterm neonates. Obstet. Gynecol. 124 (1), 47–56.

Baenziger, O., Stolkin, F., Keel, M., et al., 2007. The influence of the timing of cord clamping on postnatal cerebral oxygenation in preterm neonates: a randomised controlled trial. Pediatrics 119 (3), 455–459.

Begley, C.M., Gyte, G.M.L., Devane, D., et al., 2015. Active versus expectant management for women in the third stage of labour. Cochrane Database Syst. Rev. (3), Art. No.:CD007412, doi:10.1002/14651858.CD007412 .pub4.

Blackburn, S., 2008. Physiological third stage of labour and birth at home. In: Edwins, J. (Ed.), Community Midwifery Practice. Blackwell, Oxford, pp. 66–86.

Blouin, B., Penny, M.E., Maheu-Giroux, M., et al., 2013. Timing of umbilical cord-clamping and infant anaemia: the role of maternal anaemia. Paediatr. Int. Child Health 33 (2), 79–85.

Bose, P., Regan, F., Paterson-Brown, S., 2006. Improving the accuracy of estimated blood loss at obstetric haemorrhage using clinical reconstructions. Br. J. Obstet. Gynaecol. 113 (8), 919–924.

Brandt, M., 1933. The mechanism and management of the third stage of labour. Am. J. Obstet. Gynecol. 23, 662–667.

Brant, H.A., 1967. Precise estimation of postpartum haemorrhage: difficulties and importance. Br. Med. J. 1, 398–400.

Buckley, S.J., 2004. Undisturbed birth – nature's hormone blueprint for safety, ease and ecstasy. MIDIRS Midwifery Digest 14 (2), 203–206.

Carroli, G., Cuesta, C., Abalos, A., Gulmezoglu, A.M., 2008. Epidemiology of postpartum haemorrhage: a systematic review. Best Pract. Res. Clin. Obstet. Gynaecol. 22 (6), 999–1012.

Cernadas, J.M.C., Carroli, G., Pellegrini, L., et al., 2006. The effect of timing on cord clamping on neonatal venous haematocrit values and clinical outcome at term: a randomized controlled trial. Pediatrics 117 (4), 779–787.

Chen, M., Chang, Q., Duan, T., et al., 2013. Uterine massage to reduce blood loss after vaginal delivery. A randomized controlled trial. Obstet. Gynecol. 122 (2), 290–295.

Cook, E.L., 2007. Delayed cord clamping or immediate cord clamping? A literature review. Br. J. Midwifery 15 (19), 562–571.

Deneux-Tharaux, C., Sentilhes, L., Maillard, F., et al., 2013. Effect of routine controlled cord traction as part of the active management of the third stage of labour on postpartum haemorrhage: multicenter randomized controlled trial (TRACOR). Br. Med. J. 346, F1541.

Dixon, L., Fletcher, L., Tracy, S., et al., 2009. Midwives care during the third stage of labour: an analysis of the New Zealand College of Midwives Midwifery Database 2004–2008. New Zealand College of Midwives 41, 20–25.

Fawole, B., Awolude, O.A., Adeniji, A.O., Onafowokan, O., 2012. WHO recommendations for the prevention of postpartum haemorrhage: RHL guideline. The WHO Reproductive Health Library; Geneva: World Health Organization. Available online: <http://apps.who.int/rhl/archives/guideline_pphprevention_fawoleb/en/> (accessed 3 March 2015).

Fry, J., 2007. Physiological third stage of labour: support it or lose it. Br. J. Midwifery 15 (11), 693–695.

Gabel, K.T., Weeber, T.A., 2012. Measuring and communicating blood loss during obstetrical haemorrhage. J. Obstet. Gynecol. Neonatal Nurs. 41, 551–558.

Ghavam, S., Batra, D., Mercer, J., et al., 2014. Effects of placental transfusion in extremely low birthweight infants: meta-analysis of long- and short-term outcomes. Transfusion 54 (4), 1192–1198.

Gülmezoglu, A.M., Lumbiganon, P., Landoulsi, S., et al., 2012. Active management of the third stage of labour with and without controlled cord traction: a randomised controlled, non-inferiority trial. Lancet 379, 1721–1727.

Harris, T., 2011. Care in the third stage of labour. In: MacDonald, S., Magill-Cuerden, J. (Eds.), Mayes' Midwifery, fourth ed. Elsevier, Edinburgh, pp. 535–550.

Herman, A., 2000. Complicated third stage of labor: time to switch on the scanner. Ultrasound Obstet. Gynecol. 15, 89–95.

Herman, A., Zimerman, A., Arieli, S., et al., 2002. Down–up sequential separation of the placenta. Ultrasound Obstet. Gynecol. 19, 278–281.

Hofmeyr, G.J., Abdel-Aleem, H., Abdel-Aleem, A., 2013. Uterine massage for preventing postpartum haemorrhage. Cochrane Database Syst. Rev. (7), Art. No.:CD006431, doi:10.1002/14651858.CD006431 .pub3.

Hofmeyr, G.J., Mshweshwe, N.T., Gülmezoglu, A.M., 2015. Controlled cord traction for the third stage of labour. Cochrane Database Syst. Rev. (1), Art. No.:CD008020, doi:10.1002/14651858.CD008020.pub2.

Kanikasamy, F., 2007. Third stage: the 'why' of physiological practice. Midwives 10 (9), 422–425.

Knight, M., Nair, M., Shah, A., et al. on behalf of the MBRRACE-UK, 2014. Maternal mortality and morbidity in the UK 2009–12: surveillance and epidemiology. In: Knight, M., Kenyon, S., Brocklehurst, P., on behalf of MBRRACE-UK, et al. (Eds.), Saving Lives, Improving Mothers' Care – Lessons learned to Inform Future Maternity Care from the UK and Ireland Confidential Enquiries into Maternal Deaths and Morbidity 2009–12. National Perinatal Epidemiology Unit, Oxford, pp. 9–26.

Krapp, M., Baschat, A.A., Hankeln, M., Gembruch, U., 2000. Greyscale and color Doppler sonography in the third stage of labor for early detection of failed placental separation. Ultrasound Obstet. Gynecol. 15 (2), 138–142.

Liabsuetrakul, T., Choobun, T., Peeyananjarassri, K., Islam, Q.M., 2007. Prophylactic use of ergot alkaloids in the third stage of labour. Cochrane Database Syst. Rev. (2), Art. No.: CD005456, doi:10.1002/14651858.CD005456.pub2.

Lucas, M., 2006. Reflections on the third stage. Pract. Midwife 9 (6), 30–31.

Magann, E.F., Evans, S., Chauhan, S.P., et al., 2005. The length of the third stage of labor and the risk of postpartum hemorrhage. Obstet. Gynecol. 105 (2), 290–293.

March, M.I., Hacker, M.R., Parson, A.W., et al., 2013. The effects of umbilical cord milking in extremely preterm infants: a randomized controlled trial. J. Perinatol. 33 (10), 763–767.

McAdams, R.M., 2014. Time to implement delayed cord clamping. Obstet. Gynecol. 123 (3), 549–552.

McDonald, S.J., Abbott, J.M., Higgins, S.P., 2004. Prophylactic ergometrine-oxytocin versus oxytocin for the third stage of labour. Cochrane Database Syst. Rev. (1) Art. No.: CD000201. doi:10.1002/14651858.CD00020 .1.pub2.

McDonald, S.J., Middleton, P., Dowswell, T., Morris, P.S., 2013. Effect of timing of umbilical cord clamping of term infants on maternal and neonatal outcomes. Cochrane Database Syst. Rev. (7), Art. No.:CD004074, doi:10.1002/ 14651858.CD004074.pub3.

Medsafe, 2014a. Syntocinon: solution for injection. Available online: <http:// www.medsafe.govt.nz/profs/ Datasheet/s/syntocinoninj.pdf> (accessed 3 March 2015).

Medsafe, 2014b. Ergometrine: solution for injection. Available online: <http://www.medsafe.govt.nz/profs/ datasheet/d/DBLErgometrineinj.pdf> (accessed 3 March 2015).

Mercer, J., Vohr, B.R., McGrath, M., et al., 2006. Delayed cord clamping in very preterm infants reduces the incidence of intraventricular hemorrhage and late-onset sepsis: a randomized controlled trial. Pediatrics 117 (4), 1235–1242.

Mercer, J.S., Vohr, B.R., Erickson-Owens, D.A., et al., 2010. Seven month developmental outcomes of very low birthweight infants enrolled in a randomized controlled trial of delayed versus immediate cord clamping. J. Perinatol. 30 (1), 11–16.

Meyer, M.P., Mildenhall, L., 2012. Delayed cord clamping and blood flow in the superior vena cava in preterm infants: an observational study. Arch. Dis. Child. Fetal Neonatal Ed. 97, F484–F486.

Moore, E.R., Anderson, G.C., Bergman, N., Dowswell, T., 2012. Early skin-to-skin contact for mothers and their healthy newborn infants. Cochrane Database Syst. Rev. (5), Art. No.: CD003519, doi:10.1002/14651858.CD003519 .pub3.

Mori, R., Nardin, J.M., Yamamoto, N., et al., 2012. Umbilical vein injection for the routine management of third stage of labour. Cochrane Database Syst. Rev. (3), Art. No.: CD006176, doi:10.1002/14651858.CD006176 .pub2.

NZCOM (New Zealand College of Midwives), 2013. Consensus Statement: Facilitating the Birth of the Placenta. Available online: <http:// www.midwife.org.nz/quality-practice/ practice-guidance/nzcom-consensus -statements/> (accessed 6 September 2014).

NICE (National Institute for Health and Care Excellence), 2014. CG190 Intrapartum care: care of healthy women and their babies during childbirth. NICE, London. Available online: <www.nice.org.uk> (accessed 3 March 2015).

Odent, M., 1998. Don't manage the third stage of labour! Pract. Midwife 11 (9), 31–33.

Oladapo, O.T., Okusanya, B.O., Abalose, E., 2012. Intramuscular versus intravenous prophylactic oxytocin for the third stage of labour. Cochrane Database Syst. Rev. (2), Art. No.: CD009332, doi:10.1002/ 14651858.CD009332.pub2.

Page, D., 2007. Breastfeeding: learning the dance of latching. J. Hum. Lact. 23 (1), 111–112.

Palethorpe, R.J., Farrar, D., Duley, L., 2010. Alternative positions for the baby at birth before clamping the umbilical cord. Cochrane Database Syst. Rev. (10), Art. No.: CD007555, doi:10.1002/14651858.CD007555 .pub2.

Patel, S., Clark, E.A.S., Rodriguez, C.E., et al., 2014. Effect of umbilical cord milking on morbidity and survival in extremely low gestational age neonates. Am. J. Obstet. Gynecol. 211 (519), e1–e7.

Pena-Marti, G.E., Comunian-Carrasco, G., 2007. Fundal pressure versus controlled cord traction as part of the active management of the third stage of labour. Cochrane Database Syst. Rev. (4), Art. No.: CD005462, doi:10 .1002/14651858.CD005462.pub2.

Rabe, H., Diaz-Rossello, J.L., Duley, L., Dowswell, T., 2012. Effect of timing of umbilical cord clamping and other strategies to influence placental transfusion at preterm birth on maternal and infant outcomes. Cochrane Database Syst. Rev. (8), Art. No.:CD003248, doi:10.1002/ 14651858.CD003248.pub3.

Raju, T.N.K., 2013. Timing of umbilical cord clamping after birth for optimizing placental transfusion. Curr. Opin. Pediatr. 25, 180–187.

RCOG (Royal College of Obstetricians and Gynaecologists), 2009. Prevention and Management of Postpartum Haemorrhage. Available online: <https://www.rcog.org.uk/ globalassets/documents/guidelines/ gt52postpartumhaemorrhage0411 .pdf> (accessed 22 February 2015).

RCM (Royal College of Midwives), 2012. Evidence Based Guidelines for Midwifery-Led Care in Labour: Third Stage of Labour. Online. Available online: <https://www.rcm.org.uk/ content/evidence-based-guidelines> (accessed 27 August 2014).

Rogers, C., Villar, R., Pisal, P., Yearley, C., 2011. Effects of syntocinon use in active management of the third stage of labour. Br. J. Midwifery 19 (6), 371–378.

Rogers, C., Harman, J., Selo-Ojeme, D., 2012. The management of the third stage of labour – A national survey of current practice. Br. J. Midwifery 20 (2), 850–857.

Scheans, P., 2013. Delayed cord clamping: a collaborative practice to improve outcomes. Neonatal Netw. 32 (5), 369–373.

Sloan, N.L., Durocher, J., Aldrich, T., et al., 2010. What measured blood loss tells us about postpartum bleeding: a systematic review. Br. J. Obstet. Gynaecol. 117 (7), 788–800.

Soltani, H., Poulose, T.A., Hutchon, D.R., 2011. Placental cord drainage after vaginal delivery as part of the management of the third stage of labour. Cochrane Database Syst. Rev. (9), Art. No.: CD004665, doi:10.1002/14651858.CD004665 .pub3.

Stevenson, L., 2010. Guideline for the systematic assessment of perineal trauma. Br. J. Midwifery 18 (8), 498–501.

Takami, T., Suganami, Y., Sunohara, D., et al., 2012. Umbilical cord milking stabilizes cerebral oxygenation and perfusion in infants born before 29 weeks of gestation. J. Pediatr. 161, 742–747.

Tarnow-Mordi, W.O., Duley, L., Field, D., et al., 2014. Timing of cord clamping in very preterm infants: more evidence is needed. Am. J. Obstet. Gynecol. 211, 118–123.

Toledo, P., McCarthy, R.J., Hewlett, B.J., et al., 2007. The accuracy of blood loss estimation after simulated vaginal delivery. Anesth. Analg. 105 (6), 1736–1740.

Tolosa, J.N., Park, D.H., Eve, D.J., et al., 2010. Mankind's first natural stem cell transplant. J. Cell. Mol. Med. 14 (3), 488–495.

Upadhyay, A., Gothwal, S., Parihar, R., et al., 2013. Effect of umbilical cord milking in term and near term infants: randomized controlled trial. Am. J. Obstet. Gynecol. 208, 120e1–120e6.

Westhoff, G., Cotter, A.M., Tolosa, J.E., 2013. Prophylactic oxytocin for the third stage of labour to prevent postpartum haemorrhage. Cochrane Database Syst. Rev. (10), Art. No.: CD001808, doi:10.1002/14651858 .CD001808.pub2.

WHO (World Health Organisation), 2012. WHO recommendations for the prevention and treatment of postpartum haemorrhage. Available online: <http://apps.who.int/ iris/bitstream/10665/75411/1 /9789241548502_eng.pdf> (accessed 3 March 2015).

WHO (World Health Organisation), 2014. Guideline: Delayed umbilical cord clamping for improved maternal and infant health and nutrition outcomes. Available online: <http:// apps.who.int/iris/bitstream/10665/ 148793/1/9789241508209_eng.pdf> (accessed 3 March 2014)

Wickham, S., 1999. Further thoughts on the third stage of labour. Pract. Midwife 2 (10), 14–15.

Winter, C., Macfarlane, A., Deneux-Tharaux, C., et al., 2007. Variations in policies for the management of the third stage of labour and the immediate management of postpartum haemorrhage in Europe. Br. J. Obstet. Gynaecol. 114, 845–854.

Yoong, W., Karavolos, S., Damadaaram, M., et al., 2010. Observer accuracy and reproducibility of visual estimation of blood loss in obstetrics: how accurate and consistent are health-care professionals? Arch. Gynecol. Obstet. 281, 207–213.

Chapter 33

Principles of intrapartum skills: examination of the placenta

LEARNING OUTCOMES

Having read this chapter, the reader should be able to:

- describe the appearance and structure of the term placenta
- describe the examination of the placenta and the significance of the information obtained
- discuss how the midwife can obtain cord blood samples
- discuss the role and responsibilities of the midwife in relation to examining the placenta.

Examination of the placenta following delivery is an important skill undertaken by the midwife to reduce the occurrence of both postpartum haemorrhage (PPH) and infection. This chapter begins with a description of the appearance and structure of the placenta, discussing the significance of deviations and the procedure for undertaking examination of the placenta, followed by a discussion around obtaining cord blood samples. It concludes with a brief discussion concerning disposal of the placenta. Obtaining blood for cord blood banking is not discussed.

APPEARANCE AND STRUCTURE

The placenta is a disc-shaped structure with different appearances to the maternal and fetal surfaces. Whilst around 90% of placentae are round-to-oval in shape, the remaining 10% have an abnormal appearance, e.g. bipartite, succenturiate lobe (Baergen 2011). Hargitai et al (2004) suggest an abnormal placental shape is associated with a placenta that underwent disturbed implantation or with a uterine abnormality. The term placenta weighs approximately 500–600 g. Ryan et al (2011) suggest the baby should weigh 7–8 times the weight of the placenta. It has a mean diameter of 22 cm and thickness of 2.5 cm (Baergen 2011). A thicker diameter may be associated with diabetes, macrosomia and hydrops, whereas a thinner placenta can be associated with intrauterine growth restriction (IUGR). The placenta will be heavier if early cord clamping is used and lighter with delayed cord clamping (DCC) due to the transfusion of blood from the placenta to the baby at delivery. A larger placenta may be associated with maternal diabetes, fetal infections and multiple pregnancy and a smaller placenta with chronic IUGR and placental insufficiency. The placenta should not have an offensive smell – this is associated with intrauterine infection.

A circumvallate placenta is a rare abnormal development of the placenta resulting in an abnormal structure and appearance. This occurs because the placenta enlarges underneath the surface of the endometrium and the embryonic sac grows above it, resulting in the endometrium between them being compressed and obliterated. This results in the formation of an acellular membrane which can affect the placental attachment to the decidua and increase the risk of placental abruption. Hargitai et al (2004) question whether a circumvallate placenta is significant but advise it may be associated with IUGR and both acute and chronic maternal haemorrhage. When examining the placenta, there will be a thick grey/white raised ring around the central part of the fetal surface which is a result of the fetal membranes folding back on themselves.

Fetal surface of the placenta

The amnion, covering the fetal surface of the placenta and the chorionic plate (a thin membrane continuous with the chorion), creates a white shiny appearance to the fetal surface of the placenta. If the baby passed meconium *in utero* it may be seen on the fetal surface. Underneath the surface layer are 50–60 lobes (cotyledons) which are further divided into 1–5 lobules. These usually present as one unified group but occasionally a placenta is divided into two (bipartite) or three (tripartite) separate, distinct lobes, each having its own section of umbilical cord inserted into it. The cord presents as one cord until it is close to the placental surface where it divides to supply each lobe (Fig. 33.1).

Inspection of the fetal surface will show arteries and veins beneath the amnion spreading outwards from the point of cord insertion with the arteries crossing over the veins. The cord is usually inserted centrally or slightly off centre (Fig. 33.2A, B). A 'battledore' or marginal insertion

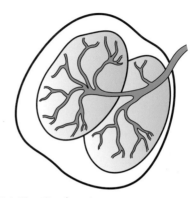

Figure 33.1 Bipartite placenta.

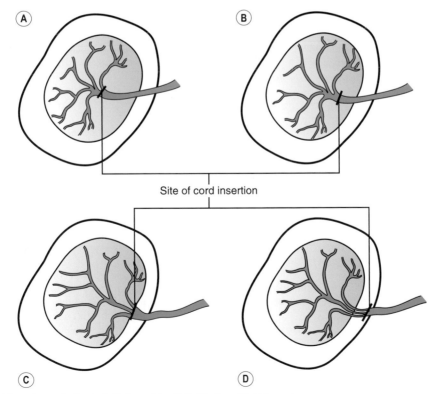

Figure 33.2 Cord insertions. **A,** Central. **B,** Eccentric. **C,** Battledore. **D,** Velamentous.

Site of cord insertion

refers to the cord that is inserted at the edge of the placenta (Fig. 33.2C); this is usually insignificant but may have a more fragile attachment, which can increase the risk of cord avulsion during controlled cord traction (CCT). Occasionally the cord is inserted into the membranes – a 'velamentous' insertion (Fig. 33.2D) – with blood vessels running from the cord through the membranes to the placental surface. In this situation the attachment of the cord can be very fragile, resulting in an increased incidence of cord avulsion during CCT. Rarely the blood vessels can lie over the cervix (vasa praevia) and have a risk of rupturing during spontaneous or artificial rupture of the membranes, resulting in massive fetal haemorrhage. A furcate cord is one that divides prior to insertion regardless of the site of insertion.

The umbilical cord

The cord contains the umbilical vein that carries oxygenated blood to the fetus and two smaller umbilical arteries that bring the deoxygenated blood from the fetus to the placenta. The blood vessels are surrounded by Wharton's jelly, which helps protect them, and are covered by the amnion. A cord with less than three vessels can be associated with a congenital abnormality and the baby should be referred to the paediatrician for review. A small portion of the cord may also be required for analysis. When examining the cord for the presence of three vessels the vein is the larger vessel with the two smaller vessels being the arteries. If the cut end of the cord has been squashed, it can be difficult to locate the vessels – cut off a small portion of the cord to make counting the vessels easier.

The average umbilical cord is 40–70 cm long, less than 40 cm is a short cord and longer than 70 cm is a long cord (Baergen 2011), although Hargitai et al (2004) suggest this should be longer than 100 cm. A short cord is usually insignificant, although if it is very short, the cord will be pulled taut as the fetus descends through the pelvis, which can lead to an abnormal fetal heart rate pattern. There is a risk of a long cord wrapping around the fetus or becoming knotted, resulting in occlusion of the vessels. There is also an increased risk of cord presentation and prolapse, particularly if the presenting part is poorly applied to the cervix, e.g. with a malposition or malpresentation. The cord is 1–2 cm wide – a thicker cord is associated with diabetes, macrosomia, and hydrops and may be difficult to secure prior to clamping, whereas a thinner cord is associated with IUGR (Baergen 2011). The cord is twisted in a spiral with one coil every 5 cm which provides some protection to the vessels from pressure and has enhanced capacity to withstand kinking, compression, and torsion. False knots may be noted in the cord and can occur when the blood vessels are longer than the cord, forming a loop in the Wharton's jelly.

The fetal membranes

Two membranes surround the fetus and form the amniotic sac – the amnion and chorion. These can appear to be fused but are not and can be separated by stripping one from the other. The amnion covers the cord and fetal surface of the placenta and is the inner lining of the amniotic sac; it is smooth, tough, and translucent. The chorion begins at the placental edge and extends around the decidua and is thick, friable, and opaque. Following delivery the membranes will have a hole in them through which the baby has been born. They should be carefully examined as a piece of membrane may be retained *in utero* and is likely to give the appearance of ragged membranes. Even a small fragment of retained membrane can result in uterine atony and PPH or be a site for microorganisms to grow, predisposing to infection. Pieces of membrane may be found in clots passed postpartum, hence the need to examine postpartum clots for the presence of membranes, particularly when the membranes were ragged.

Maternal surface of the placenta

The maternal side is composed of 15–20 cotyledons (divided by septa), which have arisen from two or more main stem villi and their branches. Fibrin deposition can occur around the villi during the second and third trimesters, resulting in isolated villi infarction. Whilst this is usually insignificant, an excessive number of infarctions can affect the exchange of nutrients and waste products between the fetal and maternal circulation resulting in IUGR. Lime salt deposition can result in small areas of calcification appearing on the surface, giving the surface a gritty feel; these are insignificant. If a cotyledon is separated from the other cotyledons, it will be seen in the membranes connected to the main part of the placenta by blood vessels – this is a 'succenturiate' lobe (Fig. 33.3). It is important to examine the membranes for unexplained

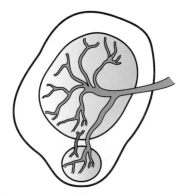

Figure 33.3 Succenturiate lobe.

holes or blood vessels in the membranes that do not connect to anything, as it is possible that the succenturiate lobe has been retained *in utero* and can predispose to uterine atony, haemorrhage, and infection. While the surface has a dark red appearance, it may appear paler if DCC or fetal haemorrhage has occurred.

PROCEDURE: examination of the placenta

- Explain the procedure to the parents and ascertain if they wish to observe the examination.
- Gather equipment:
  - non-sterile gloves and apron
  - disposable protective cover
  - disposal bag for placenta
  - placenta
  - equipment for cord blood sampling if indicated.
- Wash and dry hands, apply apron and gloves.
- Place the disposable protective cover onto a firm surface.
- Lay the placenta onto the cover fetal surface uppermost and note the size, shape, smell and colour.
- Inspect the cord, noting the length, insertion point and presence of knots.
- Count the number of vessels in the cut end of the cord.
- If cord blood is required and has not yet been obtained, the samples should be taken now (see below).
- Observe and feel the fetal surface for irregularities.
- Taking hold of the cord with the non-dominant hand, lift the placenta from the surface and examine the hole in the membranes looking to see if the membranes appear complete or ragged then replace on to the surface.
- Spread the membranes outwards, looking for extra vessel or lobes, or unexplained holes.
- Separate the amnion and chorion, pulling the amnion back over the base of the umbilical cord.
- Turn the placenta over so the maternal side is uppermost.
- Examine the cotyledons, ensuring all are present, noting the size and amount of areas of infarction or blood clots.
- Weigh or swab the placenta, if indicated.
- If the placenta is being disposed of by the hospital, dispose of it according to the hospital protocol.
- If the placenta is being taken home by the parents, securely wrap it in two plastic bags or place in an appropriate container and seal, then give it to the parents.
- Remove gloves and apron.

- Wash and dry hands.
- Discuss the findings with the parents.
- Document findings and act accordingly.

CORD BLOOD SAMPLES

The midwife may be required to obtain cord blood when the mother is Rhesus negative to ascertain the baby's blood group and Rhesus factor and determine whether or not the mother requires anti-D administration, as part of the post-mortem assessment following an intrauterine death or for cord blood gas analysis.

The sampling should be undertaken as soon as possible after birth and before the blood has clotted. For most cord blood samples the blood can be obtained from one of the cord blood vessels or from a vessel on the fetal surface of the placenta. The vein is the larger of the vessels and if only one sample is required, Armstrong & Stenson (2007) recommend using the vein, as it is easier to withdraw blood from. To prevent contamination with maternal blood, the site of sampling should be wiped with a gauze swab before obtaining the sample. For blood gas analysis, paired samples of arterial and venous blood are best taken from the cord vessels. The arterial sample reflects the fetal status whilst the venous sample reflects the maternal acid–base status and placental function.

The acid–base status of the umbilical cord blood provides an objective measurement of placental aerobic and anaerobic metabolism reflecting the fetal exposure and response to intrauterine intrapartum hypoxia (Ramin et al 2014, Wiberg et al 2008). Armstrong & Stenson (2007) suggest that with an uncomplicated labour the base excess can reduce by around 3 mmol/L overall. During a 'normal' second stage, base excess can reduce by approximately 1 mmol/L per hour but this can increase to 1 mmol/L every half hour where there are repeated fetal heart rate decelerations. Ramin et al (2014) advise that only a minority of babies with a low Apgar score are acidotic at birth and suggest depression at birth may be related to something other than prolonged intrauterine hypoxia. Wong & Maclennan (2011) agree; their study found only 13% of babies with low Apgar scores had severe metabolic acidosis and 50% had a normal pH. The risk of neonatal morbidity is inversely related to pH with a lower pH, particularly below 6.9, associated with the highest risk and with a base deficit >12 mmol/L (Ramin et al 2014, Wong & Maclennan 2011). Base deficit and pH values are higher in the vein than in the arteries. Small differences between the two may be due to impairment of the maternal perfusion of the placenta and large differences may be due to cord compression restricting umbilical blood flow (Armstrong & Stenson 2007).

Metabolism and gaseous exchange can continue within the cord and placenta following birth, which will result in different results depending on how long it takes to obtain the samples. Wiberg et al (2008) sampled cord blood at birth, 45 seconds and 90 seconds in unclamped cords and found the pH and base deficit reduced over time while the partial pressure of carbon dioxide ($PaCO_2$) and lactate levels increased. The changes were most pronounced at 45 seconds within the artery and 90 seconds within the vein. Between 45–90 seconds there was a trend towards increasing metabolic acidosis. Lynn & Beeby (2007) double clamped cords and took arterial samples at 0, 30, 60, and 90 minutes from the cord and placental surface. They found the base excess and pH values reduced significantly by 30 minutes and continued to decrease over 90 minutes (base excess ↓−4.1 at 30 minutes and −9.0 at 90 minutes, pH ↓0.05 by 30 minutes and ↓0.112 by 90 minutes). The changes in the placental surface arteries were significantly higher than the cord arterial values with changes being less predictable over time. Armstrong & Stenson (2007) agree there will be progressive changes in acid–base status in the unclamped, uncut cord, suggesting that between 60 seconds and 60 minutes the arterial and venous pH can decrease by >0.2. These changes were not found when the samples were taken from a cord that had been double clamped. They found similar changes when the vessels on the placental surface were sampled but advise the changes were larger and less predictable. Lynn & Beeby (2007) suggest the blood in the clamped section has ongoing cell metabolism but the products of metabolism cannot be removed as the blood is trapped, whereas the placental surface blood continues to be perfused until it separates, so gaseous exchange still occurs, producing different results. de Paco et al (2011), however, found no significant difference between cords clamped at birth and those clamped at 2 minutes apart except from a higher mean arterial partial pressure of oxygen (pO_2) in the delayed clamping group. When a cord blood gas analysis is required, a 10–20 cm segment of cord should be double clamped as soon as possible after birth.

Blood is collected in heparinized syringes from both vessels. The artery should be sampled first as the thicker vein provides support for the thinner arteries and from a portion of the cord that has been double clamped. To obtain the sample the cord is held by the non-dominant hand. The needle is held in the dominant hand and is inserted slowly into the vessel following a 45° angle with the bevel of the needle pointing down to reduce the risk of puncturing the posterior vessel wall. When the sample is obtained the air bubbles should be expelled by gently rolling the syringe between the fingers, as air bubbles can interfere with the results. The syringe is capped and labelled and the second venous sample is obtained in the same way. The samples should be taken to the laboratory as soon as possible, although Armstrong & Stenson (2007) advise the sample is stable at room temperature for 60 minutes.

DISPOSING OF THE PLACENTA

Within the UK the majority of women leave the placenta for the hospital to dispose of, usually by incineration (Blackburn 2008); local policy should be followed. However, the woman might want to take her placenta home. Many cultures bury the placenta on family ground; some may want to plant a tree over the top. The midwife should ascertain the wishes of the woman regarding disposing of the placenta.

The placenta and or cord are collected in some maternity units and frozen for research purposes. Histological investigation may be required in certain situations (e.g. multiple deliveries, preterm deliveries, stillbirths, suspected infection).

Beacock (2011) suggests that there has been a small revival, within both the UK and the US, of placentophagy – ingestion of the placenta. For some women this may be by ingesting the raw or cooked placenta or liquidizing it to have as a drink, but for many women it will be by encapsulation of the placenta. The placenta can be raw or cooked (usually by steaming) and is sliced and dehydrated. It is then ground and placed into capsules for easy consumption. However, the European Food Safety Authority are considering classifying human placenta as a novel food under Regulation (EC) 258/97, which would make it more difficult for encapsulation to occur. Selander et al (2013) found that woman in the US were likely to ingest the placenta for the alleged mood-enhancing benefits and unspecified health benefits. The women in their study self-reported increased mood and energy and there did not appear to be any negative effects apart from the unappealing taste or smell of the capsules.

Although not too common, some women have a lotus birth (umbilical non-severance). The cord and placenta remain attached to the baby until the cord shrivels and separates naturally (Blackburn 2008). If the woman requests a lotus birth, the midwife should leave the cord intact and if possible undertake expectant management of the third stage of labour, placing the placenta into a bowl close to the mother. Lotus Birth (2015) advocate waiting until the placental transfusion of blood to the baby is complete before handling the placenta. The placenta should be examined as normal, then washed with warm water and patted dry. Lotus Birth (2015) recommend the placenta is placed into a sieve for 24 hours to facilitate drainage, although Lotusfertility (2015) suggest keeping the placenta in an uncovered bowl close to the mother or wrapping in cloth, which is the next step advised by Lotus Birth

(2015), who also recommend placing the wrapped placenta in a placenta bag and changing the covering each day to facilitate drying. If this does not occur the placenta may develop a distinct musky smell. It is not unusual to rub the placenta with sea salt to assist with the drying process. The woman may add essential oils (e.g. lavender) with or without powdered herbs (e.g. goldenseal). The baby is fed, held, and bathed as normal and wrapped in loose clothes. Lotusfertility (2015) advise that the cord will quickly dry and shrink in diameter, usually detaching around the third day although this may be longer, up to a week, in humid indoor air conditions.

The Royal College of Obstetricians and Gynaecologists (RCOG) advised in 2008 that there was no research around lotus births and no medical evidence to demonstrate any benefit to the baby. They are concerned about the risk of infection developing within the placenta which may spread to the baby. It would seem prudent that the woman should be advised to monitor her baby for any signs of infection and seek medical help if it occurs.

ROLE AND RESPONSIBILITIES OF THE MIDWIFE

These can be summarized as:
- undertaking the examination of the placenta correctly
- recognizing the normal, identifying deviations and instigating referral
- obtaining cord blood when required
- appropriate use of personal protective equipment (PPE)
- appropriate record keeping.

SUMMARY

- The placenta has fetal and maternal components; both sides should be examined carefully.
- Examination of the placenta should be undertaken to ensure it is complete; retained products predispose to PPH and infection.
- Deviations from normal can indicate underlying problems for the baby, e.g. infection, congenital abnormality.
- PPE should always be used when handling and disposing of the placenta.
- Cord blood gases provide an accurate assessment of the acid–base status of the baby at birth.
- Women vary in how they want to dispose of their placenta and the woman's wishes should be established and facilitated.

SELF-ASSESSMENT EXERCISES

The answers to the following questions may be found in the text:
1. Describe the general appearance of the term placenta.
2. What are the differences between the fetal and maternal placental surfaces?
3. Describe the procedure for examining the placenta.
4. How would the midwife obtain cord blood for blood gas analysis?
5. What is a lotus birth?

REFERENCES

Armstrong, L., Stenson, B., 2007. Use of umbilical cord blood gas analysis in the assessment of the newborn. Arch. Dis. Child. Fetal Neonatal Ed. 92, F430–F434.

Baergen, R.N., 2011. Manual of Pathology of the Human Placenta, second ed. Springer, New York, (Ch. 3) pp. 23–42.

Beacock, M., 2011. Does eating the placenta offer postpartum health benefits? Br. J. Midwifery 20 (7), 464–469.

Blackburn, S., 2008. Physiological third stage of labour and birth at home. In:

Edwins, J. (Ed.), Community Midwifery Practice. Blackwell, Oxford, pp. 66–86.

de Paco, C.L., Florido, J., Garrido, M.C., et al., 2011. Umbilical cord blood acid-base and gas analysis after early versus delayed cord clamping in neonates at term. Arch. Gynecol. Obstet. 283 (5), 1011–1014.

Hargitai, B., Marton, T., Cox, P.M., 2004. Examination of the human placenta. J. Clin. Pathol. 57, 785–792.

Lotus Birth, 2015. Care of the Placenta. Available online: <http://www

.lotusbirth.net/index.php/care-of-the -placenta> (accessed 3 March 2015).

Lotusfertility, 2015. Common Questions About Neonatal Umbilical Integrity (Lotus Birth): A Resource. Available online: <http://www.lotusfertility .com/Lotus_Birth_Q/Lotus_Birth _QA.html> (accessed 3 March 2015).

Lynn, A., Beeby, P., 2007. Cord and placenta arterial gas analysis: the accuracy of delayed sampling. Arch. Dis. Child. Fetal Neonatal Ed. 92, F281–F285.

Ramin, S.M., Lockwood, C.J., Barss, V., 2014. Umbilical cord blood acid-base analysis. UpToDate. Available online: <www.uptodate.com> (accessed 27 July 2014).

RCOG (Royal College of Obstetricians and Gynaecologists), 2008. RCOG statement on umbilical non-severance or 'lotus birth'. RCOG, London. Available online: <www.rcog.org.uk> (accessed 3 March 2015).

Ryan, J.G., Davis, R.K., Bloch, J.R., 2011. The placenta as a research biospecimen. J. Obstet. Gynecol. Neonatal Nurs. 41 (6), 834–845.

Selander, J., Cantor, A., Young, S.M., Benyshek, D.C., 2013. Human maternal placentophagy: a survey of self-reported motivations and experiences associated with placenta consumption. Ecol. Food Nutr. 52, 93–115.

Wiberg, N., Källén, K., Olofsson, P., 2008. Delayed Umbilical Cord Clamping at Birth Has Effects on Arterial and Venous Blood Gases and Lactate Concentrations. Br. J. Obstet. Gynaecol. 115, 697–703.

Wong, L., Maclennan, A.H., 2011. Gathering the evidence: cord gases and placental histology for births with low Apgar scores. Aust. N. Z. J. Obstet. Gynaecol. 51, 17–21.

Chapter 34

Principles of intrapartum skills: perineal repair

CHAPTER CONTENTS

LEARNING OUTCOMES

Having read this chapter, the reader should be able to:
- state the aims of perineal repair
- describe the four degrees of perineal trauma
- discuss the role and responsibilities of the midwife when undertaking perineal repair
- discuss the current evidence for the choice of materials and techniques used
- describe how to infiltrate the perineum
- demonstrate tying a knot, continuous non-locked and subcuticular sutures
- list the factors that should be included with record keeping.

Approximately 85% of women who have a vaginal delivery in the UK experience some degree of perineal trauma and 60–70%, around 1000 women per day, will require suturing (Kettle et al 2012). Steen & Roberts (2011) suggest a second-degree tear is the most common spontaneous perineal injury during childbirth. Recognizing the degree of trauma and having the skills to undertake the repair is an important skill for the midwife. Perineal trauma and repair is associated with both short- and long-term problems (Beckman & Stock 2013). This chapter reviews the anatomy of the pelvic floor, the damage that may occur, the significance of correct repair, the evidence around perineal suturing, and the materials and techniques used. While care of the perineum postnatally is an important aspect of postnatal care, it is not covered within this chapter.

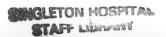

THE PELVIC FLOOR

Within the pelvis are two layers of muscles in a hammock-shaped arrangement that provide support to the pelvic organs and prevents them from prolapsing and through which the urethra, vagina, and anal canal pass (Fig. 34.1). The pelvic floor is an important component in the correct functioning of the vagina, bladder, uterus and rectum; a damaged or weakened pelvic floor may cause long-term urinary, faecal and sexual morbidity. The deep muscles provide strength to the pelvic floor and are made up of three muscles – the pubococcygeus, iliococcygeus and ischiococcygeus – collectively referred to as the levator ani muscles. The superficial muscles consist of the ischiocavernosus, bulbocavernosus and transverse perineal muscles. The perineal body is a triangular-shaped structure situated between the vagina and rectum, with its apex pointing upwards. It is composed of two superficial muscles (bulbocavernosus and transverse perineal) and one deep muscle (pubococcygeus). As the presenting part descends during the second stage, it flattens and displaces but can be damaged spontaneously during the birth of the baby or via an episiotomy.

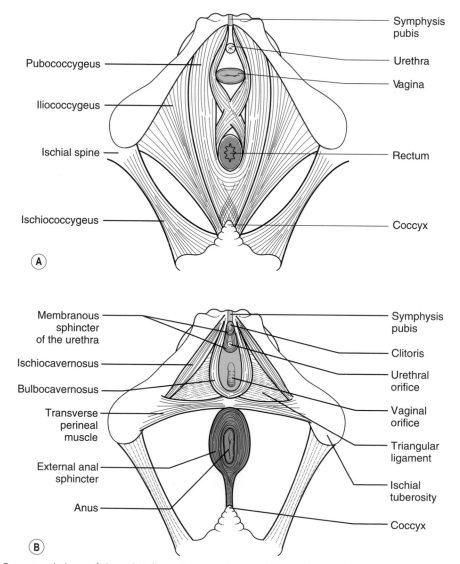

Figure 34.1 A, Deep muscle layer of the pelvic floor. **B,** Superficial muscle layer of the pelvic floor.

AIMS OF PERINEAL REPAIR

The aim of repairing the perineum is to realign the tissues into their correct anatomical position, promote healing by primary intention, and prevent haemorrhage by sealing off bleeding vessels and reducing the dead space into which bleeding can occur, causing a haematoma. Ultimately the aim is to restore the integrity of the woman's pelvic floor and maintain normal function.

PERINEAL DAMAGE

The degree of perineal trauma is classified according to which structures are involved and do not include any reference to the depth or size of the injury. The accepted definitions are:

- first-degree: only the perineal skin is torn
- second-degree (may be due to a tear or episiotomy): this affects the perineal skin, posterior vaginal wall and perineal muscles – usually superficial muscle (bulbocavernosus, transverse perineal) but occasionally deep muscle (pubococcygeus) is affected
- third-degree: this affects the same structures as a second-degree but also involves the anal sphincter and is classified further as:
  - 3a <50% of external anal sphincter torn
  - 3b >50% of external anal sphincter torn
  - 3c injury to both the external and internal anal sphincter
- fourth-degree: involving the structures with a third-degree tear and the anal sphincter complex and epithelium (NICE 2014, RCOG 2015).

Further damage may also occur to the walls of the vagina and labia while keeping the skin intact. Careful examination of the labia is required to determine if the clitoris or urethra have been damaged. Labial tears are usually described as 'grazes' or 'tears' but there is currently no accepted definition of what a labial tear or a graze is and thus this description is subjective. Jenkins (2011) suggests that labial tears are more likely to be sutured than grazes but cautions there is no evidence to support how labial trauma should be sutured.

The genital tract should be independently examined by two midwives as soon as possible post-delivery to assess the extent of perineal (and other) trauma (see p. 255) and decide whether it requires repair, by whom, in which environment and using which materials. Kettle et al (2012) emphasize the importance of skilled operators undertaking perineal repair by using the best techniques and suture materials that will result in the least amount of short- and

long-term morbidity for the woman. Extensive trauma, such as third- and fourth-degree tears, require suturing by a senior obstetrician, often in theatre under general or regional anaesthesia. Suturing by a genitourinary specialist may be indicated if the urethra has been damaged.

To prevent the labia fusing, bilateral labial grazes that would be in apposition when standing or sitting should also be sutured. Arkin & Chern-Hughes (2001) cite a case study in which the labia needed surgically parting some months following abrasions in childbirth. If the woman declines suturing of bilateral labial tears, she should be advised about the risks and encouraged to part her labia daily to reduce the likelihood of fusion.

Suturing is the most common method of perineal repair; however, there is increasing interest in the use of tissue adhesive. Adhesive is currently used widely in other areas, e.g. paediatric and ophthalmic surgery, and initially it was thought the perineum would be an unsuitable site for adhesive use due to the amount of moisture in the area. Mota et al (2009) found the use of adhesive for skin closure shortened the time taken to close the skin layer and a similar rate of complications and pain compared with subcuticular suturing. Ismail et al (2013) are undertaking a review to evaluate the different methods of perineal repair and the reader is advised to review the results when published.

To suture or not to suture?

NICE (2014) recommend that first-degree tears where the wound is not in apposition and all second-degree tears should be sutured (although if following suturing of the muscles the skin is opposed, it does not need to be sutured). However, Elharmeel et al (2011) suggest that small tears can heal well without being sutured and short-term outcomes are similar to sutured tears; long-term outcomes were not evaluated in the studies they reviewed and the sample sizes were small. They conclude there is insufficient evidence to recommend whether suturing or non-suturing is best practice and propose women should be offered information and informed choice around perineal suturing until conclusive studies are available. The Royal College of Midwives (RCM) (2008) suggest there appears to be neither benefit nor disadvantage in relation to suturing or not suturing the skin. Viswanathan et al (2005) advise it is preferable to leave both the superficial vaginal and perineal skin unsutured.

When discussing with the woman whether or not to suture, the midwife should discuss the rationale for suturing, with the advantages and disadvantages, to allow the woman to make a more informed choice. The advantages of suturing include quicker initial healing of the tissues with better wound alignment compared with not suturing (Langley et al 2006, Leeman et al 2007) and reduced urinary problems (Metcalfe et al 2006). However, suturing can be a painful procedure in itself, may require the use of lithotomy, which can be difficult for some women (e.g. those with pelvic girdle pain) and may result in increased use of analgesia (Langley et al 2006, Leeman et al 2007). Metcalfe et al (2006) found reported levels of perineal pain were similar between sutured and unsutured women.

Choice of suture material

Both non-dissolvable and dissolvable sutures have been used over the years to repair perineal trauma with the latter being more popular in recent years. Kettle et al (2010) suggest the ideal suture material should be one that causes minimal tissue reaction, be able to hold the tissues in apposition during the healing process and be absorbed once healing has occurred. While the sutures remain in the tissues, the body views them as foreign material which may cause a significant inflammatory response. If microorganisms colonize the implanted sutures or knots it can be difficult to eradicate any resulting infection which may predispose to abscess formation and wound dehiscence (Kettle et al 2010).

Catgut, made from purified collagen derived from the small intestine of cattle or sheep or from beef tendon, retains full tensile strength for 10 days. It causes an inflammatory response within the tissues causing the suture to be broken down by proteolytic enzymes and phagocytosis, although absorption times can be unpredictable, particularly in the presence of a wound infection of malnutrition (Kettle et al 2010). Subsequently, both chromic catgut (treated with chromate salts to prevent the catgut absorbing so much water, which slows down the absorption process and reduces the inflammatory reaction) and softgut (catgut impregnated with glycerol to make it remain more supple and prevent excessive drying) were introduced (Kettle et al 2010). Catgut is no longer available to the UK market, having been replaced with synthetic sutures, but is still used in non-European countries (Kettle et al 2010). Additionally, because low-cost chromic catgut is more readily available, it is likely to be continued as the preferred suture material for perineal repair in most poorly resourced settings (Peveen & Shabbir 2009).

Synthetic sutures include polyglycolic acid (e.g. Dexon), Polyglactin 910 (e.g. Vicryl) and Vicryl Rapide) and Biosyn. The polyglycolic acid suture is made of 100% glycolide and is converted into a braided suture material which is similar to Vicryl. Kettle et al (2010) advise it is designed to maintain wound support for up to 30 days and be completely absorbed by 120 days. Polyglactin 910 is a copolymer of glycolide (90%) and lactide (10%) which is derived from glycolic and lactic acids. They are also braided and coated with a copolymer of lactide, glycolide, and calcium stearate to reduce bacterial adherence and tissue drag (Kettle et al

2010). They are absorbed more quickly, by 90 days. Vicryl Rapide has the same chemical composition as Polyglactin 910 but is irradiated during the sterilization process creating a faster absorption rate of 42 days while providing wound support for 14 days (Kettle et al 2010). Biosyn is a newer monofilament product composed of glycolide (60%), dioxanone (14%) and trimethylene carbonate (26%). It provides wound support for up to 21 days and is fully absorbed between 90 and 110 days (Kettle et al 2010) although Medtronic suggest their product is fully absorbed by 56 days (Medtronic 2008). This suture has less tissue drag and less tissue reactivity and promotes better wound healing (Medtronic 2008, Kettle et al 2010).

So which is the best type of suture to use for perineal repair? Kettle et al (2010) suggest catgut increases short-term pain and wound dehiscence with an increased need to resuture compared to synthetic sutures but also advise that there is an increased need to remove synthetic sutures. For synthetic sutures, Kettle et al (2010) suggest there is little difference between Polyglactin 910 and Vicryl Rapide. Fewer sutures required removing in the first 3 months with Vicryl Rapide use but there was a slightly increased risk of superficial partial skin dehiscence causing the skin edges to gape (much less than with catgut) (Kettle et al 2010).

Wound dehiscence is associated with infection and provides a potential route for systemic infection with increased risk for septic shock. Infection causes the edges of the wound to become softened which can lead to the suture cutting out of the tissue and causing the wound to breakdown (Kettle et al 2010). Harper (2011) cites the case of a maternal death from sepsis following a second-degree tear which became infected.

Overall the fast-absorbing polyglactin sutures are currently considered to be the suture material of choice as they are associated with less perineal pain, a reduced need for analgesia, less uterine cramping at 24–48 hours and at 6–8 weeks, a significant reduction in the need for suture removal, fewer healing problems in the short term, and earlier resumption of sexual activity (Greenberg et al 2004, Leroux & Bujold 2006, Viswanathan et al 2005). Size 2/0 is indicated for perineal tissue.

Needles

Parantainen et al (2011) suggest the use of blunt needles will noticeably reduce the risk of exposure to blood and body fluids by reducing the risk of needlestick injuries and also the risk of glove perforation by 54% compared to using sharp needles. The American College of Surgeons also support the use of blunt-ended needles when suturing muscle to reduce the risk of needlestick injury (ACS 2007). However, Wilson et al (2008) found no difference in the rate of surgical glove perforation between blunt and sharp needles during perineal repair but the use of blunt needles increased the difficulty of perineal repair. Blunt needles do not penetrate the skin as easily as sharp needles and are better suited for subcutaneous wound closure (Parantainen et al 2011).

PRINCIPLES OF PERINEAL SUTURING

A successful perineal repair incorporates all of the following principles:

Effective analgesia for the woman

Pain during suturing can be greater than midwives realize for women who do not have regional analgesia (Sanders et al 2002); thus it is important to ensure effective analgesia. Where an epidural has been used effectively during labour, the infusion should be maintained if it is providing effective anaesthesia. If this does not achieve effective anaesthesia or regional analgesia has not been used, the perineum should be infiltrated using 20 mL 1% lidocaine or equivalent (NICE 2014). The use of lidocaine during childbirth by midwives in the UK does not require a Patient Group Direction as it is one of the permitted substances specified in medicines legislation under the 'Midwives Exemptions' (Department of Health 2010). Berlit et al (2013) suggest that nitrous oxide is a satisfactory and effective alternative to the use of lidocaine. Following repair, Hedayati et al (2003), Kenyon & Ford (2004) and NICE (2014) recommend a non-steroidal P.R. suppository, e.g. diclofenac 100 mg, is given (part of the Midwives Exemptions List), provided it is not contraindicated, as it is associated with reduced pain during the first 24 hours following the repair and less analgesia used within the first 48 hours.

Asepsis and standard precautions

The midwife should use a sterile suturing pack and appropriate PPE, e.g. sterile gloves, full body gown, apron and any other necessary items for infection control and protection purposes that local protocols suggest. An Aseptic Non Touch Technique (ANTT) should be used, with a Critical Aseptic Field (Chapter 10). Research into suitable fluids for perineal swabbing remains limited but water is widely used.

Swabs and sharps

All swabs and sharps opened should be counted and recorded and the count repeated after the repair is completed with an entry in the woman's notes to record they are both correct.

Alignment of the tissues to encourage granulation and healing by primary intention

Familiarity with the pelvic floor anatomy can assist with alignment of the tissues; the distinction in colour between the tissues may be helpful. For the assessment and repair it is essential to have a good light source and access to the perineum. Occasionally, further examination with the woman in lithotomy may indicate the tear is more extensive than originally thought. Decisions should be reviewed and if necessary an obstetrician is called. While the lithotomy position is still widely used in hospitals, its use is not always essential.

The woman must be comfortable and able to open her legs sufficiently. However, care must be taken to ensure that the woman's legs are not abducted excessively. Resting her legs against the lithotomy poles may be more comfortable. At home suitable alternatives can be found (e.g. sitting on the edge of the bed with legs supported on chairs). When aligned properly the process of wound healing begins (Chapter 52); sutures that are too tight or too loose may hamper this process. Tissues with a good blood supply heal rapidly. If there is tension at the wound edges, the tissue can become devascularized (Kettle et al 2010), disrupting the healing process.

Cessation of haemorrhage

This must be achieved in each part of the repair, otherwise haemorrhage can continue between the layers resulting in a haematoma or postpartum haemorrhage. When a bleeding vessel is located, it should be tied off.

Reduction of any dead space

If bleeding occurs into areas of dead space a haematoma can result; thus it is important to bring the tissues into apposition to reduce the risk of this.

Minimal amount of suture material

Foreign material in tissue can cause an inflammatory reaction which will impair healing and increase the risk of infection. Fewer knots and less suture material minimize this risk and result in improved healing.

Infiltration of the perineum for repair

Anaesthetic, usually 20 mL 1% lidocaine, is administered using an Aseptic Non Touch Technique and is infiltrated into the four aspects of the tear, along the left- and

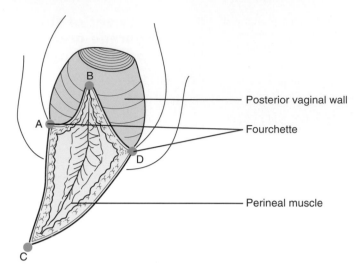

Figure 34.2 Infiltration prior to suturing.

right-hand sides of the vaginal wall and perineum. The tissue is held with tissue forceps while the needle is inserted at point A along to point B (Fig. 34.2) and the plunger withdrawn to ensure the needle has not punctured a blood vessel. If blood is seen in the syringe, withdraw the needle and recommence the procedure using a new needle, syringe, and solution (aspiration is repeated each time the position of the needle is changed). If no blood is seen, the needle is slowly withdrawn as the anaesthetic is injected along line B to A, the needle is reversed rather than removed and inserted to point C and the line C to A is infiltrated. The needle is withdrawn and inserted into point D and the process repeated B to D, C to D. Sufficient time should be allowed for the anaesthetic to work prior to commencing suturing.

Using a needle holder

The needle holder appears very similar in appearance to artery forceps; however, the grooves are designed to retain a better grip on the needle. The suture is positioned in the packet so that as the packet is torn at the right-hand side, the needle is exposed in the correct position to attach it to the needle holder without having to remove the suture from the packet. The suture is attached to the needle, the needle being appropriately shaped to reduce tissue trauma and also levelled off approximately one-third of the way along the needle to allow the needle holder to grasp it securely. The needle holder should be placed on the last third of the needle (the part closest to the thread) at right angles to the curve of the needle.

The needle holder is held by the shank with the wrist curved backwards and the needle is inserted into the tissue.

The wrist is then turned forwards to guide both the direction and depth of the needle through the tissue. The free end of the needle is secured using tissue forceps while the needle holder is removed from the needle and then reclamped on the end of the needle protruding through the tissue. With the palm facing down, the needle is pulled completely through the tissue using a flicking movement of the wrist along the curve of the needle.

Technique

Perineal repair is usually undertaken in three stages:

1. posterior vaginal wall
2. perineal muscle layer
3. perineal skin.

The use of a loose continuous suture is currently recommended for all three layers, as it results in less short-term pain than interrupted or locked sutures (Kettle et al 2012). In the past a continuous locked suture was used to repair the vaginal wall, as it was thought it would prevent shortening of the vagina by avoiding concertinaing of the vaginal wall if the continuous non-locked suture were pulled too tight; however, there is a lack of good quality evidence to support this (Kettle et al 2012) Furthermore, Kettle et al (2012) caution that stitches that are too tight can restrict the distribution of tissue oedema which can result in increased pain and advocate the use of a loose continuous suture as it enables the tension to be transferred throughout the length of the whole stitch, thereby reducing pain. Oedema can apply excessive pressure on the wound edges and capillaries, resulting in ischaemia. Consequently the wound edges necrose, resulting in a nidus for infection.

SUTURING TECHNIQUES

The basic suturing techniques described are for a right-handed midwife; a left-handed person will need to adapt these principles. Note that where there is any possible exposure to the needle, tissue forceps rather than fingers should be used to hold the tissue.

Tying a knot

The knot is tied three times, to the right with two throws, to the left (one throw) and back to the right (one throw) so that it will not slip and will lie flat:

- The needle is inserted through the tissue from the woman's left to her right side so that it is protruding through the right side (Fig. 34.3A).
- The needle holder is removed from the needle and placed on the opposite end of the needle and the needle and thread pulled through, leaving 6–8 cm of thread on the left side (Fig. 34.3B).

- Holding the needle holder in the right hand parallel to the maternal tissue, the thread is grasped on the right side between the thumb and index finger of the left hand and passed twice around the needle holder (Fig. 34.3C).
- Keeping the loops on the needle holder, open the needle holder and use it to grasp the free short end of the thread and draw/pull it through the loops (Fig. 34.3D).
- The two ends of the knot should be pulled at a 180° angle to each other to tighten the knot; encourage it to stay as flat as possible and prevent the thread pulling through to a sliding hitch (Fig. 34.3E).
- Repeat from Fig. 34.3C to Fig. 34.3E but passing the thread around the needle holder in the opposite direction once.
- Repeat again passing the thread over the needle holder once in the original direction.
- The knot ends should be cut short if this is the final knot or just the free end if suturing is to continue.

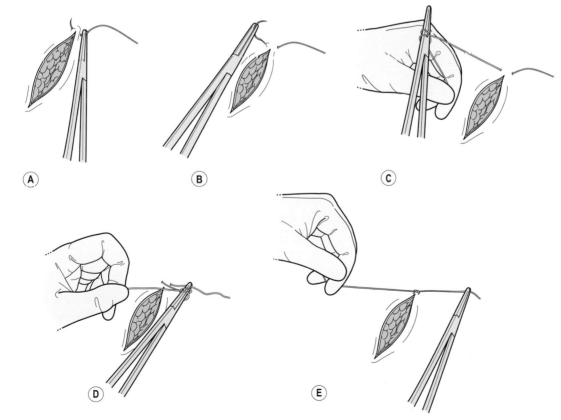

(A) (B) (C)

(D) (E)

Figure 34.3 A, B, C, D, E, Instrument-tied knot: consisting of three throws to 'lock' and prevent slippage.

If the thread is kinked or not tightened enough, the security of the knot is reduced due to breakage or slippage. Using a needle holder rather than hands to tie the knot is usually more economical on the amount of suture thread used.

Continuous non-locked suture

This is recommended for use on the posterior vaginal wall and perineal muscles. The apex of the tear is located and visualized to ensure the tear is repaired completely – inserting a lubricated tampon may assist by minimizing lochial blood loss.

- The first stitch enters the tissue above the apex and a knot tied to anchor it and the short end cut.

- The next stitch is placed below and parallel to the first one entering on the woman's left side. The left hand applies slight tension to the thread so the needle emerges below and to the far side of the thread that is held (Fig. 34.4). The needle should enter and exit at a 90° angle and traverse a vertically semi-circular course to follow the curve of the needle. It is important to visualize the needle at the trough of the wound to ensure the dead space will be closed and prevent the suture from going through the rectal mucosa. If the wound is not deep, it may be possible to enter and exit in one movement, but if it is deep, the sides may need two separate actions. The thread is pulled completely though both sides of the wound.

- Suturing is continued at approximately 1-cm intervals down the vaginal wall to the fourchette and, if

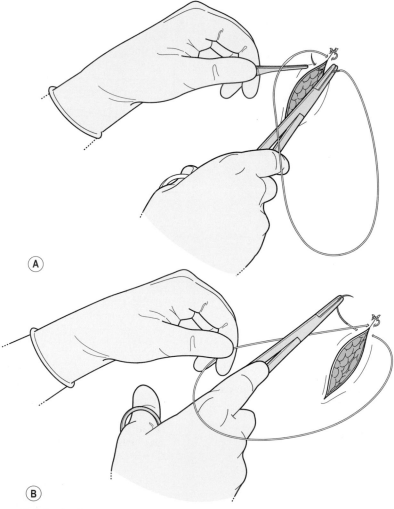

Figure 34.4 Continuous non-locked suture.

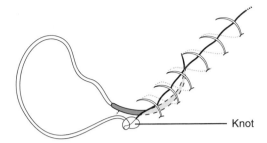

Figure 34.5 Burying a knot.

required, along the perineal muscle layer taking the same size 'bites' from each side of the wound ensuring the sutures are not pulled too tight.

- If the skin does not require suturing, the suture is tied and a loop is retained to act as the short end.
- The knot is then tied in the same way, it may be buried for comfort. Burying a knot is achieved by cutting the short end then passing the needle under the suture line to take the knot into the tissue. The long end is then cut (Fig. 34.5).

Subcuticular suture to perineal skin

A subcuticular suture is one that is just beneath the skin surface. If the perineal muscles have not been sutured or there is no thread to continue with, a new stitch is begun at the anal end with a knot tied beneath the skin. The needle is inserted deeply on the left-hand side of the tear, emerging (still on the left) superficially just below the skin and a knot tied. The needle is then reversed on the needle holder (so the point of the needle emerges in front of the needle holder). The needle is inserted superficially beneath the skin on the right-hand side of the tear, opposite the knot on the left. The needle emerges superficially (still on the right) at approximately the length of the needle and the thread pulled through. The next bite is taken along the left side of the incision, entering opposite where the last suture emerged on the right (Fig. 34.6). It is important that the bites are parallel to the skin surface, at the same depth and length to prevent an uneven vertical overlap. The process is repeated until the fourchette is reached. A loop is retained with the last suture to tie off a knot which is then buried. Both ends are cut. There should not be any suture material apparent on the outside of the perineum.

PROCEDURE: perineal repair

- Gain informed consent.
- Collect equipment and place on a cleaned dressings trolley or suitable cleaned working surface:
  - sterile repair pack (with sterile gown)
  - water/lotion/locally approved skin cleanser
  - plastic apron
  - sterile gloves
  - sterile sutures
  - 20 mL lidocaine with sterile needle (21-g green) and syringe
  - lubricant – sterile, single-use
  - diclofenac suppository (if not contraindicated)
  - alcohol handrub
  - sharps bin.
- Assist the woman into a suitable position and keep her covered. A stool should be available for the midwife to sit on and the light positioned appropriately.
- With clean hands, open the outer covering of the repair pack (an assistant can do this).
- Put on apron, wash and dry hands.
- Open the pack.
- Using an ANTT, open and place on sterile field other items required, e.g. sutures, swabs, needle, syringe, gloves, gown, diclofenac suppository, and add lotion and lubricant to bowl/gallipots (this can be done by an assistant, if present).
- If using lidocaine, open the ampoule and place within easy reach on a clean surface unless an assistant is present to open and hold the ampoule.
- Uncover the woman as necessary.
- Apply handrub.
- Put on the gown and gloves.
- Check and count the swabs, needles and instruments.
- Arrange the trolley in a way that suits.
- Draw up the anaesthetic using an ANTT – if no assistant is present, the ampoule can be held using a swab to maintain sterility.
- Cleanse the vulva using an ANTT, working from top to bottom, using each swab only once.
- Establish a sterile field beneath the woman's buttocks, over her legs and abdomen using the sterile towels and fenestrated drape.
- If required, infiltrate the perineum as described above; time is given for anaesthesia to be achieved.
- Re-examine the genital tract to establish the extent of the trauma and realign the tissues; refer if necessary.
- Insert a lubricated vaginal tampon to absorb the lochial loss so that visibility while suturing is good, attaching the tail to the sterile drapes using artery forceps.
- Locate the apex, insert the first suture just above it, and anchor with a knot.
- Complete a continuous loose non-locked suture down the vaginal wall.
- Locate the perineal muscles and suture with a continuous non-locked suture, securing with a buried knot if the skin is in good apposition (0.5 cm

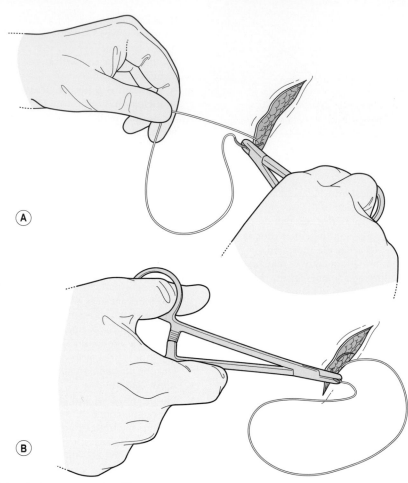

Figure 34.6 A, B, Subcuticular suture to the skin.

maximum gap). If necessary the deep and superficial muscles can be sutured in two layers.

- If the skin is not in good apposition, complete a subcuticular suture, beginning at the anal end and ending at the fourchette and burying the knot.
- Examine the vagina and perineum to establish that the tissue is in good alignment and that all bleeding has stopped.
- Remove the tampon, examine the repair gently, and insert one lubricated finger into the anus to establish the sutures have not gone through the rectal mucosa. Administer rectal analgesia if not contraindicated.
- Remove the drapes, assist the woman into a comfortable position, and cover her, placing a sanitary towel over the perineum. Advise her with regard to ongoing perineal care.
- Count the swabs, instruments and needles and dispose of sharps correctly.

- Dispose of the equipment, remove gloves and apron.
- Wash and dry hands.
- Document the repair and act accordingly.

RECORD KEEPING

The following should be included:

- time and date of the procedure
- nature and extent of the tear – a diagram can be helpful
- position of the woman, e.g. lithotomy
- amount and type of anaesthetic drugs used (also documented on the medicine administration record)
- tampon inserted and removed
- suture material used

- order of repair
- techniques used to which area
- examinations *per vaginam* and *per rectum* following the repair
- swabs, needles and instrument counted and correct
- analgesia administered following procedure (also documented on the medicine administration record)
- legible signature and name of suturing midwife
- any specific after care instructions.

ROLE AND RESPONSIBILITIES OF THE MIDWIFE

These can be summarized as:
- regular training and assessment of competency for suturing
- regular review of evidence-based practice around suturing to ensure knowledge level is up-to-date
- appropriate assessment of the wound to establish who should suture, where, with which anaesthetic/analgesia and which material
- providing the woman with evidence-based information to allow her to make an informed decision regarding suturing
- use of appropriate materials, technique, asepsis and standard precautions
- education and support of the woman before, during and following the procedure
- contemporaneous records.

SUMMARY

- The repair is a sterile procedure that uses an ANTT approach, in which the aims include alignment of the tissue, stemming haemorrhage and reduction of dead space.

- When indicated, a perineal wound should be sutured using a rapidly absorbing polyglactin suture, e.g. Vicryl Rapide, with a loose continuous unlocked suture to the posterior vaginal wall and muscle layer, bringing the skin into good apposition.
- If skin closure is indicated, a continuous subcuticular technique should be used.
- To reduce the risk of short- and long-term morbidity for the woman, perineal repair should be undertaken by a skilled operator; thus it is important the midwife is trained appropriately, updated and able to acknowledge any limitations in her ability, referring as necessary.
- Evidence-based practice should be used with regard to the materials and techniques used.

SELF-ASSESSMENT EXERCISES

The answers to the following questions may be found in the text:
1. How is perineal trauma currently classified?
2. List the aims of successful perineal repair.
3. When might a midwife ask a senior obstetrician to complete the suturing?
4. What is the current material of choice for perineal repair?
5. Describe how to successfully infiltrate the perineum prior to suturing.
6. Give a rationale for the techniques used when suturing the posterior vaginal wall and perineal muscles.
7. What technique should be used for suturing the perineal skin?
8. Summarize the role and responsibilities of the midwife in relation to perineal repair.
9. List all the aspects of the repair that should be documented.
10. Find some suitable suturing equipment and demonstrate tying a knot, continuous non-locked and subcuticular suturing.

REFERENCES

ACS (American College of Surgeons), 2007. Statement on sharps injury. Available online: <https://www.facs.org/about-acs/statements/58-sharps-safety> (accessed 3 March 2015).

Arkin, A., Chern-Hughes, B., 2001. Case report: labial fusion postpartum and clinical management of labial lacerations. J. Midwifery & Women's Health 47 (4), 290–292.

Beckman, M.M., Stock, O.M., 2013. Antenatal perineal massage for reducing perineal trauma. Cochrane Database Syst. Rev. (4), Art. No.: CD005123, doi:10.1002/14651858.CD005123.pub3.

Berlit, S., Tuschy, B., Brade, J., et al., 2013. Effectiveness of nitrous oxide for postpartum perineal repair: a randomised controlled trial. Eur. J. Obstet. Gynecol. Reprod. Biol. 170 (2), 329–332.

Department of Health, 2010. Implementation of Medicines for

Human Use (Miscellaneous Amendments) Order 2010 Midwives Exemption List. Available online: <http://www.gov.uk/government/uploads/system/uploads/attachment_data/file/213869/dh_116516.pdf> (accessed 18 December 2015).

Elharmeel, S.M.A., Chaudhary, Y., Tan, S., et al., 2011. Surgical repair of spontaneous perineal tears that occur during childbirth versus no intervention. Cochrane Database Syst. Rev. (8), Art. No.: CD008534, doi:10.1002/14651858.CD008534.pub2.

Greenberg, J.A., Lieberman, E., Cohen, A.P., Ecker, J.L., 2004. Randomized comparison of chromic versus fast absorbing polyglactin 910 for postpartum perineal repair. Obstet. Gynaecol. 103 (6), 1308–1313.

Harper, A., 2011. Sepsis. In: Centre for Maternal and Child Enquiries (CMACE). Saving Mothers' Lives: reviewing maternal deaths to make motherhood safer: 2006–08. The Eighth Report on Confidential Enquiries into Maternal Deaths in the United Kingdom. Br. J. Obstet. Gynaecol. 118 (Suppl. 1), 85–96.

Hedayati, H., Parsons, J., Crowther, C.A., 2003. Rectal analgesia for pain from perineal trauma following childbirth. Cochrane Database Syst. Rev. 2003 (3), Art.No.: CD003931, doi:10.1002/14651858.CD003931.

Ismail, K.M.K., Israfilbayli, F., Toozs-Hobson, P., Kettle, C., 2013. Suturing versus alternative closure techniques for repair of episiotomy or second degree perineal tears. Cochrane Database Syst. Rev. (4), Art. No.: CD010486, doi:10.1002/14651858.CD010486.

Jenkins, E., 2011. Suturing of labial trauma: an audit of current practice. Br. J. Midwifery 19 (11), 699–705.

Kenyon, S., Ford, F., 2004. How can we improve women's postbirth perineal health? MIDIRS Midwifery Dig. 14 (1), 7–12.

Kettle, C., Dowswell, T., Ismail, K.M.K., 2010. Absorbable suture materials for repair of episiotomy and second degree tears. Cochrane Database Syst. Rev. (6), Art. No.: CD000006, doi:10.1002/14651858.CD000006.pub2.

Kettle, C., Dowswell, T., Ismail, K.M.K., 2012. Continuous and interrupted suturing techniques for repair of episiotomy or second degree tears. Cochrane Database Syst. Rev. (11), Art. No.: CD000947, doi:10.1002/14651858.CD000947.pub3.

Langley, V., Thoburn, A., Shaw, S., Barton, A., 2006. Second degree tears: to suture or not? A randomized controlled trial. Br. J. Midwifery 14 (9), 550–554.

Leeman, L.M., Rogers, R.G., Greulich, B., Allbers, L.L., 2007. Do un-sutured second degree perineal lacerations affect postpartum functional outcomes? J. Am. Board Fam. Med. 20 (5), 451–457.

Leroux, N., Bujold, E., 2006. Impact of chromic catgut versus polyglactin 910 versus fast-absorbing polyglactin 910 sutures for perineal repair: a randomized controlled trial. Am. J. Obstet. Gynaecol. 194 (6), 1585–1590.

Medtronic, 2008. Caprosyn monofilament synthetic absorbable suture fact sheet. Available online: <http://www.medtronic.com/content/dam/covidien/library/global/english/product/wound-closure/absorbable-sutures/caprosyn-absorbable-suture-fact-sheet.pdf> (accessed 18 December 2015).

Metcalfe, A., Bick, D., Tohill, S., et al., 2006. A prospective cohort study of repair and non-repair of second degree perineal trauma: results and issues for future research. Evid. Based Midwifery 4 (2), 60–64.

Mota, R., Costa, E., Amaral, A., et al., 2009. Skin adhesive versus subcuticular suture for perineal skin repair after episiotomy – a randomized controlled trial. Acta

Obstet. et Gynecol. Scand. 88 (6), 660–666.

NICE (National Institute for Health and Care Excellence), 2014. Intrapartum care. Care of healthy women and their babies during childbirth Clinical Guideline 55. Available online: <www.nice.org.uk> (accessed 3 March 2015).

Parantainen, A., Verbek, J.H., Lavoie, M.C., Pahwa, M., 2011. Blunt versus sharp suture needles for preventing percutaneous exposure incidents in surgical staff. Cochrane Database Syst. Rev. (11), Art. No.: CD009170, doi:10.1002/14651858.CD009170.pub2.

Peveen, F., Shabbir, T., 2009. Perineal repair: comparison of suture materials and suturing. Tech. J. Surg. Pak. (Int.) 14 (1), 23–28.

RCM (Royal College of Midwives), 2008. Suturing the Perineum. Midwifery Practice Guidelines. Royal College of Midwives, London.

RCOG (Royal College of Obstetricians and Gynaecologists), 2015. Third- and Fourth-degree Perineal Tears, Management (Green-top 29). Available online: <www.rcog.org.uk> (accessed 29 August 2015).

Sanders, J., Campbell, R., Peters, T., 2002. Effectiveness of pain relief during perineal suturing. Br. J. Obstet. Gynaecol. 109, 1066–1068.

Steen, M., Roberts, T., 2011. The consequences of pregnancy and birth for the pelvic floor. Br. J. Midwifery 19 (11), 692–698.

Viswanathan, M., Hartmann, K., Palmieri, R., et al., 2005. The use of episiotomy in obstetrical care: A systematic review. Agency for Healthcare Research and Quality. Available online: <http://www.ncbi.nlm.nih.gov/books/NBK11967/> (accessed 3 March 2015).

Wilson, L.K., Sullivan, S., Goodnight, W., et al., 2008. The use of blunt needles does not reduce glove perforations during obstetrical laceration repair. Am. J. Obstet. Gynecol. 199 (6), 1097–6868.

Chapter 35

Principles of intrapartum skills: management of birth at home

LEARNING OUTCOMES

Having read this chapter, the reader should be able to:

- discuss some of the evidence that relates to safety when delivering at home
- discuss the differences in skills and attitudes that the midwife utilizes when managing birth at home
- discuss the value and principles of good preparation for all the parties concerned
- list the equipment and information that the midwife needs available
- discuss the overall role and responsibilities of the midwife when caring for labouring women at home
- discuss the initial assessment necessary if attending a birth that has already happened without medical assistance (BBA, born before arrival).

This chapter focuses on the midwife's role and management of labour and delivery in the home setting. It highlights the considerations for care at home that are different from care in hospital; the reader may find it helpful to refer to other relevant chapters (e.g. Chapters 31, 32, and 33). Safe homebirth is very much a team effort, the woman and her family are at the centre of the care, but it can only be facilitated with midwifery skills, the communication and planning of obstetric services as a whole, effective working with the ambulance service and in some instances active involvement of the general practitioner (GP). Some women will prefer to give birth in a hospital setting; this is as much their choice as home is for other women.

INCIDENCE

Homebirth is surrounded internationally by lots of debate and 'politics' within the different professional groups (Dahlen 2012, McNutt et al 2013). In 2012 in England and Wales, 2.3% of births took place at home (ONS 2012). There is however, considerable regional variation with rates of nearly 10% for some areas (BirthChoiceUK 2011), and individualized midwifery providers managing much higher rates (e.g. Collins & Kingdon 2014, 31%).

SAFETY

Safety is always the uppermost in everyone's mind. The Birthplace Study (BIECG 2011) examined the outcomes for 65 000 low-risk women in the UK between 2007 and 2010. Its findings cannot be ignored: birth is generally very safe, for multiparous women home birth is safe also, but for primiparous women a planned home birth increases the risk for the baby. This blanket statement covers the statistic that for 1000 planned primiparous homebirths there were 9.3 adverse perinatal outcomes. These were classified as birth-related injuries, stillbirth, early neonatal death, encephalopathy, and meconium aspiration syndrome. This compared to 5.3 per 1000 in obstetric units. However, while the aim of care is to achieve 0 per 1000 births (highly unrealistic), 9.3 per 1000 births remains a low figure, i.e. 0.93%. Supporters of home birth would argue that birthing at home also offers so much in the qualitative experience for women who choose it, as well as safety (Dahlen 2012). The joint RCOG/RCM work indicated lower intervention rates and higher maternal satisfaction when birthing at home compared to hospital (RCOG/RCM 2007). NICE (2014) are clear in their updated labour guideline that four birth venues are open to all women: adjoining and free-standing midwifery-led units, home and obstetric units. Women should be given the information to decide which is right for them.

The distinction is made here between planned births at home (often with low risk factors) and unexpected (for whatever reason) delivery at home.

While NICE (2014) are clear that women should be given a choice about where to give birth, they also propose medical and obstetric conditions that would affect the choice of birthing venue. It is generally considered that low-risk women can be booked for home birth, whilst those with the risk factors listed in Box 35.1 should either be booked for, or individually reviewed for, obstetric unit care. Primiparity is not included in the list; this continues to suggest that the real risk is low.

If women are encouraged to book for the venue of their choice, midwives should be alert to the women for whom home is chosen, but for whom risk factors are present. NICE (2014) identify that midwives should not disclose their personal views about the woman's choice. In the UK, Supervisors of Midwives work to support all women in their choices and to support all midwives as they care for all women. Supervisors help midwives to maintain a high standard of clinical practice; if the midwife feels less than confident with regard to any aspect of home birth or caring for a particular woman at home, the Supervisor of Midwives is able to facilitate appropriate professional development.

> ## Box 35.1 Risk factors suggesting planned birth at obstetric unit
>
> - Medical disorders: cardiac disease, hypertension, asthma that requires additional treatment, cystic fibrosis, haemoglobinopathy disease, thromboembolic disease or history, platelet disorders, atypical antibodies, infections: group B streptococcus (antibiotics in labour), HIV, hepatitis B and C, active toxoplasmosis, chicken pox, rubella, genital herpes, tuberculosis. Immune, endocrine and renal disorders, abnormal liver function tests, epilepsy or previous cerebrovascular accident, psychiatric disorder requiring current inpatient care, myomectomy/hysterotomy
> - Pregnancy/labour related issues: pre-eclampsia/eclampsia (now or previously), placenta praevia, small for gestational age, fetal death, confirmed polyhydramnios/oligohydramnios, abnormal fetal heart rate/Doppler studies, multiple birth, malpresentation, antepartum haemorrhage, substance misuse, preterm labour or rupture of membranes, Hb <8.5 g/dL, body mass index (BMI) >35 kg/m^2 at booking, induction of labour (IOL), gestational diabetes
> - Other factors warranting individual assessment: haemoglobinopathy traits, Hb 8.5–10.5 g/dL, spinal abnormalities, previous fractured pelvis, history of previous baby >4.5 kg, history of extensive perineal trauma, >35 years, parity 4 or more, cone biopsy or fibroids, some cardiovascular, endocrinal, gastrointestinal and immune disorders
>
> Adapted and summarized from NICE (2014)

If the midwife feels concerned at the woman's choice, various steps can be taken:

- Within a good relationship, verbal and written information are given regarding possible risks, how they might be managed, where, when and method and time taken for transfer if necessary.
- Working and planning with a Supervisor of Midwives and the local obstetric unit so that realistic plans are in place for care at home and if transferred in, at the unit.
- Collaborative working with the local ambulance service so that they are aware of the situation and have a care plan in place.
- Additional midwifery team members who also get to know the woman and are updated clinically with their own skills and knowledge of the woman's situation. Likely attendance of two midwives to the delivery with direct support from a Supervisor of Midwives.

- Detailed written care plan that the woman can contribute to and sign if she wishes.
- Regular review of the plans as the pregnancy progresses.

For all women, there should be ongoing assessment throughout the pregnancy and labour to ensure that the booked place of birth is appropriate.

MIDWIFERY SKILLS

There are many articles of opinion that share highly positive experiences for midwives and their practice as well as the women and families in their care (Collins & Kingdon 2014, Cook 2003, Dahlen 2012, Jones 2003, Kitzinger 2001). While many midwives may have limited experiences of home birth, those that do often regard it as a professionally enhancing experience. Some additional skills are helpful:

- Needing a full understanding and confidence in labour physiology and a woman's ability to give birth naturally. Gwillim & Charles (2013) suggest there is a danger of providing a hospital birth at home for those midwives who are not truly confident in home birth. Floyd (1995) suggests that a woman has greater 'success' if the midwife has a positive attitude, confidence, competence and willingness.
- Fundamental midwifery skills using limited equipment, e.g. Pinard stethoscope or fetal Doppler 'sonicaid' use rather than cardiotocography monitor, delivery in alternative positions, management of pain with limited availability of pharmacological preparations.
- 'Active inactivity': women who have planned their birth at home often assume a greater level of control. A midwife may feel a little superfluous but has, in fact, to remain 'with woman', to keep alert, being active in, for example, observing for signs of the labour progressing, while appearing to be relatively inactive. As a guest in the woman's home the midwife is obliged to be relaxed, tactful, blending in to the circumstances and events, while still exercising the full range of professional labour care and support. Mood and temperament of the environment affect the finely tuned hormonal interplays that are needed physiologically for labour (Russell 2008). Odent (1996) describes the midwife's role as watching, waiting, and trusting the woman's own ability to give birth. Dahlen (2012) takes her knitting! She recognizes that this helps the woman to know that the midwife feels that all is well, while as a midwife she tunes in to the woman's verbal cues better.

- Flexibility and adaptability are required, e.g. continuing to maintain standard precautions, following aseptic guidelines, or maintaining health and safety protocols while working in an unfamiliar environment. Midwives also find that their decision-making skills and professional autonomy are increased.
- Management of unexpected situations or emergencies for mothers or babies when assistance may be some miles or minutes away. As mentioned earlier, the midwife should maintain all skills, particularly the emergency drills that include resuscitation, management of haemorrhage, shoulder dystocia, and breech delivery. In the home setting these situations may have to be managed *alone* (Magill-Curden 2012).

PREPARATION

Good preparation is necessary for several agencies involved.

Maternity services

Each service, whether NHS or independent, needs to have considered home birth provision within its service as a whole, including the training and updating of midwives, budgetary provision for items such as mobile phones and birthing equipment, and issues such as midwife availability, referral, and transport systems. It is likely that risk management assessments are made frequently in relation to the service. Provision should be made for women who fall outside of the low-risk criteria but continue to choose the home birth option as discussed above. Protocols should include whether midwives are expected, for example, to site intravenous cannulae in an emergency.

The midwife

It can be helpful if the midwife knows the geography and socioeconomic demography of the area. This can highlight potential risk factors to personal safety, e.g. whether aspects of the Lone Worker Protocol need activating, whether the location is very remote and difficult to find, whether Satnav is correct. Equally, good working relationships with others in the healthcare team can make the management of problems smoother and enhance the communication that facilitates the woman's care. Knowing which second midwife to call and how to access the Supervisor of Midwives is essential information which should be easily to hand. The Royal College of Midwives (RCM 2002) rightly point out that midwives are fully equipped to manage normal birth; the essence is to manage it confidently at home with good judgements and actions.

Equipment

Equipment (Box 35.2) should be stored, used, serviced, cleaned, and restocked correctly. The midwife should be confident about its location and use, keeping items together (e.g. equipment for primary postpartum haemorrhage (PPH) management or resuscitation) means that they are readily accessible and easily moved around the home with

---

Box 35.2 Equipment suggested for managing labour and birth at home

- Antenatal equipment including Pinard stethoscope and/or fetal Doppler (waterproof) and gel, relevant spare batteries, sphygmomanometer, thermometer, venepuncture equipment, sharps box, swabs and medium, reagent sticks, blood and MSU (midstream specimen of urine) bottles, pen torch, scissors, tape measure, gloves (sterile and non-sterile), documentation such as continuation sheets, blood forms
- Labour equipment including sterile delivery, vaginal examination (VE) and suturing packs, aprons and other personal protective equipment, urinary catheters (residual and Foleys and bag), amnihook, speculum and lubricating gel, cannulation equipment, fluids and giving sets, suturing materials, torch (waterproof if possible), incontinence pads, drugs (see below), suppositories, container for placenta, rubbish bags, water thermometer, documentation for labour care including birth notification, baby ID bands and emergency management cards; mobile phone and charger.
- Drugs: According to Midwives Exemptions and locally agreed PGDs (Chapter 18): uterotonics (Syntometrine, Syntocinon [third-stage and PPH], ergometrine), lidocaine 1% for suturing, pethidine (but often supplied by the GP), naloxone, vitamin K, Entonox, oxygen, intravenous fluids: crystalloid and colloid.
- Resuscitation equipment for woman and baby including oxygen (with tubings, airways, bags and masks), suction with neonatal and maternal suckers, stethoscope, stop watch, towels, heat source, and possibly endotracheal tubes and laryngoscope depending on local protocol, blood glucose sticks, and lancets. Resuscitation Council UK (2011) has a detailed list – see the list of References for website address.
- Postnatal equipment including weighing scales, equipment for neonatal examination and documentation such as neonatal examination forms, child health record, postnatal exercises and advice, transfer of care documentation, cord clamp cutter, stitch cutter, baby labels, vitamin K.

(Adapted from RCM 2003, Dahlen 2012 & Gwillim & Charles 2013)

the woman. Access to the required drugs will be according to the locally agreed protocol and NMC standards (NMC 2007). They too should be stored correctly, in date and restocked appropriately. Pethidine is usually supplied to the woman personally via her GP (Chapter 18).

Usually by 36 weeks' gestation the midwife will have spent time at the woman's home. This allows for discussion of the practicalities including finding it in the dark. Who else will be present? Is there a mobile phone signal? Where does the woman anticipate giving birth? Will there be children or animals present? What will the plan be if transfer is needed?

It is likely that some of the equipment will be stored in the woman's home, locally agreed arrangements allow for organization of the later items, e.g. drugs. The midwife will need to supply her own food and drinks.

The woman and her family

For a planned home birth the woman is likely to be well prepared. The RCM (2003) recommend obtaining items such as plastic sheeting, towels, rubbish bags, light foods and drinks, alternative sources of heating and lighting, massaging equipment, appropriate clothing for mother and baby, pillows, pethidine, and drinking straws (Dahlen 2012), among other things. Gwillim (2009) recommends a birthing surface covering of 1×1.25 m, this being polythene covered with layers of newspaper and an old sheet, all of which is glued into place and can be disposed of afterwards. Family poverty should not be a hindrance to home birth, and as such the maternity provider may need to assist in obtaining some of the items needed. The woman should be fully aware of how and when to get hold of the midwife and the signs of labour. Family and supporting partners should also have the opportunity to ask their questions and to be reassured.

PRINCIPLES OF MANAGING BIRTH AT HOME

- Knowing how the midwife will be notified and whether there is a requirement to notify anyone else of the call out, e.g. labour ward or second midwife.
- Assessment on arrival: is labour progressing? Can the midwife leave and return later at a given time or rest in another room for a while? Is a second midwife needed for an imminent birth? This assessment should also include a history of the labour so far, with all assessments being recorded in the woman's records. Fetal and maternal wellbeing need to be established, abdominal examination is necessary;

vaginal assessment is undertaken according to the clinical indicators and the woman's wishes.

- Opportunity to establish a working area: space for equipment and resuscitation (portable, if possible), table for writing records, opportunity to inform the second midwife of the likely schedule (if not already contacted).

- Ongoing labour care: as for any labouring woman, including all assessments for labour progress, fetal and maternal wellbeing. It is likely that the woman will naturally be mobile and utilize the furniture and supporters around her for comfort and pain relief. She may also take regular baths or showers, eat and drink as she feels appropriate, pass urine as needed and use other techniques, e.g. the ironing, to help and distract. As labour progresses, the midwife is more likely to observe the 'in on self' effect as the woman has less conversation and a greater level of concentration. The midwife will utilize the 'active inactivity' described above and is likely to begin intuitively to understand how the woman is progressing. If water labour or birth is planned, the reader is encouraged to read Chapter 36.

- Second stage of labour: physiological pushing is likely to be aided using the furniture, etc. available; the midwife remains vigilant as to signs of second stage onset, fetal and maternal wellbeing and indicators of progress (see Chapter 31 for greater detail). The second midwife should ideally be called if not already present. Dahlen (2012) advocates the presence of a second midwife and Collins & Kingdon (2014) indicate that their midwives always work in pairs. The midwife should be mindful of her own care, e.g. back strain, when needing to adapt to the woman's position. This is also true of hospital births but in the home sofas, beds, etc. are at an immovable height, often low. A hot water bottle, tumble drier, or radiator can be used to warm up the towels prior to the baby's arrival (ensure the hot water bottle is removed before using the towels).

- Third stage of labour: many women may opt for expectant management at home; this requires that the midwife understands the physiology and is competent to undertake its management (see Chapter 32). The placenta remains the woman's property; however, often the midwife removes it from the home in a suitable container and disposes of it as for hospital births. If the woman wishes to keep it, she should be encouraged to bury it deeply in the garden or seek advice from the Environmental Health Department. The midwife will need to improvise to examine the genital tract with sufficient light and visibility; if suturing is required, chairs may be needed to support her legs and something firm may be needed beneath

the woman's buttocks. All equipment is dealt with as for hospital births and returned to the hospital.

- Care of the newborn: there is little difference in the care of the newborn at home. If resuscitation is required, the decision to call help is made swiftly and the midwife follows the Resuscitation Council guidelines (Chapter 56). Skin-to-skin care would be carried out as for any other birth, with early breastfeeding encouraged as the feeding cues are seen. Provision is made in the next 24–48 hours for a qualified person to undertake the neonatal examination.

- Transfer to hospital: the midwife must have referral systems and numbers in place; often referral is to the nearest consultant delivery suite or to a consultant obstetrician directly. Advice may also be sought from the Supervisor of Midwives and calls may be made directly to ambulance control on agreed numbers. Transfer to hospital is made using an ambulance (often paramedic) in the event of an emergency, a non-urgent transfer may be made using the woman's own transport, but this may depend upon local protocols. GPs are often, by agreement, bypassed in such circumstances. The woman may find referral very hard and it is appropriate to discuss the likely criteria with her in advance as well as at the time. Building a relationship, and therefore trust, with the woman antenatally is likely to make transfer a little easier for her. If an emergency transfer, it can be helpful to have a card written out (filling in the details at the last minute) that a member of the family can read from when speaking to ambulance control. Leaving the front door open and a light on can save valuable time. If a paramedic attends, the midwife should be aware that the woman is still the midwife's 'case' and that full responsibility remains with the midwife, not the paramedic.

- Documentation: this is as thorough as for any hospital birth, including all discussions, referrals and actions. Partograms, birth notifications, etc. may all be left in the woman's home in advance. The parts of the records that require computerization will be undertaken by the midwife as locally agreed.

- Other practitioners: occasionally women may bring in their own assistants such as aromatherapists. The midwife should ensure that, as the professional responsible, the woman and practitioner have sensible working limits and that if for any reason the midwife needs the therapy to stop, this is understood.

- Leaving after the birth: the midwife generally leaves when:
  - the mother's vital sign observations have been undertaken and are confirmed within normal limits

- the mother's uterus is well contracted with the expected lochial loss. Any suturing has been completed, pain relief administered, a shower may have been taken, and most probably the woman has passed urine
- the baby has been fed, has a temperature within normal limits, and has made an uncomplicated adaptation to extrauterine life. The parents are asked to note that urine and meconium are passed within the next 24 hours
- the family have been supplied with appropriate telephone numbers to call at any time with clear indications of which issues should be discussed, e.g. failure to pass urine within 6 hours, increasing pain, signs of haemorrhage or clots *per vaginam*, any baby feeding difficulties, any changes in the baby's colour (pallor/cyanosis) or tone, or any other concerns that they may have
- a time has been agreed for the next call, often later the same day or the following morning
- the midwife is confident that all is well, has completed the records, and has cleared away all necessary equipment.

It is likely that more than 1 hour has passed since the birth; 1 hour would be the minimum time that the midwife would need to be with the woman and baby.

- Communicating when there are difficulties: occasionally women choose options that the midwife feels less comfortable about, for example, poor lighting from candles only. Good preparation, continuity of care and opportunities to build a good trusting relationship with the woman in advance will smooth the management of such issues.
- Self-appraisal and audit: clinical governance ensures that the service is effective via audit, but this also aids midwives to appreciate the quality of their care and to review any areas that can be improved. Self-appraisal will help less experienced midwives to develop confidence in home birth management, along with the support of a Supervisor of Midwives.

BORN BEFORE ARRIVAL (BBA)

When unplanned births occur at home, the midwife may be called after the ambulance service. It is necessary to make some swift assessments:

- Baby: Does it need resuscitating? Is it cold? What is its gestation? Where was it born? (sometimes into the toilet). Has it been fed?
- Mother: Was it a precipitate labour? Placenta in or out? Bleeding? State of perineum? Blood group? Vital signs?

Unexpected births at home (or other locations) can cause mothers, babies, and other family members to feel a little stunned. Labour has often been rapid and there may be the danger of haemorrhage. The baby may be hypothermic and very likely the placenta is still *in situ*. The midwife should manage the prioritizing issues quickly and effectively before deciding whether transfer to hospital is necessary. This decision is made in conjunction with the woman and her family, particularly if staying at home is a possible option. The midwife takes the time to thoroughly establish that all is well before leaving this client. Records are completed as for any other birth, it is also likely that some form of audit/reporting system is undertaken.

ROLE AND RESPONSIBILITIES OF THE MIDWIFE

These can be summarized as:
- effective collaboration during pregnancy with the woman and other relevant agencies, to plan for a safe and relaxed home birth
- professional, thorough labour care planned and undertaken in an unfamiliar environment but according to all rules and protocols that govern safe and effective practice
- recognizing deviations from the norm, managing them appropriately, and instigating referral
- contemporaneous and thorough record keeping.

SUMMARY

- Providing labour care at home for healthy women with a planned home birth can be a highly satisfying experience for the midwife and the family.
- A range of new and existing skills are utilized; maintenance of skills such as resuscitation and emergency drills is essential.
- Preparation, by all parties involved, contributes to the safety and delivery of care. This includes issues such as drugs, equipment, accessibility to other healthcare professionals and referral systems.
- Many aspects of home care mirror hospital care but the midwife often needs to utilize her professional autonomy to the full. This is particularly the case when the unexpected occurs or the woman is outside of the low-risk criteria.
- Care should be taken to protect the midwife's personal safety.

SELF-ASSESSMENT EXERCISES

The answers to the following questions may be found in the text:

1. Compile a low-risk criteria to identify women suitable for home birth.
2. Discuss the skills needed by the midwife to undertake safe home births.
3. List the items needed for a home birth.
4. Summarize the differences between caring for a labouring woman at home and caring for one in hospital.
5. To whom will a midwife refer if a deviation from the norm occurs?
6. Discuss what assessments would be made initially on arrival at a BBA.

REFERENCES

BirthChoiceUK, 2011. Index of National Maternity Statistics. Available online: <http://www.birthchoiceuk.com/Professionals/statistics.htm> (accessed 1 March 2015).

BIECG (Birthplace in England Collaborative Group), 2011. Perinatal and maternal outcomes by planned place of birth for healthy women with low risk pregnancies: the Birthplace in England national prospective cohort study. Br. Med. J. 343 (d7400), 1756–1833.

Collins, M., Kingdon, C., 2014. One to One midwives: first-year outcomes of a midwifery-led model. Br. J. Midwifery 22 (1), 15–21.

Cook, M., 2003. A 'beautiful' birth. MIDIRS Midwifery Digest 13 (4), 447–448.

Dahlen, H., 2012. Homebirth: ten tips for safety and survival. Br. J. Midwifery 20 (12), 872–876.

Floyd, L., 1995. Community midwives' views and experience of home birth. Midwifery 11, 3–10.

Gwillim, J., 2009. Home birth. In: Chapman, V., Charles, C. (Eds.), The Midwife's Labour and Birth Handbook, second ed. Wiley-Blackwell, Oxford, pp. 83–92.

Gwillim, J., Charles, C., 2013. Home birth. In: Chapman, V., Charles, C.

(Eds.), The Midwife's Labour and Birth Handbook, third ed. Wiley-Blackwell, Chichester, pp. 102–116.

Jones, D., 2003. Midwifery supervision and home births. Midwives 6 (9), 386–388.

Kitzinger, S., 2001. Becoming a mother. MIDIRS Midwifery Digest 11 (4), 445–447.

Magill-Curden, J., 2012. Choosing homebirth. In: Steen, M. (Ed.), Supporting Women to Give Birth at Home. Routledge, Abingdon, p. 39 (Chapter 2).

McNutt, A., Thornton, T., Sizer, P., et al., 2013. Opinions of UK perinatal health care professionals on home birth. Midwifery 30, 839–846.

NICE (National Institute for Health and Care Excellence), 2014. Intrapartum Care: Care of Healthy Women and Their Babies During Childbirth. Clinical Guideline 190. NICE, London. Available online: <nice.org.uk/> (accessed 27 February 2015).

NMC (Nursing and Midwifery Council), 2007. Standards for Medicines Management. NMC, London.

Odent, M., 1996. Why labouring women don't need support. Mothering 80, 47–51.

ONS (Office for National Statistics), 2012. Births in England and Wales by

Characteristics of birth 2. Available online: <http://www.ons.gov.uk/ons/rel/vsob1/characteristics-of-birth-2--england-and-wales/2012/sb-characteristics-of-birth-2.html> (accessed 27 February 2015).

RCM (Royal College of Midwives), 2002. Home Birth Handbook, vol. 1: Promoting home birth. RCM Trust, London. 47.

RCM (Royal College of Midwives), 2003. Home Birth Handbook, vol. 2: Practising home birth. RCM Trust, London.

RCOG/RCM (Royal College of Obstetricians and Gynaecologists/Royal College of Midwives), 2007. Home Births Joint statement No.2. RCOG, London.

Resuscitation Council UK, 2011. Equipment used in homebirth May 2011. Available online: <https://www.resus.org.uk/quality-standards/equipment-used-in-homebirth/> (accessed 9 November 2015).

Russell, K., 2008. Watching and waiting: the facilitation of birth at home. In: Edwins, J. (Ed.), Community Midwifery Practice. Blackwell Publishing, Oxford, pp. 25–46.

Chapter 36

Principles of intrapartum skills: management of labour and birth in water

LEARNING OUTCOMES

Having read this chapter, the reader should be able to:

- discuss the benefits and safety of water use in labour
- outline low-risk criteria and indicate the situations in which water use is prohibited or dubious
- list the items of equipment necessary
- discuss the aspects of care pertinent to labouring in water
- discuss the midwife's role and responsibilities.

Water is used internationally in labour and in many instances for birth. Charles (2013) believes that all midwives should be able to assist at a water birth. Mothers and midwives can recount highly positive experiences of calm, trouble-free births. There is, however, resistance from some professional groups, e.g. American College of Obstetricians and Gynecologists (2014, cited Harper 2014) despite growing evidence of safety (Burns et al 2012, Harper 2014).

CONSIDERATIONS

Many women will choose to bath or shower in labour, the benefits of warm water bringing comfort and relief to the discomfort of uterine contractions. Immersion in deeper warm water is increasingly used for these benefits, but also for the birth of the baby into similar surroundings. Providers of maternity care should be familiar with the evidence of its efficacy and safety and have protocols that assist women and midwives if this choice is utilized. Water used in this way may be in a home or hospital setting, using pools that may be permanent or hired.

CONSIDERED BENEFITS AND SAFETY OF WATER USE

During the first stage of labour, water can (adapted from Garland 2011):

- aid descent of the fetal head and shorten the length of first stage

- promote an upright position and increased mobility
- provide a safe place which aids relaxation and coping strategies
- reduce the need for pharmacological analgesia and medical intervention
- promote a calm, less stressed and fearful environment.

During the second stage of labour, water can:

- reduce perineal trauma
- reduce birth intervention
- provide a gentle transition to extra uterine life for the baby
- more likely facilitate expectant management of the third stage of labour.

As maternity care providers, midwives can experience increased job satisfaction and the service attracts staff and clients (Garland 2011). Garland (2011) also notes that there can be some less positive aspects: costs can prevent some clients from hiring pools, this also often makes it a 'white middle class'/elite activity; midwives need training and support; midwives need additional guidance in the care of their backs. The occasional poorer outcome can cause the media to create a storm.

Both NICE (2014) and the RCOG/RCM joint statement (2006), in the light of currently available evidence, endorse labouring in water for pain relief purposes in the first stage of labour where inclusion/exclusion criteria exist. The RCOG/RCM (2006) are prepared to state, too, that 'healthy women with uncomplicated pregnancies at term... should be able to proceed to water birth if they wish'. NICE (2014) are less sure, stating that 'there is insufficient high-quality evidence to either support or discourage giving birth in water'. Garland (2011) indicates that many of the studies are robust and show positive outcomes, but are often small studies. However, Burns et al (2012) included over 8000 women in their review over an 8-year period: 58.3% were water births, just over half being to primiparous women. They concluded that pool use was associated with a higher frequency of spontaneous and normal birth, particularly among primiparous women.

PHYSIOLOGICAL DIFFERENCES

The physiological differences contribute to the safety. Babies experience an increase in prostaglandin in the 48 hours before labour commences and from 4 cm of cervical dilatation so that fetal breathing *in utero* ceases and the baby is not able to gasp or inhale during the birth process (Harper 2014). Equally the physiologically mild hypoxia that all babies have at the end of labour encourages them to swallow, none of us is able to swallow and breathe at the same time – breathing is inhibited until the first swallow has taken place. Along with these actions, the dive reflex (present until 6–9 months of age) closes off the glottis to abnormal substances so that fluids cannot be inhaled into the lungs.

The severely compromised fetus, however, will gasp; on this basis, signs of fetal compromise should exclude the woman from the water, either earlier in labour or if necessary standing out of the water at the point of delivery. The baby's face should never be reimmersed once out from the water.

Babies born into warm water are less likely to cry, they have a continued supply of oxygen through their umbilical cord and are likely to take longer to become pink all over. For this reason Apgar scoring should take place at a true 1 minute; Apgar scores taken before then are unlikely to be correct and could suggest fetal compromise when this is not the case (Garland 2011). It should be that all Apgar scores at all deliveries are assessed at 1 minute, but Garland (2011) noted that if estimating when 1 minute has passed, midwives are capable of under- and overestimating the time.

For the mother it is noted that with less gravity there is often a passive second stage. This means that sometimes the fetal head is on the perineum without signs of pushing, but it also means that there is often no faecal contamination of the water. This is an important aspect of safety.

WHO IS SUITABLE TO USE A BIRTHING POOL?

In many situations the inclusion criteria is the same as that for birthing in a midwife-led unit or at home: low-risk women suitable for intermittent auscultation in labour. However, any woman who has been given all the available information and wishes to use the pool should be considered. If the woman makes a choice that the midwife is uncomfortable with, Supervisors of Midwives can support the woman and the midwife, this and other actions that can be taken are discussed in Chapter 35.

General inclusion criteria for pool use:

- singleton fetus and cephalic presentation
- uncomplicated pregnancy of >37 weeks' gestation.

Situations in which the use of water is contraindicated include:

- maternal dislike
- maternal pyrexia
- opiate use in labour of less than 2 hours ago (NICE 2014)
- any known cause for concern for mother or fetus, particularly fetal compromise (presence of thick

meconium included), maternal haemorrhage, oxytocin induction/augmentation, epilepsy, pre-eclampsia.

Situations for which there is generally an embargo but no real evidence is available:

- known infection, e.g. group B streptococcus. The use of universally applied standard precautions and adherence to cleansing protocols make this ban questionable. The need to protect intravenous cannulae usually prevents these women from getting into the water
- the need for electronic fetal monitoring. Equipment is available to monitor continually in water but this raises a number of issues; as suggested above, the presence of fetal compromise prohibits delivery in water
- previous caesarean birth. However, McKenna & Symon (2013) record the successful use of water for women experiencing a vaginal birth after a caesarean section (VBAC)
- high body mass index; the woman may be more mobile and benefit from the buoyancy but be harder to remove from the pool in the event of an emergency
- prolonged rupture of membranes, for which no evidence is presented, although in some instances this may relate to the need for I.V. antibiotics (see above).

Despite many of the women being in the low-risk group, the midwife should always be alert to any obstetric or neonatal emergency, removing the woman from the pool swiftly and undertaking the correct management measures.

WHEN IS A GOOD TIME TO ENTER THE POOL?

Odent (1998) recognized that the relaxation offered by water and the lack of gravity could cause a non-established labour to cease. Most women were then prohibited from entering the water until 5 cm dilated. However, Garland (2006) notes that an uncomfortable woman, whatever her dilatation, is likely to relax in the water; Cluett et al (2004) noted that such labours often then progress. Garland (2006) considers that the next hour is the most critical time to observe for signs of progress; if the labour is slowing, the woman can be asked to mobilize again for a while. Water can both aid slow progress and cause labour to slow; consequently the midwife should observe for contraction length, strength and frequency as for any and every labour and respond accordingly. The water can be used intermittently if that is the woman's choice.

WHEN SHOULD THE WOMAN GET OUT OF THE POOL?

- When she chooses.
- If choosing other analgesia, e.g. epidural.
- If the midwife has a valid reason for asking her to:
  - if labour progress slows, as suggested above
  - if there are abnormalities to the fetal heart suggestive of fetal compromise
  - any signs of haemorrhage, raised blood pressure or pyrexia. In the event of ante- or postpartum haemorrhage, the woman leaves the pool immediately and the protocol is followed as for any birth
  - if the water is no longer clear. Garland (2011) suggest that clear water is a good indicator, and that when the clarity is lost the woman should be asked to leave the pool. Leaving at this point, before she feels unwell, makes leaving the pool easier. The reason for lack of clarity can be investigated (haemorrhage, bowel movement, or meconium being the most likely), if no abnormality is found the pool can be cleaned and refilled. Allowing the woman to be in a contaminated pool is potentially dangerous
  - if delivery of the shoulders does not follow in the contraction after delivery of the head. Under these circumstances the woman leaves the pool immediately and the shoulder dystocia drill is instigated. Care should be taken not to knock the baby's head on the side of the pool, and to note that the action of stepping out may cause dislodging of the fetal shoulders, rapid delivery may follow.
- For an active management of the third stage (see below).
- When ready after the delivery.

EQUIPMENT

There should be space around the pool on each side and the means to fill, reheat and empty it. A water thermometer is necessary, as is a sieve (to remove any debris from the water) and an aqua Doppler. A mirror and torch may both be useful where lighting is dim. The midwife can also benefit from a kneeler or stool and the woman may appreciate a float to rest on. Midwives should protect themselves; for example, the woman can float to the surface for fetal auscultation, reducing the risk of damage to the midwife's back. Correctly sized gauntlet gloves may also be useful.

The midwife must ensure, whether in hospital or at home, that the means to call for assistance and resuscitation equipment are all to hand. A hoist or other equipment (a net) should be available to aid the woman in leaving the pool quickly, a mattress or other means of lying down comfortably should be available, absorbent non-slip floor coverings, e.g. old towels, and a good supply of drying towels are all essential. A birthing stool may be helpful for land management of the third stage. Pool use at home should include a trial run, ensuring that birthing partners are also comfortable with their role.

PRINCIPLES OF CARE

Assessments of maternal and fetal wellbeing

As with homebirth (Chapter 35), midwives have the opportunity to exercise their autonomy in a generally low intervention environment. The need to have confidence in the physiology of labour and the woman's ability to give birth naturally are significant features. All labour observations, care and documentation are undertaken as for any other labour, just as referrals are made if there is any deviation from the norm.

- A full set of vital sign observations are undertaken prior to getting to the pool, these act as a baseline and aid the midwife to appreciate whether any change is physiological or pathological.
- The woman's temperature should be recorded hourly, as should the water temperature (see below).
- Pulse, respiration rate, blood pressure and fetal heat rate are assessed as for any dry land birth (Chapters 30–32).
- Abdominal and vaginal examinations may be undertaken in the pool or on dry land; if in the pool, the maternal abdomen is floated up to the surface.
- The woman may choose to leave the pool to pass urine, or to void, standing, into a bowl, or (as a sterile fluid) she may choose to void into the water. The midwife needs to know that the bladder has been emptied.
- The woman is encouraged to adopt positions that are comfortable but to change position regularly.
- Entonox can be used with hydrotherapy (but the woman should not be left alone), as may other complementary therapies (but no oils directly into the water).
- It is important that the woman remains well hydrated, drinking at least 500 mL per hour (Garland 2011).

- The room temperature should be maintained at 21–22°C. This allows the mother to evaporate heat and so remain normothermic in the water.

Water depth and temperature

The birthing pool needs to be able to accommodate water to the level of the woman's breasts when sitting. NICE (2014) recommend assessing and recording the water temperature hourly, it should not exceed 37.5°C. Anderson (2004) believes that women should be able to choose a comfortable water temperature, this is often the case for pain relief during the first stage of labour; water temperature for delivery remains a source of debate but should in the region of adult body temperature: 37–37.5°C. Good mixing is necessary prior to taking the water temperature.

The birth

It is advisable to have a second midwife in attendance, but this may vary according to local protocol. The woman is likely to push physiologically and is more likely to have a 'hands poised' (McCandlish et al 1998) delivery (avoiding any stimulation to the baby) with the midwife giving gentle verbal instruction (if necessary), while utilizing the mirror and possibly torch, to see advancement of the presenting part. As for all deliveries, it is not necessary to assess for the presence of the umbilical cord around the neck; interference can again cause premature stimulation. The baby should be born fully underwater; once born, the baby is brought to the surface without any unnecessary delay, where respiration can begin in air. As noted above, the baby's respiratory response is naturally slower; if, however, there are obvious respiration difficulties, it is necessary to clamp and cut the cord, removing the baby for resuscitation (Chapter 56).

When bringing the baby to the surface, care should be taken in case of a short umbilical cord. This has now been noted repeatedly over some years (Anderson 2000, Burns et al 2012). Burns et al (2012) note that of the 20 instances of cord snapping in their review, 18 of them occurred at water birth. Cord clamps should be readily available, the midwife should be alert to the need to act quickly and no undue traction should be applied to the cord on lifting the baby into skin-to-skin.

The baby should rest with its head above water (gently dried), retaining its body heat in skin-to-skin contact.

Third stage of labour

If clinically appropriate and desired by the woman, a physiological third stage can be completed in the pool with the cord clamped and cut according to maternal wishes. Blood

289

loss may be harder to estimate, and therefore the woman's clinical condition should be considered as part of the assessment.

An active management of the third stage is not advocated in the water. After a short delay in cord clamping and cutting, the woman is assisted to leave the pool prior to the intramuscular injection. Controlled cord traction, if undertaken, would be on dry land.

The mother and baby are brought out of the pool at a convenient point. Floor coverings are needed to reduce the risk of slipping on the wet floor. Care is taken to dry and keep warm, both mother and child. Examination of the mother's genital tract should take place as for any other birth, any suturing requirements should be undertaken an hour later (to allow waterlogged tissues to dry). Care of the baby is as for any other delivery.

Infection control

As for any birth, measures are taken to maintain asepsis; however, there is often less intervention and so water cleanliness becomes one of the priorities (see above, leaving the pool). Unlined pools should be thoroughly cleansed using the approved cleanser after each use, any disposable liners are thrown away. Jacuzzi-style pools should never be used.

ROLE AND RESPONSIBILITIES OF THE MIDWIFE

These can be summarized as:
- thorough, safe labour care as for any birth, but with added considerations for the comfort and safety of the woman, baby and midwife when using the medium of water for analgesia or birth
- identifying any occasions when removal from the pool is indicated and/or referral needed
- contemporaneous record keeping.

SUMMARY

- Clearer guidance now exists to support women and midwives in their use of water for the all stages of labour.
- Physiological adaptations protect the healthy infant, a compromised fetus should not be delivered in water. The mother can benefit from a number of positive effects of immersion in warm water.
- Care is taken to ensure that the pool is appropriately filled; water and maternal temperature should be recorded hourly, the water should not exceed 37.5°C. The water should remain clear.
- A water birth is a low intervention birth, the baby is brought to the surface without delay; care is taken to avoid the cord snapping.

SELF-ASSESSMENT EXERCISES

The answers to the following questions may be found in the text:
1. What is the current evidence with regard to the use of water for labour and birth?
2. Describe the positive effects of immersion in water for the labouring woman.
3. List the items of equipment necessary for birth in water.
4. Describe how the midwife would manage the second stage of labour in water.
5. How would the midwife manage a shoulder dystocia if this occurred in the pool?
6. List the considerations that a midwife should be mindful of when caring for a woman labouring in water.

REFERENCES

Anderson, T., 2000. Umbilical cords and underwater birth. Pract. Midwife 3 (2), 12.

Anderson, T., 2004. Time to throw the waterbirth thermometer away? MIDIRS Midwifery Digest 14 (3), 370–374.

Burns, E., Boulton, M., Cluett, E., et al., 2012. Characteristics, interventions and outcomes of women who used a birthing pool: a prospective observational study. Birth 39 (3), 192–202.

Charles, C., 2013. Water for labour and birth. In: Chapman, V., Charles, C. (Eds.), The Midwife's Labour and Birth Handbook, third ed. Wiley-Blackwell, Chichester (Chapter 7).

Cluett, E.R., Pickering, R.M., Getliffe, K., et al., 2004. Randomised control trial of labouring in water compared with standard of augmentation for management of dystocia in first stage of labour. Br. Med. J. 328 (7435), 314–318.

Garland, D., 2006. On the crest of a wave: completion of a collaborative audit. MIDIRS Midwifery Digest 16 (1), 81–85.

Garland, D., 2011. Revisiting Waterbirth: An Attitude to Care. Palgrave Macmillan, Basingstoke (Chapters 3, 4, 6, 7).

Harper, B., 2014. Birth, bath and beyond: the science and safety of water immersion during labor and birth. J. Perinat. Educ. 23 (3), 124–134.

McCandlish, R., Bowler, U., van Asten, H., et al., 1998. A randomised control trial of care of the perineum during second stage of normal labour. Br. J. Obstet. Gynaecol. 105 (12), 1262–1272.

McKenna, J., Symon, A., 2014. Water VBAC: exploring a new frontier for women's autonomy. Midwifery 30, e20–e25.

NICE (National Institute for Health and Care Excellence), 2014. Intrapartum Care: Care of Healthy Women and Their Babies during Childbirth. Clinical Guideline 190. NICE, London. Available online: <http://www.nice.org.uk/guidance/cg190> (accessed 3 March 2015).

Odent, M., 1998. Use of water during labour – updated recommendations. MIDIRS Midwifery Digest 8 (1), 68–69.

RCOG/RCM, (Royal College of Obstetricians and Gynaecologists/ Royal College of Midwives, 2006. Immersion in water during labour and birth. Joint Statement No. 1 RCOG/RCM, London. Available online: <https://www.rcm.org.uk/sites/default/files/rcog_rcm_birth _in_water.pdf> (accessed 3 March 2015).

Chapter | 37 |

Assessment of the baby: assessment at birth

LEARNING OUTCOMES

Having read this chapter, the reader should be able to:

- discuss how the Apgar score is undertaken and the significance of the scores
- describe the initial examination of the baby at birth, identifying how normality is confirmed
- discuss the role and responsibilities of the midwife in relation to assessment of the baby at birth.

There are two components to assessing the baby at birth – the Apgar score which is undertaken to determine how well the baby is adjusting from intrauterine to extrauterine life, and the top-to-toe physical examination that looks to confirm normality and detect any deviations from this so that referral can be made. These examinations are usually undertaken by the midwife as part of the care of the baby at birth (NICE 2014); thus it is important the midwife is competent in both of these assessments and understands the significance of what is being assessed and the findings. This chapter focuses on the assessments of the baby at birth, how they are undertaken, what is looked for, and the significance of what is found. Although in some countries the midwife will undertake a fuller examination to include looking for the red eye reflex, examining the hips for developmental dysplasia of the hip (DDH), palpating femoral pulses, listening to the heart and lungs, and palpating the abdomen for organomegaly, this is only undertaken in the UK if the midwife has had further training and thus these aspects are not discussed within this chapter.

THE APGAR SCORE

The Apgar score was formulated by Dr. Virginia Apgar in the 1950s as a way of assessing the baby's condition at birth and the need for resuscitation. Five inter-related variables, assessed at 1, 5, and 10 minutes (although these can be repeated at different time frames), are based on what happens and can be seen if the baby does not breathe effectively at birth (Pinheiro 2009). Each of the five

Table 37.1 The Apgar scoring system: the five classifications used and the criteria for scoring 0–2

Sign	0	1	2
Appearance (colour)	Blue, pale	Body pink, limbs blue	All pink
Pulse (heart rate)	Absent	<100	>100
Grimace (response to stimuli)	None	Grimace	Cry
Activity (muscle tone)	Limp	Some flexion of limbs	Active movements, limbs well flexed
Respiratory effort	None	Slow, irregular	Good, strong cry

variables is given a score of 0, 1, or 2 with a total score out of 10 (Table 37.1). The variables are breathing, heart rate, colour, tone and reflex irritability. If the baby is not breathing, there is less oxygen reaching cardiac tissue causing the heart rate to decrease which results in less oxygen reaching the tissues. This will affect the colour, muscle tone, and reflex irritability. Thus a low score will indicate the need for resuscitation. As breathing occurs, the heart rate improves resulting in the baby becoming pinker, improved muscle tone, and reflex irritability. A high score reflects a baby who does not need resuscitation and can reflect the baby who has made the adjustment well or has had a good response to resuscitative measures undertaken. However, it must be remembered that resuscitation should begin before 1 minute if indicated by the condition of the baby and an Apgar score calculated during resuscitation is not equivalent to that of a baby who is breathing spontaneously. There is no accepted standard for calculating Apgar scores for babies who are being resuscitated (Pinheiro 2009).

A low score at 1 minute does not correlate with future outcome, whereas at 5 minutes it is associated with neonatal mortality from 24 weeks' gestation, but there is conflicting evidence around neurological disability (Lee et al 2010, Li et al 2013, O'Donnell et al 2006, Pinheiro 2009). Iliodromiti et al (2014) found an increased risk of infant death for babies who had a 5-minute Apgar score of 0–3.

Dijxhoorn et al (1986) suggest changes in the fetal heart rate do not compare well with Apgar scores at delivery, making it difficult to anticipate which babies will have a low score at birth. This may account for why some emergency caesarean sections undertaken because of serious concerns regarding the fetal heart rate deliver a baby with a total Apgar score of 9 or 10. Additionally a persistently low Apgar score on its own should not be considered a specific indicator of intrapartum asphyxia. Salustiano et al (2012) undertook a retrospective study to assess risk factors associated with an Apgar score <7 at 5 minutes and found prolonged second stage of labour and repeated late decel-

erations on the cardiotocograph (CTG) were predictive but age, parity and breech birth were not. They also found these babies had an increased risk of respiratory distress, mechanical ventilation, admission to the neonatal intensive care unit, and a strong association with hypoxic–ischaemic encephalopathy (Salustiano et al 2012).

The Apgar score is vulnerable to bias, as it is a subjective score and is often undertaken retrospectively. McCarthy et al (2013) found that babies being resuscitated were given an Apgar score at 1 minute even though there was no documented evidence that the heart rate had been recorded and suggest the score does not accurately reflect the events occurring during resuscitation or when interventions are occurring. Ideally it should be undertaken by someone other than the midwife in attendance at the birth, as the midwife can be distracted by what is happening to the mother and the baby. The retrospective scoring is often based on what happened to the baby; thus a baby who had no resuscitative measures will score high. In some situations the Apgar score is jointly assigned by all midwives and doctors present at delivery but again is often retrospective and O'Donnell et al (2006) caution there is poor interobserver reliability even when undertaken independently.

There are a number of factors that can influence the score, e.g. the quality of lighting can affect the perception of the baby's colour as can skin pigmentation and haemoglobin levels. Tone can be affected by gestational age, congenital abnormality and maternal drugs. Silverton (1993) advises that skin pigmentation in non-Caucasian babies usually develops from the fifth day of life which can make these babies appear less well perfused. If the skin is darkly pigmented, colour can be assessed by observing the mucous membranes, palms of the hand, and soles of the feet, as these should be pink. The preterm baby has an immature neurological system resulting in poorer muscle tone and slower reflexes, as well as a bluish-red skin colour, which can lead to a low Apgar score, even though the baby requires no resuscitation.

Assessing the Apgar score

The five variables have been made into the acronym 'APGAR' – appearance, pulse, grimace, activity, and respiration.

- Observe the appearance, e.g. is the baby pink all over (2), is the body pink but the extremities blue (1), or is the baby pale or blue all over (0)?
- Assess the heart rate by palpating the umbilicus or placing two fingers across the chest over the apex, count the rate for 6 seconds then multiply by 10. Determine whether the heart rate is above 100 (10 beats or more over the 6-second period) (2), >100 (less than 10 beats in 6 seconds) (1), or absent (0). A baby who is pink, active and breathing is likely to have a heart rate above 100.
- The response of the baby to stimuli should be noted. This could be in response to being dried or handled or, for a baby who is being resuscitated, it may be the response to face masks or airways used. Determine whether the baby cries in response to stimuli (2), whether it is trying to cry but is only able to grimace (1), or whether there is no response (0).
- Assess the degree of muscle tone by observing the amount of activity and degree of flexion of the limbs: are there active movements using well-flexed limbs (2), is there some flexion of the limbs (1), or is the baby limp (0)?
- Finally, observe the respiratory effort made by the baby: is it good and strong (often seen in conjunction with a crying baby) (2), is respiration slow and irregular (1), or is there no respiratory effort (0)?

The scores are added and a total score is documented. Babies scoring above seven rarely need resuscitation.

PROCEDURE: Apgar scoring

- Ensure the lighting facilitates good visualization of colour and there is access to the baby, which may involve uncovering the baby briefly.
- Note the time of delivery, wait 1 minute, then undertake the first assessment, assessing the five variables quickly and simultaneously, totalling the score and recovering the baby.
- Act promptly and appropriately according to the score, e.g. a baby scoring 0–3 requires immediate resuscitation (it may already have commenced if the baby is obviously compromised at birth).
- Repeat at 5 minutes; the score should increase if previously eight or below.
- Repeat again at 10 minutes.
- Document findings and act accordingly.

BIRTH EXAMINATION

The initial birth examination is a physical examination undertaken to confirm normality and detect deviations from normal and is part of the midwife's competencies (NMC 2010). It is usually undertaken within the first couple of hours of life, having given the baby time for skin-to-skin contact with his mother and to complete his first feed (NICE 2014). The examination should be undertaken in a warm environment, free from draughts (to ensure the baby does not become cold), and with a good light source. This examination is likely to reveal obvious abnormalities but others, some of which may not be apparent at birth, will be detected during the physical examination undertaken within the first 72 hours of birth (NSC 2008) by a midwife who has undertaken further training and assessment in the examination of the newborn (NMC 2012) or a paediatrician.

The midwife will develop her own systematic approach to examining the baby, the order is less important than ensuring the examination is thorough and complete.

PROCEDURE: birth examination

- Discuss the procedure with the parents and gain their informed consent, requesting one or both are present for the examination (if the mother is unable to move from the bed, the examination can take place at the bedside or on the bed).
- Gather equipment:
  - thermometer suitable for use with a baby (p. 35)
  - scales for weighing the baby
  - disposable tape measure
  - disposable sheet
  - non-sterile gloves
  - nappy.
- Wash and dry hands and put on non-sterile gloves.
- Place the baby on to the disposable sheet which has been placed on top of a firm, safe surface with good lighting.
- Check the baby is warm by taking his temperature before beginning the procedure; to maintain the temperature only uncover the part of the baby being examined and re-cover the baby quickly.
- Examine the baby systematically and thoroughly, noting the colour, tone and activity throughout the procedure.
- Begin by examining the head, face and neck then moving onto the clavicles, arms, hands, chest and abdomen. The genitalia are then examined followed by the legs, feet, spine and buttocks. Reflexes can be assessed during the procedure (see below for more detail).

- Measure the baby's weight, head circumference, and length and note if any urine and meconium are passed.
- Place the baby skin-to-skin with his mother or dress him (the parents should be encouraged to do this).
- Dispose of disposable sheet and gloves, wash and dry hands.
- Discuss the findings with the parents during the procedure or at the end if they are not present.
- Document findings and act accordingly.

The head

The size of the head should be reviewed in relation to the rest of the baby – the head will appear large and out of proportion to the body and limbs in the preterm baby, asymmetrical growth restriction and hydrocephaly, whereas one that appears too small is associated with microcephaly and fetal alcohol spectrum disorders. Look for signs of moulding and caput succedaneum, as these may result in the head appearing asymmetrical and will influence the measurement of the head circumference. The parents should be reassured that both the moulding and caput swelling will resolve spontaneously over the next 48 hours and the head will become more rounded. On rare occasions the swelling may be due to a subgaleal haemorrhage, especially if the delivery was by ventouse extraction. The swelling will be present at birth but may not pit on pressure and will increase in size as the condition of the baby deteriorates. Urgent paediatric referral is required (Swanson et al 2011). Visible signs of trauma should be looked for, particularly if an amnihook, fetal scalp electrode, forceps, or ventouse cup has been used, as should signs of bruising which may increase the risk of physiological jaundice developing.

The suture lines and fontanelles should be palpated to assess their size and appearance. Widely spaced sutures may be indicative of a preterm baby, lack of moulding, or hydrocephalus. Narrowly spaced sutures are usually a result of moulding. The triangular-shaped posterior fontanelle should feel small and often appears closed at birth due to moulding. The diamond-shaped anterior fontanelle should be palpated; Bailey (2014) advises it should measure 3–4 cm in length and 1.5–2 cm in width (this may vary with moulding). A large fontanelle may be due to prematurity, hypothyroidism or hydrocephalus; a small one is suggestive of microcephaly. If the fontanelle is raised/bulging, this may be due to raised intracranial pressure (from birth injury, bleeding, hydrocephalus), while a depressed fontanelle is suggestive of dehydration – rarely seen at birth. Occasionally a third fontanelle can be felt between the anterior and posterior fontanelles and is suggestive of trisomy 21.

Head circumference

The occipitofrontal circumference is used to measure the head circumference which is the measurement around the occiput and forehead. However, due to the changes that can occur at birth from moulding, this measurement is likely to change over the next 48 hours. England (2014) suggests the normal measurement for a term baby is 32–36 cm, whereas Michaelides (2011) proposes it is 33–38 cm. Johnston et al (2003) suggest somewhere in-between – 33–37 cm with the average cited as 35 cm while Gardner & Hernandez (2011) cover the whole range with 32–38!

Shape of the face

There should be a symmetrical shape to the face; the size and position of the eyes, nose, mouth, chin, and ears should be noted in relation to each other. Moderate facial asymmetry may be associated with prolonged second stage, forceps delivery, macrosomia, and birth trauma, e.g. facial (Bell's) palsy (Stellwagen et al 2008). If the face appears unusual in appearance, England (2014) recommends looking at the face of both parents before expressing concern.

Eyes

If the baby's eyes are closed, gently tip the baby backwards then raise slowly as this may encourage him to open his eyes. The eyes are examined to ensure two are present with an assessment of their size, shape, symmetry, and any slanting (which may be normal). Widely spaced or narrowly spaced eyes are abnormal and may be indicative of an underlying syndrome. Epicanthic folds are normal in some ethnic groups, e.g. East, Southeast, and Central Asians, Indigenous Americans, but may also be associated with an underlying syndrome, e.g. trisomy 21. The cornea should be clear, if it is cloudy-looking it could be infection, trauma (from forceps), dystrophies, metabolic abnormality, or congenital glaucoma. While the sclera should be clear, conjunctival haemorrhage can be present, usually acquired during the second stage of labour, and should be noted. The parents should be reassured that this is likely to resolve within a few days. Any profuse or purulent discharge should be noted and a swab taken, as this is not normal and could be indicative of infection. On examination the pupils should appear round and clear, occasionally a keyhole shape is present (coloboma), which could be indicative of an underlying retinal defect. They should constrict to light. White or grey cloudiness within the pupil could indicate congenital cataracts (an early red eye reflex examination is required). White speckles on the iris, Brushfield's spots, may be indicative of trisomy 21 but can also be a normal variant.

Nose

Observe the shape of the nose and width of the bridge, which should be greater than 2.5 cm in the term baby. Two patent nares should be present, if blocked it will affect the baby's ability to breathe as babies are initially nose breathers rather than being able to use the mouth and the nose. Gardner & Hernandez (2011) suggest patency can be assessed by closing the baby's mouth and obstructing one nostril and observing breathing from the other nostril then repeating with the other side or by placing a stethoscope diaphragm under the nostrils and looking for bilateral 'fogging'. It is not unusual for the nose to be squashed at birth; if so, this should be noted, particularly if it is affecting the baby's ability to breathe. The nostrils should not flare; if they do, this is usually indicative of respiratory illness.

Mouth

The lips should be formed and symmetrical, asymmetry could be indicative of facial (Bell's) palsy. The size of the baby's mouth should be reviewed – a small mouth may be due to micrognathia, often associated with underlying abnormality. The area between the lips and the nose is then examined for the presence of a cleft lip. The inside of the mouth should be visualized using a good light source and is more easily achieved when the baby is crying or by pressing gently on the chin or the angle of the jaw to encourage him to open his mouth. The palate is then observed for intactness, particularly at the junction of the hard and soft palates where a cleft palate may occur; the palate should be high and arched. Digital examination is only undertaken if a submucous cleft palate is suspected (Habel et al 2006). The presence of white spots on the gums or palate are usually due to epithelial (Epstein's) pearls, which are of no significance, or teeth and are noted, as is the length of the frenulum to assess for tongue tie.

Ears

The ears are examined to ensure two are present which should be fully formed and in the correct position. There should be enough cartilage in the ears of a term baby to allow the ears to spring back into position when moved forwards gently. The pinna should be well formed with defined curves in the upper part. Correct positioning of the ears is determined by tracing an imaginary line from the outer canthus of the eyes horizontally back to the ears, with the top of the pinna above this line. Low-set ears may be associated with an underlying chromosomal abnormality (e.g. trisomy 21), renal abnormality or a normal variation. Gardner & Hernandez (2011) advise the ears are positioned almost vertically and suggest it is abnormal if the angle is >10°. The external auditory meatus should be examined to ensure patency. The presence of accessory skin tags or auricles should be noted and may be associated with renal abnormalities and hearing impairment (Roth et al 2008).

Neck

Babies generally have short necks, which should be examined for symmetry. The presence of swelling (e.g. cystic hygroma, sternomastoid tumour) can be detected by feeling all around the neck. The baby should be able to move his head to both sides well past the shoulder 100–110° from the midline and flex his head 50–60° laterally towards his ear. The head should also flex towards the chest so that it almost or does touch the chest and extend backwards so the back of the occiput reaches or is almost touching the back (Michaelides 2011). Limited lateral movement is associated with torticollis (Stellwagen et al 2008). Webbing is unusual and could be indicative of a chromosomal abnormality (e.g. Turner's syndrome); redundant skin folds at the back of the neck are suggestive of trisomy 21.

Clavicles

Feel along the clavicles using the index finger to ensure they are intact, particularly if there was a breech presentation that required manipulation or shoulder dystocia – both increase the risk of a fractured clavicle, resulting in little or no movement in the associated arm.

Arms

The arms should be the same length, confirmed by straightening the arms down the side of the baby and comparing the two together. Both arms should be moving freely; spontaneous arm movements can usually be elicited by stroking the forearm or hand. Lack of movement may be associated with underlying trauma (e.g. fractures, nerve damage) or poor motor control associated with neurological impairment. The number of digits are then counted and examined for webbing between them, polydactyly and/or syndactyly is noted. The palm should be straightened and the number of palmar creases noted; a single crease may be associated with chromosomal abnormality (e.g. trisomy 21) but can also be a normal variant. The nails should be examined for the presence of paronychia and hangnails; hangnails may become infected or get caught on bedding, causing them to tear and bleed.

Chest

The chest is observed for a rounded shape and symmetry of movement with respiration; asymmetrical movement may be due to unilateral pneumothorax or phrenic nerve injury, particularly if there was a shoulder dystocia at birth. The respiratory rate can be counted if it appears abnormal and signs of respiratory distress (e.g. sternal recession, intercostal recession) reported to the paediatrician immediately. The nipples and areolae are well formed in the term baby and appear symmetrical on the chest wall but not widely spaced (this may be indicative of an underlying chromosomal abnormality). Any accessory nipples should be noted. The breasts may appear enlarged; this is normal and of little significance unless there are signs of infection.

Abdomen

Observe the abdomen, which should appear rounded and move in synchrony with the chest during respiration, inspecting the area to confirm it is intact and gently palpating to ensure there are no abnormal swellings. The abdomen is usually protruding slightly, a flat or sunken abdomen may be associated with decreased tone or diaphragmatic hernia (this is likely to cause respiratory difficulty particularly when the baby is laid flat). Diastasis recti (separation of the rectus muscles) is common and may facilitate the presence of a midline hernia around the umbilicus which should resolve spontaneously within 24 hours (Michaelides 2011). Midline defects, e.g. gastroschisis, exomphalos, require covering and urgent referral. The umbilical cord should be securely clamped and inspected to ensure there are no signs of haemorrhage.

Genitalia

With boys, the length and shape of the penis should be assessed – this is usually about 3 cm and straight – and the position of the urethral meatus confirmed (easier to see when the baby passes urine). England (2014) suggests an apparently short penis is common and usually due to the presence of suprapubic fat which may reassure parents. The foreskin should not be retracted, as it is adherent to the glans penis and physically retracting it at this age can lead to phimosis. The scrotum is observed for symmetry, suggestive of two descended testicles and gently palpated to feel for both testicles, Michaelides (2011) advises they are 1.5–2 cm long and feel similar to a pea. England (2014) cautions that a dark discoloration of the scrotum, with or without swelling, is abnormal and may be indicative of testicular torsion. This should not be mistaken for the generalized darker pigmentation seen with highly pigmented skin.

For girls, the vulva should be examined by parting the labia gently to ensure the presence of the clitoris, and urethral and vaginal orifices. A mucoid discharge may be present which is normal.

Legs

The legs and feet should be observed for their symmetry, size, shape and posture. To confirm the legs are the same length straighten them together to compare the two, then flex the hips and knees and place the feet on the surface touching their buttocks. The knees should be at the same height (Galeazzi test/Allis sign); if they are not, it could be indicative of developmental dysplasia of the hip (see Chapter 40). Both legs should be moving freely; lack of movement may be associated with underlying trauma (e.g. fractures, nerve damage) or poor motor control associated with neurological impairment. The position of the feet in relation to the legs should be noted as both positional and anatomical deformities may cause the feet to be turned inwards or outwards, upwards or downwards. Some of these deformities require corrective treatment. The shape of the feet should be noted, including oedema or a 'rocker bottom' appearance and the number of toes counted and examined for webbing between them by separating them; polydactyly or syndactyly should be noted.

Spine

The spine is examined by turning the baby over, looking for any obvious abnormality such as spina bifida, swelling, dimpling, or hairy patches; these could indicate an abnormality of the spinal cord or vertebral column. Assess the curvature of the vertebral column by running the fingers lightly over the spine – the spine should feel straight with no scoliosis, lordosis or kyphosis. This may be easier to do by straddling the baby over one hand, while using the other hand to feel the spine (ensure the head is supported). Gently part the cleft of the buttocks, look for dimples or sinuses and confirm the presence of the anal sphincter. Wilson et al (2010) caution the buttocks must be parted, as a cursory examination without doing this may result in an anorectal malformation being missed.

Skin

The condition of the skin can be observed throughout the examination, particularly the colour and the presence of any rashes or marks (e.g. birthmarks, bruising). Acrocyanosis is seen when the baby's body is pink but his extremities, in particular his hands and feet, are blue or purple. It is normal during the first few hours of life, often disappearing within 24 hours and is usually physiological due to the large arteriovenous oxygen difference resulting during the slow blood flow throughout the peripheral capillary beds (Steinhorn 2008).

Any obvious swelling or spots should be examined and recorded. A Mongolian blue spot may be evident in some babies, particularly those with an Asian or African ancestry.

This appears like bruising, usually over the sacral area, and should be observed over the next few days to enable the midwife to differentiate between the possibility of the discoloration being a bruise or a Mongolian blue spot. 'Birth marks' should be noted as an infantile haemangioma may present at birth (Leonardi-Bee et al 2011).

Elimination

If urine or meconium is passed it should be recorded, as it indicates patency of the renal and lower gastrointestinal tracts, respectively.

Weight

The weight of the baby is recorded in kilograms; this can be undertaken at the beginning or end of the examination provided the baby is warm. Many parents may want to know the weight in pounds and ounces and it is useful to have a conversion chart with the scales.

Length

While the crown–heel length of the baby may be recorded, as parents are interested in 'how long' their baby is; it is not routinely undertaken and is difficult to measure accurately. The length is measured in two stages using a non-stretchable, disposable tape measure and the baby on his side: from the crown (top part of the head) to the base of the spine, and from the base of the spine to the heel. A second person may be required to straighten the legs. Length can also be measured by placing the baby on a disposable sheet and marking the paper where the top of the baby's head is. The baby's legs are then straightened without moving the paper from under the baby and a mark placed where his feet are positioned. The baby can then be lifted from the sheet and the distance between the two marks measured.

Reflexes

A number of reflexes may be seen or looked for during the examination which reflect the intactness of the neurological system. These need to be undertaken when the baby is relaxed for maximum effect. These reflexes are described below.

Rooting

When the baby's cheek is stroked he will turn his head in the direction of the stroke to search for the source of the stimulation. His head will move in gradually decreasing

arcs until the object is found and may make sucking motions. This is less evident if the baby is sleepy or not hungry.

Sucking

This is seen in response to tactile stimulation around the mouth or when an object, e.g. nipple, finger, teat, is inserted into the baby's mouth.

Snout

If gentle pressure is applied over the philtrum the baby will pucker his lips.

Moro

This response occurs if the baby's head suddenly changes position, particularly downwards or if he is startled by an unexpected sound. His legs and head will extend while his arms move up and out with his palms up and thumbs flexed. He will then bring his arms together and clench his fists. It may be accompanied by crying.

Babinski/plantar reflex

When the sole of the baby's foot is stroked firmly, the baby's big toe moves upwards and the other toes fan out.

Palmar grasp

By placing a finger on the infant's open palm, the hand will be seen to close around the finger. As an attempt is made to remove the finger, the baby will tighten his grip. The palmar grasp can be strong, almost allowing the baby to be lifted up if both his hands are grasping fingers.

Asymmetrical tonic neck

This is seen when a baby is lying on his back and has his head turned to the side. The arm on the side where the head is facing reaches away from the body with the hand partly open while the opposite arm will flex with a tightly clenched fist. If the baby's head is moved to the opposite side, the reverse happens. This position has been referred as the 'fencer's position' because of its similarity to a fencer's stance.

Stepping/walking

When the baby is held upright and the soles of his feet touch a flat surface, he will attempt to walk by placing one foot in front of the other.

ROLE AND RESPONSIBILITIES OF THE MIDWIFE

These can be summarized as:

- being able to competently assess the baby at birth, using the Apgar score, and understanding the significance of the score and factors that may influence it
- recognizing all the components that encompass the birth examination and recognizing what is normal
- undertaking the birth examination thoroughly and competently, referring as necessary
- involving the parents with the birth examination and informing them gently of any concerns found and of what will happen next, e.g. referral, diagnostic tests, treatment
- contemporaneous record keeping.

SUMMARY

- Assessment of the baby at birth is an important skill undertaken by the midwife.
- Apgar scoring is quick and easy to undertake, but is subjective and influenced by factors such as lighting and skin pigmentation.
- Birth examination is a thorough physical examination that detects obvious abnormalities; some abnormalities may not be apparent until the baby is older, thus subsequent examinations should be undertaken as required.

SELF-ASSESSMENT EXERCISES

The answers to the following questions may be found in the text:

1. How would a baby who scores one for each category of the Apgar score be recognized?
2. What factors influence the score awarded at birth?
3. Describe the top-to-toe examination of the baby undertaken by the midwife at birth.
4. Identify six reflexes that a newborn baby has and discuss how these are elicited.
5. What are the role and responsibilities of the midwife in relation to the assessment of the baby at birth?

REFERENCES

Bailey, J., 2014. The fetus. In: Marshall, J., Raynor, M. (Eds.), Myles Textbook for Midwives, sixteenth ed. Elsevier, Edinburgh, p. 120.

Dijxhoorn, M.J., Visse, G.H.A., Fidler, V.J., et al., 1986. Apgar score, meconium and acidaemia at birth in relation to neonatal neurological morbidity in term infants. Br. J. Obstet. Gynaecol. 893, 217–222.

England, C., 2014. Recognizing the healthy baby at term through examination of the newborn screening. In: Marshall, J., Raynor, M. (Eds.), Myles Textbook for Midwives, sixteenth ed. Elsevier, Edinburgh, pp. 591–609.

Gardner, S.L., Hernandez, J.A., 2011. Initial nursery care. In: Gardner, S.L., Carter, B.S., Enzman-Hines, M., Hernandez, J.A. (Eds.), Merenstein &

Gardner's Handbook of Neonatal Intensive Care, seventh ed. Elsevier, St. Louis, pp. 96–102.

Habel, A., Elhadi, N., Sommerlad, B., Powell, J., 2006. Delayed detection of cleft palate: an audit of newborn examination. Arch. Dis. Child. 91, 238–240.

Johnston, P.G.B., Flood, K., Spinks, K., 2003. The Newborn Child, ninth ed. Churchill Livingstone, Edinburgh, p. 48.

Iliodromiti, S., Mackay, D.F., Smith, G.C.S., et al., 2014. Apgar score and the risk of cause-specific infant mortality: a population-based cohort study. Lancet 384 (9956), 1749–1755.

Lee, H.C., Subeh, M., Gould, J.B., 2010. Low Apgar score and mortality in extremely preterm neonates born in

the United States. Acta Paediatr. 99 (12), 1785–1789.

Leonardi-Bee, J., Batta, K., O'Brien, C., Bath-Hextall, F.J., 2011. Interventions for infantile haemangiomas (strawberry birthmarks) of the skin. Cochrane Database Syst. Rev. (5), Art. No.:CD006545, doi:10.1002/ 14651858.CD006545.pub2.

Li, F., Wu, T., Lei, X., et al., 2013. The Apgar score and infant mortality. PLoS ONE 8 (7), e69072.

McCarthy, L.K., Morley, C.J., Davis, P.G., et al., 2013. Timing of interventions in the delivery room: does reality compare with neonatal resuscitation guidelines? J. Pediatr. 163 (6), 1553–1557.

Michaelides, S., 2011. Physiology, assessment and care. In: Macdonald, S., Magill-Cuerden, J. (Eds.), Mayes'

Midwifery, fourteenth ed. Elsevier, Edinburgh, pp. 567–599.

NICE (National Institute for Health and Care Excellence), 2014. Intrapartum guidelines: care of healthy women and their babies during childbirth. NICE, London. Available online: <http://www.nice.org.uk/guidance/cg190> (accessed 3 March 2015).

NMC (Nursing and Midwifery Council), 2010. Standards for competence for registered midwives. Available online: <http://www.nmc-uk.org/Publications/Standards/> (accessed 8 February 2015).

NMC (Nursing and Midwifery Council), 2012. Midwives rules and standards. Available online <http://www.nmc-uk.org/Publications/Standards/> (accessed 1 February 2015).

NSC (UK National Screening Committee), 2008. Newborn and Infant Physical Examination.

Available online: <http://newbornphysical.screening.nhs.uk/standards> (accessed 1 February 2015).

O'Donnell, C.P.F., Kamlin, O.F., Davis, P.G., et al., 2006. Interobserver variability of the 5-minute Apgar score. J. Pediatr. 149 (4), 486–489.

Pinheiro, J.M.B., 2009. The Apgar cycle: a new view of a familiar scoring system. Arch. Dis. Child. Fetal Neonatal Ed. 94, F70–F72.

Roth, D.A., Hildesheimer, M., Bardenstein, S., et al., 2008. Preauricular skin tags and ear pits are associated with permanent hearing impairment in newborns. Pediatrics 122 (4), e884–e890.

Salustiano, E.M.A., Campos, J.A.D.B., Ibidi, S.-M., et al., 2012. Low Apgar scores at 5 minutes in a low risk population: maternal and obstetrical factors and postnatal outcome. Rev. Assoc. Med. Bras. 58 (5), 587–593.

Silverton, L., 1993. The Art and Science of Midwifery. Prentice Hall, New York.

Steinhorn, R.H., 2008. Evaluation and management of the cyanotic neonate. Clin. Pediatr. Emerg. Med. 9 (3), 169–175.

Stellwagen, L., Hubbard, E., Chamber, C., Lyons Jones, K., 2008. Torticollis, facial symmetry and plagiocephaly in normal newborns. Arch. Dis. Child. 93 (10), 827–831.

Swanson, A.E., Veldman, A., Wallace, E.M., Malhotra, A., 2011. Subgaleal haemorrhage: risk factors and outcomes. Acta Obstet. Gynecol. Scand. 91, 260–263.

Wilson, B.E., Etheridge, C.E., Soundappen, V.S., Holland, A.J.A., 2010. Delayed diagnosis of anorectal malformation: are current guidelines sufficient? J. Paediatr. Child Health 46 (5), 268–272.

Chapter | 38 |

Assessment of the baby: daily examination

LEARNING OUTCOMES

Having read this chapter, the reader should be able to:

- describe the observations that may be made as part of the daily examination of the baby, identifying how normal progress is recognized

- discuss the role and responsibilities of the midwife in relation to the daily examination of the baby.

During the postnatal period the midwife will undertake an examination of the baby each day while the baby is in hospital and when visited at home to monitor early changes and ensure optimal progress is occurring. Whilst normality is identified, deviations from normal can also be recognized and appropriate action and referral instigated. NICE (2014) recommend the use of a postnatal care plan to guide individualized care for the mother and baby; this is updated each visit. Furthermore, parents should be given information and advice that will enable them to assess their baby's general condition so they can recognize signs and symptoms of common health problems for babies and seek appropriate help (NICE 2014). Although it is referred to as a daily examination, it is not essential to see the baby every day during the postnatal period but according to clinical need. This chapter considers how the daily examination of a baby is undertaken and the role and responsibilities of the midwife in relation to this. This chapter should be read in conjunction with a number of other chapters which are referred to within the text.

PRINCIPLES OF THE DAILY EXAMINATION

Parental care

The facilitation of optimal infant health and development relies significantly on the skills, education and care given by the parents. This process begins during pregnancy with the midwife working with families in the beginnings of infant health and wellbeing and the development of the postnatal care plan. The midwife teaches by example (e.g. handwashing) as well as with verbal (wherever possible, evidence-based) suggestions. During the daily examination of the baby, the midwife relies on communication with the parents to appreciate the complete picture of how the baby is progressing. Equally, it is a time for guiding, educating and advising parents, as well as supporting and encouraging them in their new role.

Consent

The procedure should be discussed with the parents and informed consent gained, as the baby cannot give consent for the examination. There will be times when the parents may not give consent; for example, the baby is now asleep, having been awake all night. The midwife undertakes a risk assessment, based on detailed conversation, to appreciate whether a physical examination must be undertaken or whether it can be postponed until later. The examination should ideally be undertaken when one or both parents are present, as this provides a good opportunity for discussion as issues from the examination arise.

Reducing infection risks

The baby is considered a 'compromised host' at birth, at risk from infection that can affect morbidity and mortality. Standard precautions should be utilized (see Chapter 8) and it is important to avoid cross-infection from other sources; hand hygiene should be scrupulous (see Chapter 9). If contact with body fluids is anticipated, then personal protective equipment is used (e.g. gloves, apron).

Examination of the newborn

The daily examination is not a copy of the birth examination, but an assessment of progress thereafter. It therefore relies on the fact that all body systems have been screened and deviations from normal are known about, with progress assessed accordingly. It should be undertaken methodically, in a good light and a warm environment.

INITIAL OBSERVATIONS

Observations on entering a woman's personal environment (hospital or home) can give immediate indicators as to the situation and provide the midwife with prompts when giving care advice. The midwife should observe:

- how the parents are feeling by looking at them: peaceful, tired, tearful, happy, etc.
- whether the parents immediately begin to express problems or anxieties
- how the baby is positioned and dressed within the sleeping area

- how the parent(s) handle and react to their baby
- environmental factors such as heat/cold, the presence of smoke, pets, other relatives/siblings/visitors – their reactions or concerns, general level of hygiene.

The following observations are likely to lead into more detailed discussion and provide an opportunity for reassurance, education and support:

- The baby's behaviour: is the baby active, sleepy, contented, or unsettled; does the baby cry a lot; what is the cry like; can the baby be pacified easily?
- Feeding patterns: is the baby waking for feeds and how often? What is the approximate feeding pattern? (This will vary according to feeding method.) If breastfeeding, is the mother happy that the baby latches correctly and is achieving an effective feed? (see Chapter 41) If formula feeding, are amounts taken appropriate for the age of the baby? Is the mother fully conversant with sterilizing and preparing feeds (see Chapters 43 and 44)? Is the baby settled after a feed? Is there any vomiting or posseting? In the event of vomiting green bile, or any projectile vomiting, a direct referral is made to a paediatrician.
- Elimination: do the number and nature of wet and soiled nappies suggest that feeding is progressing and body systems are functioning normally?
- Are the parents feeling confident about other aspects of baby care, e.g. skin care, managing unsettled periods?
- Do the parents have any other concerns or questions at this time?

GENERAL OBSERVATION OF THE BABY

Observing the baby before undressing it can reveal several potential problems:

- Under-/overclothed: advice may be needed as to correct temperature management when indoors to avoid problems associated with hypo- and hyperthermia.
- Position of the baby: the baby should be positioned on his back to sleep, but 'tummy time' should be encouraged when awake and someone is with him.
- Respirations: the respiratory pattern is noted (often irregular in newborn babies, see Chapter 6), with a normal respiratory rate of 30–40 per minute expected when the baby is at rest with no signs of respiratory distress. The respiratory rate can increase to 60 per minute with crying. Chest movement should be symmetrical (this is often better assessed when the baby is undressed), nasal flaring should not be seen.

- Obvious signs of vomiting or posseting (see above).
- Skin colour: the baby should appear pink all over, reflecting good peripheral perfusion. With skin that is highly pigmented, signs of peripheral perfusion can be assessed by observing the mucous membranes, the palms, and the soles. Cyanosis with or without signs of respiratory distress should be reported to the paediatrician immediately. If the baby appears pale, this should be reported, as it could be indicative of underlying illness. Physiological jaundice, seen as a yellow discoloration of the skin (and sometimes the sclera and mucous membranes) is not unusual in babies. Physiological jaundice usually appears from the third day and may deepen over the next couple of days before beginning to subside by the seventh day. If the jaundice appears severe and widespread, particularly if the baby is very sleepy or not feeding, the serum bilirubin level should be estimated. Clinical estimation of the degree of jaundice can be inaccurate and is influenced by the type of lighting, the reflective ability of objects around the baby and the peripheral blood flow (Johnston et al 2003). Arkley (2007) advises that prolonged jaundice (lasting longer than the first 2 weeks) should be considered abnormal and a split bilirubin blood test undertaken. The majority of prolonged jaundice cases will be breast milk jaundice and the parents can be reassured. However, liver disease is sometimes the underlying cause.
- Limb movement: when the baby is active, all four limbs should be moving without any signs of discomfort. If the baby was in an extended breech presentation antenatally, it is likely his legs will continue to maintain an extended position for a few days.
- Head shape: signs of birth trauma may be noted. The head is examined in greater detail as the examination progresses (see below).

Following the initial observations, discussions with the parents and general observations, the midwife then undertakes a 'top-to-toe' examination of the baby. Care is taken to only expose the parts that are being assessed so that the baby does not cool. On picking up the baby, the midwife will appreciate the baby's body temperature and whether he is irritable on handling.

PHYSICAL EXAMINATION

Head

With the fingertips, the midwife will feel along the suture lines and fontanelles; moulding should have resolved within the first 24 hours of birth. The anterior fontanelle is palpated and should be level. If raised, it could be indicative of raised intracranial pressure particularly if the baby is irritable whereas a depressed fontanelle is suggestive of dehydration. While feeling around the head, note any new swellings. A cephalhaematoma first appears between 12 and 36 hours and is likely to increase in size, taking up to 6 weeks to disappear. It is a firm swelling that does not pit on pressure and does not cross suture lines. A large cephalhaematoma may cause a deepening of physiological jaundice. Any bruised or traumatized areas noted at or since birth should be examined to ascertain that healing is occurring and there are no signs of infection.

Eyes

The eyes are inspected to ensure they are clear, with no signs of discharge. If a discharge is present, the eyes should be cleaned (see Chapter 13), a swab taken if indicated (see Chapter 11) and the parents shown how to clean the eye. The majority of discharges are not due to infection, but if concerned, referral to the paediatrician or general practitioner is warranted. Jaundice may be noted in the sclera, as discussed above.

Mouth

With a good light source inspect the mouth, which should be clean and moist. The presence of white plaques on the tongue or inner cheek could be indicative of a monilial infection (if breastfeeding, the mother's nipples should also be assessed) and so warrants further investigation. Oral candidiasis occurs in approximately 4% of babies (Dinsmoor et al 2005) and is common when the mother is taking antibiotics. If the baby has fed recently, sucking blisters may be apparent on the lips. Although this gives the appearance that the skin is peeling from the lips, no treatment is needed and the parents should be reassured this is normal.

Skin

Skin colour should be assessed as discussed above. The skin is also examined for the presence of rashes, spots, bruising, signs of infection or trauma. Erythema toxicum appears as a blotchy red rash and is of little significance, as are milia. However, septic spots should be identified early and treatment instigated if required. Areas of excoriation should be looked for, as these may occur due to friction with bedding or clothes, or in cases of excoriation of the buttocks, may be due to an irritant contact dermatitis or fungal infection. The nails should be examined for paronychia. If the baby was postmature, the skin may be dry; parents should be reassured that no treatment is necessary (see Chapter 13). On exposure of the baby's trunk (non-infective), engorged breasts may be noted in both boys and girls. Parents need reassuring that this is a physiological response to maternal hormones and that no treatment is necessary; as hormone levels fall, the problem will resolve. It is very important that the breasts are not squeezed in an attempt to reduce their size and appearance. This will not only cause discomfort and pain but may result in mastitis. In the event of redness or signs of infection, the baby should be referred to the paediatrician.

Umbilicus

The umbilical cord and umbilicus should be examined for signs of separation and to exclude infection (see Chapter 13). The cord usually separates within 5–15 days, often leaving a small stump of cord in the umbilicus, which will fall out over the next few days. Some midwives prefer to remove the cord clamp at 48–72 hours although there is no clinical indication to do so. Early signs of infection may be detected by redness around the umbilicus; the cord may also smell offensive and become sticky. This should not be mistaken for the normal process of cord separation.

Nappies

Elimination acts as a guide for neonatal health, particularly for effective feeding. In the first few days of life, term babies micturate 15–60 mL/kg/day, have a bladder capacity of 40 mL and void 2–6 times per hour (Blackburn 2013). Urine output increases over the first 4 weeks to 250–400 mL/day with one or more episodes of voiding per feed (Blackburn 2013). The midwife should ask the parents how many wet and dirty nappies the baby is having to gauge if normal output is occurring.

It can be difficult to tell if the baby has passed urine with some of the superabsorbent disposable nappies although the nappy will feel heavier. If there is any concern about whether the baby is passing urine, a folded tissue pressed in the nappy may reveal the presence of urine; alternatively the nappy can be torn open at the back to reveal urine within the crystals.

Urine is colourless in the newborn baby. If the nappy is stained yellow or darker, this could be from conjugated bilirubin due to liver disease (Arkley 2007) and should be investigated regardless of the whether or not jaundice is present.

Meconium is seen for the first 2 days, then a changing stool (greenish-brown) is present for the next couple of days, indicating patency of the upper intestinal tract, followed by a yellow stool thereafter. UNICEF UK (2014) advise the changes to a yellow stool should have occurred by day 5. During the first couple of days, babies pass one or more stools per day; on days 3–4 there are at least two stools passed each day (UNICEF UK 2014). By the end of the first week the UNICEF UK (2014) suggest the baby should be passing six or more wet nappies in a 24-hour period with at least two stools. When feeding is established, a breastfed baby may pass an inoffensive, soft, bright yellow stool every 2–3 days. The baby receiving formula tends to pass a firmer, mustard yellow, and mildly offensive stool more often but will also have a tendency towards constipation. Pale stools should always be investigated, as this could be indicative of liver disease (Arkley 2007).

Newborn babies have higher levels of uric acid which is a by-product of nucleotide breakdown (Blackburn 2013). These may sometimes be seen in the nappy, often as orange or red urate crystals and may be mistaken for blood. Parents need reassurance that this is not a major complication, but care should be taken to ensure that feeding is giving the baby sufficient fluid and nutrition. Parents may notice a tiny mucousy red bleed in the nappy of female baby which can be worrisome for them. However, this is likely to be a small pseudo-menstruation caused by the effects of maternal hormones within the baby's system and is harmless.

Weight

A healthy term baby normally loses weight in the first week of life but this is usually transient and of no significance (NICE 2014). Birth weight is generally regained by 2 weeks of age. Routine weighing of babies before this time has both benefits and harm associated (NICE 2014) and there is no high-quality evidence to base a recommendation of when to weigh babies. Crossland et al (2008) acknowledge there is little accurate knowledge known about weight changes in healthy term babies up to 2 weeks of age. In their small study, babies were weighed each day for 2 weeks. They concluded that feeding problems should be considered if weight is not increasing by 6 days, but some healthy babies took 17 days to regain their birth weight. Grossman et al (2012) found breastfed babies initially lost more weight than formula-fed babies, with over half the babies losing the most weight by day 2. They suggest more research is needed to determine if the smaller weight loss with non-breastfed babies is significant for future adverse health outcomes, e.g. predisposition to obesity in later life (Grossman et al 2012). Tawia & McGuire (2014) agree that breastfed babies lose a higher percentage of weight initially compared with the formula-fed baby; however, this is physiological and not abnormal. They found babies usually begin to gain weight from around day 4, but the median time for regaining the birth weight was 8.3 days for breastfed babies and 6.5 days for formula-fed babies (Tawia & McGuire 2014). The midwife should be guided by local protocol. It is important that correctly calibrated electronic scales are used each time. A weight loss >10% of birth weight would give cause for concern and, if accompanied by suboptimal urine and stooling, then feeding would need careful investigation, as the mother may require additional support with feeding.

Identity

If the daily assessment is being undertaken in hospital then it is important to establish that the baby is wearing identity bands according to local protocol.

SCREENING

Undertaking the examination as a whole is a form of screening for normality. Specific haematological screening, e.g. newborn blood spot screening or serum bilirubin, may be undertaken with parental consent. Newborn blood spot screening should be undertaken between days 5–8 (see Chapter 39).

AFTER THE EXAMINATION

When the examination is complete, the baby should be redressed and the findings recorded in the appropriate documentation and adjustments made to the postnatal care plan, if indicated. The findings should form the basis of advice given to the parents regarding the progress and subsequent care of the baby. Any deviations from normal should be acted on accordingly and appropriate care instigated.

PROCEDURE: daily examination of the baby

- Make a mental note of anything significant on entering the woman's personal environment (see above).
- Discuss the progress of the baby with the parents, allaying their anxieties if necessary.
- Explain the procedure and gain informed consent.
- Wash and dry hands (apply non-sterile gloves if contact with body fluids is anticipated), undertake a general observation of the baby.
- Ensure there is good light and a warm environment, undress the baby, and undertake the 'top-to-toe' examination described above.
- Weigh the baby if indicated.

- Redress the baby and give back to the parents.
- If day 5–8, newborn blood spot screening may be taken with consent. The baby would be redressed but with a foot exposed; the baby will be with a parent or with the midwife, depending on preference.
- Discuss the findings with the parents and made a date for the next visit.
- Wash and dry hands.
- Document the findings and act accordingly.

ROLE AND RESPONSIBILITIES OF THE MIDWIFE

These can be summarized as:
- reviewing and adjusting the postnatal care plan
- undertaking all aspects of the daily examination thoroughly and competently, referring as necessary
- education and support of parents
- contemporaneous record keeping.

SUMMARY

- Examination of the baby during each postnatal visit (in hospital and at home) by the midwife is an essential component of the care provided to the mother and baby during the postnatal period.
- The midwife uses skills of communication and observation to ensure that optimal infant health is achieved.
- The daily examination provides an opportunity to discuss detailed care and advice with the parents.

SELF-ASSESSMENT EXERCISES

The answers to the following questions may be found in the text:
1. Describe the different aspects of the daily examination of the baby.
2. What would the midwife do if the baby's mouth had visible white plaques?
3. How should the midwife advise a mother who has seen urates in the baby's nappy?
4. What are the role and responsibilities of the midwife in relation to the daily examination of the baby?

REFERENCES

Arkley, C., 2007. Yellow alert: identification of liver disease in neonates and their appropriate referral – the role of the midwife. MIDIRS Midwifery Dig. 14 (4), 571–573.

Blackburn, S.T., 2013. Maternal, Fetal and Neonatal Physiology: A Clinical Perspective, fourth ed. Saunders, St. Louis, p. 376.

Crossland, D.S., Richmond, S., Hudson, M., et al., 2008. Weight change in the term baby in the first 2 weeks of life. Acta Paediatr. 97, 425–429.

Dinsmoor, M.J., Viloria, R., Lief, L., Elder, S., 2005. Use of intrapartum antibiotics and the incidence of postnatal maternal and neonatal yeast infections. Obstet. Gynecol. 106 (1), 19–22.

Grossman, X., Chaudhuri, J.H., Feldman-Winter, L., Merewood, A., 2012. Neonatal weight loss at a US baby-friendly hospital. J. Acad. Nutr. Diet. 112, 410–413.

Johnston, P.G.B., Flood, K., Spinks, K., 2003. The Newborn Child, ninth ed. Churchill Livingstone, Edinburgh.

NICE (National Institute for Health and Care Excellence), 2014. Postnatal care clinical guideline 37. Available online: <https://www.nice.org.uk/guidance/cg37> (accessed 3 March 2015).

Tawia, S., McGuire, L., 2014. Early weight loss and weight gain in healthy, full-term, exclusively-breastfed infants. Breastfeed. Rev. 22 (1), 31–41.

UNICEF (United Nations Children's Fund) UK, 2014. Breastfeeding assessment form. Available online: <http://www.unicef.org.uk/Documents/Baby_Friendly/Guidance/breastfeeding_assessment_tool_mat.pdf?epslanguage=en> (accessed 9 November 2015).

Chapter | 39 |

Assessment of the baby: capillary sampling

LEARNING OUTCOMES

Having read this chapter, the reader should be able to:

- describe the procedure for obtaining a heel prick capillary blood sample
- discuss the factors that need to be considered to promote the safety and comfort of the baby
- describe in detail the specific considerations for taking a reliable newborn blood spot screening (NBS)
- discuss the role and responsibilities of the midwife in relation to capillary sampling.

This chapter considers capillary blood sampling from the baby. Obtaining blood samples from the neonate via a heel prick remains a simple, generally effective method. The midwife undertakes this as part of routine national screening in the UK, and also to detect or confirm deviations from the norm (eg serum bilirubin or serum glucose estimations).

UNDERPINNING ANATOMY

For a heel prick blood test the blood is obtained from the capillaries contained within the skin. The arterial–venous network of the skin is located at the junction of the lower dermis and upper subcutaneous tissue. The skin should be punctured only to the depth of this junction to facilitate blood flow; a deeper puncture can have serious complications. If the calcaneus (heel bone) is punctured, there is a risk of osteochondritis or osteomyelitis. The distance between the skin and bone can vary depending on where on the foot the measurement is taken (with the narrowest distance being at the posterior curve of the heel) and the weight and gestation of the baby.

Another consideration is the position of plantar arteries and nerves, which should be avoided. Puncturing the arteries can result in haemorrhage and increases the risk of introducing infection, which could result in septicaemia. Puncturing the nerves can result in permanent damage to the nerve.

Blumenfeld et al (1979) estimated the distance from the surface of the skin to the arterial–venous network to be 0.35–1.6 mm (post-mortem). Jain & Rutter (1999)

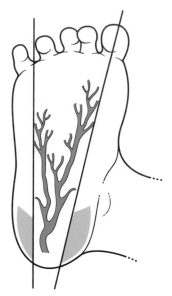

Figure 39.1 *Shaded areas:* the ideal sites for capillary sampling in the baby.

attempted to replicate this work with live babies and argue that none of the babies in their study had a distance of less than 3 mm between capillaries and skin, and thus argue that any part of the plantar surface would be suitable for pricking. However, for NBS the guidelines are clear that for a single test the sites shaded in Figure 39.1 should be used (described below), with a maximum puncture depth of 2 mm. For repeated testing the plantar surface of the whole heel may be considered but to a maximum puncture depth of 1 mm. Automated lancets vary in their puncture depth but often the greatest is 2.4 mm. Using something other than an automated device is forbidden; it is highly likely that puncture depth will be in excess of the maximum permitted.

GUIDELINES FOR SITE SELECTION

- Use the lateral and medial portions of the heel (plantar surface) as puncture sites (UKNSPC 2012).
- Draw an imaginary line from midway between the fourth and fifth toes laterally and medially from the middle of the big toe as the calcaneus rarely extends beyond these (Fig. 39.1) (these points are also furthest away from the arteries and nerves). Puncture the skin on the sole of the heel, not on the side or back of the heel.
- Select a new puncture site not previously punctured and free from bruising, for each collection.

Repeated heel pricks can also make the localized skin sore or infected and the baby is also exposed to a repeatedly painful procedure (discussed below). A consistently good sampling technique reduces the risks for the baby and limits the number of negative experiences. The midwife and parents can be confident that the result is not influenced by a poor sampling technique. If repeated sampling is required some other form of venous access, e.g. peripheral cannula, may be considered as an alternative.

NEWBORN BLOOD SPOT SCREENING (NBS)

NBS is offered to all babies in the UK and should be taken between 5 and 8 days after birth (day of birth being day 0), ideally on day 5 (this may vary internationally). Screening at this age is recommended in order to instigate diagnosis/treatment as early as possible. Currently five different disorders are screened from these blood spots:

- phenylketonuria (PKU)
- congenital hypothyroidism
- sickle cell disease
- cystic fibrosis
- medium-chain acyl coenzyme A dehydrogenase deficiency (MCADD).

In 2015 a further four rare conditions were added to the list: maple syrup urine disease, isovaleric acidaemia, glutaric aciduria, and homocystinuria. The reader is encouraged to remain up to date with constantly evolving testing schedules.

The blood spot form is accompanied by its own glassine envelope. A type of blotting paper is used for the drops of blood; this allows the blood to soak through to the required depth for accurate testing. There are four circles, each one needs to have one drop of blood in it, that fills the circle fully. Three percent of tests per year (20,000 babies) need repeating because of poor sampling or incorrect documentation. Inaccurate results may be obtained if the blood:

- is multilayered
- is multi-spotted (several smaller drops fill the circle)
- has been forced out of the heel by squeezing
- is contaminated (faeces, adult blood, alcohol, heparin, or any other substance in close proximity) or compressed
- has not soaked through.

Repeat tests are requested if:

- a specific condition, e.g. cystic fibrosis, requires it
- the test was taken before 4 days of age
- the specimen card has errors or omissions
- the test was taken less than 72 hours after transfusion of a blood product

- it is an insufficient or contaminated sample
- if there has been a delay in it reaching the laboratory (UKNSPC 2012). All specimens should be posted first class immediately.

Historically there has been guidance with regard to ingestion of milk feeds for certain days before testing, presence of antibiotics, and gestational age. The UKNSPC are clear that testing should be undertaken on day 5 irrespective of these things. For babies cared for in specialist units, blood can be taken for blood spot screening along with other specimens so long as there is no contamination of the spots. If a transfusion is anticipated, babies less than 5 days old should have a single spot specimen taken, marked 'pre-transfusion' and dispatched with the routine screening on day 5 (or specimen taken 3 days after the transfusion is completed). The date of transfusion must be recorded on the card. Babies born before 32 weeks' gestation require a second screen at 28 days of age.

One of the UKNSPC's standards (2012) is that the form should be completed fully, contemporaneously, and with the baby's NHS number (ideally a bar coded label given to parents on discharge from hospital). Parents also need to be able to give informed consent for the test; the UKNSPC recommends the booklet *Screening Tests for You and Your Baby* (downloadable) suggesting that it is given antenatally and then discussed again at least 24 hours prior to the test. In the event of declining any or all of the screenings, 'DECLINE' should be written on the form, and it should be forwarded to the laboratory and fully labelled, as for any others. Parents should receive the result before their 6–8 week paediatric assessment; the health visitor should be contacted if the result has not arrived.

BILIRUBIN ESTIMATION

A capillary sample may be taken to estimate the level of unconjugated bilirubin in the blood of a jaundiced baby. While the test may vary, often two thin pre-heparinized capillary tubes are filled with blood. Care should be taken to avoid getting air in the capillary tubes as this may result in the blood dispersing totally from the tubes during spinning, necessitating a further blood test. Alternatively blood may be collected drop by drop into a neonatal sampling bottle. Care should be taken to ensure that the correctly sized sample is collected, failure to do so often requires a repeat specimen.

BLOOD GLUCOSE ESTIMATION

This is usually undertaken as a diagnostic test when hypoglycaemia is suspected or as a screening test in babies considered to be 'at risk' of developing hypoglycaemia. The midwife should be familiar with the equipment used to estimate the level of glucose in the blood. Increasingly, blood glucose is being estimated via a venepuncture sample rather than a capillary sample as the results are more accurate. Cleansing of the skin with alcohol-impregnated wipes affects the accuracy of the results (among other things) and should not be done.

FACTORS TO CONSIDER WHEN UNDERTAKING CAPILLARY SAMPLING

Preparation

Informed consent should be gained (see above for NBS) whatever the nature of the test, along with an indication of how and when to expect the results.

The need to warm the foot in advance (with extra socks or warm water is no longer considered appropriate. UKNSPC (2012) support non-warming of the foot, noting that a warm baby is all that is needed. Barker et al (1996) found in their trial that foot warming had no effect on the time taken, baby's response or need for a second specimen. Hassan & Shah (2005) illustrate a case of scalding that occurred when a warm water nappy had been wrapped around the foot.

Comfort of the baby

Despite giving informed consent, many parents will still find these kinds of procedures difficult to cope with. Most parents will appreciate explanations of what is going to happen, the baby's expected response, and what they can do to assist. Others may choose to absent themselves and allow the midwife to continue alone. In both instances reassurances are necessary; part of the baby's comfort will come from its parents' response.

There are a number of behavioural responses to pain seen within the baby, which include facial expressions, body movements, and crying characteristics. Facial expressions consisting of brow bulge, eye squeeze, nasolabial furrow, and open lips can be seen in the majority of babies within 6 seconds of the heel prick. Facial expressions are considered more specific than body movements (which also occur in response to wiping the heel with a medicated swab) and crying (premature infants are less likely to cry) (Harrison & Johnston 2002). For many babies, however, this elicits a crying response with some becoming very distressed. This may inhibit blood flow as the leg muscles contract and impede circulation. Physiological responses including an increase in the heart and respiratory rate may also be seen, although it is not known if this is due to the pain of the procedure or the effects of being handled. The midwife should consider how the pain and discomfort can be reduced.

For the baby who is breastfeeding when the procedure is performed, very little pain symptomatology may be noticed, particularly when this is combined with skin-to-skin contact (Shah et al 2012, Gray et al 2000). If not breastfed at the time, the baby should be cuddled and spoken to gently with good eye-to-eye contact. Swaddling may also reduce the discomfort. While not supported by researched evidence, it would seem sensible to consider formula feeding (if that is the feeding choice) in skin-to-skin contact, as another possible means of promoting comfort. Massage and non-nutritive sucking are other potential physiological pain relievers.

Oral sucrose reduces the pain behaviour exhibited (Bilgen et al 2001, Overgaard & Knudsen 1999). While Stevens et al (2013) agree that sucrose is safe and effective for a single event, they suggest an optimal dose has not yet been identified and repeated use of sucrose in babies requiring several capillary samples should be investigated. Use of sucrose in the very low birthweight baby, where the condition is unstable or the baby is ventilated, also needs to be investigated further (Stevens et al 2013). Some parents may be opposed to the idea of administering sucrose to their baby. Overgaard & Knudsen (1999) found that making sure the baby was quiet and relaxed prior to the capillary sampling had a similar effect to sucrose administration.

The use of a local anaesthetic gel has been proposed for neonatal venepuncture (Moore 2001) and heel pricks (Bellini et al 2002) although Jain et al (2001) found it to be ineffective. If this is to be used, it is important to ensure it is suitable for use in neonates and will not cause vasoconstriction, as this will increase the difficulty in obtaining a sample and increase the pain felt by the baby. It is also important that the specimen is not contaminated by it.

Cleansing and puncturing the foot

For NBS the UKNSPC (2012) suggest that the heel should be cleansed with warm water and should be dried carefully. Soft paraffin preparations should be avoided. The use of automated lancets is indicated.

Safety

Non-sterile gloves should be worn for any capillary sampling. The danger of sharps injury is reduced by automated lancets that 'withdraw' after firing. A sharps box must be used at the point of care.

Facilitating blood flow

Newborn babies have a sluggish circulation or vasoconstriction (acrocyanosis) that may affect not only the amount of blood obtained but also the measurement of some blood tests. The baby should be kept warm, with only the foot exposed during the procedure. Holding the foot downwards encourages blood flow. If the blood is not flowing well, the temptation to squeeze the foot must be resisted, blood spot results are affected if the blood is diluted by interstitial fluid from squeezing and the risks of haemolysis and bruising are also increased.

Blood collection

After puncturing the foot, patience should be employed to allow a large drop of blood to collect. Permalloo & Chapple (2008) suggest that 15 seconds allows for this, longer may see the blood clotting.

- Newborn blood spot screening: ensure that one large drop of blood drops onto the top side of the card into each circle. It should soak through automatically. Allow it to air dry before placing the card in the envelope. (Some authorities require longer drying times, the reader is advised to understand their local protocol).
- Blood glucose: one large drop of blood is placed onto/into the reagent strip (depending on the type of monitor used).
- Bilirubin estimation: the end of the capillary tube is placed in the drop of blood and one finger is placed on the other end of the tube. The blood is drawn into the capillary tube and the finger removed to facilitate the passage of the blood down the tube, taking care not to allow the blood to spill out the other end or air to enter. When full, the tubes are sealed, often with plasticine.
- Placing the specimen into a blood bottle requires patience, allowing it to drip in drop by drop. The heel can be held with slight tension and released as the drop falls, but while this action appears to be squeezing and releasing, squeezing the foot is not appropriate and should not happen (see above).

Stopping the bleeding

When sufficient blood has been obtained, pressure should be applied to the site using gauze or cotton wool, to stem blood flow and decrease the risk of haematoma formation and bruising. When the bleeding has stopped, hypoallergenic tape or a plaster may be applied.

Record keeping and specimen dispatch

As well as the specimen card (discussed above), records are completed that indicate when the test was taken and for the NBS, when it was sent to the laboratory. Completed NBS cards should be sent via first class mail on the same day. All other specimens should be processed or dispatched promptly. NBS screening should also be recorded in the child's personal health record (red book). Results from the laboratory should be recorded and acted upon; NBS results should be sought by the Health Visitor if not received within 6–8 weeks.

PROCEDURE: obtaining a capillary sample

- Gain informed consent from the parents; determine if they will be present and who will hold the baby.
- Gather equipment:
  - automated lancet
  - non-sterile gloves
  - warm water
  - appropriate form/blood bottle/reagent strip or capillary tube (check expiry date if applicable)
  - cotton wool balls or gauze swabs
  - plaster /hypoallergenic tape
  - portable sharps box.
- Wash and dry hands, apply gloves.
- Ask the parent to hold/cuddle/comfort/breastfeed the baby according to chosen method of comfort, encourage a calm and relaxed atmosphere.
- Inspect the foot to select the best site (free from previous punctures or bruising), avoiding underlying nerves and bone (Fig. 39.1).
- Wipe with warm water and gauze swab, dry, ensure it is completely dry before puncturing.
- Hold the ankle with the non-dominant hand with the foot flexed.
- With the dominant hand pierce the skin with the lancet; put used lancet in sharps box.
- Hold the foot downwards, wait patiently for a large drop of blood to accumulate (approximately 15 seconds), collect the specimen as required (see above).
- If the blood clots, wipe away firmly with gauze, it is likely that it will begin flowing again. Avoid squeezing the foot. If blood does not flow, consider a second puncture using a different site on the same foot, or the other foot.
- When completed, use a cotton wool ball or gauze swab to apply pressure to the site; apply plaster/tape if required. Re-dress the baby.

- Dispose of equipment correctly and wash and dry hands. Dispatch the specimen.
- Document the taking of the specimen and relevant results, and act accordingly.

ROLE AND RESPONSIBILITIES OF THE MIDWIFE

These can be summarized as:
- recognizing the need for capillary blood sampling
- undertaking the procedure correctly and safely at the correct time
- ensuring comfort measures for the baby
- education and support of the parents
- contemporaneous record keeping
- actioning the results, where appropriate.

SUMMARY

- Obtaining a capillary blood sample from the baby should be undertaken only when required, as there are risk factors associated with this procedure. Informed consent should be gained from the parents.
- The reliability of the results partly depends upon the accuracy of the procedure. When undertaking NBS (day 5), care should be taken not to contaminate the specimen, to fill each circle with one large drop of blood, to fully complete the request card and to ensure its prompt dispatch.
- The midwife should be aware of the measures that can facilitate a non-traumatic experience for the parents and the baby.

SELF-ASSESSMENT EXERCISES

The answers to the following questions may be found in the text:
1. List the indications for undertaking capillary blood sampling.
2. When obtaining a capillary blood sample from the heel of the baby, how can the risk of damage to the underlying nerves and bone be minimized?
3. When obtaining a capillary blood sample from the heel of the baby, how can blood flow be encouraged?
4. List the factors that could contribute to needing a repeat specimen when undertaking NBS.
5. How can the amount of pain felt by the baby be reduced?
6. What are the role and responsibilities of the midwife in relation to capillary sampling?

REFERENCES

Barker, D.P., Willetts, B., Cappendijk, V.C., et al., 1996. Capillary blood sampling: should the heel be warmed? Arch. Dis. Child. 74, F139–F140.

Bellini, C.V., Bagnoli, F., Perrone, S., et al., 2002. Effect of multisensory stimulation on analgesia in term neonates: a randomised controlled trial. Pediatr. Res. 41 (4), 460–463.

Bilgen, H., Ozek, E., Cebeci, D., et al., 2001. Comparison of sucrose, expressed breast milk and breast-feeding on the neonatal response to heel prick. J. Pain 2 (5), 301–305.

Blumenfeld, T.A., Turi, G.K., Blanc, W.A., 1979. Recommended site and depth of newborn heel skin punctures based on anatomical measurements and histopathology. Lancet 1, 230–233.

Gray, L., Watt, L., Blass, E.M., 2000. Skin-to-skin contact is analgesic in healthy newborns. Pediatrics 105 (1), 460–463.

Harrison, D., Johnston, L., 2002. Bedside assessment of heel lance pain in the hospitalized infant. J. Obstet. Gynaecol. Neonatal Nurs. 31 (5), 551–557.

Hassan, Z., Shah, M., 2005. Scald injury from the Guthrie test: should the heel be warmed? Arch. Dis. Child. Fetal Neonatal Ed. 90 (6), F533–F534.

Jain, A., Rutter, N., 1999. Ultrasound study of heel to calcaneum depth in neonates. Arch. Dis. Child. 80, F243–F245.

Jain, A., Rutter, N., Ratnayaka, M., 2001. Topical amethocaine gel for pain relief of heel prick blood sampling: a randomised double blind controlled trial. Arch. Dis. Child. Fetal Neonatal Ed. 84, F56–F59.

Moore, J., 2001. No more tears: a randomized controlled double-blind trial of amethocaine gel vs. placebo in the management of procedural pain in neonates. J. Adv. Nurs. 34 (4), 475–482.

Overgaard, C., Knudsen, A., 1999. Pain-relieving effect of sucrose in newborns during heel prick. Biol. Neonate 75, 279–284.

Permalloo, N., Chapple, J., 2008. Newborn screening revisited: what midwives need to know. In: Edwins, J. (Ed.), Community Midwifery Practice. Blackwell, Oxford, pp. 107–131.

Shah, P., Herbozo, C., Aliwalas, L., Shah, V., 2012. Breastfeeding or breast milk for procedural pain in neonates. Cochrane Database Syst. Rev. (12), Art. No.: CD004950, doi:10.1002/14651858.CD004950.pub3.

Stevens, B., Yamada, J., Lee, G., Ohlsson, A., 2013. Sucrose for analgesia in newborn infants undergoing painful procedures. Cochrane Database Syst. Rev. (1), Art. No.: CD001069, doi:10.1002/14651858.CD001069.pub4.

UKNSPC (UK Newborn Screening Programme Centre), 2012. Guidelines for Newborn Blood Spot Sampling. NHS, London. Available online: <https://www.gov.uk/government/publications/newborn-blood-spot-screening-sampling-guidelines> (accessed 17 Sept. 2015).

Chapter | 40 |

Assessment of the baby: developmental dysplasia of the hips

LEARNING OUTCOMES

Having read this chapter, the reader should be able to:

- discuss the factors that contribute to developmental dysplasia of the hips (DDH)
- describe DDH and how it is classified
- describe the different tests that are used to assess for DDH
- discuss how DDH may be prevented once the baby is born
- discuss the role and responsibilities of the midwife in relation to DDH.

Developmental dysplasia of the hips (DDH) is used to describe a wide range of conditions related to the development of the hips in babies through to young children. It includes abnormal development of the acetabulum and proximal femur (the femoral head and neck, and the greater and lesser trochanter) through to mechanical instability of the hip joint (Rosenfeld et al 2014). If undiagnosed or left untreated, there is associated long-term morbidity of gait abnormalities, chronic pain, degenerative osteoarthritis, and avascular necrosis due to impairment of the blood supply, leading to hip replacement often before the age of 40 years, widening of the perineum, and hyperlordosis (Rosenfeld et al 2014, Shorter et al 2013, Wang et al 2013). DDH has also been called congenital dislocation of the hip, hip dysplasia, developmental dislocation of the hip, and acetabular dislocation. In some countries the assessment is undertaken by midwives at birth as part of the first examination, e.g. New Zealand, whereas in other countries, such as the UK, the assessment is undertaken by a paediatrician (often junior doctors rather than Registrars or Consultants) or a midwife who has undertaken further training and assessment in the examination of the newborn (NMC 2012). This chapter considers the factors that predispose to DDH, how it might be prevented, and a discussion of the tests undertaken to screen for DDH, who should undertake these and when, with reference to the management of DDH.

WHAT IS DDH?

DDH occurs when the femoral head is not sitting centrally in the acetabulum. This can occur during late pregnancy or during the neonatal period. There may be dislocation (total loss of contact between the acetabulum and the femoral head) or subluxation (the femoral head is partially within the acetabulum in a non-centric position). The hip may:

- have instability where the femoral head is reduced (meaning 'within the acetabulum') at rest but not with movement, and there is laxity within the acetabulum
- be subluxable if the femoral head is reduced at rest but can be partially dislocated with examination manoeuvres (also referred to as mild instability)
- be reducible if the hip is dislocated at rest but, with manipulation, the femoral head can be positioned into the acetabulum (Rosenfeld et al 2014).

During the neonatal period the femoral head and acetabular cartilage continue to grow, which is critical for normal hip development, as is reduction and stability of the femoral head (Hart et al 2006). It is normal for babies to have physiological laxity of the hip during the first few weeks of life; however, this usually resolves spontaneously as the acetabulum and femoral head grow and development continues normally (Rosenfeld et al 2014). Rosenfeld et al (2014) suggest that of the 60% of babies who have hip instability in the first week of life, 90% will have stabilized by 2 months.

Continued dislocation of the femoral head causes the tendons, muscles and bony structures to develop secondary adaptive changes which include stretching of the acetabular capsule, leading to the development of abnormal attachments, shortening and contracture of muscles, flattening of the femoral head and acetabular dysplasia which will eventually result in osteoarthritis in childhood (Hart et al 2006).

The degree of dislocation can be classified according to the Graf hip classification type, of which there are five (Rosenfeld et al 2014):

- Type I refers to a fully mature, normal hip that has a deep acetabular cup and an angular acetabular rim with the cartilaginous roof of the acetabulum covering the femoral head.
- Type IIa is seen in infants less than 3 months of age, reflecting the physiological immaturity of the baby's hip joint. The femoral head is situated within the acetabulum but the acetabulum is shallow and the rim is round, with the cartilaginous acetabular roof covering the femoral head. Ninety percent will resolve spontaneously (Paton et al 2014).

- Type IIb are abnormal hips seen in babies over 3 months of age and will worsen without treatment. The acetabulum is slightly shallow with a round rim and the cartilaginous acetabular roof covers the femoral head.
- Type III are dislocated hips that have a shallow acetabulum while the acetabular roof is deficient.
- Type IV are dislocated hips where the acetabulum is almost flat and the acetabular roof is significantly displaced.

Hips that 'click' do not signify DDH and the term 'clicky hips' should not be used, as it is misleading. Rosenfeld et al (2014) advise a 'clunk' (or a 'jerk', suggestive of DDH) is a different sensation to a 'click', being one of a high-pitch joint popping movement rather than the clicking or snapping sensation caused by the snapping of tendons or ligaments around the hip and knee.

RISK FACTORS

The hip is thought to develop normally during pregnancy but gradually becomes abnormal for a number of reasons (Hart et al 2006). Towards the end of pregnancy there is pressure on the hip joint forcing the femur head into an abnormal position within or outside of the acetabulum; thus many of the risk factors within the literature are related to this. However Choudry et al (2013) suggest there is a lack of known factors in 69–73% of cases.

- Family history – Stevenson et al (2009) propose the risk of DDH increases 12-fold if a first-degree relative has DDH, while the International Hip Dysplasia Institute (IHDI 2015) suggest it is a 1:8 chance, and if a sibling has DDH it is 1:7, but if both a parent and a sibling have DDH the risk increases to 1:3.
- Female gender – Schwend et al (2014) state that 78% of DDH cases occur in females. Hart et al (2006) wonder if this is because female fetuses are more susceptible to the effects of maternal relaxin. However, Bracken et al (2012) point out that cord studies have shown no correlation between relaxin concentration and DDH.
- Breech (extended) presentation ≥34 weeks' gestation (Rosenfeld et al 2014, Shorter et al 2013), although if an external cephalic version is undertaken (p. 206), the risk reduces from 9.3% to 2.8% (Lambeek et al 2013), and if the baby is born by elective caesarean section, the risk reduces further (Fox & Paton 2010). Schwend et al (2014) propose the highest risk is a female fetus in an extended breech presentation.
- Improper swaddling whereby the legs are straightened to a standing position which can loosen the joints

and result in damage to the soft cartilage of the acetabulum (IHDI 2015).

- Multiple pregnancy (IHDI 2015).
- Oligohydramnios (Paton et al 2014, Rosenfeld et al 2014).
- First-born babies (Rosenfeld et al 2014).
- Ethnicity – increased in Caucasian babies (McCarthy et al 2005).
- High birthweight babies (Dezateux & Rosenthal 2007).
- Babies with fixed idiopathic congenital talipes equinovarus are not at increased risk of DDH (Paton et al 2014), although those with congenital talipes calcaneovalgus (CTCV) are 5.2 times more likely to have DDH than babies without CTCV (Paton & Choudry 2009).
- DDH may also occur when certain syndromes are present, e.g. trisomy 21, Ehlers Danlos (Rosenfeld et al 2014).

INCIDENCE

The incidence of DDH varies according to the definition used and whether or not it is a screened population. Fox & Paton (2010) suggest the incidence is 1–3 : 1000 live births, while in the US Hart et al (2006) state the incidence is 11.5 : 1000 with frank dislocation occurring 1–2 : 1000, which Clarke et al (2012) agree with.

Bracken et al (2012) suggest the left hip is four times more likely to be affected than the right; however, Hart et al (2006) suggest the left hip is affected in 60% of cases, the right hip in 20% and both hips in 20% of cases. It is thought the left hip is affected more because the fetus is more likely to lie on the left side of the uterus, pushing the left hip against the maternal sacrum and preventing movement of the hip joint.

Late presentation can occur despite the previous tests being normal (Jaiswal et al 2010) and Schwend et al (2014) propose the incidence of this is 1 : 5000, suggesting the condition may be occult. However litigation around missed diagnosis is increasing (Clarke et al 2012) and Atrey et al (2010) found that DDH was the third most common cause of litigation in orthopaedics over a 10-year period in English Health Trusts with an average cost per case of £48,534.

WHEN TO ASSESS FOR DEVELOPMENTAL DYSPLASIA OF THE HIPS

The NSC (2008) recommend that all babies have an examination that includes screening for DDH within 72 hours of birth and repeated by 6 weeks of age. However, during the first 72 hours there will be more hips that appear to be dislocatable which could lead to over-referral for suspected DDH and possibly overtreatment (Shorter et al 2013). There is still an ongoing debate about whether DDH should be assessed at birth or when the baby is older, as the majority of cases of DDH detected at birth resolve spontaneously in the first week of life (Mahan & Kassler 2008). Isolated hip clicks are not pathological but are a frequent cause of referral and will stabilize as the baby gets older (Mahan & Kassler 2008). However, early detection and treatment is necessary to prevent serious damage to the acetabulum; thus it would seem prudent to follow the advice of the UK National Screening Committee (NSC) and screen early, ensuring practitioners are competent in assessing the hips. Midwives who do this regularly are in a better position to do this than the junior doctors who are doing a rotation to Paediatrics and who may have received little or no training in screening for DDH (Cescutti-Butler 2013, Talbot & Paton 2013). Schwend et al (2014) agree, referring to a study among US Navajo Indians where the most significant DDH cases were found by a competent practitioner regardless of their profession.

SCREENING FOR DDH

National screening in the UK was introduced in 1969 and today involves assessing the length and appearance of the legs and skin folds, manipulating the legs using the Barlow's test and or Ortolani's test while assessing the range of abduction and Klisic's sign. Screening is ideally discussed during the antenatal period and revisited prior to testing to ensure the parents can provide informed consent. The NSC (2008) recommend parents receive written information about the screening tests during pregnancy.

Length of the legs

In the presence of unilateral DDH, one leg will be shorter than the other. This is assessed by lying the baby on his back without a nappy on, flexing his hips and knees with his feet flat on the surface, and touching his buttocks. The height of the knees can be seen and should be the same if there is no DDH but this may also occur with bilateral DDH. If one knee is lower than the other, it is suggestive of unilateral DDH in the shorter leg. This is known as the Galeazzi test or Allis sign. The baby needs to be relaxed to do this which may be easier to achieve after the baby has fed.

Appearance of skin folds

When both femur heads are in the acetabulum the skin folds should be symmetrical. Bracken et al (2012) advise that isolated asymmetrical thigh and gluteal (buttock) skin folds are common during the neonatal period; nevertheless, asymmetrical skin folds may be indicative of DDH. These can be seen when the baby is on his back or his front. While Rosenfeld et al (2014) advise asymmetrical thigh skin folds are suggestive of DDH, the IHDI (2015) disagree, cautioning they are rarely indicative of DDH unless the gluteal folds are asymmetrical. These are assessed with the baby on his front. Rosenfeld et al (2014) recommend assessing whether the inguinal folds reaches beyond the anus, as they do not in the absence of DDH. If one inguinal fold extends beyond the anal, opening it is suggestive of

unilateral DDH whereas bilateral DDH is suspected if both extend beyond the anal opening.

Barlow's test

Barlow's test is a manoeuvre that attempts to push the femoral head out of the acetabulum to assess if it is dislocatable. It involves adducting the hip by bringing the thigh towards the midline and applying light pressure in a downward (posterior) direction (Fig. 40.1). A positive test occurs if the femoral head dislocates, often felt as a 'clunk'; the normal hip should not dislocate.

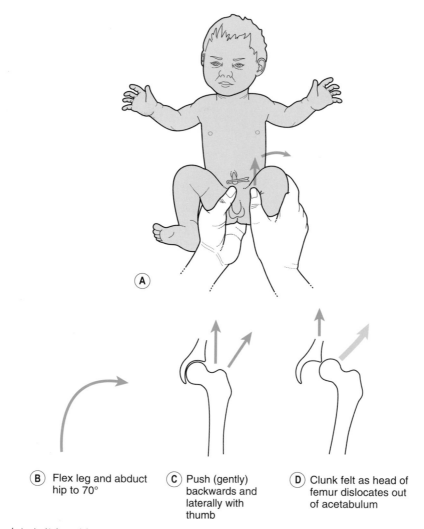

A

B Flex leg and abduct hip to 70°

C Push (gently) backwards and laterally with thumb

D Clunk felt as head of femur dislocates out of acetabulum

Figure 40.1 Barlow's test. *(Adapted from Farrell & Sittlington 2009)*

PROCEDURE: undertaking the Barlow's test

- Discuss the procedure and gain informed consent from the parents, undertaking the examination in the presence of one or both parents.
- Wash and dry hands; apply non-sterile gloves if necessary.
- Lie the baby on his back on a flat, firm surface.
- Ensure the baby is warm and relaxed, then undress the baby from the waist down, removing the nappy.
- Bring the baby's legs together with the hips and knees flexed.
- Examining the hips one at a time, hold the knee and hip in a flexed position; then abduct the hip, placing a thumb on the inner aspect of the thigh (over the inner trochanter) and the index and middle fingers over the outer part of the thigh (over the greater trochanter of the femur at the hip).
- Gently adduct the leg toward the midline while pushing down on the hip laterally towards the supporting surface then gently pulling the leg upwards to try to dislocate the hip laterally.
- Repeat with other leg.
- Redress the baby and return to parents.
- Wash and dry hands.
- Discuss the findings with the parents.
- Document the findings and act accordingly.

Ortolani's test

This manoeuvre is undertaken to relocate a dislocated or unstable femoral head back into the acetabulum by applying pressure on the back of the greater trochanter. If the femoral head relocates (reduces) a clunk may be felt (Fig. 40.2). A normal hip will not produce a clunk, as the femoral head is not dislocatable.

PROCEDURE: undertaking the Ortolani's test

- Discuss the procedure and gain informed consent from the parents, undertaking the examination in the presence of one or both parents.
- Wash and dry hands; apply non-sterile gloves if necessary.
- Lie the baby on his back on a flat, firm surface.
- Ensure the baby is warm and relaxed, then undress the baby from the waist down, removing the nappy.

- Bring the baby's legs together with the hips and knees flexed.
- Examining the hips one at a time, take hold of each leg, placing the thumb on the inner aspect of the thigh (over the inner trochanter) and the index and middle fingers over the outer aspect of the thigh (greater trochanter of the femur at the hip).
- Flex the knees and the hips 90° and gently abduct the leg (a 'clunk' is felt as the dislocated head of the femur is moved back into the acetabulum; if no clunk is felt, but the leg cannot be abducted fully, DDH is also indicated).
- Redress the baby and return to parents.
- Wash and dry hands.
- Discuss the findings with the parents.
- Document the findings and act accordingly.

Klisic's sign

With the baby positioned on his back, place the index finger on the anterior superior iliac spine and the middle finger on the greater trochanter. An imaginary line is drawn between these two points and should point towards or above the umbilicus if the hip is not dislocated and will be below the umbilicus if DDH is present (Rosenfeld et al 2014). Bilateral DDH may be suspected from this sign if both imaginary lines are below the umbilicus.

DIAGNOSIS

If there is a positive Barlow's or Ortolani's test, the baby should be referred for an ultrasound assessment of the hips. This will review the acetabulum and femoral head and measure different angles to determine if DDH is present. The ultrasound should be reviewed by an experienced orthopaedic paediatric surgeon.

TREATMENT

Depending on when DDH is diagnosed, different treatment options are available. These include using a Pavlik harness which is designed to gently reposition the baby's hips in a well-aligned and secure position so that the femoral head and acetabulum can grow and develop normally. Other splints include the Von Rosen splint and a variety of hip abduction braces. For late diagnosis, surgery may be required which is either closed or open reduction, and may also include use of a spica body cast.

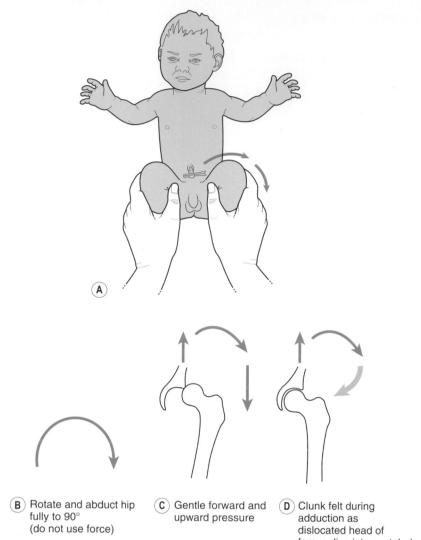

(A)

(B) Rotate and abduct hip fully to 90° (do not use force)

(C) Gentle forward and upward pressure

(D) Clunk felt during adduction as dislocated head of femur slips into acetabulum

Figure 40.2 Ortolani's test. *(Adapted from Farrell & Sittlington 2009)*

PREVENTION

Swaddling is a major cause of DDH as noted in cultures where the legs are tightly wrapped so they are positioned together and straight (as if standing). This position does not encourage the femoral head to remain in the acetabulum. This is still a common practice within areas of the Middle East and other countries and DDH rates are

high (Clarke 2014). In cultures where babies and children are carried in the straddle/jockey position, often in warmer climates such as the native sub-Saharan African population, e.g. Malawi, DDH is rarely encountered (Graham et al 2015). This style of carrying the baby is similar to the baby in a Pavlik harness. Swaddling tightly with blankets has the same effect, as babies are not able to flex their hips and knees and this is increasing in popularity in an attempt to encourage the baby to settle and sleep for longer and reduce crying. Clarke (2014) suggests that approximately 90% of babies in North America are swaddled in the first few months of life. In Japan, rates of DDH have fallen from between 1.1% to 3.5% with traditional swaddling to 0.2% when it is not done! It also happens with some car seats and baby slings where the legs are encouraged together rather than apart.

To counteract the negative effects of placing the hips into forced sustained passive hip extension and adduction while the hips are developing during the first few months of life, the IHDI (2015) suggest the baby should be positioned so the hips are slightly flexed and abducted, with knees flexed, as they would be during late fetal life. They have a video showing how to swaddle babies to facilitate this on their website: http://hipdysplasia.org/developmental-dysplasia-of-the-hip/hip-healthy-swaddling/ which the reader is encouraged to watch. IDHI also provide advice on how to choose baby carriers such as slings, car seats and bouncers to encourage the correct positioning of the baby's hips and knees. The Lullaby Trust (2015) also recommend that thin materials are used, swaddling is not used above the baby's shoulders and should not be too tight, the swaddled baby should not sleep on his front, and parents should check the baby's temperature to ensure he is not getting too hot. For further information, visit their website: http://www.lullabytrust.org.uk/swaddling-slings.

The midwife can play a vital role in reducing the rates of DDH by advising parents on how to swaddle their baby if this is what they want to do and advise them on how to choose a baby carrier to encourage good positioning of the hips and knees.

ROLE AND RESPONSIBILITIES OF THE MIDWIFE

These can be summarized as:
- discussing the DDH screening test with parents and providing suitable information for them to make an informed decision with regard to DDH screening
- being aware of the risk factors that may increase the incidence of DDH and advising parents on the care of their baby to reduce this
- being able to undertake the assessment procedures for DDH correctly and safely, when appropriately trained
- referral as necessary if the screening test is positive
- contemporaneous record keeping.

SUMMARY

- An appropriately trained and competent midwife or paediatrician should undertake the assessment for developmental dysplasia within 72 hours of birth, whether in hospital, a birthing centre or at home.
- There are two tests that can be used to assess the ability of the femur head to dislocate: Barlow's and Ortolani's along with assessing leg length, skin fold creases (Galeazzi sign) and Klisic's sign.
- If swaddling the baby, it should be done in such a way that the hips are slightly flexed and abducted and the knees flexed.

SELF-ASSESSMENT EXERCISES

The answers to the following questions may be found in the text:

1. When would the midwife undertake the test for DDH?
2. Describe the two methods of assessment.
3. What would you notice from Klisic's sign and inguinal folds that would lead you to suspect bilateral DDH?
3. What is the significance of the 'clunk'?
4. What are the role and responsibilities of the midwife in relation to the assessment of DDH?

REFERENCES

Atrey, A., Gupte, C.M., Corbett, S.A., 2010. Review of successful litigation against English Health Trusts in the treatment of adults with orthopaedic pathology: clinical governance lessons learned. J. Bone Joint Surg. Am. 92, e36.

Bracken, J., Tron, T., Ditchfield, M., 2012. Developmental dysplasia of the hip: controversies and current concepts. J. Paediatr. Child Health 48, 963–973.

Cescutti-Butler, L., 2013. Examination of a newborn: whose job – midwife or doctor? You decide… MIDIRS Midwifery Digest 23 (4), 512–515.

Choudry, Q., Goyal, R., Paton, R.W., 2013. Is limitation of hip abduction a useful clinical sign in the diagnosis of developmental dysplasia of the hip? Arch. Dis. Child. 98, 862–866.

Clarke, N.M.P., 2014. Swaddling and hip dysplasia: an orthopaedic perspective. Arch. Dis. Child. 99 (1), 5–6.

Clarke, N.M.P., Reading, I.C., Corbin, C., et al., 2012. Twenty years' experience of selective secondary ultrasound screening for congenital dislocation of the hip. Arch. Dis. Child. 97, 423–429.

Dezateux, C., Rosenthal, K., 2007. Developmental dysplasia of the hip. Lancet 369, 1541–1552.

Farrell, P., Sittlington, N., 2009. The normal baby. In: Fraser, D.M., Cooper, M.A. (Eds.), Myles Textbook for Midwives, fifth ed. Churchill Livingstone, Edinburgh, pp. 778–779.

Fox, A.E., Paton, R.W., 2010. The relationship between mode of delivery and developmental dysplasia of the hip in breech infants. J. Bone Joint Surg. Br. 92 (12), 1695–1699.

Graham, S.M., Manara, J., Chokotho, L., Harrison, W.J., 2015. Back-carrying infants to prevent developmental dysplasia and its sequelae: is a new public health initiative needed? J. Pediatr. Orthop. 35 (1), 57–61.

Hart, E.S., Albright, M.B., Rebello, G.N., Grottkau, B.E., 2006. Developmental dysplasia of the hip. Nursing implications and anticipatory guidance for parents. Orthop. Nurs. 25 (2), 100–109.

IHDI (International Hip Dysplasia Institute), 2015. Available online: <www.hipdysplasia.org> (accessed 31 January 2015).

Jaiswal, A., Starks, I., Kiely, N.T., 2010. Late dislocation of the hip following normal neonatal clinical and ultrasound examination. J. Bone Joint Surg. Br. 92 (10), 1449–1451.

Lambeek, A.F., De Hundt, M., Vlemmix, F., et al., 2013. Risk of developmental dysplasia of the hip in breech presentation: the effect of successful external cephalic version. BJOG 120, 607–612.

Mahan, S.T., Kassler, J.R., 2008. Does swaddling influence developmental dysplasia of the hip? Pediatrics 121 (1), 177–178.

McCarthy, J., Scoles, P., MacEwen, G., 2005. Developmental dysplasia of the hip (DDH). Curr. Orthop. 19 (3), 223–230.

NSC (UK National Screening Committee), 2008. Newborn and Infant Physical Examination. Available online: <http://newbornphysical.screening.nhs.uk/standards> (accessed 1 February 2015).

NMC (Nursing and Midwifery Council), 2012. Midwives rules and standards. Available online: <http://www.nmc-uk.org/Publications/Standards/> (accessed 1 February 2015).

Paton, R.W., Choudry, Q., 2009. Neonatal foot deformities and their relationship to developmental dysplasia of the hip. J. Bone Joint Surg. Br. 91 (5), 655–658.

Paton, R.W., Choudry, Q.A., Jugday, R., Hughes, S., 2014. Is congenital talipes equinovarus a risk factor for pathological dysplasia of the hip? Bone Joint J. 96-B, 1553–1555.

Rosenfeld, S.B., Phillips, W., Torchia, M.M., 2014. Developmental dysplasia of the hip. UpToDate. Available online: <www.uptodate.com> (accessed 31 January 2015).

Schwend, R.M., Shaw, B.A., Segal, L.S., 2014. Evaluation and treatment of developmental hip dysplasia in the newborn and infant. Pediatr. Clin North Am. 61, 1095–1107.

Shorter, D., Hong, T., Osborn, D.A., 2013. Screening programmes for developmental dysplasia of the hip in newborn infants. Cochrane Database Syst. Rev. (9), Art. No.: CD004595, doi:10.1002/14651858.CD004595.pub2.

Stevenson, D.A., Mineau, G., Kerber, R.A., et al., 2009. Familial disposition to developmental dysplasia of the hip. J. Pediatr. Orthop. 29 (5), 463–466.

Talbot, C.L., Paton, R.W., 2013. Screening of selected risk factors in developmental dysplasia of the hip: an observational study. Arch. Dis. Child. 98, 692–696.

The Lullaby Trust, 2015. Swaddling. Online. Available online: <http://www.lullabytrust.org.uk/swaddling-slings> (accessed 19 February 2015).

Wang, T.-M., Wu, K.-W., Shih, S.-F., et al., 2013. Outcomes of open reduction for developmental dysplasia of the hips: does bilateral dysplasia have a poorer outcome? J. Bone Joint Surg. Am. 95 (12), 1081–1086.

Chapter | **41** |

Principles of infant nutrition: breastfeeding

LEARNING OUTCOMES

Having read this chapter, the reader should be able to:

- briefly describe the anatomy of the breast and the physiology of lactation
- describe how to facilitate correct attachment at the breast using (1) the traditional approach and (2) the concept of biological nurturing
- compare and contrast the traditional and biological nurturing practices
- discuss the recognition and significance of effective attachment at the breast, feeding cues, feeding patterns and signs of effective feeding
- discuss correct expressing and storage of breast milk.

There can be no doubt as to the suitability of human milk for human infants. It is an internationally recognized fact that babies should be breastfed *exclusively* for the first 6 months of life, and then preferably (with a weaning diet) until 2 years old and onwards (WHO 2011). However, while the UK 2010 Infant Feeding Survey (HASCIC 2012) noted an increase (since the 2005 survey) in the number of babies being breastfed at 6 weeks of age, the figure still remains low at 34%. Colson (2005a) questions the advice and care given to breastfeeding women over the last few decades and suggests that the relationship of particular maternal/child positions stimulate innate breastfeeding behaviours and so significantly aid the initiation of breastfeeding (Colson 2007a). Colson (2007a) terms this new approach to breastfeeding initiation as biological nurturing (BN). This will be reviewed in this chapter as well as the traditional approach to breastfeeding practice. Also discussed are basic breast anatomy, feeding cues and patterns, assessing for effective feeding and problem solving. The chapter ends by discussing the safe expressing and storage of breast milk.

UNDERSTANDING LACTATION

Each breast functions independently. Each has a rich blood, nerve and lymphatic supply and is comprised of glandular tissue and fat. Support is provided from ligaments. The proportions of fat and glandular tissue vary for each woman, glandular tissue increases in pregnancy under hormonal influences in preparation for lactation. In some women the proportion of glandular tissue to fat is 2 : 1.

The glandular tissue is an extensive convoluted ductal network separated into lobes. These are subdivided into lobules; within each lobule are alveoli, each of which is a cavity lined with lactocytes surrounded by myoepithelial cells. Under the influence of prolactin, milk is produced in the lactocytes. When the infant suckles (under the influence of oxytocin) the milk is propelled into the network of ducts by the muscular contraction of the myoepithelial cells. The lactiferous ducts branch to join other larger ducts, eventually opening out onto the surface of the nipple. Geddes (2009) suggests that there are 4–18 ducts opening onto the nipple, the average being 9. The network of ducts has been identified much nearer to the surface of the breast than originally thought and the milk collecting areas (lactiferous sinuses) were not visualized, suggesting that milk is transported freshly through the ducts on demand, rather than being stored.

Colostrum is present from about the 16th week of pregnancy but it is the loss of placental hormones, particularly progesterone, that initiates the rise in oxytocin and prolactin and therefore the availability of increasing volumes of milk for the newborn infant. Colson (2008, 2007b) suggests that practice should protect and encourage the mechanisms that stimulate breastfeeding hormones in order to ensure effective transfer of nutrition from mother to child. These include prolonged cuddling and baby holding, skin-to-skin contact, privacy, feeding in biological nurturing positions (below), and maintaining the physical environment in a calm, warm, safe manner (minimal neocortical stimulation). Early priming of the lactocytes is essential for the long-term production of breast milk. This occurs with an early first feed after delivery, under the influence of rising prolactin levels.

Milk is supplied according to demand; consequently it is the effective removal of milk from the breast, according to the baby's appetite and feeding action, that stimulates the milk supply. Milk composition changes during the feed (and changes over time as the infant grows) so that both the hunger and thirst are satisfied. Consequently, babies require nothing other than breast milk for the first 6 months of life. As the baby comes off the breast, the second one is always offered, the baby will only take from the second one if he is still hungry or thirsty.

SUCCESSFUL ATTACHMENT AT THE BREAST USING A TRADITIONAL APPROACH

There is no doubt in any part of the literature that an incorrect attachment at the breast potentially damages the nipples and prevents effective transfer of milk.

These are the principles for achieving successful attachment at the breast:

- Encourage the mother to be comfortable.
- Ensure that the baby's body is turned in, close to the mother's body.
- Keep the baby's head and body in a line.

- The baby should be supported across his shoulders and back so that his head can extend as he attaches (to facilitate a deep attachment) and allow him to swallow.
- The mother may find it helpful to shape the breast slightly using a 'C' hold. This helps her to direct the nipple towards the roof of the baby's mouth (this is known as an exaggerated latch). Once attached, the mother can release her hold on the breast.
- The baby's nose should be level with the nipple. As the baby's top lip brushes against the nipple, his mouth will open widely.
- With a wide mouth, the baby is brought swiftly to the breast, chin leading, aiming the nipple to the back of the baby's mouth (Fig. 41.1).
- Once attached, the baby's nose should be close but clear and if any areola is visible, there should be more above the top lip than the bottom lip.

Inch (2013) states that breastfeeding is a learnt skill. This means that the midwife's role is both in educating parents (generally using a 'hands off' approach) and in enabling the mother to gain the skills and confidence for herself. Appreciating that the baby is appropriately positioned and attached at the breast allows for feeding to be relaxed and effective. These are some of the signs that the mother can look for:

- The baby has a large mouthful of breast tissue, with his lips curled out.

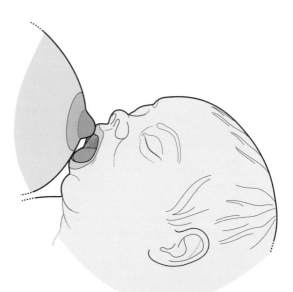

Figure 41.1 The wide gape. Note, too, the slightly extended head, proximity of top lip/nose to nipple, position of bottom lip and direction that the nipple enters the mouth.

- The baby's cheeks should be rounded and stay rounded as he feeds.
- Feeding is quiet, no sucks or clicks are heard, but audible swallowing may be heard.
- The initial drawing out of the nipple may feel momentarily uncomfortable for the mother, but thereafter feeding should be a painless experience. If continued pain is felt, the mother should be advised to break the seal from the baby's mouth using her little finger and to attach the baby again.
- Rapid sucks are seen initially, after milk has been 'let down' the sucks become deeper and slower. The baby swallows after every one or two sucks, towards the end of the feed 'flutter' sucking can be seen.
- The baby stays on the breast, pauses from sucking are seen periodically, sucking begins again spontaneously. The baby leaves the breast spontaneously and may fall asleep promptly. (The other breast is offered.)
- At the beginning of a feed the baby's arm is often held tensely upwards, as the baby feeds it relaxes and falls to the baby's side.
- The parents should see adequate urine and stool output (see below).
- From about 2 weeks of age, regular weight gain is seen.
- The breast is lighter and softer after the baby has fed with no visible change to the shape or colour of the nipple.

SUCCESSFUL ATTACHMENT AT THE BREAST: THE BIOLOGICAL NURTURING APPROACH

Biological nurturing aims to achieve the environment in which babies and mothers exhibit innate reflexes that facilitate infant feeding. The mother is encouraged to adopt a comfortable, sustainable and well-supported semi-recumbent position. Mother and baby are in skin-to-skin contact (or lightly dressed), the baby lies prone on his mother's abdomen with his head in the area of her breast. In this way the baby is fully supported by her body contours or (depending on position) his feet may be supported by the bed or pillows. It is noted that in this position, gravity holds the baby in a naturally chosen position (Batacan 2010); the more traditional approach to breastfeeding practice requires the mother to hold the baby. This difference is noted to be significant but is yet to be fully explored. The atmosphere should be relaxed and unhurried with plenty of time for caressing and cuddling. These positional interactions release the innate reflexes with which the baby is born (Colson et al 2008) (including moderately preterm

and small for gestational age infants (Colson et al 2003)). These reflexes encourage the baby, in his own time, to find the breast, self-attach and effectively feed. The baby often manoeuvres himself into the optimal position, Colson (2005b) notes that if a baby has not self-attached successfully at the breast, a modification in his body lie (the direction of his position) may then facilitate this. In her studies, babies adopted a similar lie for feeding to their *in-utero* position – longitudinal, transverse or oblique. Between feeds the baby may sleep in this position or in arms but Colson et al (2003) proposed that unrestricted access to the breast, including feeding while asleep, for at least the first 3 days of life may increase breastfeeding duration.

WHICH APPROACH SHOULD BE USED?

Skin-to-skin contact, in which immediately post-birth the baby rests against the mother's chest, skin-to-skin, has widely been recognized to facilitate several physical and emotional benefits. These include the regulation of body temperature, heart and respiration rates, stimulation of the gastrointestinal tract, introduction to friendly skin bacteria and the beginnings of emotional attachment. Moore et al (2012), after their systematic review, concluded that babies that received skin-to-skin care cried less, breastfed for longer, and had greater cardio-respiratory stability. Bergman (2013) also observed that newborns who experienced skin-to-skin care received key early neurological stimulation that particularly arose from the touch and smell of the mother. Whichever breastfeeding approach is taken, skin-to-skin contact at birth is the most important practice to support it (Barry & Murphy 2013). It can also be argued that skin-to-skin contact is the vital component that all babies need, whichever their method of feeding. Consequently, both approaches to breastfeeding should begin with uninterrupted skin-to-skin care. Thereafter, it is likely that the baby will follow the recognized nine behaviours following birth (crying, relaxation, awakening, activity, crawling, resting, familiarization, suckling and sleeping) which result in the baby self-attaching at the breast. It is recognized that mothers often have greater confidence to breastfeed where the baby can self-attach. However, biological nurturing is a technique that mothers cannot do while out or in public places and therefore the teaching of practical skills remains very important (UNICEF UK 2009). Colson (2005b) also recognizes that some mothers will still need more traditional guided but 'hands off' assistance (Inch et al 2003) to achieve correct positioning and attachment at the breast. It is noted that often babies who can self-attach adapt easily to different positions and approaches. UNICEF UK (2009) recognize the value of both breastfeeding approaches in equipping mothers to breastfeed successfully. As well as the mutual health benefits for mother and child, there is pleasure in breastfeeding – a commodity that Colson (2005a) suggests should be part of the marketing pitch for it.

FEEDING CUES

Baby-led parenting (Rapley & Murkett 2014) encourages all parents to understand the ways in which babies communicate their needs. Feeding cues are one such way; understanding these cues allows parents to respond before their baby becomes distressed, which allows for appropriate prompt care. This applies to whichever method of infant feeding is chosen. As the baby's sleep begins to lighten, rapid eye movements can be seen beneath the eyelids, this is often one of the first feeding cues. The baby may make sucking sounds, begin to 'fidget', begin to 'root' (look for the breast with their mouth), or suck his fingers. Movement of his arms and legs becomes more obvious; if there is no response to these cues, the baby begins to cry. Crying is a late feeding cue, a crying baby releases cortisol (stress hormone) and needs to be calmed before feeding can take place. If cortisol is repeatedly stimulated, brain development is affected; Entwistle (2013) discusses the evidence for this in detail.

EXPECTED FEEDING PATTERNS IN THE NEWBORN

The bioavailability of colostrum and breast milk combined with the size of the baby's stomach means that breastfed babies feed frequently. The midwife needs to establish that frequent feeding is not because of a poor latch or other breastfeeding difficulty. Frequent feeding (nutritive or non-nutritive) encourages hormonal surges, an increase in milk supply, uterine contraction and the reduction of physiological jaundice. Mothers can be reassured that such patterns, particularly in the first few days, are physiologically normal; effective feeding is achieved by 8–12 feeds in 24 hours (Mohrbacher & Stock 2003). Cluster feeding is also common – the baby feeds frequently over a short time period then may not feed for 4–5 hours (Mohrbacher & Stock 2003).

ASSESSING EFFECTIVE FEEDING

The midwife remains responsible to ensure neonatal and maternal wellbeing, whichever approach to breastfeeding

is used. The skills of observation and communication are necessary, with the ability to recognize deviations from the norm and to employ sensitive problem solving. If there is any doubt as to whether a baby is feeding effectively, the following aspects should be considered, some of which are also discussed above:

- Does the baby wake independently for feeds?
- Does the latch appear and feel to be appropriate?
- Does the baby appear satisfied on completion of the feed?
- Is there adequate urine and stooling for the baby's age? On days 1–2 there should be one or more stools, one or more voids of urine. On days 3–4 there should be two or more changing stools and 3 or more voids. The stool change through from green/brown colours to yellow should have occurred by day 5. Urine output will also increase so that by 1 week of age there should be six or more wet nappies in 24 hours and last least two stools (UNICEF UK 2014).
- Is weight gain appropriate? Greater than 10% of birthweight weight loss may be indicative of a feeding problem. Appropriate weight gain (approximately 450 g per month) is seen after 2 weeks of age (Chapter 38).
- Are the breasts and nipples problem free?
- Does the mother look any different when feeding? Colson (2007b) recognizes the role of oxytocin in creating a particular complexion for the mother. As oxytocin surges, the mother can be seen to be flushed, peaceful, relaxed, and slightly disconnected from the environment. This can be discreetly observed as an indicator of effective feeding.

PROBLEM SOLVING

A large proportion of breastfeeding problems can be traced back to a poor attachment at the breast. Insufficient milk supply, sore or cracked nipples, mastitis, and engorgement are all linked to feeding technique. If the baby is latched on correctly and permitted to demand feed, the nipples will not be traumatized, the milk will be drained properly so that engorgement and mastitis do not occur and the supply of the milk will match the demand. Hence, these problems may be overcome with further support and education to ensure that the technique is appropriate. For the mother who has not tried biological nurturing, the midwife can advocate this practice. Where there are ongoing breastfeeding difficulties, sitting and observing the feeding from the onset of the feed can provide valuable indicators as to how the problem can be overcome. The international Baby Café initiative (Rogers & Hickman 2008) provides both professional and peer support. Cup feeding (Chapter 42) may sometimes be utilized to support periods of breastfeeding difficulty or when supplementation is medically indicated. All breastfeeding women should understand how to express and store breast milk.

EXPRESSING BREAST MILK

There may be occasions when it is necessary to express breast milk, but this is not a routine part of care when the baby is attaching and feeding well. If there is separation from the baby, problems attaching the baby at the breast, a sleepy reluctant feeder, or a clinical need to increase the milk supply, then expressing may be undertaken manually by hand or by using a hand or electric pump. Hand expression is more effective and should be the method taught. It allows for the expression of colostrum, something that pumps struggle to do, due to the limited quantity of liquid.

Hand expression

Milk flow is aided by:

- the application of warmth (flannels, shower, bath) to the breasts
- relaxed peaceful environment in which the baby (or a photograph) is near
- gentle massage of the breasts using the fingers or clenched fist in a 'rolling downwards' of the breast tissue, towards the nipple
- nipple rolling.

To express the milk, the breast is cupped in the hand with the thumb above the nipple and fingers below ('C' hold), approximately 2–4 cm back from the nipple. Generally a change in texture can be easily felt by the mother; this change corresponds with the ideal place to position the fingers as it is where the glandular tissue is situated. The mother is encouraged to gently compress rhythmically, hold and then release the fingers as the milk begins to flow. When flowing well, the position of the hand should be moved around the breast to ensure all lactiferous ducts are emptied. A sterilized and wide-necked receptacle is needed to collect the milk in. A link is available from the UNICEF UK (Baby Friendly) website to a demonstration video (UNICEF UK undated). As the flow slows (after a few minutes), expressing should be switched to the other breast (unless purposely expressing one only), as that one slows, the first breast is then recommended. This pattern encourages a repeated 'let down' of the milk and should be continued until both breasts feel soft and the flow is noticeably slower. Expressed breast milk can be kept in the back of the fridge (4°C or lower) for 5 days or frozen (−19°C) for up to 6 months (DH 2013).

ROLE AND RESPONSIBILITIES OF THE MIDWIFE

These can be summarized as:

- using evidence-based practice with good communication to provide information, support, and encouragement to facilitate the woman's ability to successfully breastfeed, whichever approach is used
- generally using a 'hands off' approach that contributes towards confidence building for the mother
- monitoring of the ongoing health and wellbeing of the mother and child, employing problem-solving strategies should the need arise
- contemporaneous record keeping.

SUMMARY

- Whichever method of infant feeding is chosen, uninterrupted skin-to-skin care at birth and during the early postnatal period is the foundation to successful feeding.
- Traditional practice utilizing an upright maternal sitting position and the teaching of positioning and attachment skills has been challenged by the concept of biological nurturing. However, while there are differences, both approaches have value and both should be considered.
- Biological nurturing (Colson 2005b) encourages the mother to adopt a comfortable semi-recumbent position in which the baby lies prone on the mother and manoeuvres himself to self-attach at the breast. This action utilizes innate reflexes.
- Correct attachment at the breast is vital, both to facilitate nutrition and to prevent breastfeeding problems. Midwives need to be able to facilitate this (by whichever approach the woman uses) and to utilize problem-solving strategies accordingly.
- Understanding the feeding cues facilitate baby-led feeding. Midwives should be familiar with the ways to assess that effective feeding is taking place.

SELF-ASSESSMENT EXERCISES

The answers to the following questions may be found in the text:

1. Describe the basic anatomy and physiology of the lactating breast.
2. Discuss how this knowledge is used to promote successful breastfeeding.
3. How can the mother recognize when the baby is ready to feed?
4. Describe to a woman how to successfully attach her baby at the breast using the traditional approach.
5. Describe the features of biological nurturing.
6. Describe the markers used to assess effective breastfeeding.
7. What advice would you give to a woman who needs to hand express?

REFERENCES

Barry, M., Murphy Tighe, S., 2013. Facilitating effective initiation of breastfeeding – a review of the recent evidence base. Br. J. Midwifery 21 (5), 312–315.

Batacan, J., 2010. A new approach: Biological Nurturing and laid-back breastfeeding. Int. J. Childbirth Educ. 25 (2), 7–9.

Bergman, N., 2013. Breastfeeding and Perinatal neuroscience. In: Watson, G. (Ed.), Supporting Sucking Skills in Breastfeeding Infants, second ed. Jones & Bartlett Learning, Burlington. (Chapter 2).

Colson, S., 2005a. Maternal breastfeeding positions: have we got it right? (1). Pract. Midwife 8 (11), 24–27.

Colson, S., 2005b. Maternal breastfeeding positions: have we got it right?(2). Pract. Midwife 8 (11), 29–32.

Colson, S., 2007a. Biological Nurturing (1) a non-prescriptive recipe for breastfeeding. Pract. Midwife 10 (9), 42–48.

Colson, S., 2007b. Biological Nurturing (2) the physiology of lactation revisited. Pract. Midwife 10 (10), 14–19.

Colson, S., 2008. Bringing nature to the fore. Pract. Midwife 11 (10), 14–19.

Colson, S., Meek, J., Hawdon, J., 2008. Optimal positions for the release of primitive neonatal reflexes stimulating breastfeeding. Early Hum. Dev. 84 (7), 441–449.

Colson, S., de Rooy, L., Hawdon, J., 2003. Biological nurturing increases duration of breastfeeding for a vulnerable cohort. MIDIRS Midwifery Digest 13 (1), 92–97.

DH (Department of Health), 2013. Off to the best start. DH, London.

Entwistle, F., 2013. The evidence and rationale for the UNICEF UK Baby Friendly Initiative standards. UNICEF UK, London. (Chapter 4). Available online: <http://www.unicef.org.uk/BabyFriendly/Resources/Guidance-for-Health-Professionals/Writing-policies-and-guidelines/The-evidence-and-rationale-for-the-UNICEF-UK-Baby-Friendly-Initiative-standards/> (accessed 19 September 2014.).

Geddes, D., 2009. Ultrasound imaging of the lactating breast: methodology and application. Int. Breastfeed. J. 4 (4), 1746–1758.

HASCIC (Health and Social Care Information Centre), 2012. Infant feeding survey 2010. Health and Social Care Information Centre, London.

Inch, S., 2013. Feeding the newborn baby: breast milk and breast milk substitutes. In: Hall Moran, V. (Ed.), Maternal and Infant Nutrition and Nurture: Controversies and Challenges, second ed. Quay Books, London. (Chapter 4).

Inch, S., Law, S., Wallace, L., 2003. Hands off! The Breastfeeding Best Start project (1). Pract. Midwife 6 (10), 17–19.

Mohrbacher, N., Stock, J., 2003. The breastfeeding answer book. La Leche League International, Illinois, pp. 36, 75–76, 82, 285.

Moore, E., Anderson, G., Bergman, N., Dowswell, T., 2012. Early skin to skin contact for mothers and their healthy newborn infants. Cochrane Database Syst. Rev. 2012 (5), Art. No.: CD003519, doi:10.1002/14651858.CD003519.pub3.

Rapley, G., Murkett, T., 2014. Baby-Led Parenting. Vermillion, London.

Rogers, M., Hickman, I., 2008. Organisation of a Baby Café: an innovative approach. Pract. Midwife 11 (5), 40–43.

UNICEF (United Nations Children's Fund) UK, 2009. Baby Friendly Initiative Position Statement on Biological Nurturing. Available online: <http://www.unicef.org.uk/BabyFriendly/News-and-Research/News/The-Baby-Friendly-Initiatives-position-on-Biological-Nurturing/> (accessed 19 September 2014.).

UNICEF (United Nations Children's Fund) UK, 2014. Breastfeeding assessment form. Available Online: <http://www.unicef.org.uk/Documents/Baby_Friendly/Guidance/breastfeeding_assessment_tool_mat.pdf?epslanguage=en> (accessed 9 November 2015.).

UNICEF (United Nations Children's Fund) UK, 2014. Hand Expression. Available online: <http://www.unicef.org.uk/BabyFriendly/Resources/AudioVideo/Hand-expression/> (accessed 19 September 2014.).

WHO (World Health Organisation), 2011. Exclusive breastfeeding for six months best for babies everywhere. Available online: <http://www.who.int/mediacentre/news/statements/2011/breastfeeding_20110115/en/> (accessed 27 October 2014.).

FURTHER READING

Helpful tips for staff and parents can be
gained from:

Mother's guide, published periodically,
always consistent with the Baby
Friendly Initiative (UNICEF).
Further information at
www.mothersguide.co.uk

Chapter | 42 |

Principles of infant nutrition: cup feeding

LEARNING OUTCOMES

Having read this chapter, the reader should be able to:

• discuss the advantages, disadvantages and indications for cup feeding
• describe the correct technique
• summarize the midwife's role and responsibilities in relation to cup feeding.

Cup feeding is considered to be a viable alternative to using a teat for a breastfed baby but it is important that the technique is correct. This chapter considers the indications for cup feeding, the potential dangers and the correct technique. It should be read in conjunction with Chapter 43, sterilization of equipment, and Chapter 41, breastfeeding.

ADVANTAGES

The undisputed ideal way for a newborn baby to feed is to be effectively breastfed. However, when this is not possible,

for whatever reason, cup feeding provides a method of feeding that:

• promotes tongue action consistent with breastfeeding
• removes the possibility of nipple/teat confusion
• allows the baby to pace the feed and therefore avoid overexertion
• encourages initial digestion of the milk in the mouth that would not occur if fed via a nasogastric tube.

Samuel (1998) notes that less is taken from a cup than a bottle; the newborn baby's stomach is therefore not overdistended and the feeding pattern is likely to be similar to a baby-led breastfeeding pattern. Yilmaz et al's (2014) randomized controlled study (522 participants) added to the literature that advocates cup feeding for preterm infants (32–35 weeks' gestation in this study). Those cup fed were more likely to be exclusively breastfeeding on discharge and at 3 and 6 months of age than those who were fed with a bottle. This conflicted with earlier work by Flint et al (2007), who concluded that at 3 and 6 months of age it made no difference to breastfeeding status whether the baby had been fed with a cup or a teat. UNICEF (UNICEF UK 2007) consider that this latter study was flawed and continue to uphold the principle that teats should be avoided (WHO/UNICEF 1989).

DISADVANTAGES

It is recognized that term babies can become addicted to cup feeding if not put regularly to the breast and that they can also lose the skills needed to breastfeed if the cup feeding technique is incorrect. Aspiration may also occur with an incorrect technique (Thorley 1997) and while milk wastage may be higher, the length of feed can also be longer.

INDICATIONS

Cup feeding is recognized to have three valuable uses:

1. As an interim measure for full-term babies when breastfeeding is not yet established (e.g. birth trauma, use of opiates in labour, maternal infant separation, mild palate deformities), or if supplementation is medically indicated. Samuel (1998) describes the way in which babies mature their sucking action and cites examples of the ways in which cup feeding aided term babies that initially lacked the skill. Equally, the breastfeeding mother may prefer her baby to use a cup during periods of absence, e.g. on return to work, rather than a bottle and teat.

2. For the preterm infant without sufficient suck/swallow coordination, who can easily tire if breastfed or bottle fed. Lang et al (1994) suggest that cup feeding is appropriate for babies from 30 weeks' gestation. However, Freer (1999) demonstrated that preterm infants underwent greater physiological instability when cup feeding than breastfeeding and so encourages caution. Yilmaz et al (2014) recognized the value of cup feeding for preterm infants as a transition method prior to breastfeeding.

3. Cups are easier to sterilize than bottles and teats and can provide a safe feeding method in an emergency (ABA 2012).

The baby should be supported in an upright position and should lap or sip, rather than having the milk poured into their mouth. The procedure should not be hurried. Parents can be taught to cup feed easily and may gain greater confidence in relation to their subsequent feeding method, having had the opportunity to learn (Samuel 1998). Parents may choose to feed in skin-to-skin contact and should be supported to do so as a precursor to effective breastfeeding. Term babies often dribble, calculations of the amount taken should consider this, and parents need to be aware that this is normal.

Cup-feeding babies need regular review. As an interim feeding method, observations should be made as to whether there are signs that the baby is ready to breastfeed. There should be a coordinated suck–swallow reflex and parents are encouraged to look out for mouth opening, rooting reflex and evidence of hands moving to mouth (UNICEF UK 2010). It should also be established that sufficient nutrition is being achieved with cup feeding (see stool and urine output, Chapter 38) and that the baby is not being physiologically compromised or excessively tired by the process.

The cups should be made of food-grade plastic and should be cleaned and decontaminated as for any other feeding equipment used for a baby (Chapter 43), but as noted above, they are easier to clean.

Staff training should also be undertaken, as for any skill, both when new to it and with regular revision.

PROCEDURE: cup feeding

- Ensure that the baby is alert and interested. In many circumstances the baby will have been put to the breast first.
- Gather equipment:
  - expressed breast milk (ideally)
  - sterilized cup (often small, open, slightly shaped and made from polyethylene or similar)
  - bib/napkin
  - baby's records.
- Wash and dry hands.
- Sit comfortably with the baby in an upright sitting position, cuddled in close to the parent's body. Consider swaddling the top half of the baby (to prevent hands knocking the cup) and using a suitably placed bib. Parents may choose to feed in skin-to-skin contact.
- Place the cup (about half full, if possible) lightly on the baby's bottom lip, reaching the corners of his mouth, with the level of milk touching his lips. Begin slowly.
- Retain the cup in this position (throughout any pauses) allowing the baby to lap with tongue forwards. Avoid the temptation to pour the milk in.
- The baby will determine the pace and cease feeding when no longer hungry.
- Ensure that the feed time has been relaxed and pleasurable with lots of comfort and social interaction for the baby. Return the baby to a safe environment once finished.
- Wash and sterilize the cup, wash and dry hands.
- Complete documentation, noting the volume of liquid ingested, the time taken and the effect for the baby.

ROLE AND RESPONSIBILITIES OF THE MIDWIFE

These can be summarized as:

- recognizing the value of cup feeding as a significant interim measure to support breastfeeding, in babies of various gestations from 30 weeks onwards
- learning and teaching a safe and correct technique
- support and encouragement of parents
- record keeping.

SUMMARY

- Cup feeding is a valuable interim measure; it is important that the baby and the cup are both positioned correctly and that the baby laps at his own pace.

SELF-ASSESSMENT EXERCISES

The answers to the following questions may be found in the text:

1. Discuss the advantages and disadvantages of cup feeding.
2. List the circumstances when cup feeding is indicated.
3. Describe how to correctly cup feed a baby.
4. Summarize the role and responsibilities of the midwife when cup feeding.

REFERENCES

ABA (Australian Breastfeeding Association), 2012. Cup feeding in emergencies. Available online: <http://www.breastfeeding.asn.au/bf-info/cupfeedemerg> (accessed 4 March 2015.).

Flint, A., New, K., Davies, M., 2007. Cup feeding versus other forms of supplemental enteral feeding for newborn infants unable to fully breastfeed. Cochrane Database Syst. Rev. (2), CD005092 doi:10.1002/14651858.CD005092.pub2.

Freer, Y., 1999. A comparison of breast and cup feeding preterm infants. J. Neonatal Nurs. 5 (1), 16–20.

Lang, S., Lawrence, C., Orme, R., 1994. Cup feeding: an alternative method of infant feeding. Arch. Dis. Child. 71, 365–369.

Samuel, P., 1998. Cup feeding. Pract. Midwife 1 (12), 33–35.

Thorley, V., 1997. Cup feeding: problems created by incorrect use. J. Hum. Lact. 13 (1), 54–55.

UNICEF (United Nations Children's Fund) UK, 2007. Cup feeding versus other forms of supplemental enteral feeding for newborn infants unable to fully breastfeed. Available online: <http://www.unicef.org.uk/BabyFriendly/News-and-Research/Research/Miscellaneous-illnesses/Cup-feeding-versus-other-forms-of-supplemental-enteral-feeding-for-newborn-infants-unable-to-fully-breastfeed/> (accessed 4 March 2015.).

UNICEF (United Nations Children's Fund) UK, 2010. Care Pathways: Feeding a preterm baby. Available online: <http://www.unicef.org.uk/BabyFriendly/Health-Professionals/Care-Pathways/Breastfeeding2/Overview/> (accessed 4 March 2015.).

WHO/UNICEF (World Health Organisation/United Nations Children's Fund), 1989. Protecting, Promoting and Supporting Breastfeeding: The Special Role of Maternity Services. A Joint WHO/UNICEF Statement. WHO, Geneva.

Yilmaz, G., Caylan, N., Karacan, C.D., et al., 2014. Effect of cup feeding and bottle feeding on breastfeeding in late preterm infants: a randomized controlled study. J. Hum. Lact. 30 (2), 174–179.

Chapter | **43** |

Principles of infant nutrition: decontamination of feeding equipment

LEARNING OUTCOMES

Having read this chapter, the reader should be able to:

- describe all of the ways in which effective sterilization can be undertaken
- discuss the role and responsibilities of the midwife.

Utmost care should be taken to protect babies against any potential sources of infection because of the immaturity of their immune system. Differences in gut flora also make formula-fed babies at higher risk of infection. All feeding equipment should be carefully cleaned and 'sterilized'; traces of milk can harbour and multiply bacteria quickly (Redmond & Griffith 2009a). This chapter considers the correct use of the different decontamination techniques and the role of the midwife in relation to this.

STERILIZATION ADVICE

The parents of new babies need to be familiar with safe and appropriate sterilizing, regardless of method of infant feeding (UNICEF UK 2014). Mainstone (2004) argues that this advice should be a part of general home infection control measures and so should be taught in the parent's usual domestic residence. In hospital, advice is often given as part of antenatal education and prior to postnatal discharge. Particular care should be taken if the woman's first language is not the same as the midwife's; an interpreter should be used.

All the equipment used should be compatible with the chosen sterilizing method and should also be examined on a regular basis. Bacteria can be harboured in cracks or grooves in older bottles or teats, and bottles with a pattern can make it harder to see if the bottle is clean (Redmond & Griffith 2009a). In 2012 the chemical bisphenol A (BPA) was banned in Europe in food-related plastics. Older feeding equipment, particularly if damaged or scratched, can cause BPA to leak into the milk (Anon 2011).

Hancock & Brown (2010) advocate that in the US an electric dishwasher using safe chlorinated water is a sufficient method of sterilization for feeding equipment.

Current practice in the UK continues to use additional sterilizing equipment in the home.

CLEANING FEEDING EQUIPMENT

All equipment needs to be thoroughly cleansed before being sterilized, regardless of sterilization method. While ESGE (2008) are referring to gastroscopy equipment, they are clear that the process of manual cleaning is paramount in ultimately achieving sterilization. If this step is missed or performed badly, then retained milk may harbour bacteria that survive the sterilization process. Equally, Redmond & Griffith (2009a) indicate that hypochlorite disinfectants are inactivated by food debris, among other things. This is the recommended cleaning technique (adapted according to equipment used, e.g. cup or breast pump):

- Dispose of any leftover feed immediately.
- Dismantle the bottle completely.
- Wash all parts using hot soapy water and a clean bottle brush.
- Turn the teats inside out and use a teat brush to clean all surfaces
- Squeeze water through the teat holes.
- Rinse items thoroughly under running cold water to remove soap (DH 2012).

METHODS OF STERILIZATION

It should be noted that Redmond & Griffith (2009a) suggest that using the term 'sterilization' is incorrect. Surgical instruments and the like may be sterilized, that is, undergo a process that removes all viable microorganisms and spores, but the methods below used in the home are more akin to disinfection or decontamination. Midwives have a responsibility to help parents to understand that items will not be completely sterile and that therefore, greater care should be taken to carry out these procedures correctly. Which method is chosen may vary according to ease, convenience, and costs, both of the initial outlay and of ongoing use. There are four different methods of decontamination (Redmond & Griffith (2009a):

1. boiling
2. chemical (sodium hypochlorite)
3. steam: microwave
4. steam: electrical.

Boiling

Boiling in the home can be a hazardous activity and therefore should be done with great care. Prolonged use of boiling may destroy the teats; they should be examined regularly. A large saucepan with a lid is required and a trivet in the base of the pan prevents the bottles from burning. A good volume of water is required so that the bottles stay under the surface, but care should be taken to ensure that the pan does not boil over or boil dry.

PROCEDURE: decontamination by boiling

- Immerse the clean equipment fully in cold water in the saucepan, ensuring that there are no air pockets.
- Put the lid on the pan and place on the heat; bring to the boil.
- When clearly boiling, time for at least 10 minutes (DH 2012), avoid adding anything else to the pan.
- After 10 minutes, turn off the heat; leave undisturbed in the saucepan until required.
- Wash and dry hands and remove items carefully when cool enough to handle, but within 12 hours.

Chemical

Various preparations – tablets, liquids, and crystals – are commercially available for chemical decontamination, usually using cold tap water. Disinfection is only achieved if the solution is prepared correctly and if the cleaned items are correctly immersed. Anything metallic must not be placed in the fluid, but should be boiled. The manufacturer's instructions should be followed carefully, but they generally use similar principles.

PROCEDURE: chemical decontamination

- A large enough container should be available with a well-fitting lid and floating cover.
- Have thoroughly washed and dried hands and a clean working surface.
- Prepare the sterilizing solution using the correct amounts of water and chemical to produce fluid of the correct concentration.
- Fully immerse the clean utensils, ensuring there are no trapped air bubbles; put on the cover and lid, ensuring that all items stay fully immersed.
- Leave the container undisturbed for the required number of minutes (often 15 or 30); if anything needs to be added to or removed from the solution during this time the timing starts again from the time of addition/removal.

- Leave the container undisturbed until required.
- When the equipment is required, wash and dry hands, remove the items carefully, handling them by the aspects that will not come into contact with the baby or milk.
- Either shake the excess off the equipment (Redmond & Griffith 2009a) or rinse them with recently boiled, cooled water (DH 2012).
- Use them immediately.
- Change the sterilizing solution every 24 hours.

Microwave

Non-metallic equipment can also be sterilized in a microwave using a specific microwave sterilizer, prescribed amount of tap water and suitable feeding equipment. Models vary, and so the manufacturer's instructions should be followed carefully. It should be noted that the length of time needed is dependent upon the wattage of the microwave, and it should be remembered that the timings often include standing time. The length of time that the undisturbed items are sterile for varies according to sterilizer model. Decontaminating in a microwave without the recommended equipment is inappropriate. All items should be placed in the sterilizer with the openings facing downwards so that there is maximum exposure to the steam for the inside of the items.

Electric steam sterilizers

Feeding equipment can be decontaminated by steam using an electric sterilizer, for which the manufacturer's instructions should be followed carefully. The equipment does need to have complete contact with the steam and so, as above, should be loaded with open ends facing downwards. The cycle length varies (3–15 minutes); the items should be used immediately unless the manufacturer's guidance suggests otherwise. Electric steamers often need descaling monthly to maintain their efficiency.

RECONTAMINATION

There are many ways in which feeding equipment can be recontaminated after decontamination. Clean hands are essential, especially after changing nappies and toileting, food preparation, and nose blowing (Chapter 9). Redmond & Griffith (2009b) recognize that drying hands thoroughly also contributes to reducing the transfer of microorganisms. Equally, care should be taken at home to use clean hand towels; otherwise, bacteria can be transferred from

towel to hand to equipment. The work surface should be clean and uncluttered and, as the feeds are prepared it is essential that no part of the equipment that will have contact with the milk or baby should be touched.

ROLE AND RESPONSIBILITIES OF THE MIDWIFE

These may be summarized as:
- careful education of the parents, demonstration, or observation may be included. Written approved guidance in an appropriate language should be given
- appropriate documentation and ongoing review
- practising with research-based evidence.

SUMMARY

- There are four effective methods of sterilization/decontamination: boiling, chemical, microwave and electrical steam. Items must be compatible for the chosen method of sterilization and must be thoroughly cleaned before sterilizing.
- It is important that the technique is undertaken correctly whichever method is chosen; babies need to be protected from potential infection.

SELF-ASSESSMENT EXERCISES

The answers to the following questions may be found in the text:
1. Discuss why sterilization of feeding equipment is necessary.
2. Is true sterilization achieved at home? Give reasons for your answer.
3. Describe how to decontaminate feeding equipment when boiling.
4. Demonstrate how to decontaminate feeding equipment using chemical sterilization.
5. Discuss the different methods of steam decontamination.
6. Summarize the role and responsibilities of the midwife in relation to effective equipment preparation.

REFERENCES

Anon (Anonymous), 2011. News: EU bans bisphenol A from babies' bottles. Pract. Midwife 14 (1), 15.

DH (Department of Health), 2012. Guide to Bottle Feeding. Department of Health, London.

ESGE (ESGENA), 2008. ESGE-ESGENA guideline: cleaning and disinfection in gastrointestinal endoscopy – update 2008. Available online: <http://www.esge.com/esge-guidelines.html> (accessed 5 March 2015.).

Hancock, M., Brown, J., 2010. Formula-Feeding Safety: what nurses need to teach parents who choose to formula feed. Nurs. Women's Health 14 (4), 302–309.

Mainstone, A., 2004. Domestic hazard analysis of infant feeding utensils. Br. J. Midwifery 12 (6), 368–372.

Redmond, E., Griffith, C.J., 2009a. Disinfection methods used in decontamination of bottles used for feeding powdered infant formula. J. Fam. Health Care 19 (1), 26–31.

Redmond, E., Griffith, C.J., 2009b. The importance of hygiene in the domestic kitchen: implications for preparation and storage of food and infant formula. Perspect. Public Health 129 (2), 69–76.

UNICEF (United Nations Children's Fund) UK, 2014. A guide to infant formula for parents who are bottle feeding: health professionals' guide. UNICEF, London. Available online: <http://www.unicef.org.uk/Documents/Baby_Friendly/Leaflets/HP_Guide_for_parents_formula_feeding.pdf> (accessed 5 March 2015.).

Chapter | **44**

Principles of infant nutrition: formula feeding

LEARNING OUTCOMES

Having read this chapter, the reader should be able to:

• discuss the principles of correct powdered formula milk preparation and the dangers of incorrect preparation
• discuss in detail the advice and education that new parents need when choosing to formula feed
• summarize the role and responsibilities of the midwife.

When a baby is not being breastfed, the midwife has an important role in facilitating safe and effective infant nutrition using formula milk. This chapter considers the significance of correct powdered infant formula reconstitution both within and outside of the home, appropriate feeding technique and the midwife's role and responsibilities. This chapter needs to be read in conjunction with Chapter 41 (breastfeeding) and Chapter 43 (sterilization/decontamination of feeding equipment).

FORMULA FEEDING

Time has passed since the World Health Organization (WHO 2007) gave new guidance regarding the safe preparation of powdered infant formula at home. Nevertheless, the UK 2010 Infant Feeding Survey (McAndrew et al 2012) suggested that only 49% of mothers in England using formula milk had prepared it correctly during that week. While this is an improvement, this still leaves a large number of babies receiving an inaccurately prepared formula feed. It is a requirement in Baby Friendly Accredited Care (UNICEF UK 2014a) that women who are using formula milk should be shown how to correctly prepare a feed postnatally before transfer home. All parents of new babies need to understand effective sterilization/decontamination of feeding equipment (Chapter 43). Redmond & Griffith (2009) state that for various reasons, the domestic kitchen is not a good place for safe food preparation and therefore healthcare practitioners should take seriously their role in educating parents in these matters.

What are the risks?

The digestive tract of newborn infants varies in its pH according to feeding method. The formula-fed infant has a more alkaline intestine and therefore has less protection

335

against harmful microorganisms. The Department of Health are clear in their guidelines (DH 2012) that formula milk powder itself may contain microorganisms; consequently care should be taken in its reconstitution, the formula-fed baby being at a greater infection risk to begin with. Minchin (2000) and Inch (2013) both suggest that the production and manufacture of artificial milk has many unanswered questions – its composition, the role of genetically modified ingredients, the potential hazards in manufacture (and to the environment (Inch 2013)), to name but a few. Marchant & Rundall (2008) would agree, adding their concerns over misleading advertising claims as well. The health benefits to mothers and babies of breastfeeding are well documented, while the long-term consequences of a formula-fed population are not yet fully realized, but can be anticipated to show poorer health outcomes. Parents may also not appreciate the dangers of choking, overfeeding, or poor feeding technique, alongside feed preparation inside and outside of their home environment.

FORMULA MILKS

Powdered infant formula milks suitable for newborn babies are modified cow's milk and are either whey or casein dominant. There are variations in the constituents of the milk according to manufacturers; some are suggested for vegetarians, for example. Parents can find guidance about formula milks from UNICEF UK (2010). However, it is clear (Crawley & Westland 2013) that, for whichever milk is chosen, it must be an age-suitable formula. Equally, where (often because of probiotic additives) the manufacturers suggest preparation at a lower water temperature, this advice should be disregarded (DH 2013). Powdered infant formula milk should be prepared with water at 70°C (or higher, but not boiling). Each packet of formula milk powder is supplied with a plastic scoop that is suitable for use with that packet only.

EQUIPMENT REQUIRED

The following equipment is suggested:

- handwashing and drying facilities, clean towel where possible
- infant feeding bottles with tops, covers and teats (BPA free (Anon. 2011)). Wide-necked bottles are often easier to clean. The scale on the side should be clearly visible. Standard flow teats are acceptable (drip rate of 1 drop per second). The woman may make different choices later, according to her baby's needs
- sterilizing equipment (Chapter 43)

- bottle and teat brushes (non-metallic), hot water and washing-up liquid
- plastic spatula or leveller if not integral in milk packet
- a safe water supply with kettle or means of boiling water, 1 L of water at least (Crawley & Westland 2013)
- age-appropriate powdered infant formula, within 'use by' guidance
- equipment for use out of the home, e.g. flask and container for milk powder, (possibly a cool bag, depending on the situation).

FEEDING PREPARATION

Potential hazards

The dangers of reconstituting formula feed include:

- Use of unclean equipment that has been not been properly cleaned and sterilized and is (potentially) recontaminated (see Chapter 43).
- An incorrectly reconstituted feed. This is a breeding ground for microorganisms and so each feed needs to be:
  - Prepared freshly at the time of need.
  - Prepared with fresh tap water that has been boiled only once, then left to cool for a maximum of 30 minutes. Cooling the water is necessary, feeds made with boiling water may be nutritionally compromised due to the clumping of some of the ingredients. Crawley & Westland (2013) advocate boiling at least 1 L of water; the temperature of the water after 30 minutes can vary according to the amount of water boiled. Ideally, the water temperature will still be about 70°C, this is considered appropriate to kill the maximum amount of bacteria. In the event of an unsafe water supply, bottled water may be used, but it should be boiled as for tap water (DH 2012). Crawley & Westland (2013) suggest that it should contain less than 200 mg sodium and less than 250 mg sulphate.
  - Carefully reconstituted, placing the water into the bottle first and adding the correct number of loosely packed level scoops of powder (often one scoop to 30 mL water, but encourage parents to read the packet and use only the scoop with that packet). Too much powder may result in hypernatraemia, constipation and obesity, while too little can cause malnutrition.
  - Cooled under cold running water to the required temperature quickly, both to feed the waiting baby and to restrict bacterial growth.

Formula feeding away from home

If feeding outside of the home, pre-prepared formula is recommended. A less safe, but acceptable occasional practice would be to carry a freshly sterilized bottle with the powder in a sterilized container and freshly boiled water in a clean, full and sealed flask. The feed would still need to be cooled under cold running water (DH 2012).

Storage of prepared feeds

Preparing a powdered feed and then storing it is strongly discouraged (DH 2012). If this was necessary, e.g. prior to going to the childminder:

- the feed should be prepared correctly
- cooled quickly under cold running water
- stored at the back of a fridge at 5°C for an hour
- transported using a cool bag with ice blocks
- used within 4 hours.

It should be prepared as near to the time to leave as possible (while working within these guidelines), e.g. that morning rather than the night before. If it is transported without a cool bag, the feed should be used or disposed of/discarded within 2 hours, as for all non-refrigerated infant feeds. If rewarming a feed, warm water can be used for up to 15 minutes, either by placing the bottle in the water, or by holding it under a running tap. Microwaves should not be used due to the inconsistent action of reheating. Once commenced, the feed must be completed or thrown away within 2 hours.

PROCEDURE: preparation of a powdered formula milk feed

- Fill the kettle with 1 L of fresh cold water, put on to boil. Once boiled, leave to cool for a few minutes undisturbed, but a maximum 30 minutes.
- Wash and dry hands, work on a clean, uncluttered surface without distractions. Stand the sterilized feeding bottle on the work surface, leaving the top and teat in the sterilizer. If using chemical sterilization, the items may be shaken (Redmond & Griffith 2009) or rinsed with cooled boiled water (DH 2012).
- Pour the water into the bottle to the appropriate level, this is best judged at eye level.
- Take a scoop of powder without compressing it, level it using the leveller and add to the water. Continue to add scoops of powder until the correct number has been added. Do not add anything else.
- Place the teat over the bottle handling it only at the bottom edge. Place the screw ring over and tighten (if this is difficult, sterilized tongs or tweezers can be

used), put on a sterilized bottle cover. Shake the milk gently to ensure appropriate mixing of the contents; the powder should be fully dissolved and not show any signs of clumping together.
- Hold the bottle under cold running water until the feed is cooled to an appropriate temperature. Check it by testing a few drops on the inside of the parent's wrist. The milk should be warm, but not hot.
- Use immediately. Discard unfinished feeds straight away and thoroughly wash all equipment used in hot soapy water prior to sterilizing.

FEEDING TECHNIQUE

The principles of baby-led feeding should be upheld: the baby will feed when hungry, taking as much or as little as desired. All parents should be taught to recognize and understand the feeding cues (see p. 324) and so feed their baby when the early cues are seen. Entwistle (2013) suggests ways in which the feeding experience can be enhanced. These include feeding times that are enjoyable and relaxed, in which the baby feels loved. The baby should be held securely, close to his parent in a reasonably upright sitting position (head supported) so that breathing and swallowing are easy. Eye contact should be maintained. UNICEF (2014b) recommend that the number of carers feeding the baby is limited, and that they all use a similar technique. Ideally, the mother is the carer of choice, and in the early days, both she and the baby will benefit from feeding in skin-to-skin contact (UNICEF 2011). A baby should never be left unattended to feed.

As the teat brushes against the baby's lips the baby will open his mouth wide and take in the teat. The teat needs to be over the baby's tongue and the bottle just tipped sufficiently for air to be excluded from the teat. The teat should administer regular drops, rather than a stream of milk (Ellis & Kanneh 2000). The baby will suck and pause, retaining the teat in his mouth. The pace of the feed should allow for small interruptions that can break the suction that sometimes builds in the teat (move it to the side of the baby's mouth briefly), to wind the baby (gentle back rubbing or patting) or to allow the baby to appreciate whether he needs to continue or stop feeding at that time.

The baby will cease feeding when he has had sufficient milk. Volumes will be smaller initially, but by 1 week of age babies feed 150–200 mL/kg/day, until 6 months of age. Parents should be helped to understand the signs that suggest effective feeding is taking place: the baby should be settled between feeds, gaining a correct amount of weight and passing urine and stools normally (Chapter 38). The stool may be firmer and slightly more offensive than that of a breastfed baby.

337

ROLE AND RESPONSIBILITIES OF THE MIDWIFE

These can be summarized as:

- using evidenced-based knowledge and application of best practice advice with regard to formula milks, their reconstitution and storage
- education and support of parents to ensure safe infant nutrition and feeding technique
- recognition of a healthy formula-fed infant
- contemporaneous record keeping.

SUMMARY

- It is important that powdered formula milk is reconstituted correctly according to WHO guidance (2007) for each individual feed.
- As well as this, care should be taken to use sterilized feeding equipment, a safe water supply, and, if needed, appropriate storage and transport of a reconstituted feed.

- The midwife has an important role in facilitating parents to develop a loving and safe feeding technique, and in recognizing a healthy formula-fed baby.

SELF-ASSESSMENT EXERCISES

The answers to the following questions may be found in the text:

1. Describe how to correctly reconstitute powdered infant formula at home.
2. List the times/ways in which bacterial growth could occur whilst reconstituting a feed or during the feeding process.
3. Demonstrate how to hold the baby and bottle when formula feeding.
4. Prepare a leaflet for new mothers detailing the equipment needed for safe formula feeding.
5. Summarize the midwife's role and responsibilities when caring for a woman and her baby when the baby is being fed with formula milk.

REFERENCES

Anon (Anonymous), 2011. News: EU bans bisphenol a from babies' bottles. Pract. Midwife 14 (1), 15.

Crawley, H., Westland, S., 2013. Infant Milks in the UK A Practical Guide for Health Professionals. First Steps. Nutrition Trust, London.

DH (Department of Health), 2013. Preparation of infant formula (letter). Available online: <https://www.gov.uk/government/uploads/system/uploads/attachment_data/file/127411/update-from-the-Chief-Medical-Officer-and-Director-for-Public-Health-Nursing.pdf.pdf> (accessed 6 March 2015.).

DH (Department of Health), 2012. Guide to Bottle Feeding. Department of Health, London.

Ellis, M., Kanneh, A., 2000. Infant nutrition: part two. Paediatr. Nurs. 12 (1), 38–43.

Entwistle, F., 2013. The Evidence and Rationale for the UNICEF UK Baby Friendly Initiative Standards. UNICEF UK, London, p. 76. Available online: <http://www.unicef.org.uk/BabyFriendly/Resources/Guidance-for-Health-Professionals/Writing-policies-and-guidelines/The-evidence-and-rationale-for-the-UNICEF-UK-Baby-Friendly-Initiative-standards/> (accessed 6 March 2015.).

Inch, S., 2013. Feeding the newborn baby. In: Hall Moran, V. (Ed.), Maternal and Infant Nutrition and Nurture: Controversies and Challenges. Quay Books, London. (Chapter 4).

Marchant, S., Rundall, P., 2008. Safe and appropriate infant nutrition: why does it matter? MIDIRS Midwifery Digest 18 (4), 566–570.

McAndrew, T., Thompson, J., Fellows, L., Renfrew, M., 2012. Infant Feeding Survey 2010. Health & Social Care Information Centre, London.

Minchin, M., 2000. Artificial feeding and risk. Pract. Midwife 3 (3), 18–20.

Redmond, E., Griffith, C.J., 2009. Disinfection methods used in decontamination of bottles used for feeding powdered infant formula. J. Fam. Health Care 19 (1), 26–31.

UNICEF (United Nations Children's Fund) UK, 2010. A Guide to infant Formula for Parents Who are Bottle Feeding. UNICEF UK, London. Available online: <http://www.unicef.org.uk/BabyFriendly/Resources/Resources-for-parents/A-guide-to-infant-formula-for-parents-who-are-bottle-feeding/> (accessed 5 March 2015.).

UNICEF (United Nations Children's Fund) UK, 2011. Changes to the

UNICEF UK Baby Friendly Maternity Standards. Pract. Midwife 14 (3), 33–36.

UNICEF (United Nations Children's Fund) UK, 2014a. Moving from the current to the new Baby Friendly Initiative Standards. Available online: <http://www.unicef.org.uk/ Documents/Baby_Friendly/Guidance/ transition_guidance.pdf> (accessed 5 February 2015.).

UNICEF (United Nations Children's Fund) UK, 2014b. The Health Professional's Guide to: 'A Guide to Infant Formula for Parents Who are Bottle Feeding'. UNICEF UK, London. Available online: <http://www.unicef .org.uk/Documents/Baby_Friendly/ Leaflets/HP_Guide_for_parents _formula_feeding.pdf> (accessed 5 March 2015.).

WHO (World Health Organisation), 2007. Safe Preparation, Storage and Handling of Powdered Infant Formula: Guidelines. WHO, Geneva.

Chapter 45

Principles of infant nutrition: nasogastric feeding

LEARNING OUTCOMES

Having read this chapter, the reader should be able to:

- highlight the potential risks of nasogastric/orogastric feeding tubes
- detail the steps that are taken to ensure that the tube is correctly placed
- describe how one is inserted and removed safely
- describe how a baby is fed using a nasogastric tube
- summarize the role and responsibilities of the midwife.

Nasogastric (NG) tubes may be used in both adults and babies. They are, as the name suggests, a tube which passes through the nose (or mouth, orogastric), into the oesophagus and through into the stomach. They have two main uses:

- placing food or medication into the stomach
- removing substances from the stomach.

Adult NG tubes are rarely seen in maternity, occasionally one is used to empty the stomach prior to a rapid caesarean section in which a general anaesthetic is to be administered, or women who are nil by mouth with a complication, e.g. paralytic ileus, may need continuous drainage of the stomach. Inserting a tube into an adult is very similar to that in a neonate, except that the woman (if permitted) assists by taking sips of water so that as she swallows, the tube is advanced into her stomach. This chapter considers neonatal NG tube insertion: safety, feeding and removal. Safety is an issue of particular concern.

CONSIDERATIONS

Feeding via a nasogastric (NG) tube is the most unnatural method of feeding. Wherever possible, a baby is breastfed. Breastfed preterm infants were able to move to enteral feeds faster than formula-fed infants, the breast milk providing better nutritional and developmental properties (Entwistle 2013). If the gestation or clinical condition is such that feeding the baby at the breast is not possible, then expressed breastmilk should be given via a suitable alternative route, e.g. cup or tube. There are many important aspects to feeding – sociability, opportunity to show love and affection, close physical and eye contact, appetite control, to name but a few. If tube feeding is the principal means of nutrition, wherever possible, the parents are encouraged to feed with these aspects in mind. In some instances tube feeding may be accompanied by, for example, short spells of breastfeeding or cup feeding. Spells at the breast aid the milk supply and make the transition to full breastfeeding easier.

An important part of digestion begins in the mouth, this is unfortunately missed when using a tube. Jones & Spencer (1999) also note that significant fat globules can adhere to the inside of the tube and so render lesser nutrition than is expected. These and other disadvantages (unsightly, easily removed, damage to the skin) often make it a short-term measure.

There have also been several alerts in the last decade from the National Patient Safety Agency (NPSA) about the positioning and safe use of NG tubes. A number of deaths have been caused by misplacement of the tube. The alert applies to all age groups, but in 2005 they released an alert specifically for use with neonates (NPSA 2005). In 2012 they reiterated their advice, suggesting that tubes that are misplaced and cause harm or death are 'never events', events that should never happen in modern healthcare. Misplaced tubes, i.e. misplaced into the lungs instead of the stomach, can cause death, even minor incidents can cause aspiration pneumonia (NPSA 2012).

The midwife is most likely to encounter tube feeding in special care baby units, the midwife also has a role in educating and supporting parents who may need to undertake NG tube feeds safely at home.

NASOGASTRIC/OROGASTRIC TUBES

Small (fine-bore) tubes are used for neonates. They are sterile, radiopaque and have visible external markings. Those used for older children or adults may have a guide wire that is used for insertion and can be cleaned, dried, and stored (name labelled) for future use. Tubes made from PVC should be changed after 7 days, polyurethane after 30 days. The tube is always checked to make sure it is complete before insertion. It may be lubricated with sterile water before insertion, but not any other lubricant. A tube that appears blocked should have 1–2 mL of air put down it, if this does not solve the problem, it is removed and replaced.

Traditionally the NEX – nose to ear to xiphisternum measuring system – has been used for neonates to determine the appropriate length for tube insertion. However, Cirgin Ellett et al (2011) propose that this distance is regularly too short and that the newer NEMU (nose to ear to midpoint between xiphisternum and umbilicus) should be used. They point out that other studies are yet to report on other measurements, including body weight, but agree that NEX is an inappropriate measure. The reader should consider their local protocol; this text currently demonstrates NEX as its guideline.

SAFETY CONSIDERATIONS

As mentioned, feeding tubes can migrate, or may not have been placed correctly to start with. As well as the lungs, tubes can sometimes be found in the oesophagus or duodenum or coiled or kinked within the oral cavity. There are several methods previously advocated to check NG tube placement; they are no longer valid. These methods should **not** be used to assess an NG tube position (NPSA 2005):

- Auscultation (listening over the stomach with a stethoscope as air is inserted down the tube). Sounds may be heard even if the tube is in the lungs.
- Placing the end of the tube in water and watching for bubbles. Air may come from both the stomach and lungs.
- Blue litmus paper. Its sensitivity to detect between pH variations of gastric and bronchial secretions is insufficient.
- The baby's condition. Respiratory distress is not necessarily seen if the tube is in the lungs.
- The presence of aspirate in the tube. This may be still there from the last feed; it is also difficult to assess visually the differences between gastric and bronchial aspirate.
- Presence of securing tape in the same place. A tube can migrate without causing changes to the tape, the tube may also not have been placed correctly on insertion.

The only recommended method of checking that the tube is in the stomach is the aspiration and testing of gastric aspirate (see below). The NPSA (2005) have issued specific guidance for the use of NG and orogastric tubes in neonates. Their guidance surrounds the critical issues:

- Is the tube in the correct place (the stomach)?
- Is this confirmed by gastric aspirate of pH 5.5 or below?

Their decision-making flow charts problem solve what to do if no aspirate is obtained and what to do if it has a pH higher than 5.5.

NPSA (2005) GUIDELINES

- The position of the tube should be checked on insertion; before administering any feed or medication; following any episodes of vomiting, retching, or coughing; or if there is any visible indication that the tube may have moved, e.g. loose tape, change in length of visible tube. All tubes should have markings and be marked on insertion. If continuous feeds are happening, tube checking should be undertaken 15–30 minutes after the end of the feed, before the next one is commenced.

- It should be assessed using aspirate withdrawn from the stomach using pH indicator strips or paper. Only one sort of paper should be available, not different types or from different manufacturers. It should be stored correctly (in a sealed container) and should read either pH 0 to 6 or 1 to 11. It is used by placing the aspirate onto the paper, not drawing the paper through the aspirate. The result should be clearly distinguishable and appear within 10–15 seconds. This is the only test used in everyday clinical practice to confirm NG tube placement. No fluids of any description should be put down an NG tube until placement is confirmed.
- The gastric aspirate should be *pH 5.5 or below*. A raised gastric aspirate (above pH 6) may be found in the presence of amniotic fluid in a baby less than 48 hours old, in the presence of gastric acid reducing medications and if milk is in the baby's stomach (taking 1- or 2-hourly feeds). In the event of a raised pH the NPSA (2005) flow chart should be followed. Broadly this consists of waiting 15–30 minutes before aspirating again, considering re-passing the tube, checking previous X-rays (same tube? same length?), clinical review (feeds, medicines) and senior medical staff involved in the decision making.
- It is noted that some babies may consistently have a raised pH. A multidisciplinary approach is needed in assessing their risks of not feeding with the chances of tube displacement. All decisions should be clearly documented. The NPSA (2005) flow chart for decision making details the steps that are taken (see reference list for website address).

When unable to aspirate

- In the event of not being able to aspirate from the tube, the baby should be turned onto his left side and the aspiration attempted again. If none is obtained, 1–2 mL of air may be injected and a further attempt to aspirate is made. If again no aspirate is obtained the tube may be retracted or advanced slightly. These measures aim to dislodge a tube that is caught in the gastric mucosa. If aspiration is still not possible repassing the tube may be considered. *Under no circumstances is anything flushed down an NG tube before placement in the stomach is confirmed* (NPSA 2012).

- X-ray is the only other method used to confirm NG tube placement, but it is only to be used if the aspirate cannot be obtained (or cannot confirm pH 5.5 or lower) despite trying the other techniques discussed above. Equally, an X-ray would not be undertaken unless the baby was being X-rayed for some other reason.
- If an X-ray is performed, it should be read by a competent practitioner prior to permission to use the tube is given. It should also be noted that if deemed to be correct, it is only correct at the time of the X-ray and so pH aspirate screening would still be undertaken.

Despite careful checking, Wilkes-Holmes (2006) is clear that there is no completely reliable bedside method to confirm tube position, and midwives should always be alert to this. Documentation indicating every action and decision taken should be contemporaneous, dated and signed. In many places an NG tube placement record is used detailing issues such as clinical indication, the tube (size, make, batch no., etc.), ease and confirmation of placement, length inserted, length visible externally and date/time/reason for removal. A testing chart may also be used that keeps an ongoing record of each pH at each aspiration.

PROCEDURE: inserting a neonatal nasogastric tube

This should be undertaken in an environment that has working resuscitation equipment (oxygen and suction as a minimum) readily accessible.

- Gain informed consent from the parents and gather equipment:
  - sterile radiopaque NG tube size FR 6 (for a baby weighing >1.7 kg) with line markings (straightened if curved in the packaging)
  - sterile water and 2-mL syringe
  - sterile 20-mL syringe
  - tape
  - pH indicator paper with comparison chart
  - non-sterile gloves and apron
  - indelible marker pen.
- Position the baby in a good light and a safe place, e.g. in the cot or held by an assistant; swaddle tightly so that hands are kept from the face.
- Wash and dry hands and apply apron and non-sterile gloves.
- Without touching the skin, hold the tip of the tube near to the nose, measure the distance from the nose to the ear and then from the ear to the xiphisternum (Fig. 45.1), noting the distance markers on the tube, marking the spot with the pen.

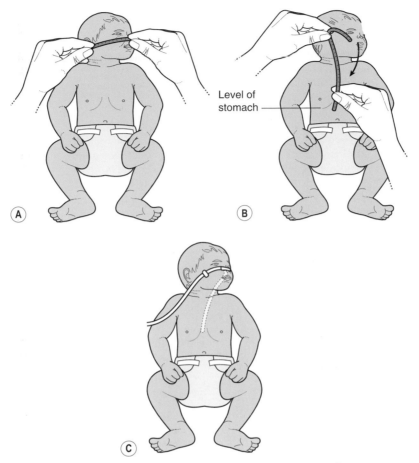

Figure 45.1 Measuring the length of the nasogastric (NG) tube prior to insertion: measure from nose to ear, then from ear to xiphisternum (NEX measuring), noting the distance markers on the tubing. Nose to ear to midpoint between xiphisternum and umbilicus (NEMU) measuring would extend to the midway point between the xiphisternum and the umbilicus.

- Pass the tube through the smaller nostril, gently but smoothly; if resistance is felt, stop and try the other nostril, observing the condition of the baby throughout. Stop and remove the tube if there is any gasping, coughing, pallor or cyanosis.
- Once the tube has been passed through the appropriate length (pen mark at the nose) hold the tube in place, attach the 20-mL syringe, and withdraw approximately 0.5 mL of gastric aspirate.
- Test the aspirate with the pH indicator paper; the result should be pH 5.5 or below. If the aspirate is hard to withdraw, the tube may have been occluded by mucus on insertion; 1–2 mL air may be injected first (using a 2-mL syringe) and then the aspirate withdrawn.

- Once the position is confirmed, tape the tube in place across the baby's cheek, flush the tube using an appropriate amount of sterile water for the tube size (1–2 mL), followed by the same amount of air.
- Dispose of equipment correctly.
- Remove gloves and apron, wash and dry hands.
- Document and act accordingly.

ADMINISTERING A TUBE FEED

Ideally the mother's expressed breast milk is used, alternatively donor milk should be accessed (Entwistle 2013) (see Chapter 41 for correct breast milk storage). The amount may be specifically prescribed or calculated based on the baby's daily requirements according to weight, gestation, and age. The World Health Organization (WHO 2011) in its review of the evidence for very low birth weight babies recommended bolus feeds rather than continuous feeds, and suggested that if less than 3 hours have passed, the baby could be fed according to his hunger cues. The tube is flushed with sterile water after each administration, followed by a small amount of air to clear the tube of water. Some guidelines will also suggest that once placement is confirmed the tube is flushed with water before feeding and medicine administration as well as afterwards, this may depend upon the baby's fluid balance.

Parents are supported to undertake the feed themselves if this is appropriate, if not, a good feeding technique is modelled, taught and encouraged.

PROCEDURE: administering a bolus tube feed

- Gain informed consent from the parents, wash hands and gather equipment:
  - 1 × 30-mL sterile syringe and 2 × 5-mL syringes
  - pH indicator paper (with comparison chart)
  - milk, at room temperature
  - non-sterile gloves
  - sterile water for oral use.
- Position the baby in a good light and a safe place; the baby should be cuddled by one of his parents and interaction should take place as for any other kind of feed (see p. 337).
- Wash and dry hands and apply non-sterile gloves.
- Establish that there are no obvious signs of the tube having moved.
- Attach a 5-mL syringe and withdraw 0.5–1 mL of gastric aspirate, place it onto the paper, and await the result. If pH 5.5 or less, continue. If pH is greater than 5.5, follow the guidelines discussed above, do not flush or feed.
- If confident the tube is correctly placed, remove the plunger from the 30-mL syringe, attach the syringe to the tube, but occlude the tube by compressing it gently. (Some protocols will flush the tube using 1–3 mL of water before feeding.)
- Pour the required amount of milk into the syringe, holding it in an upright position.
- Release the occlusion on the tube so that the milk begins to flow into the stomach.
- Regulate the flow by occluding and pausing if it is too fast, or by raising or lowering the syringe height. The feed should be leisurely and enjoyable, as for any other feed.

- Observe the baby's condition throughout and stop the procedure if necessary, e.g. coughing, vomiting, hypoxic or bradycardic episodes.
- Follow the feed with approximately 1–3 mL of sterile water drawn up using the other 5-mL syringe to cleanse the tube once the feed is completed (Naysmith & Nicholson 1998), followed by sufficient air (1–2 mL) to clear the tube of water. Water in the tube can affect the pH of the next aspirate tested.
- Close off the tube, ensure the baby is in a safe place, dispose of the equipment. Remove gloves and wash and dry hands.
- Complete the records.

REMOVAL OF A NASOGASTRIC TUBE

This takes place when clinically indicated, or if the tube needs a routine change, repositioning or replacing because of blockage. To avoid the trauma of unnecessary re-insertion, ensure that removal is definitely indicated before removing it. Unfortunately, babies frequently remove their own NG tubes unless the tube is well secured.

PROCEDURE: removal of a nasogastric tube

- Obtain informed consent; position the baby in a good light and a safe place.
- Wash and dry hands and apply non-sterile gloves.
- Remove the tape from the baby's face.
- Pull out the tube smoothly and quickly, place into a bag for disposal (the baby may sneeze), wipe the baby's nose with soft tissue.
- Check the tube is complete, dispose of equipment correctly, and wash hands.
- Complete documentation and act accordingly. Ensure that the baby feeds normally following the procedure.

ROLE AND RESPONSIBILITIES OF THE MIDWIFE

These can be summarized as:
- undertaking all the techniques safely and competently in line with current best practice
- appropriate support and education of parents
- observation of the baby during and following all the procedures; referral if indicated
- contemporaneous record keeping.

SUMMARY

- Nasogastric tubes have a role in feeding babies when oral feeding is limited or not possible.
- The tube must be confirmed to be in the stomach on every occasion. The currently advocated method is the use of pH indicator paper, the aspirate should have a pH of 5.5 or less. The tube is not used unless this is confirmed.
- The condition of the baby must be observed throughout. Efforts should be made to make feed times pleasurable.

SELF-ASSESSMENT EXERCISES

The answers to the following questions may be found in the text:

1. Discuss the possible risks of feeding via an NG tube.
2. Describe how to safely insert an NG tube and confirm its position.
3. Describe how to undertake a milk feed using an NG tube.
4. Describe how to remove an NG tube.
5. Summarize the role and responsibilities of the midwife in relation to each of these aspects of care.

REFERENCES

Cirgin Ellett, M., Cohen, M., Perkins, S., et al., 2011. Predicting the insertion length for gastric tube placement in neonates. J. Obstet. Gynecol. Neonatal Nurs. 40 (4), 412–421.

Entwistle, F., 2013. The evidence and rationale for the UNICEF UK Baby Friendly Initiative standards. UNICEF, UK, p. 103.

Jones, E., Spencer, A., 1999. Successful preterm breastfeeding. Pract. Midwife 2 (1), 54–57.

NPSA (National Patient Safety Agency), 2005. Patient Safety Alert: Reducing the Harm Caused by Misplaced Naso and Orogastric Feeding Tubes in Babies under the Care of Neonatal Units. NPSA, London. Available online: <http://www.nrls.npsa.nhs.uk/resources/?EntryId45=59798> (accessed 25 February 2015.).

NPSA (National Patient Safety Agency), 2012. Rapid Response Report: Harm from Flushing of Nasogastric Tubes before Confirmation of Placement. NPSA, London. Available online: <http://www.nrls.npsa.nhs.uk/alerts/?entryid45=133441&q=0%c2%acnasogastric+tubes%c2%ac> (accessed 25 February 2015.).

Naysmith, M.R., Nicholson, J., 1998. Nasogastric drug administration. Prof. Nurse 13 (7), 424–427.

Wilkes-Holmes, C., 2006. Safe placement of nasogastric tubes in children. Paediatr. Nurs. 18 (9), 14–17.

WHO (World Health Organisation), 2011. Optimal Feeding of Low Birth-Weight Infants in Low and Middle-Income Countries. WHO, Geneva. Available online: <www.who.int/> (accessed 26 February 2015.).

Chapter 46

Principles of phlebotomy and intravenous therapy: maternal venepuncture

LEARNING OUTCOMES

Having read this chapter, the reader should be able to:

- discuss the indications for venepuncture
- describe how venepuncture is undertaken safely and positively using an Aseptic Non Touch Technique (ANTT) (Rowley & Clare 2011)
- discuss the rationale for the choice of vein and equipment used
- highlight the possible complications and how they can be avoided
- summarize the role and responsibilities of the midwife.

Venepuncture is the puncturing of a vein with a needle, usually to obtain specimens of blood for laboratory analysis, but may also include the administration of drugs intravenously in an emergency. The ability of a midwife to undertake venepuncture facilitates individualized and holistic care for the woman from the same practitioner. This chapter considers the indications for venepuncture, the rationale for correct preparation, and the procedure. The role and responsibilities of the midwife are summarized. This chapter should be read alongside Chapters 8 and 10 for a fuller understanding.

INDICATIONS

- Antenatal 'booking' bloods
- Assessment of full blood count and presence of Rhesus antibodies during pregnancy. Further repeats if rhesus negative blood group, with Kleihauer test after delivery
- Other tests may be taken if there is an existing disease, e.g. thyroid function tests, blood glucose monitoring or tolerance testing, anti-epileptic drug levels; or if other conditions are suspected, e.g. sickle cell anaemia, pre-eclampsia, thalassaemia, hepatitis B, hyperemesis gravidarum
- Antenatal screening tests for fetal normality, e.g. alphafetoprotein
- Cross-matching prior to blood transfusion, or 'group and save' prior to operative delivery.

This is not an exhaustive list, but it does indicate that women are often asked to give blood specimens. Fear of needles or of fainting can be real fears; midwives should be sensitive to both the physical and psychological aspects of the skill. Care and time should be taken to gain an informed consent and measures used to improve the experience (see below) if the woman is very anxious. An ANTT technique should be used (Chapter 10); bloodstream infections are serious (RCN 2010), debilitating and expensive.

SUITABLE SITES

Blood is always taken from a vein, never an artery. Arterial blood is only ever sought by medical staff in specific circumstances (e.g. for blood gas analysis). The physiological additional blood volume during pregnancy and the general body warmth of the pregnant woman both create vasodilatation, making venepuncture easier than with many other groups of people. As healthy women, their veins are also often in a good condition. The midwife should appreciate the anatomy of the arm below the elbow. The basilic, median cubital and cephalic veins are all appropriately placed in the antecubital fossa and are suitable sites for effective venepuncture (Fig. 46.1). The skin should be free from infection, inflammation and bruising.

CHOOSING A VEIN

Clearly visible veins are often nearer to the skin surface but are often smaller and so are harder to obtain blood samples from. Both visual inspection and palpation should be used when choosing a vein. On palpation a vein can be assessed for its size, mobility and suitability. A vein that has been repeatedly used for venous access may be thrombosed and will not feel 'bouncy' and full. The veins in the antecubital fossa are often supported by subcutaneous tissue and so are less likely to move or 'roll' when venepuncture is attempted. The application of a tourniquet that obstructs the venous return only (arterial pulse should still be felt) increases venous filling and so makes the choice of vein easier. Scales (2008) indicates that tourniquet use should be for a maximum of 1 minute. Lavery & Ingram (2005) agree, suggesting that tourniquet use for greater than 90 seconds damages the vein and therefore causes potentially inaccurate results. This means that it will be released while the other preparations are made and then reapplied once ready to puncture. The woman can also be asked to clench and unclench her fist a couple of times, but this is not always necessary and can also affect the results. The technique of 'tapping' the veins to increase their prominence should be avoided; it can cause bruising and pain (Brooks 2014). Often women will know from past experience which

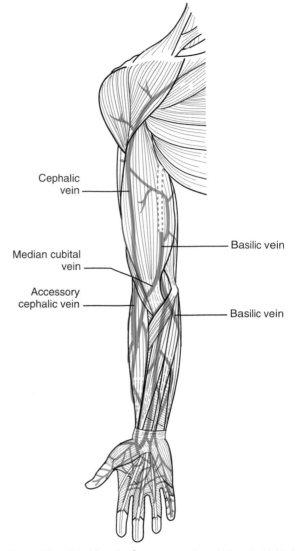

Figure 46.1 Suitable veins for venepuncture *(Adapted with kind permission from Williams 1995)*

are their 'good' veins. Palpating the vein also allows the midwife to avoid three other structures:

- valves, which are seen as 'nodules' within the vein and make specimen collection both very difficult and painful if venepuncture is attempted below the valve
- arteries, which have a palpable pulse
- nerves, which often run close to arteries.

It is also necessary to avoid recent puncture sites, existing bruising, areas of skin infection, incapacitated limbs, or those with limited lymphatic drainage, and an arm with an intravenous infusion.

PAIN RELIEF

Many authors now advocate the 'cough' technique to decrease pain on venepuncture (Lavery & Ingham 2005). This involves asking the woman to look away and to cough, as she coughs the venepuncture is undertaken. It does require the midwife to be ready. The mechanism is unclear but success is reported. Other types of distraction may be employed and local anaesthetic creams may also be prescribed. If they are used, it is necessary to wait for the required time in order for the full effect, this is 1–2 hours depending on which one is used.

ASEPSIS AND SKIN PREPARATION

Venepuncture can introduce microorganisms either locally into the tissues at the site, or into the systemic circulation. Using an ANTT approach, the skin is the Key-Site – this should be cleansed using the locally approved skin cleanser – often a 70% alcohol-based wipe, for 30 seconds using the up-and-down, side-to-side approach (friction), and then left to air dry (for at least 30 seconds). The vein is palpated before cleaning and not touched after cleaning. Non-sterile gloves are worn and all equipment is sterile, the Key-Parts are the needle, vacuum system and blood bottles. A disposable tourniquet is used (Brooks 2014) wherever possible. A reusable tourniquet should not be used if it has visible signs of soiling, it should be socially clean (Brooks 2014). The locally agreed policy should be consulted for these issues.

EQUIPMENT

Equipment should be:

- sterile and used in such a way as to maintain asepsis (discussed above)
- ideally a closed vacuum system that also protects the midwife from contact with body fluids (see below)
- chosen according to the vein and the practitioner's competence.

Closed systems are closed between the point of entry of the needle and the collecting specimen bottle. The blood bottle is vacuumed so that as it is inserted onto the needle (with the correct attachment, according to which system is used), the blood bottle fills with blood without any leakage or user contact with body fluids. A 21-g needle should be used; this has an appropriate diameter for the viscosity of blood. Other equipment may be chosen, e.g. winged devices; the procedure is adapted according to the equipment used; midwives are advised to work within their local protocols.

Syringes and needles increase the risk of contamination and needlestick injuries. Their use for venepuncture should be avoided wherever possible. Should a syringe and needle be used they must both be sterile, a needle defence system should be used and the sharps deposited safely into a sharps bin at the point of care on completion. Venepuncture using a syringe and needle requires the midwife to hold the syringe so that as the plunger is drawn back on the syringe, the needle is not withdrawn out of the vein but remains there. It is still necessary to fill the blood bottles in the correct order (see below).

Not all specimen bottles are standard in their colours and uses, local knowledge is necessary, along with knowledge regarding safe and swift transport and specimen request forms.

Portable sharps boxes should be used at the point of care, a used needle should *never* be resheathed (see Chapter 8). Needle defence systems are increasingly available and should be used wherever possible. There is variation with different designs, but in principle the shield is moved manually or activated automatically as soon as the needle is withdrawn so that the needle is covered and cannot again pierce the skin.

Blood specimens should also be drawn in the correct order, cross-contamination of the additives can occur otherwise (Brooks 2014). The order should be:

1. sterile tubes, e.g. blood culture
2. coagulation tubes
3. serum tubes
4. EDTA (ethylenediaminetetraacetic acid) tubes
5. glycolytic inhibitor.

If in doubt as to the order for drawing, the laboratory should be consulted.

POSSIBLE COMPLICATIONS (ADAPTED FROM SCALES 2008)

- Pain: increased by poor choice of site, poor technique (puncturing arteries, valves or nerves), skin cleanser that has not been left to dry and too large a needle. All of these complications can be avoided with a good choice of site, adequate preparation and a competent technique.
- Bruising: this may be caused if the tourniquet is not released at the appropriate time, if the bleeding is not arrested, if the arm is bent up, or if the needle is advanced too far (puncturing the posterior wall of the vein). The application of an ice pack (after the

bleeding has stopped) is indicated. Care should be taken with a woman with a known or suspected clotting disorder to ensure that haemorrhage does not occur after venepuncture. The woman should maintain a straight arm after the procedure for a couple of minutes until bleeding is confirmed to have stopped.

- Accidental puncture of an artery: red oxygenated blood is seen, the needle should be removed and pressure applied for at least 5 minutes with the arm in a straight position. Document the error. Avoid this with careful vein selection and a needle entry degree of 40° or less.
- Failure to obtain the specimen: if the midwife has tried once but not succeeded, or is in doubt before beginning that an appropriate venepuncture can be achieved, then referral should be made to a senior or more experienced practitioner. Repeated attempts are inappropriate both for the woman (e.g. pain, bruising) and because usable veins should be preserved in case they are required in the near future for lifesaving intravenous access.

PROCEDURE: maternal venepuncture

- Decontaminate hands, put on non-sterile gloves.
- Clean a plastic receiver using the locally approved wipes. Leave it to dry, remove gloves and wash and dry hands.
- Gather equipment:
  - vacuumed system with 21-g needle (often green) or sterile alternative with safety device (if appropriate)
  - appropriate specimen bottles
  - approved skin cleanser, often 70% alcohol-based
  - non-sterile gloves
  - antiseptic handrub
  - sterile gauze
  - disposable tourniquet
  - adhesive plaster (if not allergic)
  - specimen request form
  - portable sharps box.
- Gain informed consent; ensure correct specimen is being taken from correct woman by asking her to state her name and date of birth and checking this information against the request form. When the woman is comfortable, support her arm in an accessible position; good light is required.
- Apply the tourniquet approximately 5–7 cm above the antecubital fossa; encourage the woman to clench and unclench her fist a couple of times if necessary.
- Identify the chosen vein by palpation, retaining the site of entry in the 'mind's eye'. Release tourniquet.
- Decontaminate hands and put on non-sterile gloves.

- Cleanse the skin (Key-Site) thoroughly using an up and down, left to right approach (>30 seconds); wait for it to dry (>30 seconds).
- Assemble the needle and appropriate parts of the vacuumed system ready using an ANTT approach (see Chapter 10) for all Key-Parts, reapply the tourniquet, gently unsheath the needle.
- Using the non-dominant hand, apply slight tension to the skin below the point of entry (this will anchor the vein).
- Insert the needle into the vein at a 30° angle with the bevel (slanted edge) uppermost; be decisive but not too firm.
- Fill the blood bottles in order and according to system used. Gently mix those that require it.
- If blood does not appear the needle may be 'nudged' a little further in, or withdrawn a small amount (if no blood is seen, or the woman is in acute pain, remove the needle, collect new equipment, and try another site).
- Release the tourniquet, withdraw the needle fully and immediately apply pressure (Brooks 2014) to the puncture site using the gauze for the next minute (the woman should be encouraged to do this, if able). Keep the woman's arm horizontal. Activate the safety device (if applicable) and place the used sharps straight into the sharps bin.
- Apply plaster if required, once the bleeding has stopped.
- Remove gloves and wash and dry hands.
- Label the specimen bottles and request form while with the woman; send the specimen to the laboratory. Ensure that the results are acted upon on return.
- Dispose of other equipment correctly, clean the receiver as before.
- Document and act accordingly.

Brooks (2014) includes a useful practice checklist (appendix 1, Brooks 2014) that details the significant steps in the venepuncture process.

ROLE AND RESPONSIBILITIES OF THE MIDWIFE

These can be summarized as:
- identifying when venepuncture is necessary, keeping this to a minimum for the woman
- undertaking the procedure competently and safely using an ANTT approach
- education and support of the woman
- referral if necessary
- contemporaneous record keeping.

SUMMARY

- Venepuncture is a skill that all midwives should be able to complete competently.
- It is an aseptic procedure that ideally uses a closed vacuum system so that there is no contact with body fluids.
- Specimens should be in the correct bottles, labelled, and dispatched, and the results acted upon accordingly.

SELF-ASSESSMENT EXERCISES

The answers to the following questions may be found in the text:

1. List the occasions when a woman may be asked to supply a blood specimen.
2. Describe how to locate a suitable vein for venepuncture.
3. Discuss the techniques that can be employed to make this a positive procedure for the woman.
4. What equipment is required to complete the technique safely?
5. Demonstrate how to undertake venepuncture correctly using an ANTT approach.
6. Discuss the possible complications that can occur, and the techniques used to reduce them.
7. Summarize the role and responsibilities of the midwife when undertaking venepuncture.

REFERENCES

Brooks, N., 2014. Venepuncture and Cannulation: A Practical Guide. M&K Publishing, Keswick (Chapter 3).

Lavery, I., Ingram, P., 2005. Venepuncture: best practice. Nurs. Stand. 19 (49), 55–65.

RCN (Royal College of Nursing), 2010. Standards for Infusion Therapy, third ed. RCN, London.

Rowley, S., Clare, S., 2011. ANTT: an essential tool for effective blood culture collection. Br. J. Nurs. 20 (14), S9–S14.

Scales, K., 2008. A practical guide to venepuncture and blood sampling. Nurs. Stand. 22 (29), 29–36.

Williams, P.L. (Ed.), 1995. Gray's Anatomy, thirty-eighth ed. Churchill Livingstone, Edinburgh.

Chapter | 47 |

Principles of phlebotomy and intravenous therapy: intravenous cannulation

LEARNING OUTCOMES

Having read this chapter, the reader should be able to:

- discuss the indications for cannulation
- describe how the site is selected and the equipment chosen
- describe a safe cannulation technique
- describe the correct removal of an intravenous cannula
- summarize the role and responsibilities of the midwife.

When consistent or repeated intravascular access is needed, a cannula is inserted and secured. Some cannulas, e.g. central venous access, are beyond the scope of this text, but fairly commonly midwives insert and care for peripheral cannulae. The terminology changes; the term 'vascular access device' (VAD) can refer to a number of different devices (Dougherty 2011). In this book the term 'peripheral intravenous cannula' (PIC) will be used to describe the intravascular device placed in the hand or lower arm (generally) for the purposes of administering intravenous fluid(s), medication or blood/blood products.

Performing the skill requires training, supervised practice, and ongoing maintenance of the skill. Depending on local protocol, cannula insertion is often undertaken only by qualified staff. PICs feature highly in the nursing and midwifery literature partly because of the risks of localized and systemic infection from their incorrect insertion, use or removal. Insertion, removal and ongoing care of the PIC are all considered within this chapter. The midwife's role and responsibilities are also considered.

CONSIDERATIONS FOR THE CHILDBEARING WOMAN

The additional blood volume in pregnancy and higher body temperature usually mean that the veins are prominent and are therefore easier to gain access to. PICs should be inserted only when there is a clinical indication, and should be removed as soon as that aspect of care is completed. Complications such as infection or occlusion make the therapy more difficult to administer, increase patient discomfort, increase length of hospital stay, and potentially have a financial consequence. Undertaking an assessment prior to insertion of a cannula, and during its insertion, aids the process and reduces the risks (see below).

INDICATIONS

There are a number of potential occasions when a PIC may be required:

- fluid replacement or drug administration in an emergency
- administration of whole blood or blood products
- for drugs requiring intravenous administration
- in preparation for a potential complication or operative delivery, e.g. caesarean section, previous caesarean section labouring and aiming for vaginal delivery, multiple or breech labour, antenatal *per vaginam* bleed
- administration of patient-controlled analgesia
- intravenous fluid administration, e.g. when nil by mouth, with epidural analgesia, postoperatively, care with hyperemesis gravidarum, etc.

ASSESSMENT PRIOR TO PIC INSERTION

Prior to PIC insertion it is appropriate to assess:

- the woman – has she given informed consent? Does she have any prior experience of PIC insertion or similar, e.g. needle phobia may be revealed? Does she have any known allergies? Is she well? Are there any obvious factors that may make PIC insertion difficult or uncomfortable?
- the chosen site (see below)
- the nature and duration of medication to be administered; this can determine which size cannula is used and may also determine that a different VAD is needed.

CHOICE OF SITE

Correct choice of site considers:

- Structures to avoid:
  - the dominant arm
  - areas that are painful, bruised, tortuous, thrombosed, inflamed or with existing skin infection, e.g. eczema

- areas with compromised circulation or sensation, oedema or fracture
- joints, valves in the vein (seen as bulges), bone, ligaments, muscle, nerves or tendons
- arteries, particularly those that run in unexpected directions.
- Try to choose:
  - a vein (identified by its lack of pulse and the ability to empty and fill by occluding and releasing it digitally)
  - a vein in good condition (often described as 'bouncy' (Dougherty 2011)) that can be palpated in the lower half of the arm, e.g. dorsal venous network (back of the hand) and cephalic and basilic veins of the forearm (Fig. 47.1).

Preparation

Venous access is improved if the practitioner and woman are relaxed and if certain physical measures are undertaken. A tourniquet (ideally disposable) should be placed 7–8 cm above the chosen site, heat may be applied (heat pack or warm water), gravity or vein filling may be utilized (clenching/unclenching fist) and gentle stroking of the vein may increase its prominence (Brooks 2014). Topical analgesia can be prescribed in some situations, particularly if the woman requests it, or if a large bore cannula is being inserted. It may take 30 minutes to 1 hour to take effect. A small amount of local anaesthetic such as lidocaine (lignocaine) may be injected intradermally (see Chapter 20) at the proposed puncture site. This needs only 3–5 minutes to take effect. This is often agreed locally under a Patient Group Directive (PGD) (see Chapter 18).

ASEPSIS AND USE OF STANDARD PRECAUTIONS

The RCN (2010) are clear that infection control measures are very important for the insertion and ongoing care of PICs. The Aseptic Non Touch Technique (ANTT) approach (Rowley & Clare 2011) has a specific standard for cannulation (www.antt.co.uk), using a non touch technique for all Key-Parts and Key-Sites and a general aseptic field with the use of Micro Critical Aseptic Fields. (see Chapter 10). All equipment should be sterile and for single use only; a sterile dressing pack is used, as is appropriate personal protective equipment (PPE), e.g. a plastic apron and non-sterile gloves. All sharps should be disposed of at the point of use in a portable sharps box. If continual use of a PIC is needed, it should be renewed after 72–96 hours (RCN 2010), or sooner if no longer required, or if complications are suspected.

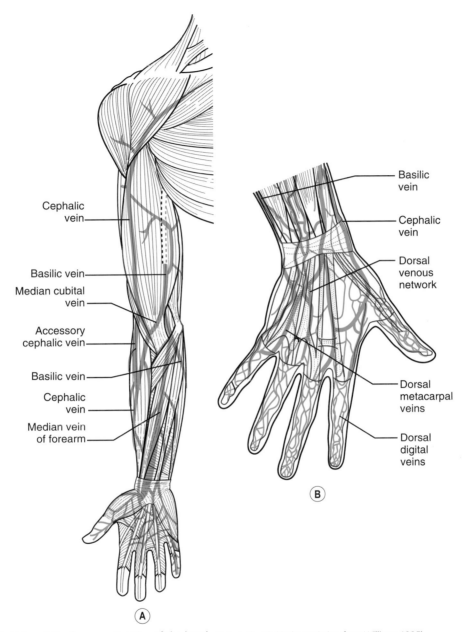

Cephalic
vein

Basilic vein

Median cubital
vein

Accessory
cephalic vein

Basilic vein

Cephalic
vein

Median vein
of forearm

Basilic
vein

Cephalic
vein

Dorsal
venous
network

Dorsal
metacarpal
veins

Dorsal
digital
veins

A

B

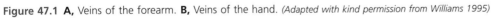

Figure 47.1 A, Veins of the forearm. **B,** Veins of the hand. *(Adapted with kind permission from Williams 1995)*

Skin cleansing (Key-Site) should be undertaken using the locally agreed wipes/solution, often 70% alcohol with 2% chlorhexidine (Loveday et al. 2014). Friction is generated using the up-and-down, right-to-left approach, cleansing for at least 30 seconds. The skin should then air dry for at least 30 seconds, the vein should not be repalpated once the skin has been cleansed. If repalpation is necessary, sterile gloves should be worn.

CHOICE OF EQUIPMENT

In the UK, cannulae are colour-coded according to size, the size is both the gauge and the length, and it determines the flow rate per minute. The one chosen should suit the site and the fluid to be infused. The smallest possible that is

353

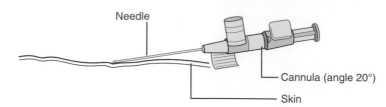

Figure 47.2 Intravenous cannulation. *(Adapted with kind permission from Nicol et al. 2000)*

appropriate should be chosen, as this improves patient comfort (RCN 2010). A larger bore cannula – 16 g (grey) or 14 g (brown) – is often chosen for the childbearing woman in an emergency.

Cannulae may vary slightly according to the manufacturer, but generally consist of a polyurethane piece of tubing with a hub, in which there is a bevelled needle (stylet), also with a hub. Wings may be attached for ease of securing the cannula and there may or may not be a needleless injection port (Fig. 47.2). Once inserted, a closed system is maintained. Any extension tubing or needleless hubs are added and used in an ANTT way. A transparent polyurethane dressing helps the cannula to stay in place, allows for observation of the site, permits the woman to bathe, but does take skill to apply correctly (Lavery & Ingram 2006). A poorly dressed cannula increases the risks of leaking, extravasation, infection, air embolism and trauma; this is unacceptable (Moureau 2013). Whichever type of dressing is used, it should be assessed every 24 hours and if contaminated or peeling, changed (RCN 2010). Otherwise it may be left in place for 48 hours.

DOCUMENTATION

As part of the overall strategy to reduce hospital-acquired infections, cannula care is subjected to standards of good practice principles, including documentation. Local arrangements may include specific forms/stickers (see Raynor 2010, p. 60, for an example) to be used alongside a detailed record of care written in the woman's notes. It should include:

- nature of information given prior to consent being granted
- date, time and site of cannula insertion with details of the site preparation and actual vein used
- clinical indication, cannula type and size (in the UK the manufacturer's printed label with the batch number, etc. is stuck into the woman's medical records)

- anything of note during the insertion procedure, including adherence to infection control protocols and number of attempts made (Raynor 2010)
- drugs administered including any local anaesthetic, flushing agent, or other medication given
- type of dressing applied and appearance of the insertion site afterwards
- proposed plan, particularly removal time
- name and signature of midwife with date and time of documentation

(Adapted from Lavery & Ingram 2006, Brooks 2014 and RCN 2010).

ONGOING CARE

Dougherty (2011) is clear that a cannula should be flushed before and after use (and every 24 hours if not being used) with 0.9% sodium chloride. This is undertaken by a suitably qualified midwife only. The pulsation technique is used, this involves a repeated push/pause action which disturbs any adhering substances and so lessens the infection risk (Lavery & Ingram 2006, Moureau 2013). A second technique, applying positive pressure requires that as the syringe is disconnected from the port, pressure is maintained on the plunger so that blood does not flash into the tip. There is less likelihood then of the cannula occluding. This technique is achieved by closing off the lock on some needleless ports while injecting the last millilitre.

Flushing the cannula serves a number of functions:

- confirms patency
- clears medications
- clears blood and adherents
- reduces the risk of occlusion (Moureau 2013).

The sodium chloride for flushing is often a locally agreed PGD (see Chapter 18) and medicine administration charts have space for signing as for any other medication. An ANTT is used; the volume prescribed is often 10 mL but it should be double the volume of the cannula and any attachment (RCN 2010).

COMPLICATIONS

On insertion of the PIC, care should be taken to stabilize the vein by applying gentle traction to the skin. It is possible to cannulate alongside a vein rather than into it. Equally, veins can be punctured out through the back wall of the vein if the angle of insertion is too great. Pain and bruising will be experienced (Ingram & Lavery 2007). In the event of a failure to insert the cannula, the circumstances may dictate whether one further attempt is made or whether a more senior colleague is called. Repeated failed attempts are distressing for the woman and reduce the number of suitable veins available.

If an artery has been punctured, bright red pulsating oxygenated blood will be seen. The cannula should be removed and firm pressure applied to the puncture site for at least 5 minutes. The arm should be straight. There should be clear documentation of this incident in the notes.

Once inserted the midwife needs to be alert to several other possible complications:

- Phlebitis: inflammation of the vein may be caused by the presence of the cannula or its movement in the vein (mechanical phlebitis); by the drugs or fluids infused through it (chemical phlebitis) and by the presence of infection (infective phlebitis). VIP (visual infusion phlebitis) scoring (Jackson 1998, cited by RCN 2010 and www.vipscore.net) uses visual indicators, e.g. redness, pain, swelling, etc., and allocates a score accordingly. For example, a healthy PIC site scores 0, while one that has slight pain or redness scores 1. At a scoring of 2 (two of the three are present: pain, redness or swelling) the cannula should be re-sited. The scoring continues to 5, at which point advanced thrombophlebitis is present. VIP scoring is undertaken every time the cannula is used, otherwise 24-hourly, the information is documented and acted upon.
- Infiltration: if the PIC is dislodged, non-vesicant (non-blistering) fluids are inadvertently administered into the surrounding tissue rather than the vein. The PIC should be removed and resited if still required.
- Extravasation: vesicant (blistering) fluids are inadvertently administered into the surrounding tissue. Vesicant drugs can cause tissue necrosis and therefore significant morbidity (Dougherty 2011). Examples include phenytoin, sodium bicarbonate, 50% dextrose, potassium, and cefotaxime. Both this and infiltration can be avoided with a good site choice, good insertion technique, and correct fixation of the cannula (Brooks 2014).

PROCEDURE: intravenous cannulation

If topical analgesia is to be used, the vein would be selected, the cream applied and covered. The procedure would commence 30 minutes to 1 hour later (depending on which medication was applied). If using intradermal lidocaine, the prescribed amount is drawn up using an ANTT as part of the preparation described below.

- Confirm identity by asking the woman to state her name and date of birth. Gain informed consent, ensure privacy and prepare the area, e.g. good lighting, free from draughts, etc.
- If appropriate, the woman is invited to wash her hand and arm using antimicrobial soap and water. It is dried using paper towels and alcohol handrub may be applied.
- In the clinical room, wash and dry hands, put on disposable plastic apron, and gather equipment onto the bottom shelf of a recently cleaned dressings trolley:
  - appropriately sized (for vein and fluid) sterile cannula with extension/needleless port set (often two arms, both with a gate clamp)
  - sterile dressing pack
  - semi-permeable occlusive dressing and hypoallergenic tape
  - approved cleansing solution/wipe (70% alcohol/2% chlorhexidine generally for skin) for both skin and equipment
  - portable sharps box
  - clean plastic tray
  - disposable tourniquet
  - two pairs non-sterile gloves and alcohol handrub
  - approved flushing solution (0.9% sodium chloride) with two sterile needles and two 5-mL syringes
  - intradermal lidocaine with appropriate sterile needle and syringe, if using
  - disposable sheet.
- Decontaminate hands, put on non-sterile gloves, and clean the tray with the approved wipes, allowing it to dry then place on the top of the trolley.
- Remove gloves and wash and dry hands.
- Open the outer wrapper of the pack and 'drop' the dressings pack onto the tray, open it using the technique shown on p. 90 (holding corners only).
- Add the sterile cannula, extension set, the dressing, the tourniquet, skin wipe and equipment wipe (both in their packets).
- Connect the first needle and syringe using an ANTT, draw up 5 mL 0.9% sodium chloride.
- Discard the needle into the sharps box and place the syringe in its wrapper on the tray.

- Open the wrapper of the extension set, connect the syringe using an ANTT, prime the extension set with the 0.9% sodium chloride and close off the gate clamp(s), then place it on the tray.
- Draw up the other 5 mL 0.9% sodium chloride, leave in its wrapper on the tray.
- Discard gloves and wash and dry hands.
- Take the trolley to the woman.
- Position the arm so that it is supported with the disposable sheet and sterile towel (from the pack) beneath it. Begin to identify a possible vein.
- Apply the tourniquet approximately 7–8 cm above the intended site so that the veins can fill, but arterial flow is not obstructed; ask the woman to clench her fist a few times to encourage the veins to fill.
- Select the most likely vein by palpation; identify a marker, e.g. a freckle, to recall the intended puncture site and release the tourniquet.
- Use handrub and apply gloves.
- Open the skin wipe, cleanse the skin thoroughly for at least 30 seconds using an up-and-down, side-to-side action, creating friction. Allow it to air dry for at least 30 seconds, reapply the tourniquet.
- Immobilize the vein by supporting the skin below the insertion point, with slight tension, using the non-dominant hand.
- Insert the cannula at an angle of approximately 20°, bevel uppermost; as the vein is entered a flashback of blood may be seen in the hub (this will vary according to the device used).
- Reduce the angle of insertion almost to skin level, advance the cannula slowly a few millimetres further, pause and withdraw the needle halfway; a second flashback may be seen along the cannula.
- Gradually advance the cannula into the vein, up to the hub, while simultaneously withdrawing the needle until almost withdrawn, remembering to remain at the same depth, following the direction of the vein. Release skin traction.
- Release the tourniquet, place a piece of gauze under the hub, gently occlude the vein above the cannula, and withdraw the needle completely. Dispose of needle into sharps box.
- Remove the cap off the extension set and secure it using an ANTT into the cannula (often needs to be screwed in).
- Secure the cannula using the tape, usually vertically over the wings, but this may vary according to the cannula type.
- Wipe the end of the needleless port/extension set, use the four corners and the middle of the wipe, scrubbing approximately for 5 seconds each time, use another part of the wipe around the sides of the port for a further 5 seconds.

- Open the gate clamp on the port, insert the syringe and flush through using the prepared flush with a pulsation method, ending with positive pressure (see above). (Often syringes are secured in extension sets using a quarter turn.)
- Secure the cannula in place with the dressing, ensuring that the puncture site can be visualized. Record the date and time, attach label to the dressing if an agreed action locally. Tape the extension set to the arm.
- If required, blood specimens would be taken before connecting the extension/flushing the cannula or adding an infusion line.
- Ensure the woman is aware of ongoing care of the cannula, asking her to report any adverse effects.
- Dispose of the equipment correctly, clean the tray, remove gloves, apron and wash and dry hands.
- Complete records – written (see above), sticker (if appropriate), and commence VIP chart (see above).
- Ensure that ongoing care of the cannula and/or infusion (see Chapter 48) is maintained.

REMOVING A PERIPHERAL CANNULA

Cannula removal is much less unpleasant for the woman than insertion. The midwife should ensure that it is clinically indicated before removing it. An ANTT is maintained, a sterile dressing should be applied to the puncture site following removal, and observations for wound healing should be undertaken in the days following. The midwife adheres to PPE use and should wear an apron and non-sterile gloves.

PROCEDURE: removal of a peripheral intravenous cannula

- Confirm the woman's identity, gain informed consent and gather equipment:
  - non-sterile gloves and apron
  - sterile gauze
  - disposable sheet
  - portable sharps box
  - alcohol handrub.
- Wash and dry hands and apply apron.
- Position the arm so that it is supported, with the disposable sheet beneath it.
- Loosen the tape around the cannula.
- Open the gauze, apply handrub and then the gloves.
- Begin to withdraw the cannula from the vein; prepare to place the gauze immediately over the puncture site as the cannula is withdrawn.

- Fully withdraw the cannula, apply continuous pressure to the puncture site for at least 1–2 minutes.
- Examine the cannula to confirm that it is complete, dispose of it correctly.
- Once the bleeding has stopped, remove the gauze and cover the wound using a sterile adhesive dressing.
- Ensure the woman is comfortable.
- Dispose of remaining equipment correctly, remove gloves and apron, wash and dry hands.
- Ask the woman to call if any signs of bleeding appear.
- Complete documentation clearly stating date and time of removal, appearance of site, whether the cannula was complete, nature of dressing applied and any further plan of care.

ROLE AND RESPONSIBILITIES OF THE MIDWIFE

These can be summarized as:
- correct selection of site and equipment, careful insertion and removal of peripheral cannula
- appropriate training and maintenance of the skill, assessment of competence
- education and support of the woman
- ongoing care and observation of the site
- correct documentation.

SUMMARY

- Peripheral intravenous cannulation is an uncomfortable, invasive technique that may result in localized or systemic infection.

- The midwife should be appropriately trained and able to maintain the skill.
- It is an Aseptic Non Touch procedure, using the correct-sized cannula for the vein and nature of the fluid.
- The site is chosen with care, avoiding arteries and joints but choosing the basilic or cephalic veins of the hand and forearm.
- Complications may arise both on insertion and in the following days. Vigilant care is needed to prevent them.
- Documentation is thorough and contemporaneous, both on insertion and removal.
- Removal is generally quick and easy; it is still an Aseptic Non Touch procedure.

SELF-ASSESSMENT EXERCISES

The answers to the following questions may be found in the text:
1. Discuss the indications for cannula insertion.
2. Describe how to choose a suitable site for a PIC.
3. Discuss the type of equipment selected, with a rationale for each.
4. Describe and demonstrate how a cannula is inserted correctly.
5. Discuss the complications that may arise following cannula insertion.
6. Describe how to remove a cannula correctly.
7. Summarize the role and responsibilities of the midwife when inserting and removing a PIC.

REFERENCES

Brooks, N., 2014. Venepuncture and Cannulation: A Practical Guide. M&K Publishing, Keswick, (Chapter 3).

Dougherty, L., 2011. Vascular access devices: insertion and management. In: Doughty, L., Lister, S. (Eds.), The Royal Marsden Hospital Manual of Clinical Nursing Procedures, 8th ed. Wiley Blackwell, Chichester, pp. 1079–1164.

Ingram, P., Lavery, I., 2007. Peripheral intravenous cannulation: safe insertion and removal technique. Nurs. Stand. 22 (1), 44–48.

Lavery, I., Ingram, P., 2006. Prevention of infection in peripheral intravenous devices. Nurs. Stand. 20 (49), 49–56.

Loveday, H., Wilson, J., Pratt, R.J., et al., 2014. Epic3: national evidence-based guidelines for preventing healthcare-associated infections in NHS hospitals in England. J. Hosp. Infect. 86 (Suppl. 1), S1–S70.

Moureau, N., 2013. Safe patient care when using vascular access devices. Br. J. Nurs. 22 (2), S14–S21.

Nicol, M., Bavin, C., Bedford-Turner, S., et al., 2000. Essential Nursing Skills, second ed. Mosby, Edinburgh.

Raynor, M., 2010. Peripheral intravenous cannulation. In: Marshall, J., Raynor, M. (Eds.), Advancing Skills in Midwifery Practice. Elsevier, Edinburgh, pp. 57–66.

Rowley, S., Clare, S., 2011. ANTT: an essential tool for effective blood culture collection. Br. J. Nurs. 20 (14), S9–S14.

RCN (Royal College of Nursing), 2010. Standards for Infusion Therapy, third ed. RCN, London.

Williams, P.L. (Ed.), 1995. Gray's Anatomy, thirty-eighth ed. Churchill Livingstone, Edinburgh.

Chapter | 48 |

Principles of phlebotomy and intravenous therapy: intravenous infusion

LEARNING OUTCOMES

Having read this chapter, the reader should be able to:

- discuss the indications for an intravenous infusion
- describe the different types of fluid solution commonly used for an intravenous infusion
- describe the formula for calculating the flow of an intravenous infusion
- discuss the complications associated with infusion therapy and how these are recognized and managed
- discuss how fluid balance is monitored and the significance of this.
- discuss the role and responsibilities of the midwife in relation to intravenous infusion therapy

Women may require intravenous infusion therapy for a variety of reasons but this can be debilitating for the woman, affect her mobility, body image and independence; consequently she may require assistance in caring for herself and for her baby. Intravenous infusion therapy is not without risk ranging from localized complications to more serious systemic ones. Zheng et al (2014) suggest 20–70% of patients receiving an intravenous infusion will develop infusion phlebitis. This chapter focuses on the skills involved with the setting up, monitoring and discontinuation of an intravenous infusion, including reference to the types of solution commonly used and the monitoring of fluid balance. These are skills primarily used in the hospital setting for the childbearing woman and occasionally the baby.

DEFINITION

An intravenous infusion is the introduction of sterile fluid into the venous circulation through the use of pressure. Access to the circulation is usually via the veins of the back of the hand, wrist or lower arm if intravenous therapy is expected to be short term; the subclavian vein or internal jugular vein is the preferred access site if long-term therapy is required (lasting several days or weeks). The latter is rarely used in midwifery. Infusions can be continuous or intermittent (which may be as a secondary infusion).

INDICATIONS

- Prevention of fluid and electrolyte disturbances particularly when oral fluids/food are withheld or not tolerated, e.g. pre- and postoperatively, vomiting, diarrhoea.
- Restoring fluid and electrolyte balance, e.g. hypovolaemia, haemorrhage, shock, dehydration.
- Administration of drugs, e.g. oxytocin.

EQUIPMENT

Intravenous administration set ('giving set')

These are sterile pre-packed sets consisting of a long piece of air-filled tubing with a trocar at the top end that is inserted into the bag/bottle of fluid, a drip chamber (which may contain a filter), and a nozzle at the bottom end that connects to a cannula. The tubing has an adjustable roller clamp around it that adjusts the fluid flow (Fig. 48.1) which should be positioned on the upper third of the tubing. The position of the clamp should be changed periodically to prevent the tubing from kinking, as it may then attempt to straighten out, pushing the clamp open (Ansell & Dougherty 2011). There are two main types used in midwifery – one for the administration of clear fluids and one for blood transfusion (Chapter 49), the latter having a double chamber and a filter. The tubing has needleless ports through which drugs can be administered.

Calibrated burette sets (volume control devices) can be used when a medical infusion device is unavailable to obtain greater control over the flow rate. Calibrated burette sets allow for very small amounts of fluid to be administered and are more likely to be used in the neonatal unit than the maternity unit or to administer diluted drugs.

The use of a closed system of infusion will reduce the risk of infection; with each connection that is added to the infusion line, the infection risk increases (Ansell & Dougherty 2011). For example, three-way taps (stopcocks) used between the cannula and infusion line are difficult

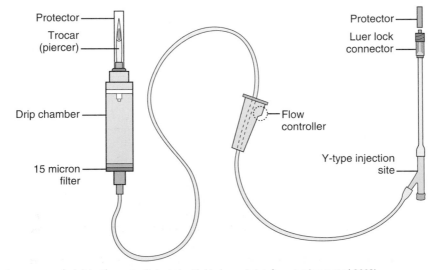

Figure 48.1 An intravenous administration set. *(Adapted with kind permission from Jamieson et al 2002)*

to keep clean and can act as a reservoir for microorganisms, which multiply in the warm, moist environment, increasing the risk of infection (Ansell & Dougherty 2011, Felver 2015).

Medical infusion devices

There are a variety of infusion devices available that allow the infusion flow to be regulated electronically, administering a prescribed amount of fluid over a set time. The midwife should know how the infusion devices work and ensure they are properly cleaned and maintained. Whenever possible, the pump should be connected to a power source to maintain the battery charge. Relying on the battery to continue the infusion for many hours is not best practice. Aceves et al (2013) suggest the battery can die around 2 minutes after the low-battery alarm sounds.

Most of the pumps are smart pumps which can be pre-programmed to create a library of fluids and drugs commonly used in the clinical setting. These bypass the requirement to input the infusion rate and volume manually. Each programme can have predetermined limits which can be set as 'hard' – that is, they cannot be overridden – as going above that level would administer a toxic dose or cause harm (Thimbleby & Cairns 2010), or 'soft' which can be overridden (Upton & Quinn 2013). Independent double checking of the programme should occur to reduce user error (NPSA 2007).

When pre-programmed pumps are unavailable, the midwife should calculate the rate of infusion (mL/hour) using the manufacturer's instructions. Generally the formula used is:

$$\text{Rate (mL/hour)} = \frac{\text{Volume (mL)}}{\text{Time (hour)}}$$

For example, if an infusion pump is to administer 500 mL Hartmann's solution over 4 hours, the rate should be set at:

$$\frac{500}{4} = 125 \, \text{mL/hour}$$

The use of medical infusion devices does not remove the problem with infusion errors. There are still around 250 patient safety incidents concerning the use of medical infusion devices reported to the National Patient Safety Agency (NPSA) each month (NPSA 2010). The Medicines and Healthcare Products Regulatory Agency (MHRA 2013) found, from their investigation of 1085 incidents between 2005 and 2010, that no cause could be found in 68% of cases (which may be due to insufficient information, incorrect reporting or the device was working as intended). However, user error was the cause for 21% of incidents and 11% were device-related issues.

Syringe pumps

Syringe pumps can be used for the administration of drugs (e.g. insulin, opioids) and are useful when a small volume (50 mL or less) of a highly concentrated drug is required (see Chapter 23) or the drug is to be administered over a set period of time. The fluid/drug is contained within a syringe which is connected to the syringe pump and the plunger is depressed by the pump to deliver at the required rate. A 60-mL syringe is usually the largest size that can be used, with smaller syringes being used for the majority of pumps.

Volumetric pumps

Volumetric pumps are electronic devices that can accurately measure the volume of fluid to be infused and administer at preset rates; different pumps may require different administration sets. An alarm will sound if there is a blockage preventing flow of the fluid, when the fluid volume has been delivered, increased pressure is required (e.g. infiltration) and when the battery is low. Some pumps will alarm if infiltration occurs and obstructs the flow, although deWit & O'Neill (2014) caution that the infiltration can be extensive before it is detected.

Many of the pumps have air detectors to detect and prevent the passage of single bubbles (approximately 100 mcg/L) although they are very sensitive and will alarm more frequently if they detect 'champagne bubbles' (MHRA 2013).

Calculating the flow rate of the intravenous fluid when no infusion device is used

When there is no infusion device available, the infusion can be administered using gravity and the flow rate calculated and set manually. The midwife should refer to the administration set being used for details of the number of drops per millilitre, referred to as the drop factor. Commonly the drop factor is 20 for clear fluids, although this can vary between 10–60 drops/mL (Piper 2013) and 15 for blood. The drop factor is determined by the size of the tubing lumen; micro-drips administer 60 drops per millilitre and are useful for the administration of small fluid volumes whereas a macro drip is usually used for rates greater than 75 mL/hour (Bowen 2014). The following formula is used to calculate the number of drops per minute:

$$\frac{\text{Volume of solution (mL)} \times \text{drop factor}}{\text{Required infusion time (minutes)}}$$

Table 48.1 Intravenous infusion solutions commonly used in midwifery

Solution	Example	Indication for use
Crystalloid: isotonic solutions (same tonicity as blood)	0.9% sodium chloride Hartmann's, Plasmalyte	To compensate for fluid loss by expanding the circulating volume
Crystalloid: hypotonic solutions (lower particle concentration)	0.45% sodium chloride	To compensate for fluid loss by moving fluid into intracellular spaces
Crystalloid: hypertonic solutions (higher tonicity than plasma)	20% albumin 20% glucose/dextrose	To compensate for fluid loss by moving fluid from intra- to extracellular spaces
Colloids: undissolved particles (protein, starch, sugar) too large to pass through capillary walls	5% or 25% albumin	Draws fluid from interstitial and intracellular spaces. Used when crystalloids ineffective
Plasma expanders: Colloid fluids	Dextran, gelofusine, voluven	To expand plasma volume by drawing fluid from interstitial spaces
Blood and blood products	Whole blood Packed cells	To maintain circulatory volume, increase particular blood components

For example, if 500 mL Hartmann's solution is prescribed over a 4-hour period, using an administration set with a drop factor of 20, the flow rate will be:

$$\frac{500 \times 20}{240} = 41.67 = 42 \text{ drops per minute}$$

It is important to ensure the fluid is infused over the correct period of time to prevent over- or under-infusion, both of which can have serious consequences. The flow rate should be checked regularly to ensure it is still running at the correct rate. Piper (2013) suggests every 15 minutes, then when stable, hourly. The flow rate is influenced by a number of factors, e.g. height of fluid in relation to the insertion site, the fluid type, the woman's blood pressure, movements and position, patency of the cannula and kinks in the tubing (Bowen 2014). Ansell & Dougherty (2011) advise the fluid container can be hung 1–1.5 m above the infusion site for adequate pressure within the infusion to overcome venous pressure and facilitate the flow of the fluid into the circulation. If it is higher, they suggest the intravenous pressure can be too great which can cause infiltration (Ansell & Dougherty 2011). Bowen (2014) suggests that half of the initial flow rate can be lost during the first hour of infusion highlighting the importance of checking and readjusting the rate regularly.

If the infusion is switched on to free-flow, the volume of fluid delivered in a specific time frame will vary. Pierce et al (2013) found that 250 mL phenylephrine placed at 80 cm and running through a micro-drip and an 18-gauge cannula would empty in <10 minutes whereas a 1000 mL bag of crystalloid at 100 cm through a 14-gauge cannula would empty in less than 30 minutes. This again highlights the importance of regularly checking the flow rate.

INTRAVENOUS FLUID

A variety of solutions can be administered intravenously (Table 48.1); crystalloids are the commonest. Crystalloids are iso-, hypo-, or hypertonic solutions, depending on their tonicity. Isotonic solutions have the same tonicity as the body's internal environment with a very similar sodium concentration (e.g. 0.9% sodium chloride, Hartmann's, Plasmalyte). Isotonic fluids will expand the extracellular fluid volume (ECV) without moving water in or out of cells. Hypotonic solutions have a lower tonicity; thus they attract water from the ECV into the cells (e.g. dextrose 5%) and hypertonic solutions have increased tonicity which draws water from the cells by osmosis into the ECV (e.g. albumin 20%).

The fluid is usually contained within a soft plastic bag but may also be in a glass bottle or semi-rigid plastic container (polyfusor); these may have calibrations on the side to indicate how much fluid is in the container. However, Nowicki (2013) cautions that the fluid bag gradations are inaccurate and do not represent the amount of fluid left in the bag. The soft bags have a double plastic layer that is pulled apart or twisted off and the trocar inserted though the opening. Glass containers have a rubber bung covered with a sterile seal. Once the sterile seal is removed, the trocar is inserted through the bung along with a sterile air inlet needle for venting, to equalize pressure within the bottle and facilitate fluid flow. The semi-rigid bag requires opening using sterile scissors and the trocar inserted into the tube. Soft and semi-rigid containers do not require venting.

Prior to use, glass containers should be checked for cracks and chips, and plastic containers squeezed to ensure there are no leaks (Piper 2013). The fluid should be looked at to ensure there is no discoloration, cloudiness, particles or precipitate present. If in doubt, do not use.

Checking the infusion solution prior to administration

In the UK a doctor must prescribe the solution which is checked by two people, one of whom should be a qualified midwife, nurse or doctor to ensure the correct infusion is given to the correct woman. The midwife should check:

- the woman's name and hospital number
- the medicine administration chart – type of infusion fluid and amount to be infused, which should be accurately written up and signed, and ensure the method of administration, route and timing are appropriate to the choice of fluid being administered
- the fluid bag is checked that it is the correct solution and volume and that it has not expired
- the fluid should be examined for signs of discoloration, cloudiness, or sediment and the container examined for signs of contamination
- the flow rate should be calculated if an infusion device is not available
- if an infusion device is used, that the programme is the correct one
- the batch number should be recorded on the medicine administration chart.

PROCEDURE: commencing an intravenous infusion using a fluid bag

- Due to the risk of infection, it is important to use an Aseptic Non Touch Technique (ANTT) throughout (see Chapter 10).
- Confirm the identity of the woman (ask her to verbally state her name and date of birth) and confirm details on her identity band against the medicine administration chart and gain informed consent (some NHS Trusts also require the woman to state her address).
- Ensure a patent cannula is *in situ*.
- Decontaminate hands by washing and drying or applying handrub.
- Clean a large plastic or metal tray to create an aseptic field with locally approved cleanser, often 70% alcohol/2% chlorhexidine solution/wipe and allow to dry for at least 30 seconds.
- Gather equipment:
  - plastic apron
  - administration set
  - infusion solution (checked as above)
  - sterile or clean receiver
  - handrub plus non-sterile gloves
  - infusion stand
  - medical infusion device if required
  - locally approved skin cleanser, often 70% alcohol/2% chlorhexidine.
- Wash hands and dry hands or apply handrub and allow to dry.
- Apply plastic apron and non-sterile gloves.
- Open the administration set and close the roller clamp below the drip chamber and place on the tray.
- Unwrap the infusion solution and place on the tray.
- Remove the cover from the trocar at the top end of the tubing and from the infusion bag, without touching either opening (both ANTT Key-Parts).
- Invert the fluid bag and insert the trocar into it.
- Suspend the fluid bag from an infusion stand.
- Gently compress the drip chamber to half fill it and reduce the risk of air bubbles in the tubing.
- Place the other end of the tubing over the receiver.
- Slowly release the flow control clamp to fill the tubing with fluid (priming) with no air bubbles.
- Close the roller clamp.
- Connect to the medical infusion device if being used.
- Remove gloves if contaminated and apply handrub, then reglove.
- Scrub the cannula port tip with the locally approved cleanser using the four corners and the middle of the wipe, each for approximately 5 seconds then cleaning away from the tip, in a side-to-side, up-and-down direction, creating friction.
- Allow to dry for 30 seconds.
- Occlude the vein if a needle-free connector has not been applied to the cannula end, remove the cover from the end of the tubing, and connect the tubing to the cannula using an ANTT. Key-Parts are the cannula/connection into it and the tubing to be connected.
- Remove gloves and apron and decontaminate hands.
- Adjust the flow rate accordingly using the roller clamp.
- Label the tubing with time and date infusion commenced. If two infusions are running, each line should be labelled with the contents of the infusion solution and (if any) drugs.
- Dispose of equipment correctly and wash and dry hands.
- Commence a fluid balance record.
- Document and act accordingly.

AIR BUBBLES

Air bubbles have the potential to damage tissue immediately by causing an obstruction leading to ischaemia or in the longer-term by provoking a thromboinflammatory response (Wilkins & Unverdorben 2012). However, it is not known how much air in the tube is 'safe'. Bakan et al (2013) and Wilkins & Unverdorben (2012) suggest a small amount of air will be absorbed spontaneously with no adverse effect, often within 30 minutes. Wilkins & Unverdorben (2012) cite the International Electrotechnical Commission standard that 1 mL of air, with a 12.4 mm diameter, infused within 15 minutes is not considered a safety issue. For this calculation they excluded any bubbles in the 1 mL of air if they were less than 50 mcg and 4.6 mm diameter. Bakan et al (2013) further state that the amount of air considered to be a lethal volume is 200–300 mL or 3–5 mL/kg for adults (which Wilkins & Unverdorben 2012 agree with).

Although small amounts are probably insignificant, there have been fatal cases reported from very small air bubbles, particularly with neonates (Wilkins & Unverdorben 2012). As it can be very difficult to estimate the size of air bubbles in tubing, it is best practice to avoid the infusion of air bubbles. Wilkins & Unverdorben (2012) recommend aspirating air from stopcocks and needle-free connectors and caution that even small volumes of air should be considered as potentially having adverse effects.

CHANGING THE ADMINISTRATION SET

Ullman et al (2013) suggest the administration set can be changed every 96 hours, as this is not associated with an increased risk of infection; Felver (2015) agrees if the infusion has been continuous but advises every 24 hours if it is intermittent. The exceptions to this are if a blood transfusion has been administered (every 12 hours, see Chapter 49), lipids have been administered (every 24 hours, Felver 2015) or the administration set has had a number of manipulations. The tubing should be changed immediately if it becomes occluded or damaged, if it becomes disconnected from the cannula and each time the cannula is replaced (at least every 72 hours). The procedure is the same as above. The tubing should be labelled with the date and time its use began to enable it to be replaced within the required timeframes (Baldwin et al 2013).

CHANGING THE INTRAVENOUS SOLUTION

The next bag of fluid should be checked and ready for use before the current bag empties completely; deWit & O'Neill (2014) recommend this should be when there is 50 mL of solution left to infuse. The solution should be checked as above. Close the roller clamp ensuring the drip chamber is half full before changing the solution. With cleaned, gloved hands, the midwife removes the trocar from the fluid bag and inserts it into the newly opened solution using the ANTT approach. The roller clamp should be opened and the flow rate adjusted. Record keeping is completed as appropriate. Ansell & Dougherty (2011) advise the bag of solution should hang for no more than 24 hours.

Bakan et al (2013) found there is a risk of air embolism occurring with collapsible intravenous fluid bags that do not have a self-sealing outlet if the closed system has broken down, such as may occur when a pressure bag is used for rapid infusion. Thus when a pump is not used, and especially when a pressure bag is used for rapid infusion of fluid, keep checking the amount of fluid remaining in the bag and change the infusion before air empties from the infusion bag.

ONGOING CARE OF THE INTRAVENOUS INFUSION

- The flow rate should be checked regularly to ensure it is still running at the correct rate. Piper (2013) suggests every 15 minutes, then when stable, hourly.
- If the infusion is not running as required, do not infuse a large amount to 'catch up' – the infusion rate should be recalculated (deWit & O'Neill 2014).
- deWit & O'Neill (2014) suggest the infusion site should be checked at least hourly although Baldwin et al (2013) propose twice a day and Piper (2013) recommends at least once a day. This will facilitate early detection of complications. Felver (2015) recommends the cannulation site should be palpated through the dressing to assess for tenderness in addition to the visual inspection of the site and arm.
- Ensure the tubing does not touch the ground, as this will increase the risk of contamination (Felver 2015).
- If the infusion is completed but the cannula remains *in situ* it should be flushed as discussed on p. 354.
- The dressing over the cannula site should be changed every 24–72 hours, as moisture or a non-adherent dressing increase the risk of bacterial contamination (Bowen 2014). Felver (2015) suggests the transparent

dressing should be replaced when the tubing is replaced or when it is damp, soiled, or loose; if a gauze dressing is used, it should be changed every 48 hours. Transparent dressings are preferable as they allow visualization of the site.

- If the woman's clothing needs to be changed while an infusion is in progress, do not disconnect the tubing but pass the bag of fluid and tubing through the clothing. This is easily achieved if the arm without the tubing is removed from the clothing first, followed by the arm with the infusion *in situ*. When putting on clothes, the fluid bag and tubing are passed through the sleeve (in the same direction the arm is placed through it) followed by the arm with the infusion *in situ* and then the unaffected arm through the other sleeve.
- If the woman is mobilizing, e.g. to walk to the toilet, the infusion/medical infusion device should be placed onto a pole with wheels and the woman encouraged to hold onto the pole using the hand with the infusion *in situ* to push the pole while walking (Felver 2015).

SECONDARY AND CONCURRENT INFUSIONS

There may be times when a second infusion is connected to the infusion running (primary infusion), often for the purpose of medication administration. It is important that the second administration set and all connectors are primed as above to prevent the administration of a large amount of air into the circulation. A secondary infusion ('piggy-back') usually refers to two infusions running through the same pump with the second infusion connected into the primary infusion. Cassano-Piché et al (2012) recommend the secondary infusion bag should be at a higher height than the primary infusion bag to prevent the contents of the secondary infusion bag back-flowing into the primary infusion tubing. Alternatively the primary infusion should be clamped whilst the secondary infusion is running. It is important the fluids in both tubing sets are compatible (in case there is mixing of fluid) to prevent precipitates forming and obstructing the flow. A concurrent infusion refers to two infusions running through a single IV port, e.g. Y-connector, both with their own infusion device to control the rates of flow individually. Where more than one administration set is used, it is vital to label each as to its contents.

COMPLICATIONS

A number of complications can develop from intravenous infusions, these include the following:

Infection

If infection occurs at the cannula site the area may be red, warm, tender and swollen.

Phlebitis

This is inflammation of the vein and occurs if the vein is injured or irritated from the cannula or infused drugs/fluids. Felver (2015) suggests phlebitis is also associated with hypertonic solutions and a rapid infusion rate. The area will be painful, swollen, and inflamed along the vein (seen as a red streak), which may feel hard and warm to touch. A warm, moist compress applied to the affected site can reduce discomfort (deWit & O'Neill 2014, Felver 2015) and the infusion should be re-sited.

Infiltration

deWit and O'Neill (2014) advise infiltration is the commonest complication. If the cannula gets dislodged or has penetrated the vessel wall, the solution flows into the surrounding tissues causing increasing pain and swelling, the site may feel cool and the arm may become oedematous with sensation eventually affected. The infusion rate slows down and there will be no blood in the tubing when it is held below the level of insertion (Piper 2013). The infusion should be discontinued and restarted at a new site. The woman should be advised to limit the movement of the limb with the infusion running through (Bowen 2014).

Thrombus

A blood clot can form around the traumatized tissue at the cannula site. The area will appear similar to phlebitis and the infusion may stop if the clot occludes the cannula. Bowen (2014) suggests applying a warm compress and re-siting the infusion but cautions against rubbing or massaging the affected area.

Speed shock

This occurs when a large volume of fluid is administered quickly, if the roller clamp is too loose or if the flow rate is too rapid. The body recognizes the substance as foreign and a systemic reaction occurs. The woman will develop a flushed face, pounding headache, feel light-headed, with tightness in her chest, and become tachycardic (pulse may be irregular) and hypotensive. As the reaction increases, she will become shocked, lose consciousness, and cardiac arrest can follow. If these signs and symptoms develop, the infusion should be turned off, urgent medical assistance sought, vital signs monitored and symptoms treated.

Fluid/circulatory overload

This occurs when excessive amounts of isotonic fluids are given. The extracellular volume increases in proportion to the amount of fluid administered and is not drawn into the intracellular compartment. This may occur if the fluid rate is too fast or the amount required miscalculated. The woman will develop engorged neck veins (jugular), hypertension, tachypnoea, dyspnoea, tachycardia (pulse may be bounding), elevated central venous pressure measurement and peripheral oedema. The fluid balance chart will show a high positive balance. If this develops, the infusion should be stopped or slowed, the woman sat upright, oral fluids may need to be withheld, medical assistance sought, vital signs monitored and the symptoms treated.

Air embolism

The woman will develop sudden dyspnoea and be short of breath, wheezing, coughing with tachycardia (may be weak), hypotension, raised central venous pressure, level, distended jugular veins and may lose consciousness. Treatment is to occlude the cannula, sit the woman up, call for urgent medical assistance, monitor vital signs and treat the symptoms.

Sepsis

This may occur if sterility is not maintained during insertion of the cannula or connecting/changing fluids and equipment. Bowen (2014) suggests frequent dressing changes may be a cause of sepsis. The insertion site will appear red and be tender. The woman can develop fever, malaise, headache, nausea, vomiting, tachycardia and tachypnoea. If suspected, medical assistance is called for, the infusion site changed, blood cultures obtained and, if indicated, antibiotics administered.

MONITORING FLUID BALANCE

A fluid balance chart should be started at the beginning of the infusion and maintained throughout to ensure the woman is tolerating the amount of fluid being infused. A fluid balance chart records all fluids taken into the body through the intravenous and oral routes (and very rarely for the adult via a nasogastric tube) and all fluid lost from the body mainly in urine but includes vomit, wound drainage, diarrhoea, nasogastric drainage, blood loss. Normally intake and output balance; however, if the amount of fluid taken in exceeds the amount excreted, circulatory overload can result. Cardiac failure can ensue, characterized initially by increasing dyspnoea and peripheral oedema, unless fluid intake is restricted. A reduction in plasma osmolarity

and oedematous cells can also result in convulsions and coma if the brain cells swell. If output exceeds intake, dehydration with shrinkage of cells and tissues can occur.

It is important the midwife carefully measures the amount of fluid actually drunk by the woman and the amount of solution infused, keeping a cumulative total of the intake. All forms of fluid output should be measured carefully and recorded, again with a cumulative total. Keeping the cumulative totals up-to-date enables a very quick assessment of the fluid balance status of the woman and any change such as decreasing urinary output should be notified to the doctor. These charts do not usually take into account fluid obtained from food (although some food such as yoghurt may be included) or insensible fluid loss; however, Bowen (2014) suggests these two usually balance each other out. Intake and output are totalled at the end of each 24-hour period and a calculation as to whether the woman is in balance or has a positive (excess intake) or negative (excess output) balance with this documented in the appropriate records and acted on accordingly. The overall balance should be carried forwards to the next 24-hour period as the intake–output balance may not be achieved for 2–3 days (Bowen 2014).

ROLE AND RESPONSIBILITIES OF THE MIDWIFE

These can be summarized as:

- maintaining competency in the setting up and ongoing monitoring of the intravenous infusion
- minimizing the risk of infection during all procedures which includes using an ANTT
- being familiar with the medical infusion devices available, ensuring they are properly used and maintained
- identifying complications and how to treat them, referring as necessary
- recognizing the significance of fluid balance and maintaining accurate fluid balance charts
- contemporaneous record keeping.

SUMMARY

- An intravenous infusion is a means of giving fluid or drugs directly into the venous circulation.
- Medical infusion devices are used to administer the infusion at a set rate; their use is not without risk.
- Intravenous infusion is associated with a number of complications and regular monitoring of the woman is required during the procedure.
- It can be debilitating for the woman who may require assistance in caring for herself and her baby.

SELF-ASSESSMENT EXERCISES

The answers to the following questions may be found in the text:

1. What are the indications for an intravenous infusion?
2. When would an isotonic solution be used rather than a hypo- or hypertonic solution?
3. What is the formula for calculating the flow rate of an intravenous infusion when a medical infusion device is not used?
4. Identify four complications associated with intravenous infusion therapy and how you would recognize and manage these.
5. Describe how an intravenous infusion is set up and commenced.
6. What are the ongoing responsibilities of the midwife during the infusion?
7. How is fluid balance recorded and why is this important?

REFERENCES

Aceves, A.M., Oladimeji, P., Thimbleby, H., Lee, P., 2013. Are prescribed infusions running as intended? Quantitative analysis of log files from infusion pumps used in a large acute NHS hospital. Br. J. Nurs. July (CareFusion Suppl), 15–21.

Ansell, L., Dougherty, L., 2011. Medicines management. In: Dougherty, L., Lister, S. (Eds.), The Royal Marsden Hospital Manual of Clinical Nursing Procedures, eighth ed. Wiley Blackwell, Chichester.

Bakan, M., Topuz, U., Esen, A., et al., 2013. Inadvertent venous air embolism during cesarean. Rev. Bras. Anestesiol. 63 (4), 362–365.

Baldwin, W., Murphy, J., Shakespeare, D., et al., 2013. Campaign for best practice in intravenous therapy. Nurs. Times 109 (33/34), 22–23.

Bowen, L., 2014. Fluid, electrolyte and acid-base balance. In: Dempsey, J., Hillege, S., Hill, R. (Eds.), Fundamentals of Nursing and Midwifery, second ed. Lippincott, Williams & Wilkins, Philadelphia, pp. 1268–1278.

Cassano-Piché, A., Fan, M., Sabovitch, S., et al., 2012. Multiple intravenous infusions phase 1b: practice and training scan. Ont. Health Technol. Assess. Ser. 12 (16), 1–132.

deWit, S.C., O'Neill, O., 2014. Administering intravenous solutions and medications. In: Fundamental Concepts and Skills for Nursing, fourth ed. Elsevier, St. Louis, pp. 698–725.

Felver, L., 2015. Fluid, electrolyte and acid-base balance. In: Potter, P.A., Perry, A.G., Stockert, P.A., Hall, A. (Eds.), Essentials for Nursing Practice, eighth ed. Elsevier, St. Louis, pp. 482–488.

Jamieson, E.M., McCall, J.M., Whyte, L.A., 2002. Clinical Nursing Practices, fourth ed. Churchill Livingstone, Edinburgh.

MHRA (Medicines and Healthcare Products Regulatory Agency), 2013. Infusion systems. Available online: <https://www.gov.uk/government/uploads/system/uploads/attachment_data/file/403420/Infusion_systems.pdf> (accessed 9 November 2014).

Nowicki, R.W.A., 2013. Inaccuracy of fluid container volume markings. Anaesthesia 68, 640–654.

NPSA (National Patient Safety Agency), 2007. Patient Safety Alert 20: Promoting safer use of injectable medicines. Available online: <http://www.nrls.npsa.nhs.uk/resources/?entryid45=59812> (accessed 27 December 2014).

NPSA (National Patient Safety Agency), 2010. Design for patient safety: A guide to the design of electronic infusion devices. Available online: <http://www.nrls.npsa.nhs.uk/resources/?entryid45=68534> (accessed 27 December 2014).

Pierce, E.T., Kumar, V., Zheng, H., Peterfreund, R.A., 2013. Medication and volume delivery by gravity-driven micro-drip intravenous infusion: potential variations during 'Wide-Open' flow. Anesth. Analg. 116, 614–618.

Piper, K., 2013. Meeting fluid and electrolyte needs. In: Koutoukidis, G., Stainton, K., Hughson, J. (Eds.), Tabbner's Nursing Care, sixth ed. Elsevier, Chatswood, pp. 546–550.

Thimbleby, H., Cairns, P., 2010. Reducing number entry error: solving a widespread serious problem. J. R. Soc. Interface 7 (51), 1429–1439.

Ullman, A.J., Cooke, M.L., Gillies, D., et al., 2013. Optimal timing for intravascular administration set replacement. Cochrane Database Syst. Rev. (9), Art. No.: CD003588, doi:10.1002/14651858.CD003588.pub3.

Upton, D., Quinn, C., 2013. Smart pumps – good for nurses as well as patients. Br. J. Nurs. July (Carefusion Suppl.), 4–8.

Wilkins, R.G., Unverdorben, M., 2012. Accidental infusion of air a concise review. J. Infus. Nurs. 35 (6), 404–408.

Zheng, G.H., Yang, L., Chen, H.Y., et al., 2014. Aloe vera for prevention and treatment of infusion phlebitis. Cochrane Database Syst. Rev. (6), Art. No.: CD009162, doi:10.1002/14651858.CD009162.pub2.

Chapter | 49 |

Principles of phlebotomy and intravenous infusion: blood transfusion

LEARNING OUTCOMES

Having read this chapter, the reader should be able to:

- define blood transfusion, listing its likely uses in the maternity care setting
- discuss why O Rhesus-negative blood is the universal donor and AB-positive the universal recipient
- discuss in detail the role of the midwife with regard to safe transfusion practice.

This chapter examines the safe administration of a blood transfusion for women (not the fetus or baby) and the midwife's role and responsibilities.

DEFINITION

Whole blood or components of blood are introduced into the venous circulation, usually for the purposes of treating a clinical abnormality. Shortage of red blood cells results in hypoxia and the circulatory system needs to have sufficient blood within the vessels to sustain blood pressure, heart rate and all other circulatory functions. The DH (1994) recommend using whole blood quickly for the management of massive obstetric haemorrhage. UK maternity units have 2 units of O Rhesus-negative blood available for immediate transfusion to any woman while awaiting cross-matched blood, such is the significance of blood transfusion in saving lives.

Blood transfusion can be a controversial treatment: it is the transfer of live tissue from one person to another – a transplant. Some people will refuse transfusion; Lewis (2005) includes guidelines for the management of obstetric haemorrhage in women who decline blood transfusion. Despite careful screening, there is the possibility of disease or antibody transmission and blood is an expensive treatment that may vary in its availability.

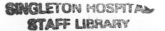

There is a duty for UK Hospital Trusts to report transfusion incidents to the Medicines and Healthcare products Regulatory Agency (MHRA). This is done by the recognized person, often the transfusion practitioner or haematologist. While voluntary, >99% of UK Healthcare facilities also submit adverse (potential or actual) transfusion incident reports (anonymized) to the haemovigilence scheme, SHOT (Serious hazards of transfusion). Their annual report aims to improve practice standards and to educate practitioners (Hurrell 2014).

The responsibility for safe and effective transfusion rests with the multidisciplinary team, but especially with those directly administering it, e.g. the midwife. The stages of safe transfusion practice are considered in detail below.

INDICATIONS FOR MATERNAL TRANSFUSION

Indications for transfusion include:

- hypovolaemia, e.g. after a significant haemorrhage
- low haemoglobin
- some clotting disorders and blood diseases.

Blood can be administered in different forms: whole blood, packed red cells (plasma removed), platelet concentration, fresh frozen plasma, white blood cells and cryoprecipitate (clotting factors) (Jones & Heyes 2014, Watson & Hearnshaw 2010). Anti-D immunoglobulin is also a human blood product. Cell salvage and techniques such as autologous donation or erythropoiesis-stimulating agents are all aiming to reduce the need for external blood transfusion. The midwife should be aware of developing techniques; the inappropriate use of blood transfusion has a significant effect, both in human and financial terms. The midwife has a responsibility in the provision of effective antenatal care, and in the management of the third stage of labour, as well as obstetric haemorrhage emergencies, all to ensure that the need for transfusion is minimized. The need for transfusion should be reviewed on an individual and careful basis.

UNDERSTANDING BLOOD GROUPS

Blood groups are defined as A, B, AB, or O Rhesus negative or positive. The group is determined by the presence of an antigen on the red cell surface and an antibody in the serum. Individuals with group A, for example, have A antigens on their surface and B antibodies in the serum (Table 49.1). Eighty-five percent of the population has an additional antigen on their red cells, the Rhesus factor. If Rhesus-positive blood is introduced into a Rhesus-negative

Table 49.1 Antibodies/antigens of the blood groups

Group	Antigen	Antibody
A	A	B
B	B	A
AB	AB	None
O	None	AB

person, antibodies then form, with a haemolyzing effect on the next introduction of Rhesus-positive blood. Blood group O is known as the universal donor (having no antigens for antibodies to fight), while group AB is known as the universal recipient (having no antibodies to fight foreign antigens). Therefore the true universal donor is O Rhesus negative (Rh−) and the true universal recipient is AB Rhesus positive (Rh+).

An incompatible blood donation initiates the antigen–antibody reaction, causing red blood cells to agglutinate (clump together); this is a serious transfusion reaction, potentially leading to kidney failure and death.

MATERNAL ANTIBODIES

The presence of maternal antibodies (e.g. anti-D, anti-Kell, etc.) means that cross-matching should be undertaken carefully to ensure a safe match. Maternal antibodies can have life-threatening consequences to the fetus. In the UK, blood group and Rhesus factor screening of maternal blood should take place at booking and, if the woman is Rhesus negative, prophylactic anti-D (single dose, 1500 IU) is offered at 28–30 weeks' gestation (Norfolk 2013 p. 113). SHOT (Bolton-Maggs et al 2014) reported that in 2013, 277 pregnant Rhesus-negative women in the UK developed, or were at risk of developing, anti-D antibodies because of delayed or omitted prophylaxis. If postnatal administration of anti-D is required it should be administered within 72 hours. SHOT should be informed if a woman develops a new immune anti-D at any time during maternity care (Bolton-Maggs et al 2014).

SAFE TRANSFUSION PRACTICE: PRINCIPLES AND PROCEDURES

There are potentially significant dangers associated with blood transfusion (see below). While many of them are avoidable, not all of them are (Hurrell 2014), those that are, are largely associated with human error (Bolton-Maggs 2014). The standard of care is set by the British Committee for Standards in Haematology (BCSH 2009), the standards are underpinned by:

- patient identification
- good documentation
- excellent communication.

PRE-TRANSFUSION PREPARATION

- A full history must be taken of any previous transfusions, transplants, pregnancies and current medication to identify any possible risk factors for this transfusion. The antenatal booking history will include this information, but it should be discussed again if transfusion is being considered.
- A physical examination (or re-assessment of condition) should be undertaken to establish that a transfusion is necessary. The need for transfusion should not be based on laboratory results alone (Norfolk 2013). Lives are also lost if transfusion is necessary but is overlooked or delayed.
- Women should be fully informed of the risks, benefits and alternatives, both verbally and with written information so that consent, if given, is fully informed. In an emergency situation the next-of-kin are asked to give consent, the woman should be fully informed retrospectively. The reason for transfusion and a summary of the information given is recorded in the woman's medical records.
- Blood is not a medicine and is therefore not prescribed but authorized (it will be called a prescription in this text). The qualified authorizer completes the locally approved 'prescription' chart indicating specifically:
  - what is to be transfused
  - the date/when it is to be transfused and over what duration/rate
  - the volume/number of units
  - any special requirements, e.g. an irradiated specimen.
- In hospital the woman must be wearing an identification band (or other ID, e.g. photocard) that accurately shows (as a minimum) her full name, date of birth and unique identification number, e.g. NHS number. Positive identification also includes asking the woman to state her name and date of birth. Where the patient is unable to do this, e.g. if unconscious, relatives at the bedside are asked to confirm it.

- The blood sample taken for cross-matching (group and screen specimen) is taken from the woman:
  - after informed consent has been given
  - after she has been positively identified
  - when she is the only woman being bled at that time
  - when the practitioner is uninterrupted
  - when the correct bottles are not prelabelled but are filled and labelled fully and legibly, by hand, in the presence of the woman
  - when the specimen request form is fully completed and signed by the practitioner who took the sample.

The 'wrong blood in the bottle' is a persistent incident reported to SHOT (Bolton-Maggs et al 2014); in 2013 in the UK, 643 such incidents occurred. Some such errors will have been identified in the laboratory but if the woman does not have a blood history recorded, there could be fatal consequences. The taking of booking bloods and of this cross-matching specimen are both a critical part (Oldham 2014) in the safety of the woman being transfused. The prescriber who requests the transfusion (preferably in writing) must be clear about what is required, where and when it is required and for whom, including the diagnosis and any other relevant clinical information.

PRACTICALITIES

Establish, before the blood is collected, that the environment is prepared ready:

- Are there adequate staffing levels for the woman to be appropriately supervised throughout the transfusion? Ideally non-urgent transfusions take place during the day.
- Has the woman given her consent? Is she ready for the transfusion to happen? Does she have a wristband or other ID in place?
- Is the prescription completed correctly?
- Have a set of vital sign observations been completed? This should be undertaken as a baseline reading before transfusion commences, but no more than 1 hour before. A dedicated transfusion or MEOWS (Maternal Early Obstetric Warning Score) chart (Chapter 6) is used.
- Is the appropriate equipment ready and does the woman have patent venous access? A single lumen standard intravenous cannula can be used for blood unless a rapid transfusion is needed. A large bore cannula (14 g) is often selected. An intravenous blood administration set is used, the integral mesh (170–200

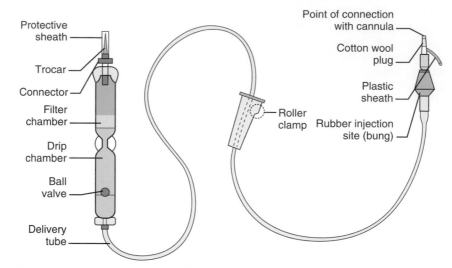

Figure 49.1 Blood transfusion administration set; note the filter and double chambers.
(Adapted with kind permission from Jamieson et al 2002)

microns) acts as a filter (Fig. 49.1), warming is not necessary for standard rate transfusions. The medical infusion device should be maintained as for any medical device and the rate checked throughout the transfusion. It is not necessary to prime the administration set with any other intravenous fluids, just the blood to be administered.

- When ready, the blood is collected from the laboratory fridge by a trained, competent practitioner. Local operating procedures are followed, often including bar coding and electronic checking, but the principles include:
  - taking a written form of the woman's ID, e.g. medicine administration chart, to the blood storage facility
  - comparing closely to ensure that all the ID and blood details match exactly. If any discrepancies are found, the blood is left in the fridge and the haematologist is contacted
  - completing the laboratory register (written or electronic)
  - signing/confirming the identity of the person removing the blood from the fridge.
- Only 1 unit of blood is collected at a time (unless in a major haemorrhage situation); it is taken promptly to the ward in the approved carrier.
- The transfusion should commence within 30 minutes of leaving the laboratory fridge (blood that has been out of the fridge for longer should be reported to the haematologist for their decision as to whether to proceed).

COMMENCING THE TRANSFUSION

- At the woman's bedside, the checking procedure is commenced. If two practitioners are checking then they should do this independently. The woman is asked to state her name and date of birth (see above), each aspect of her ID band is checked against the label on the unit of blood. If there are any discrepancies the transfusion does not go ahead and the haematologist is contacted. The donor number on the bag and card should both also match exactly.
- The midwife screens the blood visually before the transfusion commences, the expiry date is checked, and colour changes, bubbles, leakage and clotting are all checked for and excluded. Nothing should be added to a unit of blood. If other medication is required, it is administered separately.
- Strict asepsis using an Aseptic Non Touch Technique (ANTT, Chapter 10) and the use of personal protective equipment is adhered to as for any intravenous administration (Chapter 48).
- Rate of transfusion is according to the prescription but is often 90–120 minutes per unit, but must be completed within 4 hours of the unit leaving the laboratory fridge.
- The prescription is signed, including the date and time the transfusion commenced along with the donation number, and later the rate/time of completion.

MONITORING THE TRANSFUSION

- The dangers of blood transfusion are discussed below; the midwife must be vigilant in observing for signs and symptoms throughout. Ideally the woman is positioned where she is easily seen, the call bell should be within easy reach.
- Where applicable, the woman is encouraged to notify the midwife of any unexpected reactions: anxiety, pain, breathlessness, shivering or flushing.
- Serious reactions can occur within the first few mL/min, vital sign observations should be taken after 15 minutes, and then repeated if any changes were noted from the baseline, or if the woman reports any changes in how she is looking or feeling, or if MEOWS scoring was initiated.
- Each new unit is treated in this way and another set of vital sign observations is undertaken on completion of each unit.
- An unconscious woman will not be able to report any reactions and so additional vigilance is needed (vital signs, non-verbal observations and urine output).
- The administration set is changed after 12 hours and at the end of the transfusion.

COMPLETING THE TRANSFUSION

- Once completed, the time is recorded with the vital sign observations, the next unit may be commenced or the transfusion discontinued if no further blood is needed. The NHS Blood Transfusion Patient Blood Management group (NHSBT 2014) advocate the 'Don't give two without review' campaign, suggesting that reassessment of the woman's clinical condition should take place before any further units are prescribed.
- If there have not been any reactions observed the blood bag is disposed of into the appropriate clinical waste.
- The woman should remain aware of the possibility of reaction within the following 24 hours particularly. If hospitalized, vital sign observations should be completed 4-hourly.
- Documentation must be thorough at every stage of the process, it is legally necessary in the UK that each blood component can be traced through from donor to recipient(s) and, should an adverse reaction occur, that the process can be scrutinized.

- Haematological screening is completed, often the following day, e.g. full blood count and urea and electrolytes.

DANGERS OF BLOOD TRANSFUSION

Transfusion incompatibility

Signs of haemolytic reactions in the conscious woman include flushing, shivering, loin and abdominal pain (Watson & Denison 2014), headache, chest pain, tachycardia, tachypnoea, hypotension, haematuria, haemorrhage, oliguria, anxiety and possible death. Usually it is a rapid reaction, occurring within a few millilitres of transfusion. An unconscious woman is likely to demonstrate hypotension, tachycardia and a bruised appearance – bleeding into the skin (Norfolk 2013). *Action:* stop transfusion, maintain venous access with 0.9% normal saline (new cannula), call medical aid urgently, resuscitate the woman using the ABC approach (Chapter 55). Intensive care may be required. Thorough checking quickly, again, of the woman's identity and matching details on the blood is necessary, if the wrong blood is being transfused another patient may also be at risk (Norfolk 2013).

Circulatory overload

Women have an increased blood volume in pregnancy (1.5 L extra) making it easier to overload their circulatory system if they are not hypovolaemic; fluid gathers in the lungs (pulmonary oedema) resulting in dyspnoea, hypertension, tachycardia, cough and raised central venous pressure. May be seen during or after transfusion. *Action:* stop transfusion, call medical aid, administer oxygen and diuretic. Transfusion-associated circulatory overload (TACO) is a major cause of morbidity and mortality (Bolton-Maggs et al 2014) and is on the increase.

Febrile reaction

As much as possible, white cells are removed from donated blood, but after a large transfusion, women can have a significant febrile reaction. This includes hyperpyrexia, rigors, sweating and tachycardia. Onset is often within 30–90 minutes and it can mimic a haemolytic reaction. *Action:* stop transfusion, call medical aid, exclude haemolytic reaction. If transfusion is to continue, antihistamines and steroids may be needed. A mild febrile reaction (temperature rise of up to $1.5°C$) is often seen; antipyretics may be given, and care should always be taken to ensure that a 'mild' reaction is not the onset of a major reaction.

Allergic reaction

The severest type of reaction is anaphylaxis (Chapter 18); it can occur within 30 minutes, exhibiting rash, wheezing, shortness of breath and hypotension. *Action*: stop transfusion, call medical aid (urgently if clearly anaphylaxis), resuscitate using adrenaline (epinephrine) and steroids.

Other reactions

Thrombophlebitis, air embolism, iron overload, hypothermia, excess potassium and reduced calcium are other dangers that can occur, either with or following the transfusion. For any untoward sign, medical aid is called.

ROLE AND RESPONSIBILITIES OF THE MIDWIFE

These can be summarized as:
- Undertaking the procedure competently at every stage, maintaining up-to-date knowledge and skills with regard to safe transfusion practice
- Contemporaneous and thorough record keeping at every stage
- Instigating appropriate referral when necessary.

SUMMARY

- Blood transfusion is valuable in saving lives; the whole process of blood transfusion should be robust; for the midwife this starts with the booking history and initial blood taking. Thorough checking, particularly of patient identity is highlighted at every stage.
- There are dangers associated with blood transfusion; the midwife should maintain careful observation of the woman.

SELF-ASSESSMENT EXERCISES

The answers to the following questions may be found in the text:
1. What is a blood transfusion?
2. When may a blood transfusion be necessary?
3. Which blood group and Rhesus factor is the universal donor? Why is this?
4. Describe the process that protects the woman from receiving an incompatible transfusion.
5. Describe how the midwife would recognize that haemolysis was occurring.
6. When does the midwife assess vital sign observations during a transfusion?

REFERENCES

BCSH (British Committee for Standards in Haematology), 2009. Guideline: the administration of blood components. Available online: <http://www.bcshguidelines.com/documents/Admin_blood_components_bcsh_05012010.pdf> (accessed 7 January 2015).

Bolton-Maggs, P. (Ed.), Poles, D., Watt, A., et al. (on behalf of the Serious Hazards of Transfusion (SHOT) Steering Group), 2014. The 2013 Annual SHOT Report. Available online: <www.shotuk.org> (accessed 7 January 2015).

DH (Department of Health), 1994. Report on Confidential Enquiries into Maternal Deaths in the United Kingdom 1988–1990. HMSO, London.

Hurrell, K., 2014. Safe administration of blood components. Nurs. Times 110 (38), 16–19.

Jamieson, E.M., McCall, J.M., Whyte, L.A., 2002. Clinical Nursing Practices, fourth ed. Churchill Livingstone, Edinburgh.

Jones, A., Heyes, J., 2014. Processing, testing and selecting blood components. Nurs. Times 110 (37), 20–22.

Lewis, G. (Ed.), 2005. The Confidential Enquiry into Maternal and Child Health (CEMACH). Why Mothers Die: 2000–2002 Report on confidential enquiries into maternal deaths in the United Kingdom. RCOG Press, London.

Norfolk, D., 2013. Handbook of Transfusion Medicine, fifth ed. TSO, Norwich. (Chapters 4 and 5).

NHSBT (NHS Blood Transfusion), 2014. Guidance for the use of blood components. Available online: <http://hospital.blood.co.uk/media/27079/140820-1-25595-patient-blood-management-single-unit-a5-flyer.pdf> (accessed 7 January 2015).

Oldham, J., 2014. Blood transfusion sampling and greater role for error recovery. B. J. Nurs. (IV therapy supplement) 23 (8), S28–S34.

Watson, D., Denison, C., 2014. Recognising and managing transfusion reactions. Nurs. Times 110 (39), 18–21.

Watson, D., Hearnshaw, K., 2010. Understanding blood groups and transfusion in nursing practice. Nurs. Stand. 24 (30), 41–48.

Chapter | 50 |

Principles of manual handling

LEARNING OUTCOMES

Having read this chapter, the reader should be able to:

- identify situations that place the midwife at increased risk from a moving and handling injury
- describe the anatomy of the spine and related structures, relating this to the mechanics of moving and handling
- discuss the different factors that should be considered before undertaking a manual handling task
- discuss how lifting should occur, should it be required
- adopt a good posture with good understanding of why it is important
- discuss the responsibilities of both the employer and employee in reducing the risk of injury occurring when moving or handling.

Manual handling refers to the moving of items/people either by lifting, lowering, carrying, pushing or pulling. While the weight of an object handled can be a cause of injury, the frequency with which the movement is repeated, the distance which an item is carried or moved, and the height at which an object is picked up/put down from are also sources of injury. Manual handling injuries occur not only through incorrect lifting techniques and inappropriate moving and lifting, but also through poor posture, prolonged standing, twisting, bending and stretching (Kay & Glass 2011). Injury may also occur when undertaking visual display unit (VDU) computer keyboard work, writing, pushing wheelchairs, pulling beds, as well as procedures such as delivery and assisting with breastfeeding, all of which can involve adopting an awkward posture, and lifting laundry bags and food trays (Carta et al 2010).

This chapter provides an overview of manual handling, focusing on the principles of moving and handling, considering how the risk of injury can be minimized, and employers' and employees' responsibilities in relation to this. Relevant anatomy of the spine is discussed and related to both lifting and posture, and how injury can occur. It is acknowledged that there is a vast amount of literature and legislation relating to manual handling which is added to regularly, hence it is not possible to cover this in detail. The reader is advised to read other texts and visit the Health and Safety Executive (HSE) website (www.hse.gov.uk) for further information.

Musculoskeletal disorders (MSDs) are the most common occupational disease in the European Union accounting for 42–58% of all work-related illnesses with a high occurrence among hospital workers (Magnavita et al 2011). Health and social care had the highest number of reported handling injuries in 2013–2014 in the UK with an incidence rate of 190 : 100 000 employees (HSE 2014). Anderson et al (2014) suggest injuries arising through moving and handling incidents are the most common cause of staff absence for >3 days in the health and social care setting. There are far-reaching implications of MSD, not just in terms of the pain and disability experienced by the injured worker, but also financial for the midwife who is unable to work in the short term and sometimes the long term, and also for employers in terms of staff absenteeism and presenteeism (reduced on-the-job productivity as a result of health problems, Letvak et al 2012) and large compensation packages paid to their injured employees (Barnes 2007, RCN 2004, Rinds 2007a, Stevens 2004). In 2004 the Royal College of Nursing obtained £4 million compensation for members who were injured at work (Nursing Standard News 2007). Staff requiring time off from work to recover from a back injury and who experience a recurrence are likely to require longer periods of time off to recover than they needed initially (Wasiak et al 2006).

Back injuries appear to be more common in newly qualified and very senior staff. Blue (1996) suggests this may be due to acute trauma in newly qualified staff, but could be a result of the cumulative effect of smaller traumatic episodes, combined with reduced physical fitness, for older, more senior staff. Cheung (2010) found MSDs were common among student nurses, which may also contribute to the incidence of MSDs in newly qualified staff. Both employers and employees have a responsibility to make every effort to reduce the risk of injury occurring. For employers it could include early manual handling training for all new staff and ensuring they are familiar with the devices available in their clinical area. For employees this could include maintaining their own fitness levels; Blue (1996) suggests back injuries occur less frequently in people who are physically fit and undertake high-energy activities on a regular basis such as swimming and running.

ANATOMY OF THE SPINE

The spine, or vertebral column, is responsible for maintaining the upright posture of the body, provides flexibility of movement and protects the spinal cord. The spine consists of 33 separate bones or vertebrae: 24 moveable and 9 fused vertebrae (Fig. 50.1):

- seven cervical vertebrae: C1–C7 (the neck)
- twelve thoracic vertebrae: T1–T12 (the upper trunk)

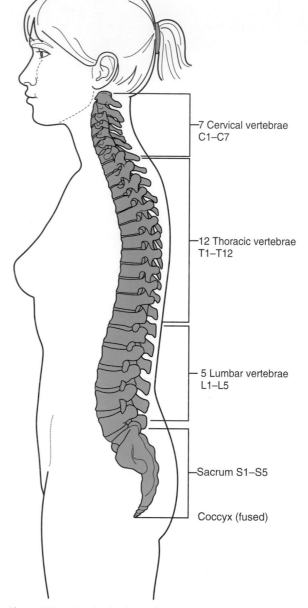

Figure 50.1 Vertebral column: bones and curves.
(Adapted with kind permission from Wilson & Waugh 1996)

- five lumbar vertebrae: L1–L5 (the lower trunk)
- five fused sacral vertebrae: S1–S5 (the sacrum)
- four fused coccygeal vertebrae (the coccyx).

The vertebrae articulate with their immediate neighbours, with muscles attached, and the thoracic vertebrae meet with the ribs. The coccyx articulates with the sacrum at the sacrococcygeal joint. Each vertebra has a main body, situated anteriorly, that acts as a shock absorber as the posture changes. The size of the vertebral body varies throughout the vertebral column, beginning small with the cervical vertebrae, increasing in size to the lumbar vertebrae. Behind the body is the vertebral foramen, a large central cavity that contains the spinal cord, with nerves and blood vessels passing out through spaces between the vertebrae.

A flexible intervertebral disc connects the vertebral bodies to each other. These discs, which have a fibrocartilage outer layer surrounding an inner semi-solid centre, assist with absorbing shock from movement and affect the flexibility of the spine. The vertebrae and discs are supported by ligaments that help to maintain the vertebrae in position and limit the amount of stress transmitted to the spine by restricting excessive movement. The ligaments do not produce as much support for the lumbar vertebrae, creating an inherent weakness in this area. The lumbar vertebrae experience higher levels of stress when the back is bent and the knees kept straight while lifting than when keeping the back straight and the knees bent (Kroemer & Grandjean 1997). This stress increases significantly if the back is twisted, as can occur when leaning over a bed.

The vertebral column is not straight, but has four curves (see Fig. 50.1):

- cervical curve (convex curve anteriorly)
- thoracic curve (concave curve anteriorly)
- lumbar curve (convex curve anteriorly)
- sacral curve (concave curve anteriorly).

The first three curves are important in relation to posture; when they meet in the midline centre of balance, weight distribution is balanced and a healthy posture ensues, protecting the supporting structures from injury (Blue 1996).

CONSIDERATIONS FOR MOVING AND LIFTING

The HSE (2004) suggest there are four important categories to consider in relation to moving and lifting; these can affect the likelihood of an injury occurring:

1. the task
2. the load
3. the working environment
4. the individual.

These four areas can be made into an acronym to assist with recall, e.g. TILE (task, individual, load, environment) (Anderson et al 2014), LITE.

The task

Does the task involve:

- holding an object or load away from the trunk?
- reaching upwards?
- twisting or stooping?
- using large vertical movements?
- carrying an object for a long distance?
- strenuous pushing or pulling?
- repetitive handling?
- insufficient rest or recovery?
- unpredictable movement of an object, e.g. carrying fluids?

Stress on the lower back increases as the load is moved away from the trunk; e.g. if a load is held at arm's length, the stress can be approximately five times higher than if it were close to the trunk (HSE 2004). Reaching up and using large vertical movements places extra stress on the arms and back with a load that is more difficult to control, as is an object with unpredictable movement, e.g. baby bath filled with water. The further the distance for which the load is held, the more it is that the grip on the load will need to be changed, which increases the risk of injury occurring. The HSE (2004) state carrying a load further than 10 metres will place more demand on the body than lifting and lowering. With repetitive movements, insufficient rest, and strenuous pushing or pulling, muscle fatigue can occur which increases the likelihood of an injury. The back, neck, and shoulders can be injured with pushing and pulling, e.g. a bed, wheelchair, with the risk increasing if the surface of the floor is poorly maintained. The HSE (2004) advise that when pushing or pulling a load, hands should be kept above the waist and below the shoulders demonstrating the importance of having the bed at the correct height when being manoeuvred around.

The load

Is the load or object:

- heavy?
- bulky?
- difficult to hold?
- unstable, e.g. fluid?
- intrinsically harmful, e.g. sharp?

If the load is deemed heavy, consideration should be given to using lifting equipment or having someone to assist with the task. A load that measures >75 cm carries an increased risk of injury as it can be difficult to maintain a suitable grip and can obscure the view in front of and beneath the person carrying it.

The working environment

Within the environment, are there:

- constraints on posture?
- poor or slippery floors?
- variations in levels?
- poor lighting conditions?

Where the moving of a load involves going through doors, the HSE (2004) recommend the use of doors that open automatically rather than having to stop to open doors or holding them open as the load passes through. This may be difficult within the maternity unit when passage through locked doors is required. When transferring a load on a slope, e.g. bed/wheelchair along a ramp, additional force is required which places further strain on the body. Consideration should be given to the number of people who should assist with moving a heavy load up or down a slope.

The individual

Does the job:

- require an unusual capability, e.g. in relation to weight of load?
- cause a hazard to anyone with a health problem?
- cause a hazard to anyone who is pregnant, or who has had a baby within the past 2 years?
- require special information or training?

A risk assessment should be undertaken if there is a positive answer to any of the questions above prior to any moving or lifting activities, to reduce the risk of injury as far as possible. The risk assessment involves identifying hazards and risks, including the potential to cause harm not only to the midwife but also the woman, as well as the likelihood and severity of harm occurring (Rinds 2007b).

An individual's ability to move a load can vary according to age, gender (in general women have a lower lifting strength than men), physical health, fitness and childbirth. The HSE (2004) suggest there is a significant decrease in physical ability from the mid-forties onwards, with the risk of manual handling injury being highest 'for employees in their teens and fifties and sixties'. Older workers often tire more quickly and take longer to recover from a musculoskeletal injury. Individuals who are anxious, depressed or have high job strain (where there are high work demands with little control over the job) are more likely to develop an MSD (Magnavita et al 2011). Extremes of temperature can significantly affect both the development and the exacerbation of MSDs (HSE 2004, Magnavita et al 2011).

The maximum weight one should lift is also affected by whether the individual is standing or sitting, with the latter lifting a significantly lower weight than the former. It is also influenced by whether the elbows are bent or straight and the position of the object to be lifted – higher weights are more permissible if at waist height than if at head or feet height. Pregnancy will also affect the maximum weight a woman should attempt to lift (Tolley 2000). MacDonald et al (2013) point out that as pregnancy progresses the pregnant woman will not be able to hold an object close to her body, and a longer arm reach is required to hold the load in place as gestation increases, placing more strain onto her arms and back. There are also physiological changes that predispose the pregnant worker to MSDs. It is therefore important to take these factors into account when undertaking a risk assessment.

PRINCIPLES OF LIFTING

While it is inevitable that some lifting will occur, mainly relating to equipment, lifting people is not usually part of the midwife's role. Rinds (2007b) and Stevens (2004) point out, however, that no-lift policies imposed by employers are, in several circumstances, illegal. For example, the midwife has a duty of care to manually lift an immobile woman away from danger such as fire if this is the only method of removal available, or to move the woman if she is unable to relieve pressure on her body and is at increased risk of pressure-ulcer formation (see Chapter 53). It is important the midwife understands the principles of lifting to reduce the risk of injury. Wherever possible, women should be encouraged to be mobile and move themselves independently rather than be reliant on midwifery staff (Barnes 2007).

There is an imaginary 'centre of gravity' for the human adult that lies approximately anterior to the second sacral vertebra when standing in an upright symmetrical position, but will vary according to positional changes adopted. In the upright symmetrical position, the feet form the base, and a vertical line drawn through the centre of gravity will reach the floor halfway between the feet, between the balls and heels (the baseline). This determines the person's balance and how far the position can be altered by leaning or reaching before balance is lost (Pheasant 1991). Prolonged periods of imbalance may result in stress and strain to the muscles of the trunk and abdomen, and – if not relieved – injury and pain (Jamieson et al 2002). Imbalance can be reduced by keeping the centre of gravity within the baseline, achieved by widening the foot stance – the feet should be shoulder distance apart. This also creates a circle of stability and moving out of this circle places the individual at risk of injury.

The weight of the head, neck, arms, hands, and upper trunk are supported by the vertebral column. As the weight of the upper body increases, so does the force placed on the spine. The spine is compressed further if an object is being carried. Thus the acts of walking, bending and twisting the trunk also increase the force placed on the spinal column, particularly the intervertebral discs. So, considerable force is placed on the intervertebral discs when moving an object in addition to walking, bending or twisting. It is important that when moving while lifting, the feet are pointing in the direction of movement; this will also help to reduce the risk of twisting.

The risk of injury occurring when lifting a load can be reduced by straightening the spine and ensuring it is in alignment with the head (which should be raised), relaxing the knees, tightening the abdominal muscles, and widening the base. The compression forces increase with both the weight of the object and the further away from the body it is held, and directly affects the amount of stress placed on the lumbar spine (Kroemer & Grandjean 1997). Thus an object being lifted should be kept as close to the body as possible by keeping the elbows tucked in close to the body and avoiding reaching (Fig. 50.2). Movements should be smooth throughout the lifting episode. If lifting is undertaken with a rounded back, curvature of the lumbar spine results, applying asymmetrical pressure on the intervertebral discs. If continued, the pressure can cause the disc to erode, resulting in a 'slipped' disc. This is where the outer layer ruptures and the centre of the disc herniates through the gap to press on the spinal nerves or their roots. Damage

to the surrounding tissues can also occur. In severe cases, the prolapsed discs can compress the spinal column.

The safe biomechanical principles used when moving people or objects, discussed above are:

- stand in a stable position
- get a firm footing
- avoid twisting
- bend the knees
- keep the elbows tucked in
- tighten the abdominal muscles
- lift with the legs, not the weaker back muscles
- keep the back upright
- keep the head up
- move smoothly.

Blue (1996) recommends using the entire hand when lifting as this encourages a better grip on the object and reduces the need for unnecessary movements to re-adjust the grip. The use of handles can also encourage a better grip on an object.

Most women within the maternity setting are mobile, with a very small minority requiring assistance with mobility, although Mander (1999) suggests immobility and impaired mobility will increase due to changes in obstetric practice (e.g. epidural analgesia, increasing caesarean section rates). Mobility should be encouraged as far as possible, as this not only reduces the incidence of injury to the

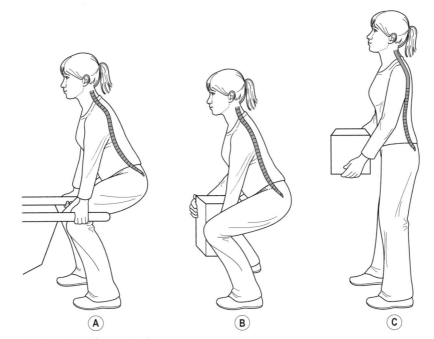

Figure 50.2 Position of spine when lifting a load.

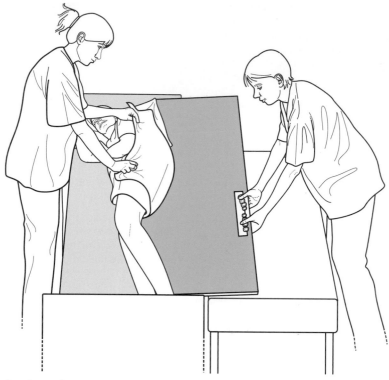

Figure 50.3 Slide placed underneath woman.

midwife, but also promotes physical wellbeing in the mother. This can be facilitated with the use of electrical profiling beds (Rinds 2007b). Profiling beds allow for variable positioning by having sections under the mattress that raise and lower by pressing a button – thus allowing women to raise the head of their bed to bring them to a sitting position or provide a knee break to stop them sliding down the bed (Fernandes 2007). They also result in less assistance with repositioning by the midwife.

If women are immobile or not able to move themselves, the use of appropriate moving and handling equipment is important. Devices such as monkey poles and sliding sheets are useful for assisting the women to move up the bed. The woman should be encouraged to bend her knees and flex her head towards her chest to reduce the shearing effect when lifting herself. The midwife can assist the woman by placing a slide sheet under the woman and pressing against her feet to prevent them slipping while she is moving up the bed. It is useful to discuss this with the woman prior to surgery whenever possible and to watch her practice moving herself up the bed following these principles. When women need to be moved from one bed to another (e.g. following caesarean section), sliding devices and sheets should be used. These are slid underneath the woman and allow her to slide between the two surfaces with minimal effort from the midwives (Fig. 50.3). When getting out of bed, the woman should be advised to turn onto her side and push herself upright with her hand, using the elbow nearest the bed as a prop. Once sitting upright, it will be easier for the woman to get up from the bed unaided, particularly if the bed is lowered so that her feet are placed on the floor.

There will be times when a woman will need assistance to roll in the bed, e.g. when changing the bed sheets for a woman who is unable to get up from the bed (see Chapter 12). The procedure should be discussed with the woman before starting so that she knows what to expect and what her role is. Prior to commencing the roll, the woman should be asked to turn her head in the direction she will be turning. The arm that is on the side she is turning towards should be moved from the side of her body or folded across her chest so that she does not roll onto it. The outside knee should be flexed and the arm brought across her chest in the direction of the roll (the woman may need assistance flexing her knee if she cannot do this herself, e.g. with regional anaesthesia. The woman should then roll on to her side by pushing with her outside foot and reaching across her body or holding onto the bed rail with her outside hand. If necessary, the midwife can help direct the roll by placing her hands on the woman's outside shoulder and hip while in a lunge position. Using the verbal prompts 'ready', 'steady', 'roll', the woman is rolled on to her side as the midwife transfers her weight to her back foot, keeping her arms straight.

When moving a woman using a hoist, sling or sliding device, it is important to ensure she feels safe and her dignity is maintained. D'Arcy et al (2011) found there were fewer MSDs when lifting devices were available. Communication throughout the procedure is vital as this will encourage cooperation from the woman and ensure all members of the team are working together (Blood 2005, Pellatt 2005).

Therefore, when lifting or moving is unavoidable, the midwife should ensure that:

- mechanical aids are used whenever possible
- the feet are widened to maintain balance
- the back is straight to prevent unnecessary pressure on the intervertebral discs
- the knees are bent to reduce the pressure on the vertebral column
- the object being lifted is kept close to the body, grasping the object between the knees if being lifted from the floor
- the body is not twisted or rotated when lifting or lowering the object
- sufficient numbers of people are involved to ensure the maximum load per person is not exceeded. All involved should understand the correct technique and be able to work as a team, with one person acting as the coordinator and directing the proceedings.

CORRECT POSTURE

Injury may occur through bad posture, particularly if prolonged, when strain is placed on the muscles of the back. Jaromi et al (2012) suggest bad posture is the most frequent cause of chronic low back pain (persisting pain >12 weeks). Situations where this can occur include:

- sitting for long periods (including driving)
- supporting a labouring woman
- delivery
- perineal suturing
- assisting with breastfeeding
- making beds.

Sitting

Sitting up with a straight back can cause the pelvis to tilt forwards causing the posture to be maintained by the muscles, which tire quickly. The pressure on the

intervertebral discs is increased when sitting compared with a standing position. To reduce the need for muscle effort, slouching can occur, allowing the pelvis to rotate backwards so the posture and weight of the trunk are maintained more by the ligaments than the muscles. While this is effective in reducing the workload on the muscles, it doubles the force placed on the intervertebral discs, compared with the upright position (Pheasant 1991). Using a chair with a good back rest can reduce this pressure; the pelvis rotates backwards, as for the slouched position, but the spine flexes again when it comes into contact with the back of the chair. This results in less pressure being placed on the intervertebral discs, which can be reduced further by the use of a pad in the lumbar region, possibly to a pressure that is 30–40% lower than when in a standing position (Pheasant 1991).

Stooped posture

During situations such as birth and breastfeeding, the midwife may have a stooped posture, where the trunk is inclined forwards. In this situation the weight of the upper body is supported by postvertebral muscles. Contraction of these muscles can result in compression of the intervertebral discs.

Asymmetric posture

An asymmetric posture, involving side bending, is sometimes adopted by the midwife when delivering a woman in an alternative position, particularly if she is upright or on all-fours and the midwife is on the floor. This again increases pressure on the spine, predisposing to injury. Whenever the midwife is required to adopt an unusual position, careful consideration should be given to maintaining a symmetric posture and not to maintain the position for long periods to avoid undue pressure on the muscles and ligaments.

EMPLOYERS' RESPONSIBILITIES

The Manual Handling Operations Regulations 1992 (HSE 2004) and Management of Health and Safety at Work Regulations (1999) require employers to avoid manual handling as far as is reasonably practicable if there is a possibility of injury. However, this is not always possible, in which case employers must reduce the risk of injury occurring as far as is reasonably practicable.

Specifically, employers should:

- avoid hazardous manual handling operations so far as reasonably practicable

- assess any hazardous manual handling operations that cannot be avoided
- reduce the risk of injury so far as reasonably practicable.

Furthermore, if an employee is complaining of discomfort, any changes employed to avoid or reduce manual handling should be monitored to determine if they are having a positive effect. If this is not the case, then alternatives must be considered.

Thus a risk assessment should be undertaken for any situation in which manual handling may be required, ideally before the situation arises so that they have sufficient time to take measures to reduce the risk of injury, e.g. use of appropriate equipment. When the risk assessment is around moving patients, a multi-staged risk assessment system may be required (HSE 2014). This includes ensuring staff are appropriately trained for their patient/client group and individual patient assessment where there are significant mobility needs. The assessment should clearly identify the tasks that are necessary, who should undertake them, and how. This also requires knowledge of the patient's ability to assist with moving and of the handling equipment available, e.g. slide sheets. Each employer should have a safer handling policy.

EMPLOYEES' RESPONSIBILITIES

Employees are required to:

- cooperate with their employers in relation to safe manual handling and be familiar with the manual handling policy
- inform their managers of any situation that could put them at risk of injury
- ensure they know how to use the equipment properly
- attend training sessions to update and maintain their knowledge and skills
- ensure their activities do not put others at risk.

Cornish & Jones (2010) found that staff who have experienced a moving and handling-related injury were more compliant with safe manual handling principles and were also more likely to maintain good back care in daily life.

ROLE AND RESPONSIBILITIES OF THE MIDWIFE

These can be summarized as:

- being familiar with the manual handling policy and attending regular training sessions
- informing the employer of any situations in which a risk assessment should be undertaken
- using moving and handling equipment correctly
- knowing how to lift a load correctly
- being able to achieve a good posture in whichever position is adopted
- recognizing the situations in which the midwife is at risk of injury from poor posture and taking steps to reduce the risk of injury.

SUMMARY

- Assessment of the manual handling task can help to reduce the risk of injury occurring.
- Incorrect moving and handling techniques can cause serious damage to the physical health of the midwife and may cause physical and psychological harm to the person being handled.
- The midwife should not be involved in lifting another person, but should use appropriate equipment for this purpose.
- A poor posture increases the risk of physical injury.

SELF-ASSESSMENT EXERCISES

The answers to the following questions may be found in the text:

1. Describe the anatomy of the spine and associated structures that are involved in the mechanics of moving and handling.
2. Identify five situations from clinical practice that place the midwife at increased risk from a manual handling injury and discuss how the midwife can reduce the risk.
3. When lifting a load, how can the risk of injury be reduced?
4. How can the midwife achieve a good posture and what is the significance of a poor posture?
5. What are the responsibilities of the midwife and the employer in relation to moving and handling?

REFERENCES

Anderson, M.P., Carlisle, S., Thomson, C., et al., 2014. Safe moving and handling of patients: an interprofessional approach. Nurs. Stand. 28 (46), 37–41.

Barnes, A.F., 2007. Moving and handling. Erasing the word 'lift' from nurses' vocabulary when handling patients. Br. J. Nurs. 16 (18), 1144–1147.

Blood, R., 2005. Safe moving and handling of individuals. Nurs. Residential Care 7 (10), 439–441.

Blue, C.L., 1996. Preventing back injury among nurses. Orthop. Nurs. 15 (6), 9–19.

Carta, A., Parmigiani, F., Roversi, A., et al., 2010. Training in safer and healthier patient handling techniques. Br. J. Nurs. 19 (9), 576–582.

Cheung, K., 2010. The incidence of low back problems among nursing students in Hong Kong. J. Clin. Nurs. 19, 2355–2362.

Cornish, J., Jones, A., 2010. Factors affecting compliance with moving and handling policy: student nurses' views and experiences. Nur. Educ. in Prac. 10 (2), 96–100.

D'Arcy, L.P., Sasai, Y., Stearns, S.C., 2011. Do assistive devices, training and workload affect injury incidence? Prevention efforts by nursing homes and back injuries among nursing assistants. J. Adv. Nurs. 68 (4), 836–843.

Fernandes, T., 2007. Suitable moving and handling equipment: a guide. Int. J. Ther. Rehabil. 14 (4), 187–191.

HSE (Health and Safety Executive), 2004. Manual handling. Manual handling operations regulations 1992; guidance on regulations ed 3. Available online: <http://www.hseni.gov.uk/l23 _manual_handling.pdf> (accessed 26 January 2015).

HSE (Health and Safety Executive), 2014. Handling injuries in Great Britain 2014. Available online: <http:// www.hse.gov.uk/statistics/causinj/ handling-injuries.pdf> (accessed 26 January 2015).

Jamieson, E.M., McCall, J.M., Whyte, L.A., 2002. Clinical Nursing Practices, fourth ed. Churchill Livingstone, Edinburgh.

Jaromi, M., Nemeth, A., Kranciz, J., et al., 2012. Treatment and ergonomic training of work-related lower back pain and body posture problems for nurses. J. Clin. Nurs. 21, 1776–1784.

Kay, K., Glass, N., 2011. Debunking the manual handling myth: an investigation of manual handling knowledge and practices in the Australian private health sector. Int. J. Nurs. Pract. 17, 231–237.

Kroemer, K.H.E., Grandjean, E., 1997. Fitting the Task to the Human: A Textbook of Occupational Ergonomics, fifth ed. Taylor and Francis, London.

Letvak, S.A., Ruhm, C.J., Gupta, S.N., 2012. Nurses' presenteeism and its effects on self-reported quality of care and costs. Am. J. Nurs. 112 (2), 30–38.

MacDonald, L.A., Waters, T.R., Napolitano, P.G., et al., 2013. Clinical guidelines for occupational lifting in pregnancy: evidence summary and provisional recommendations. Am. J. Obstet. Gynecol. 209 (2), 80–88.

Magnavita, N., Elovainio, M., de Nardis, I., et al., 2011. Environmental discomfort and musculoskeletal disorders. Occup. Med. 61 (3), 196–201.

Management of Health and Safety at Work Regulations, 1999. Available online: <http://www.legislation.gov .uk/uksi/1999/3242/pdfs/uksi _19993242_en.pdf> (accessed 23 February 2015).

Mander, R., 1999. Manual handling and the immobile mother. Br. J. Midwifery 7 (8), 485–487.

Nursing Standard News, 2007. HCAs bear brunt of workplace injuries. Nurs. Stand. 22 (14–16), 9.

Pellatt, G.C., 2005. Safe handling: the safety and dignity of patients and nurses during patient handling. Br. J. Nurs. 14 (21), 1150–1156.

Pheasant, S., 1991. Ergonomics, Work and Health. Macmillan, Basingstoke.

RCN (Royal College of Nursing), 2004. Safer Patient Handling. RCN, London.

Rinds, G., 2007a. Moving and handling: part one. Nurs. Residential Care 9 (6), 260–262.

Rinds, G., 2007b. Moving and handling, part two: risk management. Nurs. Residential Care 9 (7), 306–309.

Stevens, D.R., 2004. Manual handling and the lawfulness of no-lift policies. Nurs. Stand. 18 (21), 39–43.

Tolley, 2000. Health and Safety at Work Handbook 2000, thirteenth ed. Tolley, Croydon.

Wasiak, R., Kim, J., Pransky, G., 2006. Work disability and costs caused by recurrence of low back pain: longer and more costly than in first episodes. Spine 31 (2), 219–225.

Wilson, K.J.W., Waugh, A., 1996. Ross and Wilson Anatomy and Physiology in Health and Illness, eighth ed. Churchill Livingstone, Edinburgh.

Chapter | 51 |

Principles of perioperative skills

LEARNING OUTCOMES

Having read this chapter, the reader should be able to:

- discuss thorough preoperative care prior to elective and emergency caesarean section (CS)
- summarize the general principles of intraoperative care
- discuss recovery and post-CS care
- summarize the midwife's responsibilities in each role.

A surgical procedure is that in which there is excision of tissue, penetration of the skin or closure of a previous wound. It takes place in an operating theatre (a 'sterile' environment) (WHO 2009). Midwives care for and support women and their families who deliver by caesarean section (CS), but women may also undergo procedures such as manual removal of placenta, perineal repair, abscess drainage, and cervical suture removal. In 2013, Birth Choice UK reported that CS births accounted for 25% of deliveries in England, of which 10% were planned CSs and 15% emergencies (BirthChoiceUK 2013). The US has an even higher rate, the Centers for Disease Control and Prevention (CDC 2013) recorded a CS rate of 32.7% in 2013. The midwife has a significant role in caring safely for the woman before, during and after surgery.

This chapter considers care prior to elective and emergency surgery, intraoperative care and postoperative recovery care. It focuses largely upon CS, but the principles may be applied to other types of surgery.

Care in theatre is specialized care, requiring cooperative teamwork between all the professional groups involved (Yentis & Clyburn 2014). The midwife may take on a number of different roles (e.g. pre- or postoperative care, theatre scrub nurse or runner, recovery care) for which competency should be assessed and maintained.

REDUCING CS RATES

No surgery is without risks. The postnatal complications of pain and immobility can affect the woman's early parenting skills and attachment with her baby (NCT 2011). Thromboembolism, infection and haemorrhage all feature as significant causes of maternal death (for which the risks are increased after CS) (Knight et al 2014). A uterine scar can affect future pregnancies (increased risks of uterine rupture and placenta praevia), and the baby, too, can experience adverse effects, e.g. lacerations, poor respiratory response and less effective temperature control (NICE 2011). These issues are just a snapshot; delivery by CS should have the decision made with a consultant obstetrician and a clear clinical reason documented (NICE 2011). Reducing the CS rate reduces the overall risks for the woman and her baby, as well as the financial and other demands on the service.

NICE (2011) recommend several factors that can reduce the incidence of CS:

- the positive role of continuous support in labour, preferably from a woman
- induction of labour at 41 + weeks with an uncomplicated pregnancy
- the use of partograms in high-risk labours that incorporate a 4-hour action line
- inclusion of the consultant obstetrician in the decision-making process
- less use of electronic fetal heart rate monitoring. Suspected abnormal fetal heart rate patterns should instigate fetal blood sampling (where possible and appropriate) to confirm whether early delivery is required or not
- Other measures such as an increase in homebirth, use of birthing centres, supporting women who choose vaginal birth after caesarean (VBAC), and the use of external cephalic version for breech presentations can also reduce the incidence of CS.

CATEGORIZING CS

In the UK, CS is categorized in one of four ways:

- Category 1: where there is an immediate threat to life
- Category 2: where there is compromise but not an immediate threat to life
- Category 3: where there is no compromise, but needs early delivery
- Category 4: timing of delivery to suit the woman or staff.

For the purposes of audit, a category 1 CS should take place within 30 minutes of the decision, category 2, 75 minutes (NICE 2011).

INDICATIONS FOR PLANNED CS (NICE 2011)

- Breech presentation at term if external cephalic version (ECV) was inappropriate, declined or unsuccessful at 36-37 weeks' gestation
- Multiple pregnancy where the presenting twin is not cephalic
- Placenta praevia
- Morbidly adherent placenta
- HIV without retroviral treatment and/or viral load of 400 + copies per millilitre
- Presence of primary infection with genital herpes simplex virus
- Maternal request after extensive exploring of other birth options.

There are other reasons why CS is considered, these include previous pelvic floor or anal sphincter damage, previous shoulder dystocia, and previous CS with a classical scar. Wherever possible, planned CS is undertaken after 39 weeks' gestation. The list above, and the reasons often cited for category 1 and 2 CS (pre-eclampsia, fetal compromise antepartum haemorrhage, failure to progress, previous CS etc.), would suggest that there are often risk factors present before surgery takes place. Good preparation for surgery, whether rushed or completed at leisure, aims primarily to facilitate uneventful surgery and smooth postoperative recovery.

PREPARATION FOR SURGERY

For planned surgery the woman should be given the opportunity to discuss the practicalities, i.e. preparations beforehand, what to bring, when to come, what will happen at each different stage of the process, and have the opportunity to have her questions answered. Given that approximately one in four babies are delivered by CS, antenatal education should help all prospective parents to understand delivery in this way, whether planned or unexpected.

Consultation with obstetrician and anaesthetist

Each woman should be seen by a consultant obstetrician (see above). It is in conjunction with the woman and after detailed discussion of the risks and benefits of CS that the decision is made. The woman is asked to sign a consent form (verbal consent may be acceptable in some circumstances); this may be relatively stress free for planned surgery, but may be very difficult if surgery is being contemplated hurriedly. The midwife should work to support the woman in making her decision, whatever that may be (Charles 2013). The woman should also see an anaesthetist prior to surgery. The woman's health, reason for surgery and suitability for chosen anaesthetic are all assessed (ASA 2007, AAGBI & OAA 2005). NICE (2011) recommend offering all women regional anaesthesia (spinal or epidural), the risks being less than with a general anaesthetic.

A full blood count will confirm the haemoglobin level. Other haematology screening (group and saving of serum, cross-matching, and clotting screening) and ultrasonic location of the placenta are not routinely required (NICE 2011) for healthy women with uncomplicated pregnancies. If heavy blood loss is anticipated, e.g. placenta praevia, cross-matching would take place prior to surgery. This and other high-risk CS must take place in a location where blood transfusion services are readily available. Other investigations may be ordered as indicated (e.g. chest X-ray). The midwife will undertake an antenatal assessment and baseline vital sign observations. These are charted on a Modified Early Obstetric Warning Score (MEOWS) chart in preparation for postoperative assessment and comparison. Allergies (e.g. to latex, antibiotics, etc.) should be carefully documented and the whole team made fully aware.

Care of the gastrointestinal tract

Fasting prior to surgery is indicated so that the risk of aspiration is reduced; however, it is advisable to continue to take prescribed medication with clear fluid unless contraindicated (Crenshaw & Winslow 2006). It takes approximately 6–8 hours for the stomach to be empty from food, and 2–3 hours for fluids (ASA 2007, Scott et al 1999). However, pregnancy, labour, some drugs (e.g. pethidine) and anxiety can all delay gastric emptying; nevertheless, starvation for periods of longer than 6 hours is unnecessary and distressing for the woman. Antacid therapy or H_2 antagonists are given so that the gastric acid will be less acidic and reduced in volume, respectively. NICE (2011) recommend that all women should be offered this therapy. Often the woman takes these medications orally the evening before and the morning of surgery. An anti-emetic may also be included to reduce nausea. An intravenous (I.V.) infusion will be sited prior to the surgery, particularly if preloading is required for regional anaesthesia to reduce the risk of hypotension (ASA 2007). Good hydration also reduces the risks of thromboembolism.

Premedication

Premedication are drugs administered prior to surgery in preparation for, or as part of, the anaesthetic. They may be prescribed in any form according to need – relaxant, antiemetic, analgesic, etc. The most likely premedication in the maternity setting are the antacid/H_2 antagonists and/or anti-emetics described above. Other drugs would be administered with caution, anticipating their transfer across the placenta. It becomes important, therefore, that a premedication is given at the prescribed time, and that the anaesthetist is informed if for some reason the surgery is then delayed.

Skin preparation

In an attempt to reduce postoperative wound infections, preoperative skin preparation is indicated. This is discussed in Chapter 52 but remains a largely inconclusive science. The woman, as a minimal requirement, should take a shower. She will wear a gown, without any underwear, particularly noting that bras may reduce chest expansion and have metal components that may interact with other theatre equipment. She is asked not to use deodorant or talcum powder, both of which may be flammable. All make-up is removed, so that the actual colour of her nail beds and mucous membranes may be seen in order to recognize any cyanosis.

Hair removal from the wound site remains controversial; it is considered that if the hair is interfering with the wound or adhesive dressing then it should be removed. Shaving causes microabrasions on the skin that microorganisms can then colonize; shaving should be avoided (Jose & Dignon 2013). Better methods for hair removal are disposable head electric clippers or depilatory creams. NICE (2013) recommend that if hair does need removing, electric clippers with a single-use head should be used on the day of surgery by healthcare personnel. Women should be made aware that they themselves should not undertake any pubic hair removal.

Bladder care

An indwelling catheter is used to prevent any trauma or overdistension to the bladder during surgery and is sometimes inserted prior to transfer to theatre, or at the time of surgery (Chapter 14), where possible in accordance with the woman's wishes. It remains indwelling until mobile post-surgery.

Thromboembolic prophylaxis

Chapter 54 discusses this in detail. It is crucial that all women undergoing delivery by CS experience thromboprophylaxis according to their risk factors. Scoring systems are widely implemented and should be actioned before, during and following surgery.

Identity and removal of prosthesis

All prostheses are removed prior to surgery (e.g. contact lenses, false limbs, dentures, etc.). Hearing aids may be retained depending upon the surgeon/anaesthetist. Capped teeth are noted if general anaesthesia is to be administered due to the risk of being dislodged and inhaled. Metallic jewellery is removed (all kinds, including piercings), but wedding rings can be taped securely in place. Identity bands are worn, some hospitals require two identity bands for surgical cases – one on the wrist, one on the ankle. It is important to use allergy alert bands should an allergy be present.

Record keeping

As for all situations, record keeping should be thorough and contemporaneous (NMC 2009). The World Health Organization (WHO) Surgical Safety Checklist (WHO 2009) is a part of the record keeping but it is not a 'tick box' exercise. Its implementation is designed to increase patient safety and improve collaborative team working. The adapted checklist for maternity (WHO 2009) incorporates a 'sign in', 'time out', and 'sign out' set of criteria that are said out loud (and established to be correct) at each stage of the process.

EMERGENCY SURGERY

Preparation for emergency surgery should include all of the above, but is often carried out much more quickly. If a general anaesthetic is being considered, it may be necessary to empty the stomach. A wide bore nasogastric tube may be used for this purpose. Sometimes the speed required means that the preparation may be seen to be less thorough than for elective surgery, and therefore there are higher intraoperative and postoperative risks from emergency surgery.

INTRAOPERATIVE CARE

The midwife's role will vary in this setting depending upon which of the roles is undertaken. Theatre care is very detailed; general principles are summarized below, but the reader is encouraged to consider other literary sources. The following general principles should be upheld in theatre:

- The most important person present is the woman. Her dignity and safety should be maintained whether awake or anaesthetized, her preferences should be accommodated wherever possible.

- Her safety is paramount, whether that is her internal safety:
  - maintenance of her airway and respirations: with a general anaesthetic this includes using preoxygenation, a cuffed endotracheal (ET) tube, cricoid pressure (Fig. 55.4), rapid sequence induction and mechanical ventilation. A protocol will exist should intubation fail; the anaesthetist and operating departmental practitioner (ODP) will instigate this.
  - Pulse oximetry monitoring is used throughout to detect any hypoxia regardless of type of anaesthesia (Chapter 6)
  - the theatre table should have a tilt of 15° to avoid aortocaval occlusion (NICE 2011)
  - blood pressure is monitored throughout and generally maintained by adjusting the fluid volume; fluid balance is essential
  - asepsis is maintained throughout to reduce the risk of infection; I.V. antibiotics are offered to reduce postoperative infection, they should be administered prior to skin incision for greater effectiveness (NICE 2011)
  - maintenance of normothermia – recording the woman's temperature every 30 minutes during surgery, use of fluid warming devices and other specialist equipment as required. Particular care should be taken to avoid hypothermia if significant haemorrhage is happening
  - known allergies should be accommodated; a latex-free trolley should be available in theatre for affected women.
- Or her external safety:
  - care of the immobile or unconscious woman: safety upon the operating table, care of numb limbs and pressure areas (Chapter 53), attention to temperature maintenance, prevention of burns from diathermy equipment, care of infusion lines, monitors, etc.
- Theatre work is teamwork, for which all members of the team should be able to recognize their limitations and call in more senior or expert help if needed. The DH (1998) indicates that often consultant level expertise is either not called or called too late, and that sometimes the severity of the situation is not recognized by junior staff. Anaesthetists should be supported by skilled help, e.g. ODP. Communication should be good between all team members, especially if laboratory or haematology support is required (DH 1998).
- Theatre is a sterile environment in which strict surgical asepsis is maintained. Scrubbed persons wear sterile gowns and gloves, all of which are applied after scrupulous hand hygiene (Chapter 9). The rear of the

gown is handled at the edges by the person fastening it, but the front remains totally sterile. Disposable drapes are used to establish a sterile field; these are only touched by a scrubbed person. All items within the sterile field should be sterile and are opened and transferred in such a way as to retain their sterility. Everyone in the theatre environment moves around in such a way as to maintain the integrity of the sterile field; movement in and out of theatre is kept to a minimum (NICE 2013). The air is scavenged and as a restricted area – only people wearing theatre clothing and footwear are permitted. External sources of potential infection, e.g. shoes, are prohibited.

- Theatre should also be appropriately stocked with all necessary equipment: drugs and anaesthetic gases, anaesthetic machine, monitors, resuscitation equipment, I.V. fluids and infant Resuscitaire, among other things. All of this is checked thoroughly prior to the surgery commencing (WHO 2009).

- Staff should also protect themselves, working under the protection of the health and safety legislation, use of extensive standard precautions – e.g. masks with visors, aprons, wellingtons, etc. – and moving and handling requirements.

- Swabs, needles and instruments are all counted initially with the circulating midwife and the number of needles and swabs are recorded on a board where the scrub midwife can see them. Any additional items opened during the surgery are added to the information on the board. As the wound is closed, swabs, needles and instruments are checked and counted; the scrub midwife uses the circulating midwife again to establish that the final count equates with the original one. This ensures that nothing has been retained inside the wound and the skin should not be closed until the final count is completed and correct. Contemporaneous records should be completed; these may include a theatre register or anaesthetic record.

- CS under regional anaesthesia means that the woman will be able to appreciate fully all that is happening. Her wishes and her partner's wishes should be respected, e.g. silence may be requested so that the mother's voice is the first one heard by the baby; immediate skin-to-skin contact and early breastfeeding should be encouraged (NICE 2011). Equally, being awake can be a time of heightened anxiety. Care should include preparing her for the environment and the sensations (pushing and pulling, but not pain) that she may experience. As for any birth setting, care includes that of the supporting partner, who may also feel very anxious.

- The woman having a general anaesthetic will require repeated and ongoing reassurance as she recovers, drifting in and out of sleep.

- Specific guidance is given within the NICE guidelines (NICE 2011) as to the surgical techniques that reduce pain, haemorrhage and infection. These include issues such as transverse abdominal incision using the Joel Cohen incision (Mathai & Hofmeyr 2007) – a straight skin incision undertaken 3 cm above the symphysis pubis, blunt incision of the uterus and other layers (using scissors, not a knife, to extend if required), avoiding forceps, use of I.V. oxytocin (5 IU) and controlled cord traction for placental delivery (Anorlu et al 2008), uterine suturing in two layers within the abdomen, non-suturing of the visceral or parietal peritoneum or subcutaneous tissue (unless >2 cm) and avoidance of superficial or routine wound drains (Gates & Anderson 2005). Skin closure does not have sufficient evidence to suggest the use of one closure above another.

- Care of the baby: resuscitation equipment and personnel should be on hand if there has been a general anaesthetic or fetal compromise. Care should be taken to label the infant and maintain body temperature. Delayed cord clamping should be employed as for any other delivery, when appropriate (Chapter 32).

- The placenta and membranes are examined as for any other delivery (Chapter 33).

- Cord blood is taken if the woman is Rhesus negative and an umbilical artery and venous pH is performed if there was fetal compromise.

POSTOPERATIVE CARE

This should be completed in a recovery area where there is immediate access to oxygen, suction, resuscitation equipment, monitors, emergency call bells and appropriately trained one-to-one staff. Recovery care continues until airway control is regained, cardiovascular observations are stable, and the woman is able to communicate (NICE 2011).

After a general anaesthetic a Guedel airway is usually inserted following extubation by the anaesthetist; the woman removes this spontaneously as she regains consciousness.

Postoperative care, particularly that given during the recovery period, encompasses all of the following, whichever type of anaesthetic has been administered:

- maintenance of the airway, with or without oxygen therapy

- assessment of respirations, heart rate, blood pressure and temperature
- use of pulse oximetry for oxygen saturation with assessment of colour
- correct positioning, care of numb limbs and pressure areas
- assessment of consciousness/sedation
- assessment of levels of pain, administering analgesia as indicated, care of patient-controlled analgesia (PCA) (Chapter 23).
- care of I.V. infusion/blood transfusion/uterotonics and fluid balance
- care of wound (and drain if appropriate)
- observation of loss *per vaginam*/continued assessment of estimated blood loss and measures for the prevention of postpartum haemorrhage
- care of urinary catheter/urinary output
- return of sensation following regional anaesthesia
- time with the baby and opportunities for skin-to-skin contact and feeding
- appropriate thromboprophylaxis measures.

Observations

- All vital sign observations should be completed at regular short intervals initially and recorded on a MEOWS chart. The timings are dictated by clinical condition and locally agreed policy, but are often 5-minute intervals initially. As time passes and observations remain within normal limits, the frequency of observations may be reduced to every 15 minutes, 30 minutes, etc. They should be half-hourly for at least 2 hours and hourly thereafter until satisfactory (NICE 2011).
- When intrathecal morphine has been administered hourly assessment of the respiration rate, sedation and pain scores must take place for 24 hours (12 hours if diamorphine was used).
- When opioids have been administered via epidural or PCA, hourly assessment of respiration rate, sedation, and pain scores should continue until 2 hours post-discontinuation (NICE 2011).
- After approximately 1 hour, the woman should be conscious, comfortable, semi-recumbent if appropriate and, if she desires, able to tolerate oral fluids. She will remain in recovery until the recovery staff, in consultation with the anaesthetist, are satisfied that she may be transferred elsewhere. All of the care listed above is ongoing throughout recovery care, all observations should be within normal limits before recovery care is ended. All aspects of record keeping are maintained contemporaneously. The midwife/recovery staff should have access to calling

the anaesthetist and/or obstetrician at any time if any deviations from the norm are noted.

The baby

The baby is cared for accordingly, noting that babies born in theatre:

- are often cooler
- need to be fed as soon as possible
- may have had skin-to-skin care with birthing partner but needs skin-to-skin care with the mother
- should be labelled before leaving theatre
- are more likely to experience respiratory distress.

ONGOING CARE

Psychologically, there is relief and enjoyment of the new baby, but it may be tinged by pain, immobility, distress (if rapid emergency or major complications were present) and frustration that progress appears slow. In the days following the surgery, the woman will appreciate sensitive and individualized midwifery care and should have the opportunity to review her care and future pregnancies with her obstetric team.

Postoperative care, whilst individualized, will probably include attention to hygiene and oral care, thromboembolic prophylaxis (Chapter 54), vital sign observations, pressure area care, urinary output and effective analgesia.

For analgesia, NICE (2011) recommend intrathecal or epidural diamorphine as the initial analgesic of choice, noting that PCA offers the woman good pain relief also. Non-steroidal anti-inflammatory drugs can also be given concurrently (unless contraindicated) and continued after the opioids have stopped. Effective and regular pain relief is essential to the woman's recovery.

The woman may eat or drink as she wishes (NICE 2011). I.V. infusion is discontinued when appropriate, usually when the woman is tolerating fluids although the cannula may be left in situ until the woman is mobile (often the following day but it will require flushing to maintain patency, see Chapter 47). The urinary catheter is removed when appropriate and voiding encouraged (see Chapter 14); this should be at least 12 hours after the last regional analgesia. Early mobilization is encouraged and naturally the woman will require support and care with her baby, particularly to establish breastfeeding. While this is often a motivating factor for the woman after CS, the midwife should ensure that the woman is having sufficient rest and is not over-tired.

The wound dressing is removed after 24 hours, the midwife maintains observations for any signs of wound infection (Chapter 52), the wound is kept clean and dry.

Haemoglobin estimation may be completed on the third postoperative day after postnatal diuresis has occurred. The midwife should be sensitive to the woman's emotional state, noting that she has undergone two significant life experiences – having a baby and major surgery. Standard postnatal assessment is a part of each day's care in conjunction with specific postoperative needs.

Debriefing is recommended prior to leaving hospital so that women can discuss the reasons why the CS took place and the implications for future childbearing (Baxter 2007, NICE 2011).

Discharge from hospital will depend upon the woman's progress and social support; it may be from 24 hours to 3–4 days. Postsurgery advice includes pain management, importance of rest and nutrition, what to do should complications arise, avoidance of lifting (Gould (2007) advises the amount lifted in the first 6 weeks should be no more than the weight of a full kettle) and driving until free of discomfort, effective contraception and attendance for assessment (often with the obstetrician) at the end of the puerperium.

Audit of CS care is recommended in order that healthcare providers can both provide quality care and reduce the CS rate. The NICE audit (2011) is accessible online at www.nice.org.uk/guidance/cg132/resources under 'Electronic audit tool'.

ROLE AND RESPONSIBILITIES OF THE MIDWIFE

These can be summarized as:
- evidence-based practice throughout
- preoperative care to reduce intra- and postoperative complications
- skilled care within theatre and recovery
- comprehensive postoperative care
- effective multidisciplinary teamwork and recognition of limitations where appropriate
- referral when indicated
- contemporaneous record keeping.

SUMMARY

- Theatre care is detailed and specialized; childbearing women have increased risk factors including aspiration, aortocaval occlusion and thromboembolism.
- Preoperative preparation should include consent, identity, care of the gastrointestinal and urinary tracts, skin preparation, removal of prostheses, thromboprophylaxis and psychological support; good preoperative care can reduce the intra- and postoperative risks.
- Intraoperative care considers the woman to be the highest priority for maintaining her internal and external safety. This comprises many aspects of care.
- Postoperative care focuses on vital sign observations, airway and consciousness, pain relief, assessment of wound and haemorrhage, care of infusions, bladder care, adaptation to parenthood and feeding and psychological support.

SELF-ASSESSMENT EXERCISES

The answers to the following questions may be found in the text:
1. Discuss the requirements and rationale for preoperative preparation prior to emergency CS. Compare and contrast this with preparation for elective surgery.
2. Summarize the general principles of conduct and care in the theatre environment.
3. Discuss the midwife's role and responsibilities to the woman before, during and following CS.
4. Describe the care that the woman needs in the immediate and ongoing recovery period after a CS under regional anaesthesia.
5. List other occasions when it may be necessary for childbearing women to undergo surgery.

REFERENCES

AAGBI, OAA (The Association of Anaesthetists of Great Britain and Ireland and Obstetric Anaesthetists' Association), 2005. OAA/AAGBI Guidelines for Obstetric Anaesthetic Services, second ed. AAGBI and OAA, London.

Anorlu, R.I., Maholwana, B., Hofmeyr, G.J., 2008. Methods of delivering the placenta at caesarean section. Cochrane Database Syst. Rev. (3), Art. No.: CD004737, doi:10.1002/14651858.CD004737. pub2.

ASA (American Society of Anesthetists), 2007. Practice guidelines for obstetric anesthesia. Anesthesiology 106, 843–863.

Baxter, J., 2007. Do women understand the reasons given for their caesarian sections? Br. J. Midwifery 15 (9), 536–538.

BirthChoiceUK, 2013. National Statistics, Caesarean section. Available online: <http://www.birthchoiceuk.com/> (accessed 24 February 2015).

CDC (Centers for Disease Control and Prevention), 2013. Births: final data for 2013. Available online: <http://www.cdc.gov/nchs/fastats/delivery.htm> (accessed 24 February 2015).

Charles, C., 2013. Caesarean section. In: Chapman, V., Charles, C. (Eds.), The Midwife's Labour and Birth Handbook, third ed. Wiley Blackwell, Chichester, pp. 179–192.

Crenshaw, J.T., Winslow, E.H., 2006. Actual versus instructed fasting times and associated discomforts in women having scheduled cesarean birth. J Obstet. Gynecol. Neonatal Nurs. 35 (2), 257–264.

DH (Department of Health), 1998. Why mothers die: Report on Confidential enquiries into Maternal Deaths in the United Kingdom 1994–1996. The Stationery Office, London.

Gates, S., Anderson, E.R., 2005. Wound drainage for caesarean section. Cochrane Database Syst. Rev. (1), Art. No.: CD004549, doi:10.1002/14651858.CD004549.pub2.

Gould, D., 2007. Caesarean section, surgical site infection and wound management. Nurs. Stand. 21 (32), 57–66.

Jose, B., Dignon, A., 2013. Is there a relationship between preoperative shaving (hair removal) and surgical site infection? J. Perioper. Pract. 23 (1), 23–25.

Knight, M., Nair, M., Shah, A., et al., 2014. Maternal mortality and morbidity in the UK 2009-12: surveillance and epidemiology. In: Knight, M., Kenyon, S., Brocklehurst, P., On behalf of MBRRACE-UK, et al. (Eds.), Saving Lives, Improving Mothers' Care – Lessons Learned to Inform Future Maternity Care from the UK and Ireland Confidential Enquiries into Maternal Deaths and Morbidity 2009–2012. National Perinatal Epidemiology Unit, Oxford (Chapter 2).

Mathai, M., Hofmeyr, G.J., 2007. Abdominal surgical incisions for caesarean section. Cochrane Database Syst. Rev. (1), Art. No.: CD004453, doi:10.1002/14651858.CD004453.pub2.

NCT (National Childbirth Trust), 2011. NCT Briefing for Journalists: Caesarean Birth. NCT, London. Available online: <http://www.nct.org.uk/sites/default/files/related_documents/B3%20Caesarean%20Birth%20briefing%202011.pdf> (accessed 24 February 2015).

NICE (National Institute for Health and Clinical Excellence), 2011. Caesarean Section: NICE Clinical Guideline 132. NICE, London. Available online: <www.nice.org.uk> (accessed 6 March 2015).

NICE (National Institute for Health and Care Excellence), 2013. Surgical Site Infection NICE Quality Standard 49. NICE, London. Available online: <www.nice.org.uk/Guidance/QS49> (accessed 9 November 2015).

NMC (Nursing and Midwifery Council), 2009. Record Keeping Guidance for Nurses and Midwives. NMC, London.

Scott, E., Earl, C., Leaper, D., et al., 1999. Understanding peri-operative nursing. Nurs. Stand. 13 (49), 49–54.

Yentis, S., Clyburn, P., On behalf of the MBRRACE-UK Anaesthetic chapter writing Group, et al., 2014. Lessons for anaesthesia. In: Knight, M., Kenyon, S., Brocklehurst, P., On behalf of MBRRACE-UK, et al., (Eds.), Saving Lives, Improving Mothers' Care – Lessons Learned to Inform Future Maternity Care from the UK and Ireland Confidential Enquiries into Maternal Deaths and Morbidity 2009–2012. National Perinatal Epidemiology Unit, Oxford (Chapter 6).

WHO (World Health Organisation), 2009. WHO Surgical Safety Checklist. Available online: <http://www.nrls.npsa.nhs.uk/resources/?entryid45=59860> (accessed 24 February 2015).

Chapter | 52 |

Principles of wound management: healing and care

LEARNING OUTCOMES

Having read this chapter, the reader should be able to:

- describe the process of wound healing, identifying the factors that can affect it
- discuss the current evidence which underpins the care of surgical wounds, particularly caesarean section
- describe an Aseptic Non Touch Technique (ANTT) and apply the principles to the dressing of wounds, drains and the removal of wound closures.

A wound is any break in the skin and underlying tissues. Wound classifications mainly consider the extent, depth and causative factor. Midwives will be familiar with surgical clean contaminated wounds (caesarean section), lacerations (perineal tears or trauma to nipples) and punctures (cannulation, venepuncture, capillary sampling). Wound care is underpinned by an appreciation of the physiology of wound healing. This chapter considers wound healing and the factors that influence it, the care of caesarean section wounds, and the removal of wound closures. The reader will gain a holistic understanding by reading this chapter in conjunction with asepsis (Chapter 10) and perioperative skills (Chapter 51).

PHYSIOLOGY OF WOUND HEALING

Healing of wounds begins following any injury to the body; an intact skin provides an efficient first line of defence against invading microorganisms. Wounds whose edges are in apposition (e.g. surgical wounds) heal quickly by first intention. Deeper, gaping wounds take longer to heal by secondary or tertiary intention. The process of wound healing is well documented, but sometimes the terminology used can vary (Nobbs & Crozier 2011). There are four phases of wound healing, using commonly recognized terms:

1. haemostasis
2. inflammation
3. proliferation
4. maturation.

The length of time to progress through these phases varies for each wound and can be influenced by factors such as wound size, suturing, the clinical condition of the person, and the presence/absence of infection.

Haemostasis

This vascular phase begins immediately there is tissue damage. Vasoconstriction occurs to minimize bleeding (also initiating the coagulation process) and forming an obstacle to potential microorganism invasion. A fibrin clot forms, temporarily closing the wound. While the clot is forming, blood or serous fluid may exude from the wound as the body tries to cleanse the wound naturally.

Inflammation

The blood vessels around the wound dilate, causing localized erythema, oedema, heat, discomfort, throbbing, and sometimes functional disturbance. Macrophages clear the wound of debris in preparation for new tissue growth. A small necrotic area forms around the wound margin where the blood supply was interrupted. Epithelial cells from the wound margin move under the base of the clot, the

surrounding epithelium thickens and a thin layer of epithelial tissue forms over the wound. As the clinical signs of the inflammation phase are similar to those of infection (see below), it is important the midwife can distinguish between a wound that is healing normally and one that is infected. Provided the wound is clean, this phase lasts between 1–3 days, but is prolonged in the presence of infection or necrosis (Sharp & Clark 2011).

Proliferation

This phase begins within 3 days in acute wounds and involves the growth of new tissue through three processes:

- granulation
- wound contraction
- epithelialization.

During granulation, capillaries from the surrounding vessels grow into the wound bed. At the same time, fibroblasts produce collagen fibres, providing the framework for new connective tissue formation. Collagen increases the tensile strength and structural integrity of the wound. Healthy granulation tissue has a bright red, moist, shiny appearance, a 'pebbled' looking base and does not bleed easily.

Once the wound is filled with connective tissue, fibroblasts collect around the edges of the wound and contract, pulling the edges together. A firmer, fibrous epithelial scar forms as the fibroblasts and collagen fibres begin to shrink, resulting in contraction of the area and obliteration of some of the capillaries. This only occurs with healthy tissue that has not been sutured.

During epithelialization, new epithelial cells grow over the wound surface to form a new outer layer, recognized by the whitish-pink, translucent appearance of the wound. The process is enhanced in a moist, clean environment.

Maturation

Once epithelialization is complete, the new tissue undergoes a time of maturation when it is 're-modelled' to increase the tensile strength of the scar tissue. In lightly pigmented skin, the scar initially appears red and raised, and then with time changes to a paler, smoother, flatter appearance. Scar tissue in darkly pigmented skin has a lighter appearance initially when compared with lightly pigmented skin. Mature scar tissue is avascular and contains no sweat or sebaceous glands or hairs. Boyle (2006) suggests that scar tissue has 80% strength of the original tissue. The maturation phase begins after about 21 days and can take up to 2 years to complete. This may be the reason why some wounds that appear to have healed suddenly break down (Keast & Orsted 1998).

This healing process also occurs around sutures. When the sutures are removed, the epithelial cells can be dislodged and may be visible on the sutures as debris.

Assessing a wound identifies which of the healing stages the wound is in, as well as the appearance of the surrounding tissue and any observations for abnormalities, e.g. swelling, heat, pain, etc.

Wound healing by secondary intention occurs with deeper, wider wounds, whose edges cannot be brought into apposition. Inflammation may be chronic, with more granulation tissue forming at the expense of collagen during proliferation. Granulation tissue gradually fills the wound with re-epithelialization beginning at the edges. Healing by secondary intention takes longer, resulting in more scar tissue forming.

FACTORS THAT AFFECT WOUND HEALING

- Temperature: a fall and a rise in wound temperature both cause vasoconstriction and so impair wound healing. Dixon et al (2014) found that the surgical site skin temperature post caesarean section was much lower than for other surgical interventions. The origins of this are as yet unknown, but they theorize that this is one reason for the higher incidence of surgical site infection for this group, a startling 10% (Wloch et al 2012). Milne et al (2012) also suggest that body temperature should remain above 36°C for the duration of the surgery.
- Infection: infection causes increased inflammation and necrosis, which delays wound healing. Many factors appear to contribute to infection, these are a few: poor surgical techniques (with an increased risk of haematoma (Olsen et al 2008)), poor dressing techniques, a larger number of people in theatre (Reilly 2002), inadequate or mistimed antibiotic prophylaxis (Kaimal et al 2008) and wounds that are too dry or too wet predispose to colonization or infection. A wound that is critically colonized has sufficient bacteria competing for oxygen and nutrients at the expense of healthy cells. It may not appear infected but will fail to heal.
- Nutritional status: an adequate intake of protein, carbohydrate, fats, vitamins A, B, C and E, copper, zinc and iron are required. Proteins supply amino acids, essential for tissue repair and regeneration. Vitamins A and B and zinc are required for epithelialization, and vitamin C and zinc are necessary for collagen synthesis and capillary integrity. Iron is required for the synthesis of haemoglobin which combines reversibly with oxygen to transport oxygen around the body.
- Psycho-social factors: good management of pain will reduce the woman's anxiety, improve her acceptance of the wound, and so reduce stress. Anxiety, isolation, and altered body image all reduce wound healing (South et al 2008).
- Increasing age: this affects all phases of wound healing due to impaired circulation and coagulation, slower inflammatory response, and decreased fibroblast activity.
- Medical disorders: particularly those which impair circulation or tissue perfusion can delay wound healing. Diabetes mellitus includes the additional risk of hyperglycaemia, this can inhibit phagocytosis and predispose to fungal and yeast infection. Malignancy or the need for chemotherapy was also shown to have an adverse influence on wound infection rates (Reilly 2002).
- Drugs: anti-inflammatory drugs suppress protein synthesis, inflammation, wound contraction, and epithelialization. Corticosteroids (from stress, steroid therapy or disease) delay both the inflammatory and immune responses.
- Impaired oxygenation: a low arterial oxygen tension may alter collagen synthesis and inhibit epithelialization. Poor tissue perfusion may occur in the presence of hypovolaemia, anaemia, obesity, smoking, poor mobility, and alcohol. Oxygen is necessary for fibroblast activity. Johnson et al (2006), Olsen et al (2008), the Joint Commission Perspectives on Patient Safety (JCPPS) (2008), and Nobbs & Crozier (2011) all relate obesity particularly with an increased risk of wound infection.
- Surgery-related care: NICE (2011) suggest specific surgical techniques for caesarean section surgery. Failure to undertake these procedures increases the risk of poor healing post-surgery.
- Wound stress: prolonged or violent vomiting, abdominal distension or laboured respirations may cause sudden tension on the wound, inhibiting the formation of collagen networks and connective tissue.

The factors listed above are sometimes categorized as either intrinsic or extrinsic factors. These refer to the internal issues that relate to the woman, e.g. age, health, smoking, out of normal parameters for body mass index, presurgical rupture of membranes and those that relate to the external issues such as surgical technique, wound care, environmental hygiene, planned surgery and antibiotic prophylaxis. It becomes clear that the factors affecting wound management are considerable, significant and multidisciplinary.

COMPLICATIONS OF WOUND HEALING

Haemorrhage

Haemostasis usually occurs within several minutes of an acute wound occurring. However, bleeding may occur if a bleeding point is not tied off, as a result of the clot or suture dislodging or infection, and may occur internally and externally. Internal bleeding can lead to haematoma formation.

Infection

Infection usually appears within 2–3 days following a traumatic injury or 4–5 days following a surgical wound. The wound site will appear red (often a spreading or tracking cellulitis), hot, swollen and painful. There may also be weeping from the wound, usually a yellow, green or brown discharge (depending on the infecting organism), it may also be malodorous. The woman may have pyrexia, tachycardia, a raised white cell count and a general malaise (Boyle 2006).

Dehiscence

If an acute wound does not heal properly the layers of skin and tissue can separate, usually during the proliferation phase. Separation can be partial or complete. It occurs more commonly where there is greater strain on the wound and decreased vasoconstriction (e.g. obesity), and particularly with abdominal wounds, if a sudden strain is placed on the wound (e.g. coughing, sitting up).

Evisceration

This is a rare medical emergency that occurs when the visceral organs begin to protrude through the separated wound layers.

Fistula

A fistula is a channel that tracks through the tissue and can harbour microorganisms and cause recurring infection. It usually occurs as a result of poor wound healing.

WOUND MANAGEMENT

Wound management aims to promote healing of the tissue and also to prevent any of the possible complications listed above. Infection is one of the most common and costly complications: for example (depending on the severity), the woman experiences pain, oozing, malodour, it affects her mobility and ability to care for her baby, and she can feel systemically unwell. She may have ugly scarring forever and may be reluctant to consider surgery or childbirth again. For the healthcare provider the costs are significant, the reputation is damaged, practice is questioned, and antibiotic use is increased further. Wloch et al (2012) suggest that nationally in England 15 000 women per year experience wound infection after caesarean section, for which 960 of them will require re-admission to hospital.

Preoperative considerations

Childbearing women who are healthy and enter hospital only a short time before their planned surgery have a lesser risk of wound healing complications than those who are unwell, anaemic, have a longer hospital admission, emergency surgery or presurgical rupture of the membranes. Other measures that can optimize health before surgery should be taken; these include:

- normal range blood glucose levels
- screening for and treating existing infections, e.g. groin swabs for methicillin-resistant *Staphylococcus aureus* (MRSA) (p. 95)
- reducing obesity
- smoking cessation (JCPPS 2008).

Preoperative skin preparation

Currently in the literature this consists of:

- actions that the woman can take
- hair removal
- skin cleanser prior to surgery
- skin cleansing technique.

Actions that the woman can take

For planned surgery the woman is encouraged to bath or shower on the day using soap (NICE 2008). Toiletries or make-up should be avoided after the bath/shower.

Hair removal

This remains debatable, NICE (2008) suggest that routine hair removal is not necessary but it is considered appropriate where the hair may interfere with the surgery or application of a dressing (Jose & Dignon 2013). NICE (2008) recognize that hair can increase microorganism contamination. Jose & Dignon (2013) also cite studies where neurosurgery was undertaken without shaving, which suggests that the practice of removal is questionable.

If hair is to be removed, the method chosen should impact the minimum of damage to the skin. Razors cause microabrasions into which microorganisms can colonize. Razors should be avoided (NICE 2008). The recommendation is that single-head-use electric clippers should be used as near to the operation time as possible (but not in theatre) by healthcare personnel (NICE 2013). Depilatory creams may also be considered, but their use can cause skin irritation and allergy, and the time required is longer.

Skin cleanser prior to surgery

In the theatre the skin site should be cleansed prior to incision using povidone iodine or chlorhexidine (NICE 2008). Silva (2013) reviewed the literature and concluded that 2% chlorhexidine in 70% alcohol was the most effective. This is consistent with Loveday et al (2014), who recommend this solution for a number of skin-cleansing procedures.

Skin-cleansing technique

ANTT (Rowley et al 2010) recommend that skin cleansing for a range of aseptic procedures should be undertaken using sterile equipment, a non touch technique, and a friction-generating approach. The skin should be cleansed for at least 30 seconds, the swab/wipe should work backwards and forwards across the area (like a grid, left to right, up and down) and then left to dry for at least 30 seconds. Silva (2014) identifies that historically surgical sites have been cleansed using a concentric circles approach but that a back-and-forth action reaches deeper layers of the skin and so reduces the bacterial count.

Intraoperative care

Strict surgical asepsis should be maintained, with all standard precautions and personal protective equipment used as per the local protocol. Now well supported, including NICE (2011), is the use of a single dose of prophylactic antibiotics, intravenously and before skin incision.

Chapter 51 highlights some of the other specific issues at surgery which can reduce the incidence of healing complications, e.g. avoidance of superficial wound drains, nature and positioning of incision, secured haemostasis to prevent haematoma formation.

WOUND CLOSURE

Closure of the wound aims to bring the skin edges in neat apposition so that healing may begin by first intention. Gurusamy et al (2014) found little conclusive evidence as to the value of continuous or interrupted sutures in reducing surgical site infection (SSI). There was less wound breakdown when subcuticular suturing was used but the quality of studies was limited and none of them were obstetric surgery. Wetter et al (1991) and Johnson et al (2006) both recommend the use of subcuticular suturing and Ward et al (2008) found that wound infection was higher with staples than with a continuous suture. Olsen et al (2008) agreed.

Mangram et al (1999) highlighted that a monofilament suture carried less infection risk than a multifilamented one. Reilly (2002) found that if sutures were left in place for longer than 10 days infection rates were greater. Gould (2007) recommends that for a transverse wound the sutures or staples can be removed after 4 or 5 days, once the new epithelium has become intact. Seven to ten days is the recommended length of time for removal from a vertical incision. NICE (2011) indicate that superficial wound drains should be avoided for caesarean section wounds. If one is used, it should be removed as soon as drainage ceases, ideally the next day (Gould 2007).

WOUND DRESSINGS

It is now well accepted that a moist wound environment promotes wound healing. There are various types of dressings available for a range of wound types. The wound dressing performs several important functions:

- protects the wound from injury, hypothermia and external infection (until natural healing has begun)
- absorbs any wound secretions, maintaining the moisture balance
- minimizes pain, odour and bleeding.
  (Adapted from Doran-Williams et al 2011)

Generally, after caesarean section an absorbent nonadherent dressing is applied. This varies; however, it is often locally agreed and can be based on cost as well as effectiveness. In the event of haemorrhage a pressure dressing may be applied to aid haemostasis.

POSTOPERATIVE WOUND CARE

Cleaning and dressing wounds

A carefully sutured incision that has achieved haemostasis will be sealed by fibrin within 24 hours (Reilly 2002). At this point the dressing may be removed and the wound assessed, although Milne et al (2012) indicate that dressings should remain in place for 3–5 days, but at least for 48 hours. NICE (2011) indicate that dressing removal should take place at 24 hours and that after that the woman and wound are assessed regularly for potential infection. The woman is encouraged to wear cotton underwear and loose clothing. The wound should be cleaned and dried daily. Suture or staple removal (if necessary) is undertaken from day 5 onwards. In instances where dressings need changing, an ANTT technique should be used (Chapter 10).

CAESAREAN SECTION WOUNDS – SUMMARY

For a woman with a lower segment caesarean section (LSCS) wound, the following principles are suggested, but the reader is encouraged to be aware of the evolving audits and evidence:

- The theatre dressing can be removed after 24–48 hours.
- The woman should shower daily, the wound being gently patted dry. A dry dressing can be applied to offer protection against clothing rubbing against the wound; otherwise, it may be left uncovered. The woman should wear cotton underwear and loose clothing.
- The wound should be assessed at every postoperative/ postnatal assessment.
- Suture/staple removal is planned for the correct day, often day 5 onwards.
- If the wound is exuding fluid or shows any other signs of potential complications it should be swabbed (see Chapter 11 for technique), cleansed and re-dressed. Referral may be necessary for antibiotic therapy.
- If a wound requires cleansing and re-dressing, an ANTT is used.

LONGER-TERM CARE

Gould (2007) indicates that women need to be aware that wound healing involves several layers of tissue and that it takes time for the maturation phase to be completed (1–2 years). In both the short and the long term, women need to be aware of what constitutes impairment or complications of wound healing and so seek appropriate referral.

PERINEAL WOUNDS

Perineal wounds heal by first intention, provided that the skin edges are in apposition. Hygiene is one of the significant aids to healing, with handwashing before and after any perineal contact, being an essential part of care (NICE 2014). Perineal wound care is discussed in further detail in Chapter 12.

Aseptic wound dressing

Chapter 10 discusses the principles of asepsis which are then applied to each situation. In many instances cesarean section wounds do not require re-dressing but for a wound that does, an ANTT approach (Rowley et al 2010) should be used. Wounds that need an aseptic dressing usually require cleansing. This removes bacteria, exudate and debris, among other things. However, unnecessary cleaning may disturb the healing process. 0.9% sodium chloride (at room temperature) or warm tap water is used (Doran-Williams et al 2011). Sterile gauze, foam or a 10-mL syringe is used according to availability and suitability.

The question of when a wound dressing should be changed remains unanswered. It would appear sensible to make a daily *assessment*, but not to disturb the wound by cleaning or re-dressing it unless necessary.

PROCEDURE: aseptic dressing technique

- Confirm identity, gain informed consent and establish that re-dressing is indicated.
- Decontaminate hands, collect a clean-dressings trolley. Put on non-sterile gloves and clean the trolley with the locally approved surface wipes. Remove gloves and wash and dry hands.
- Gather the equipment onto the lower shelf:
  - alcohol handrub and non-sterile gloves
  - apron
  - sachet of 0.9% sodium chloride at body temperature
  - sterile dressing pack (in date) (should contain disposable bag and suitable dressing)
  - 10-mL syringe.
- Position the woman appropriately, maintaining privacy and dignity.
- Wash and dry hands, apply apron, loosen the existing dressing, but keep the wound covered and decontaminate hands.
- Open the outer layer of the pack, dropping it carefully onto the top shelf of the trolley.
- Open the inner wrapper of the pack touching only the edges of the paper; slide the other sterile items onto the sterile field and pour the saline into the gallipot, all with an ANTT, protecting Key-Parts.

- Loosen the existing dressing, place the disposable bag over the hand and remove the dressing (see Nicol et al 2008).
- Invert the bag, with the dressing inside, and attach it to the side of the trolley as a refuse bag.
- Use handrub and apply non-sterile gloves.
- If appropriate, place a sterile field under the wound.
- Assess the wound; if irrigation is indicated, draw up the saline in the syringe.
- Cleanse the skin around the wound with gauze.
- Then either (depending on local protocol):
  - clean the wound with gauze and gloved hands ensuring that it is only the sterile gauze that touches the wound (Key-Part and Key-Site). Use each swab to wipe once only, wiping from areas of discharge outwards. Discard the swab, repeat as necessary; OR
  - hold a piece of gauze at the dirtier end of the wound and irrigate with the syringe, from clean to dirty, catching the fluid in the gauze (this is the preferable method).
- Dry the surrounding skin.
- Apply and secure the dressing.
- Remove gloves and apron; wash and dry hands.
- Ensure the woman is comfortable; discuss findings and ongoing care with her.
- Dispose of equipment correctly, clean the trolley.
- Return the trolley to the clean area.
- Decontaminate hands.
- Document findings, including the appearance of the wound and the future plan of care. Take action accordingly.

Removal of sutures or staples

The decision to remove sutures or staples is taken according to the assessment of healing of the wound. Removal is often 4–5 days after the surgery. Sutures that are retained for too long increase the infection risk and delay wound healing. Suture removal is an aseptic procedure, a receptacle is required to place staples in so that they can be disposed of correctly in the sharps bin. If the wound gapes after any of the sutures/staples have been removed, the midwife will refer the woman before removing them all, and may apply an adhesive suture and sterile dressing in the meantime. Obviously, only non-absorbable sutures need to be removed.

Removing sutures

The aim of correct suture removal is to ensure that no part of the external suture is taken through internally. It is an aseptic procedure for which a dressings trolley is prepared and used as above, to which sterile scissors/stitch cutter or staple remover are added accordingly. Suture removal packs are sometimes available containing forceps; if unavailable, then individual sterile forceps are used.

Principles of suture removal

- Clean the wound as described above.
- Lift and hold the external part of the suture with forceps using the non-dominant hand.
- Cut beneath the knot as near to the skin as possible using scissors or stitch cutter in the dominant hand.
- Remove the suture by pulling it gently through the skin.

This last principle applies whether the sutures are interrupted or subcuticular. Subcuticular suturing is sometimes held in place with a bead, the bead should be removed at the distal end of the wound so that on removal the suture is pulled from the end nearest to the midwife. The removal should be smooth; the woman may experience the pulling sensation rather than discomfort.

Removing staples

- Clean the wound as described above.
- Hold the staple remover as if a pair of scissors.
- Insert the lower blade directly under the staple.
- Squeeze the handles together; the staple will be lifted from the skin as it concertinas.
- Lift clear, place into sterile receptacle on the trolley, dispose into a sharps box when finished completely.

The removing of sutures/staples must be recorded, including whether the removal was partial or complete. If some sutures/staples still need to be removed, a clear plan of care (including referral if needed) should be documented. Wound assessment should be completed; in some instances this is on a locally agreed wound chart.

WOUND DRAINS

Wound drains are seen infrequently in maternity care. NICE (2011) recommend that superficial drains are not used for caesarean section, the incidence of wound infection or haematoma is not reduced with their use. A wound may be drained by using either an open or a closed drainage system; a closed system is usually vacuumed (which 'pulls' the exudate from the tissues) whereas an open drain drains with gravity. The nature of the surgery determines whether a drain is inserted, and if so, which type.

Postoperatively, wound drains are observed for their drainage and must be kept positioned so that they are able to drain correctly and do not pull or fall to the floor. Any drainage from the wound drain should be recorded on the fluid balance chart. Removal is according to the obstetrician's instructions but is often 24 hours post-surgery.

Emptying a wound drain

Care should be taken to maintain the integrity of the closed drainage system to reduce infection risks, whichever type of drain is used. The drain should be emptied if the vacuum is reduced or lost, or if it is to be retained for longer than 24 hours.

Drains vary; the midwife will need to be familiar with individual types. Most drains have the vacuum mechanism integral to them, usually by compressing the drain. The principles of emptying a wound drain are:

- ANTT is used and the midwife wears non-sterile gloves.
- The emptying port is cleansed using a locally approved alcohol wipe using the four corners and centre for approximately 5 seconds each, creating friction.
- The contents are emptied into a sterile receiver. Once the drain is emptied the vacuum is initiated and the drain sealed.
- There is minimal disruption for the woman.
- The procedure and volume are documented.

Dressing a wound drain

If required for longer than 24 hours, the drain may require re-dressing. ANTT is used; the skin around the drain is cleansed with sterile 0.9% sodium chloride and a hole is cut (with sterile scissors) into the non-adherent dressing so that it sits snugly around the drain and is secured with tape.

Removal of a wound drain – principles

- After confirming that the drain should be removed, the woman's consent is sought. She does need to understand that while not a painful procedure, it can be accompanied by a strange sensation as the drain is drawn through the tissues. Analgesia may be needed pre- or post-procedure according to the timing of the previous dose.
- ANTT is used and the midwife wears non-sterile gloves.

- The skin around the drain is cleaned as per wound dressing above.
- The suture is cut using a sterile stitch cutter, as described above for any suture. The vacuum is released, the non-dominant hand supports the skin around the drain, and the drain is removed smoothly, but not too quickly.
- The site is cleaned and a non-adherent dressing is applied and secured. The site is then assessed as for any other wound.
- The amount that has drained is recorded on the fluid balance chart and the drain is disposed of in the clinical waste.
- The tip of the drain may be sent for laboratory investigation if required.

ROLE AND RESPONSIBILITIES OF THE MIDWIFE

These can be summarized as:
- understanding the physiology of wound healing and application of this to practice
- application of evidence-based care
- undertaking all procedures correctly with an ANTT approach when indicated
- referral if indicated
- contemporaneous record keeping.

SUMMARY

- Surgical wounds heal mainly by primary intention; the four phases of wound healing can be affected by various factors, e.g. nutritional status, wound temperature, diabetes, obesity, smoking.
- Evidence-based perioperative and wound care aim to reduce the possible complications, infection being one of the biggest risks.
- An Aseptic Non Touch Technique is required if a wound needs dressing or sutures/staples removing.
- Caesarean section wounds are often uncovered after 24 hours, ongoing assessment of the wound should be undertaken at each consultation. Wound infections after caesarean section are known to be 1:10 (Wloch et al 2012) in England.

SELF-ASSESSMENT EXERCISES

The answers to the following questions may be found in the text:

1. Describe the four phases of wound healing.
2. How would the midwife distinguish between a wound that is healing normally and one that is infected?
3. Discuss the factors that enhance or impair wound healing.
4. Describe the management of the wound following caesarean section.
5. Describe how to remove sutures correctly. Compare and contrast the removal of staples with sutures.
6. Describe how to clean, dress and remove a wound drain.
7. What complications are associated with wound healing?

REFERENCES

Boyle, M., 2006. Wound Healing in Midwifery. Radcliffe, Oxford, pp. 31–36.

Dixon, M., Yakub, R., Isdale, M., 2014. Surgical site skin temperature. A comparison between caesarean section and other surgical procedures. Arch. Dis. Child Fetal Neonatal Ed. 99 (Suppl. 1), A128.

Doran-Williams, P., Jackson, B., Tinne, N., 2011. Wound management. In: Doughty, L., Lister, S. (Eds.), The Royal Marsden Hospital Manual of Clinical Nursing Procedures, eighth ed. Wiley Blackwell, Chichester, pp. 1166–1202.

Gould, D., 2007. Caesarean section, surgical site infection and wound management. Nurs. Stand. 21 (32), 57–66.

Gurusamy, K., Toon, C., Allen, V., Davidson, B., 2014. Continuous versus interrupted skin sutures for non-obstetric surgery. Cochrane Database Syst. Rev. (2), Art.No. CD010365, doi:10.1002/14651858. CD010365.pub2.

JCPPS (Joint Commission Perspectives on Patient Safety), 2008. Preventing surgical site infections (SSI). Jt. Comm. Perspect. Patient Saf. 8 (9), 8–11.

Johnson, A., Young, D., Reilly, J., 2006. Caesarean section surgical site infection surveillance. J. Hosp. Infect. 64 (1), 30–35.

Jose, B., Dignon, A., 2013. Is there a relationship between preoperative shaving (hair removal) and surgical site infection? J. Perioper. Pract. 23 (1), 23–25.

Kaimal, A.J., Zlantnik, M.G., Cheng, Y.W., et al., 2008. Effect of a change in policy regarding the timing of prophylactic antibiotics on the rate of postcaesarean delivery surgical site infections. Am. J. Obstet. Gynaecol. 199 (3), 310, e1–5.

Keast, D.H., Orsted, H., 1998. The basic principles of wound care. Ostomy Wound Manage. 44 (8), 24–31.

Loveday, H., Wilson, W., Pratt, R.J., et al., 2014. epic3: national evidence-based guidelines for preventing healthcare-associated infections in NHS hospitals in England. J. Hosp. Infect. 86 (Suppl. 1), S1–S70.

Mangram, A.J., Horan, T.C., Pearson, M.L., et al., 1999. Guideline for prevention of surgical site infection. Am. J. Infect. Control 27 (2), 97–134.

Milne, J., Vowden, P., Fumarola, S., et al., 2012. Postoperative incision management. Wounds UK Suppl. 8 (4), 1–4.

NICE (National Institute for Health and Clinical Excellence), 2008. Surgical Site Infection: NICE Clinical Guideline 74. NICE, London. Available online: <www.nice.org.uk> (accessed 6 March 2015).

NICE (National Institute for Health and Clinical Excellence), 2011. Caesarean Section: NICE Clinical Guideline 132. NICE, London. Available online: <www.nice.org.uk> (accessed 6 March 2015).

NICE (National Institute for Health and Care Excellence), 2013. Surgical Site Infection: NICE Quality Standard 49. NICE, London. Available online: <www.nice.org.uk> (accessed 6 March 2015).

NICE (National Institute for Health Care Excellence), 2014. Postnatal Care: NICE Clinical Guideline 37. NICE, London. Available online: <www.nice.org.uk> (accessed 6 March 2015).

Nicol, M., Bavin, C., Cronin, P., et al., 2008. Essential Nursing Skills, third ed. Elsevier, Edinburgh.

Nobbs, S., Crozier, K., 2011. Wound management in obese women following caesarean section. Br. J. Midwifery 19 (3), 150–156.

Olsen, M.A., Butler, A.M., Willers, D.M., et al., 2008. Risk factors for surgical site infection after low transverse cesarean section. Infect. Control Hosp. Epidemiol. 29 (6), 477–484.

Reilly, J., 2002. Evidence based surgical wound care on surgical wound infection. Br. J. Nurs. 11 (16), S4–S12.

Rowley, S., Clare, S., Macqueen, S., Molyneux, R., 2010. ANTT v2: an updated practice framework for aseptic technique. Br. J. Nurs. 19 (5), S5–S11.

Sharp, A., Clark, J., 2011. Diabetes and its effects on wound healing. Nurs. Stand. 25 (45), 41–47.

Silva, P., 2013. An evidence based protocol for preoperative skin preparation. J. Perioper. Pract. 23 (4), 87–90.

Silva, P., 2014. The right skin preparation technique: a literature review. J. Perioper. Pract. 24 (12), 283–285.

South, C., Tanay, A.M., Tinne, N., 2008. Wound management. In: Doughty, L., Lister, S. (Eds.), The Royal Marsden Hospital Manual of Clinical Nursing Procedures, Student Edn. Wiley Blackwell, Oxford, pp. 1097–1162.

Ward, V.P., Charlett, A., Fagan, J., Crawshaw, S.C., 2008. Enhanced surgical site infection surveillance following caesarean section: experience of a multicentre collaborative post-discharge system. J. Hosp. Infect. 70, 166–173.

Wetter, L.A., Dinneen, M.D., Levitt, M.D., Motson, R.W., 1991. Controlled trial of polyglycolic acid versus catgut and nylon for appendicectomy wound closure. Br. J. Surg. 78 (8), 985–987.

Wloch, C., Wilson, J., Lamagni, T., et al., 2012. Risk factors for surgical site infection following caesarean section in England: results from a multicentre cohort study. Br. J. Obstet. Gynaecol. 19 (11), 1234–1333.

Chapter | 53 |

Principles of restricted mobility management: pressure area care

LEARNING OUTCOMES

Having read this chapter, the reader should be able to:

- discuss how pressure ulcers occur
- identify factors that increase the risk of pressure ulcer formation
- describe the classification of pressure ulcers
- undertake assessment of the skin, recognizing normal and abnormal changes resulting from pressure
- discuss the principles of pressure area care.

Restricted mobility can occur for a variety of reasons, e.g. during and following regional or general anaesthesia, postoperatively, increasing the risk of a pressure injury occurring. This risk increases further in the unwell woman. It is not just women who are at risk but babies, too. While the occurrence of pressure injuries within the maternity setting is low, they do occur and every patient is potentially at risk of developing a pressure ulcer if risk factors are present (Butcher 2004, McInnes et al 2011, NICE 2014). Thus it is important the midwife understands why they occur and how they can be prevented and, if they occur, contact the Tissue Viability Nurse for advice. Bennett et al (2004) caution that pressure ulcers could be indicative of clinical negligence with evidence that litigation could occur as it has in the US. Dimond (2003) agrees, suggesting that while patients and relatives have traditionally accepted that pressure ulcers were unavoidable, they are now being viewed as evidence that a reasonable standard of care and action has not been met as a reason to claim compensation. Pressure ulcers are often reportable as an incident and an investigation initiated to determine if there were any omissions in care. This chapter focuses on the principles of pressure area care including a discussion of the aetiology and classification of pressure ulcers. The factors that influence the development of pressure ulcers are given, followed by a discussion of the assessment of skin integrity.

DEFINITION

A pressure ulcer is a skin ulceration that forms due to localized tissue necrosis, commonly found on the parts of the body that have received unrelieved pressure. It has previously been referred to as a 'decubitus ulcer', 'pressure sore' or (less commonly) a 'bedsore'.

COMMON SITES FOR PRESSURE ULCER FORMATION

Although pressure ulcers can form on any part of the body, the commonest sites are the sacrum, buttocks, trochanter, and calcaneus (heels) (Bowen & Noble 2014, McGinnis & Stubbs 2014) with toes, knees, ischial tuberosities, shoulders, elbows and ears also having the potential to be affected (Fig. 53.1). Pressure may also occur from drainage tubes, indwelling catheters (against labia), nasogastric tubes (nasal passages), nasal oxygen cannulae and graduated compression stockings. Babies may also develop a pressure ulcer in the occipital region.

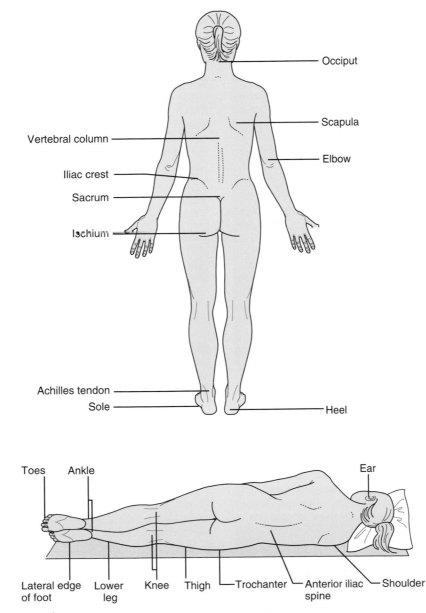

Figure 53.1 Pressure area sites.

EFFECTS OF PRESSURE

When sitting or lying, pressure is transferred from the external surface to the underlying bone via the different skin layers. This results in compression of the skin, subcutaneous fat, muscle and blood vessels. The pressure is directed downwards in an inverted cone shape and has a pressure gradient with the highest pressure at the apex. The pressure within these deep tissues is up to five times greater than within the epidermis (Dolan 2011). Consequently the pressure within the blood vessels increases. Normal capillary pressure is 12–32 mmHg; when the pressure exceeds this, the blood vessel becomes distorted and occludes (Colwell 2015). Blood flow is reduced and ischaemic injury can occur. Additionally the lymphatic supply can be occluded with accumulation of toxic substances that further increase cell damage (Hosking 2013). For the majority of people, once the pressure is removed reactive hyperaemia occurs as blood flow begins again and reperfuses the area. The area then becomes red and warm with the redness lasting up to 50–75% as long as the time the pressure prevented blood flow (deWit & O'Neill 2014). It can be difficult to detect hyperaemia in darkly pigmented skin. Bowen & Noble (2014) advise touching the skin to detect warmth. If the redness resolves or the area blanches under fingertip pressure, it is unlikely damage has occurred to the underlying tissues. However, a cycle of ischaemia and tissue reperfusion during periods of prolonged pressure is thought to contribute to tissue damage (Hosking 2013).

If the pressure is not relieved, the risk of ischaemic injury increases so that when the pressure is removed non-blanchable hyperaemia occurs. No blanching is seen with fingertip palpation – this is the first stage of skin injury and indicates deep tissue injury, although it may still be possible to reverse the damage at this stage (Colwell 2015). The cells rub together causing the cell membranes to rupture, releasing toxic intracellular material and normal skin colour is not restored. Damage can occur within 1–2 hours of continued pressure but generally is affected by the duration and amount of pressure, skin integrity, and ability of supporting structures to redistribute pressure (Bowen & Noble 2014, Colwell 2015). A deep pressure ulcer can arise when the lymphatic vessels and muscle fibres tear. In the healthy adult with full sensation, this will result in pain causing the individual to move (Benbow 2008). Where sensation is impaired (e.g. epidural anaesthesia) the change of position does not occur spontaneously.

Shearing can compound the effects of pressure. A shearing force is the pressure exerted against the skin in a direction parallel to the body's surface, occurring when the body moves up or down the bed while in an upright position. As the layers of muscle and bone slide in the direction of the body movement, the skin and subcutaneous layers stick to the bed surface, causing the bone to slide down into the skin, with a force exerted onto the skin. This can happen if the woman is pulled up the bed rather than lifted. A shearing force results at the junction of the deep and superficial tissues. The microcirculation is compressed, stretched and damaged, causing microscopic haemorrhage and necrosis deep within the tissues. This is compounded by the decreased capillary blood flow resulting from the external pressure against the skin. Eventually, a channel opens through the skin and the necrotic area drains through this (tunnelling). The areas commonly affected by shearing forces are the sacrum and coccygeus.

The skin can also be damaged by friction but this is no longer considered a cause of pressure ulcers. Friction is the mechanical force exerted when the skin is dragged across a coarse surface (e.g. bedding). Antokal et al (2012) suggest friction may cause mechanical damage to the superficial tissue cells; thus damage is due to excessive deformation rather than ischaemia. The epidermis is rubbed away, giving the appearance of a shallow abrasion injury, often on the elbows and heels. The effects of friction are exacerbated by moisture (as for shearing) (Benbow 2008).

Deep tissue necrosis often occurs first at the bony interface as a result of this pressure, and the fact that muscle tissue is more sensitive and less resistant to pressure than the skin. Pressure exerted at the bony interface then emerges at a point in the surface of the skin. A small, inflamed area, over a bony prominence, may indicate tissue breakdown that is much deeper and wider than indicated at the surface of the skin.

CLASSIFICATION OF PRESSURE ULCERS

Pressure ulcers are classified using the International National Pressure Ulcer Advisory Panel/European Pressure Ulcer Advisory Panel (NPUAP/EPUAP) pressure ulcer classification system (NPUAP/EPUAP/PPPIA 2014). This has four recognized stages related to the depth of tissue damage and involvement of associated structures. The stages can be referred to as a grade, stage or category.

- Grade 1: intact skin showing non-blanchable erythema – the early sign of potential ulcer formation. The skin may also be warm or cool, discoloured, show signs of oedema, induration, or hardness, or feel boggy. There may be pain or itching at the site. In darkly pigmented skins the area will be a persistent red/blue colour with purple hues (Bowen & Noble 2014) and the colour may differ from the surrounding tissue (Hosking 2013). This will heal slowly within 7–14 days without epithelial loss (Colwell 2015).

- Grade 2: partial-thickness skin loss of epidermis and/or dermis – a superficial ulcer that presents as a shiny or dry abrasion, blister (ruptured or intact) or shallow crater. There is a red-pink wound bed without slough (Hosking 2013). No bruising is noted (indicates deep tissue injury, Colwell 2015). Healing is through re-epithelialization.
- Grade 3: full-thickness skin loss and damage/necrosis of subcutaneous tissue which does not extend through the underlying fascia – presents as a deep crater that can also undermine adjacent tissue. The depth varies by anatomical position. Slough should not be present. Healing is through re-epithelialization and granulation.
- Grade 4: damage/necrosis to underlying tissue, muscle, bone or supporting structures, e.g. tendon with or without full-thickness skin loss. Healing is through re-epithelialization and granulation.

There are two further stages that are ungraded:

- Suspected deep tissue injury: localized area of purplish/maroon discoloured intact skin or a blood-filled blister. Prior to this being seen, pain may be felt and the area can appear firm, mushy, soft, warmer or cooler than the adjacent tissue. It can be difficult to detect in darkly pigmented skin but it may present with a thin blister over a darker wound bed. This stage occurs before the appearance of a grade 1 pressure ulcer. The depth of this is unknown.
- Unstageable: there is full-thickness tissue loss with the ulcer base covered by slough (ranging in colour from yellow, tan, grey to green or brown) and/or eschar (tan, brown, or black) which may or may not have a scab over the top of it. The depth and grade of the pressure ulcer cannot be determined until the wound has been debrided.

Undermining refers to deeper tissue destruction where the skin has separated from the underlying wound margins or granulation tissue. This results in large areas of tissue damage just below the skin, with less skin damage at the surface (Colwell 2015). With continued pressure the destruction continues with larger areas of necrotic tissue and tunnelling.

FACTORS INFLUENCING DEVELOPMENT

- Impaired sensory input: an altered sensory perception resulting in decreased or no experience of pressure

and pain, with no awareness of the need to move, e.g. regional analgesia

- Impaired motor function produces an inability to move despite the presence of pain or pressure, e.g. epidural analgesia
- Immobility, e.g. regional anaesthesia
- Decreased circulation
- Altering levels of consciousness
- Severe/chronic illness
- Previous history of pressure damage
- Oedema reduces blood circulation in affected tissues and impairs clearage of waste products
- Anaemia affects tissue oxygenation
- Poor posture increases the risk of shearing and friction
- Infection increases metabolic demands causing hypoxic tissue to be more susceptible to ischaemic injury (Colwell 2015)
- Obesity may accelerate the development; adipose tissue may have an inadequate blood supply and be more susceptible to ischaemia
- Inadequate dietary intake of protein which is required for all stages of healing, enzyme synthesis, cell multiplication, and collagen and connective tissue synthesis (Dorner et al 2009) and to maintain a positive nitrogen balance (Bowen & Noble 2014)
- Inadequate dietary intake of vitamin C making capillaries more fragile (Bowen & Noble 2014). Vitamin C is also involved in tissue repair and regeneration (Dorner et al 2009)
- Inadequate dietary intake of zinc which is required for collagen formation, protein synthesis and cell proliferation (Dorner et al 2009)
- Dehydration – fluid administration may increase low tissue oxygen and so promote wound healing (Dorner et al 2009)
- Excessive moisture on the skin (e.g. urine, sweat, liquor, wound exudate, faeces) softens the skin and decreases resistance to physical factors such as shearing forces and pressure
- Increasing temperature increases the cells' oxygen requirements, but vasodilation can reduce circulation
- Immunosuppression
- Increasing age resulting in loss of subcutaneous fat and skin elasticity and generalized skin atrophy
- Use of equipment that provides no pressure relief, e.g. lithotomy straps.

PRESSURE AREA CARE

This is undertaken to reduce the incidence of pressure ulcer formation. It involves undertaking an assessment of the risk

Table 53.1 Plymouth maternity pressure sore risk assessment scale

Skin type Visual risk areas		Continence		Special risks	
Dry	1	Incontinent	1	**Neurological deficit**	
Oedamatous	1	Spontaneous rupture of membranes	1	e.g. motor/sensory/paraplegia including epidural analgesia	4–6
Clammy (pyrexia)	1	**Appetite**		Peripheral neuropathy, multiple sclerosis	2–6
Discoloured	2	Poor	1	**Tissue malnutrition**	
Broken area	3	Fluids only	2	Anaemia	2
Mobility		Anorexic	3	Smoking	1
Restless/fidgety	1	**Build/weight for height**		Unstable diabetes	2
Apathetic	2	Above normal	1	Surgery	2–4
Restricted	3	Obese	2		
Inert	4	Below normal	3		
Chairbound	5				

Women: add 2 to total score   Aged 14–49: add 1 to total score
Total score: 10 + At risk   15 + High risk   20 + Very high risk

of pressure ulcers developing, assessing the skin for signs of pressure injury, and taking steps to reduce the effects of pressure.

The ideal risk assessment tool would correctly identify those at risk of developing a pressure ulcer and those who are not at risk and do so consistently with each successive assessment irrespective of who undertakes the assessment (Guy 2012). The NPUAP/EPUAP/PPPIA (2014) advise that although there is no worldwide agreement as to the best approach for conducting a risk assessment, it should be one that is structured. There are a variety of structured risk assessment tools available for use in the clinical setting (e.g. the remodified Norton Scale, Braden Scale, RAPS scale) with varying degrees of success – these are designed for the nursing environment. However, of the tools available, Pancorbo-Hidalgo et al (2006) found the Braden Scale offered the best balance between specificity and sensitivity, the best risk estimate for pressure ulcer formation and concluded that both this scale and the Norton Scale were more accurate than nurses' judgement in predicting the risk of pressure ulcer formation. NICE (2014) recommend a risk assessment is undertaken on all in-patients although Moore & Cowman (2014) suggest there is no reliable evidence to demonstrate that using these tools can reduce the incidence of pressure ulcers. The NPUAP/EPUAP/PPPIA (2014) caution that the risk assessment tool should not be used in isolation when assessing individual risk. Morison & Baker

(2001) have adapted the nursing-based risk assessment tool to create one that is more suitable for use in the maternity setting – the Plymouth maternity pressure sore risk assessment scale, now used in maternity units across the UK (Table 53.1). The scores gained are compatible with the Waterlow risk assessment scale.

Regardless of whether a risk assessment tool is used, it is important to identify individuals at risk of developing pressure ulcers by considering the woman's or the baby's general medical condition, undertaking an assessment of their skin, mobility, moistness (including level of continence), nutrition and pain levels. For those identified as being at increased risk, appropriate interventions should be utilized.

ASSESSMENT OF SKIN INTEGRITY

The midwife, using good (preferably natural) lighting, should inspect the skin and potential pressure ulcer sites. The frequency is determined by individual needs and influenced by the presence of risk factors. For those women who are willing and able, the midwife can show them how to inspect their own skin and that of their baby. The condition of the skin, particularly over the bony prominences (e.g. sacrum, heels, hips, ankles, elbows, occiput) should be assessed initially to determine whether it is intact, dry, oedematous, red, indurated or cracking. The NPUAP/EPUAP/PPPIA (2014) recommend that all skin folds on a bariatric woman should be examined, as pressure injuries can also arise from tissue pressure across the buttocks and other areas of high adipose tissue.

The presence of hyperaemia should be noted when it first appears and steps taken to minimize pressure on the affected area. The area should be rechecked after 1 hour to determine if hyperaemia is still present. The midwife should look for persistent erythema and the absence of blanching on fingertip pressure in lightly pigmented skin by depressing the skin firmly but gently with a clean fingertip. When the pressure is removed the colour of the skin is noted. In darkly pigmented skin the colour should be observed; purplish/bluish discoloration that is darker than the surrounding skin is abnormal. The location, size and colour of the affected area should be recorded; Colwell (2015) recommends using a marker pen to outline the area to make re-assessment easier and more accurate. Photographs or tracing of the pressure ulcer with a ruler by the side of it may be required to enable accurate assessment of how the pressure ulcer is changing.

The skin is also assessed for other signs of potential damage:

- localized heat over the affected area; with further tissue damage this heat is replaced by coolness, a sign of tissue devitalization
- localized oedema: the area will feel spongy and the skin may appear shiny and taut
- localized induration
- break in the skin integrity, e.g. blister, pimple.

Where signs of pressure ulcer formation are seen, it is important the midwife documents:

- the cause (if known)
- site/location
- dimension (measured with a ruler/tape measure)
- grade of pressure ulcer
- amount and type of exudate
- signs of local infection
- wound appearance
- presence of sinus tracts or tunnelling
- pain score
- description of surrounding skin and any odour emitted.

For women at risk of a pressure ulcer or for those with a grade 1 pressure ulcer, a plan should be developed and implemented to prevent any deterioration in the condition (e.g. using high-specification foam mattresses and pressure-relieving devices, positioning and repositioning regimen). It should be fully documented using the approved assessment tool.

PRINCIPLES OF PRESSURE AREA CARE

The aim is to prevent the development of pressure ulcers by:

- identifying those who are either vulnerable to or at an elevated risk of pressure ulcer development and undertake a risk assessment within 8 hours of hospital admission (NPUAP/EPUAP/PPPIA 2014)
- regular assessment of the skin, noting the colour, integrity, presence of blanching, oedema, tissue consistency, pain or heat
- changing the woman's position if non-blanching erythema is noted and re-examining the skin at least 2-hourly until it has resolved (NICE 2014)
- relieving pressure by assisting the woman or baby to change position on a regular basis (Moore & Cowman 2012). NICE (2014) advise this should be at least 6-hourly. A turning chart may be used to record the time of turning and the positions used
- ensuring there is no pressure from tubing, e.g. indwelling urethral catheters, drains
- using high-specification foam mattresses with pressure-relieving properties for women and babies at elevated risk (McInnes et al 2011)
- raising the bedclothes from the body, e.g. bedding should be loosened at the end of the bed or left untucked, or using a bed cradle
- placing a pillow between the knees of the woman when lying laterally to reduce the pressure from the top leg
- encouraging a 30–40° position when side lying rather than 90° to distribute the pressure
- placing a foam cushion underneath the full length of the calves and flexing the knees 5–10° if elevating the heels – check regularly that the leg has not slipped off the pillow onto the bed as this will increase pressure on the heels (Clegg & Palfreyman 2014)
- removing all creases, crumbs, etc. from the bedding as these can exert unnecessary pressure
- increasing circulation by passive or active exercises (see Chapter 54)
- ensuring the woman or the baby is adequately hydrated; a fluid balance chart may be required
- ensuring the diet is well-balanced, referring to the dietician if there are any difficulties
- using appropriate equipment for manual handling to prevent shearing
- good hygiene, especially if incontinent or sweating profusely, using water-based and pH neutral cleansers

after washing and drying the skin with gentle patting motions

- using moisturizers for dry skin areas – not one that contains dimethyl sulfoxide (this is not approved for human use in the US (NPUAP/EPUAP/PPPIA 2014)
- using barrier creams to maintain hydration and protect the skin from excessive moisture which can damage it (NPUAP/EPUAP/PPPIA 2014)
- using soft cotton bedding in preference to synthetic fibres
- using medical grade rather than synthetic sheepskin
- avoiding contact with plastic surfaces
- NOT using ring cushions, water-filled gloves or donut-shaped devices as they move the pressure to another body surface (Bowen & Noble 2014, Hosking 2013)
- NOT massaging reddened skin. To restore the circulation to a deprived area gently rub around the area using circular outward movements (deWit & O'Neill 2014).

If a pressure ulcer is found, it should be cleaned with tap water or normal saline and a suitable dressing applied to facilitate moist wound healing (see Chapter 52) (Bowen & Noble 2014). Areas with necrotic tissue may need debridement, as necrotic tissue is a barrier to tissue healing.

ROLE AND RESPONSIBILITIES OF THE MIDWIFE

These can be summarized as:

- being aware of how pressure ulcers develop
- identifying women and babies who are vulnerable to and at elevated risk of developing pressure ulcers
- undertaking appropriate assessment of the skin to look for evidence of pressure damage
- assisting the woman and baby with measures to reduce pressure ulcer formation
- referral as appropriate
- correct documentation.

SUMMARY

- Pressure ulcers develop as a result of unrelieved pressure.
- The majority of pressure ulcers are avoidable; the midwife needs to be aware of who is vulnerable or at elevated risk and able to assess the skin condition regularly.
- There are a number of measures that can be taken to reduce the likelihood of pressure ulcer formation; the midwife should be familiar with these.

SELF-ASSESSMENT EXERCISES

The answers to the following questions may be found in the text:

1. How do pressure ulcers arise?
2. What factors predispose to pressure ulcer formation?
3. Describe the different stages of pressure ulcer formation and how these are recognized.
4. What is the midwife looking for when an assessment of the skin is undertaken?
5. How can the midwife provide pressure area care to reduce the risks of pressure ulcers forming?

REFERENCES

Antokal, S., Brienza, D., Bryan, N., et al., 2012. Friction induced skin injuries – are they pressure ulcers? A National Pressure Ulcer Advisory Panel White Paper. Available online: <www.npuap.org/resources/white -papers> (accessed 4 January 2015).

Benbow, M., 2008. Pressure ulcer prevention and pressure-relieving surfaces. Br. J. Nurs. 17 (13), 830–835.

Bennett, G., Dealey, C., Posnett, J., 2004. The cost of pressure ulcers in the UK. Age. Ageing 33 (3), 230–235.

Bowen, L., Noble, D., 2014. Skin integrity and wound care. In: Dempsey, J., Hillege, S., Hill, R. (Eds.), Fundamentals of Nursing and Midwifery, second Australian and New Zealand ed. Lippincott Williams & Wilkins Pty Ltd, Sydney, pp. 921–936.

Butcher, M., 2004. Risk of pressure damage for women using maternity services. Nurs. Times 100 (41), 46–47.

Clegg, R., Palfreyman, S., 2014. Elevation devices for the prevention of heel pressure ulcers: a review. Br. J. Nurs. 23 (20), S4–S11.

Colwell, J.C., 2015. Skin integrity and wound care. In: Potter, P.A., Perry, A.G., Stockert, P.A., Hall, A. (Eds.),

Essentials for Nursing Practice, eighth ed. Elsevier, St. Louis, pp. 1060–1110.

deWit, S., O'Neill, P., 2014. Fundamental Concepts and Skills for Nursing, fourth ed. Elsevier, St. Louis.

Dimond, B., 2003. Pressure ulcers and litigation. Nurs. Times 99 (5), 61–63.

Dolan, S., 2011. Risk management. In: Dougherty, L., Lister, S.E. (Eds.), The Royal Marsden Hospital Manual of Clinical Nursing Procedures, eighth ed. Blackwell Publishing, Chichester. (Chapter 4).

Dorner, B., Posthauer, M.E., Thomas, D., 2009. The role of nutrition in pressure ulcer prevention and treatment: National Pressure Ulcer Advisory Panel White Paper. Available online: <www.npuap.org/resources/white-papers> (accessed 4 January 2014).

Guy, H., 2012. Pressure ulcer risk assessment. Nurs. Times 108 (4), 16–20.

Hosking, G., 2013. Skin integrity and wound care. In: Koutoukidis, G., Stainton, K., Hughson, J. (Eds.), Tabbners' Nursing Care, sixth ed.

Elsevier, Chatswood, pp. 613–622 (Chapter 27).

McGinnis, E., Stubbs, N., 2014. Pressure-relieving devices for treating heel pressure injuries. Cochrane Database Syst. Rev. (2), Art. No.:CD005485, doi:10.1002/14651858.CD005485 .pub3.

McInnes, E., Jammali-Blasi, A., Bell-Syer, S.E., et al., 2011. Support surfaces for pressure ulcer prevention. Cochrane Database Syst. Rev. (4), Art. No.: CD001735, doi:10.1002/14651858.CD001735.pub3.

Moore, Z.E.H., Cowman, S., 2012. Repositioning for treating pressure ulcers. Cochrane Database Syst. Rev. (9), Art. No.: CD006898, doi:10 .1002/14651858.CD006898.pub3.

Moore, Z.E.H., Cowman, S., 2014. Risk assessment tools for the prevention of pressure ulcers. Cochrane Database Syst. Rev. (2), Art. No.: CD006471, doi:10.1002/14651858.CD006471 .pub3.

Morison, B., Baker, C., 2001. How to raise awareness of pressure sore

prevention. Br. J. Midwifery 9 (3), 147–150.

NICE (National Institute for Health and Care Excellence), 2014. CG179 Pressure ulcers: prevention and management of pressure ulcers. Available online: <www.nice.org.uk> (accessed 4 January 2014).

NPUAP/EPUAP/PPPIA (National Pressure Ulcer Advisory Panel/European Pressure Ulcer Advisory Panel/Pan Pacific Pressure Injury Alliance), 2014. Prevention and treatment of pressure ulcers: Quick reference guide. Available online: <www.npuap.org/resources/educational-and-clinical-resources/prevention-and-treatment-of-pressure-ulcers-clinical-practice-guideline/> (accessed 4 January 2014).

Pancorbo-Hidalgo, P.L., Garcia-Fernandez, F.P., Lopez-Medina, I.M., Alvarez-Nieto, C., 2006. Risk assessment scales for pressure ulcer prevention: a systematic review. J. Adv. Nurs. 54 (1), 94–110.

Chapter 54

Principles of restricted mobility management: prevention of venous thromboembolism

LEARNING OUTCOMES

Having read this chapter, the reader should be able to:

- discuss the physiological changes that predispose the pregnant women to venous thromboembolism formation
- identify risk factors for VTE in childbearing women
- describe the leg and breathing exercises that can be undertaken during periods of immobility
- discuss how graduated compression stockings are correctly applied and worn
- discuss the use and application of sequential compression devices.

Restricted mobility can influence the development of a venous thromboembolism (VTE) which affects morbidity and mortality. During 2010–2012 VTE was the highest direct cause of maternal mortality in the UK with 26 women dying during 2010–2012 (Knight et al 2014) – almost a 50% increase in numbers since 2006–2008. The majority of deaths were from pulmonary embolism (PE), with two due to cerebral vein thrombosis. This chapter focuses on the principles of VTE prevention, discussing the physiological changes that occur during pregnancy and the risk factors which increase the likelihood of VTE developing and prophylactic measures that can be used – exercises, graduated compression stockings (GCS) and sequential compression devices.

VENOUS THROMBOEMBOLISM

A thrombosis (clot) forms in response to stasis of blood flow, altered coagulation status and/or damage to the blood vessel walls (known as Virchow's triad), all of which are present at some point during pregnancy, labour and the postnatal period. Pregnancy is a state of hypercoagulability; there is a progressive change in the balance between anticoagulant and prothrombotic factors, an increase in fibrin deposition and decreased fibrinolysis, which create a procoagulant state (Arya 2011, Blackburn 2013). Blood flow in the lower limbs is reduced by up to 50% and venous distension during pregnancy can result in vessel wall damage, with further trauma occurring at delivery (Arya 2011). The changes to the coagulation factors begin with conception and may not return to their prepregnancy levels until 8 weeks following delivery (James 2011). The clot that forms is referred to as a deep vein thrombosis (DVT). If a part of the DVT breaks away, it is carried in the circulation to the major organs where it may lodge in a smaller vein causing ischaemia and may be referred to as an embolism.

During pregnancy the risk of a DVT increases four- to sixfold (Arya et al 2011, RCOG 2015) with the risk of a PE being 1.3 per 1000 pregnancies (RCOG 2015). While DVTs are often symptomatic, Meyer (2010) suggests the rates of asymptomatic DVT following surgery range from 10% for minor surgery, e.g. repair of third-degree tear, to 10–40% for major surgery, e.g. caesarean section. It is more common for a DVT to form in the left leg during pregnancy because of the increased pressure from the gravid uterus on the left common iliac vein but postnatally it can occur in either leg (Virkus et al 2013). Many antenatal VTEs occur during the first trimester (RCOG 2015), although Chan et al (2012) consider the incidence does not vary much across the trimesters. The Royal College of Obstetricians and Gynaecologists (RCOG 2015) advise the first 3 weeks postpartum is the highest risk period for VTE and PE formation, with the risk increased 22-fold.

COMPLICATIONS OF DVT

The most serious complication is death; 3.5% of women who develop a PE during pregnancy through to the puerperium will die (RCOG 2015). Approximately 89% of the women who died during 2006–2008 had risk factors and care was substandard for 56% of women (Drife 2011). Thus it is important to identify women who are at high risk of VTE and manage them appropriately.

Post-thrombotic syndrome (PTS) is thought to occur in 20–50% of DVT events (Wik et al 2012). This develops from valve incompetence causing venous stasis resulting in chronic swelling and discomfort in the affected limb, with some limbs becoming ulcerated (Roswell & Law 2011). The use of GCS worn for 2 years following the DVT can reduce the incidence of PTS by 50% (Wik et al 2012).

RISK FACTORS

The RCOG (2015) present a very comprehensible list of risk factors for VTE:

Pre-existing factors

- Previous venous thromboembolism
- Thrombophilia inherited, e.g. factor V Leiden, or acquired, e.g. persistent lupus anticoagulant
- Medical comorbidities, e.g. sickle cell disease
- Age >35 years
- Obesity – BMI >30
- Parity ≥3
- Smoking
- Gross varicose veins (symptomatic or above knee or with associated phlebitis, oedema/skin changes)
- Paraplegia.

Obstetric factors

- Multiple pregnancy
- Assisted reproductive therapy
- Pre-eclampsia
- Caesarean section
- Prolonged labour
- Mid-cavity rotational operative delivery
- Postpartum haemorrhage (PPH) (>1 L) requiring transfusion.

New-onset/transient factors

- Surgical procedure in pregnancy or puerperium, e.g. evacuation of retained products of conception (ERPC), appendicectomy.

Potentially reversible factors

- Hyperemesis, dehydration
- Ovarian hyperstimulation syndrome

- Admission or immobility (≥3 days' bed rest), e.g. symphysis pubis dysfunction restricting mobility
- Systemic infection (requiring antibiotics or admission to hospital), e.g. pyelonephritis, postpartum wound infection
- Long-distance travel (>4 hours).

Additionally, Roswell & Law (2011) advise dehydration can also predispose women to VTE formation and Arya (2011) suggests women of black race are at increased risk.

RISK ASSESSMENT

The RCOG (2015) recommend that all women have a documented assessment of risk factors for VTE in early pregnancy or, if possible, before pregnancy (Table 54.1). They advise the assessment should be repeated each time the woman is admitted to hospital or, if she develops other problems, in labour and following delivery, as her risk status may have changed (RCOG 2015). The Department of Health (2010) produced a national guideline for the National Health Service (NHS) Trusts to use for all patients on admission to hospital but do not include pregnancy-specific risk factors. The risk assessment should identify women at increased risk of developing a VTE and the RCOG (2015) recommend prophylactic treatment based on the degree of risk. However Bennett-Day (2011) argues the amount of high-grade evidence around the unique risk factors associated with VTE and the benefit of thromboprophylaxis is limited. Thus many women will be advised to have prophylactic treatment if they deliver in hospital, and Bennett-Day (2011) questions the value of this. The reader is advised to read her article for further detail.

PREVENTING VTE FORMATION

While some factors, e.g. age, are unchangeable, other factors may be modifiable or preventable. For example, advice on smoking cessation and weight reduction can be given where appropriate. Dehydration should be prevented and immobilization kept to a minimum. Encouraging women to remain active is important; however, for some women, e.g. those with severe pelvic girdle pain, postoperative immobility may be unavoidable; thus specific exercises, both passive and active, should be encouraged to assist with venous blood flow. An obstetric physiotherapist can assist with these, but the midwife is also in a good position to support and encourage these exercises.

EXERCISES

Both passive and active exercises can be undertaken and involve moving the muscles and joints through their normal range of motion to promote circulation. They also assist in maintaining and improving muscle tone and can prevent joint contracture developing with long-term immobility. Tritak (2015) advises they can also prevent thrombophlebitis developing and refers to them as 'anti-embolic' exercises, suggesting they should be undertaken each hour the woman is awake.

Passive exercises are rarely needed and are undertaken when the woman cannot do them herself, e.g. if she is unconscious. Active exercises are undertaken by the woman until she is fully ambulatory:

- Ankle pumps: the woman should be sitting or lying comfortably with straight knees and alternate dorsiflexion and plantar flexion by flexing her feet towards her body then extending them towards the bed (Tritak 2015). This can be done at least 10 times (Fig. 54.1).
- Foot circles: the woman should be sitting or lying comfortably with straight knees, then circle her ankles by moving her feet in a clockwise direction at least 10 times, then an anticlockwise direction for 10 times, keeping her hips and knees still (Fig. 54.2).
- Leg tightening: the woman should sit or lie on the bed with straight legs and pull her toes towards her legs pressing the back of her knees down towards the bed, holding the position for 4 seconds, then relaxing. This should be repeated five times.

Deep breathing exercises

Venous return is improved with each deep breath taken but additionally the secretions within the lungs can be removed preventing hypostatic pneumonia that can occur with decreased activity (deWit & O'Neill 2014). It is particularly useful following a general anaesthetic.

Two to three deep breaths should be taken while sitting up; this can be repeated often. The expiration of each breath should be followed by a short forced expiration, referred to as 'huffing', to loosen secretions.

Anticoagulation

Following the risk assessment, women may be advised to commence low molecular weight heparin prophylactically (RCOG 2015). This is a subcutaneous injection that is administered once or sometimes twice a day, usually into the abdomen (see Chapter 20). The woman should be shown how to self-administer it if she will require it at

Table 54.1 Risk assessment for venous thromboembolism (VTE) (RCOG 2015)

Pre-existing risk factors	Tick	Score
Previous VTE (excluding single event related to major surgery)		4
Previous VTE – provoked by major surgery		3
Known thrombophilia (high risk)		3
Medical comorbidities, e.g. sickle cell disease, current intravenous drug user		3
Family history of VTE – unprovoked or estrogen related		1
Known thrombophilia (low risk, no VTE)		1
Age (>35 years)		1
Obesity		1/2*
Parity ≥3		1
Smoker		1
Gross varicose veins		1
Obstetric risk factors		
Pre-eclampsia (current pregnancy)		1
In vitro fertilization/assisted reproductive technology use first trimester		1
Multiple pregnancy		1
Caesarean section in labour		2
Elective caesarean section		1
Mid-cavity or rotational forceps		1
Prolonged labour (>24 hours)		1
Postpartum haemorrhage (>1 L or transfusion)		1
Preterm birth (current pregnancy)		1
Stillbirth (current pregnancy)		1
Transient risk factors		
Surgical procedure in pregnancy or ≤6 weeks postpartum excluding perineal repair post-delivery		3
Hyperemesis		3
Ovarian hyperstimulation syndrome (first trimester)		4
Current systemic infection		1
Immobility/dehydration		1
TOTAL		
If total score ≥4 antenatally – consider thromboprophylaxis from first trimester		
If total score ≥3 antenatally – consider thromboprophylaxis from second trimester		
If total score ≥2 postnatally – consider thromboprophylaxis for at least 10 days		
If admitted to hospital antenatally, prolonged admission (≥3 days) or readmission during the puerperium – consider thromboprophylaxis		
*Score 1 for body mass index (BMI) >30 kg/m²; 2 for BMI >40 kg/m² (BMI based on booking weight)		

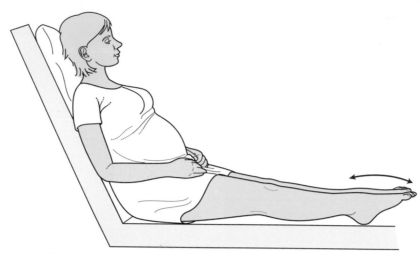

Figure 54.1 Foot exercises – flexing the feet.

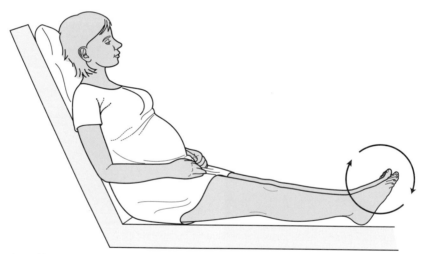

Figure 54.2 Circling the ankles.

home. As with any anticoagulation therapy, the woman should be alert to signs of haemorrhage and know who to contact if this occurs.

Graduated compression stockings

GCS are used as a passive mechanism to reduce VTE formation (Roswell & Law 2011) and may be recommended as an adjunct to anticoagulation therapy. Caprini (2010) suggests that while studies have demonstrated the effectiveness of GCS in preventing DVT compared to a placebo, there is no evidence they reduce the incidence of pulmonary embolism.

GCS are made of 82% polyamide and 18% elastane, are latex-free, and come as knee- or thigh-length stockings with an open toe. Although they come in a variety of colours, the most commonly used colour in hospitals is white. They work by improving venous emptying, increasing blood flow, and decreasing the cross-sectional area of the limb, thus reducing oedema, counteracting stasis and high venous pressure, and restoring valve function (Miller 2011, Sajid et al 2012). GCS deliver a gradient of compression across the limb with highest pressure, 18 mmHg, exerted at the ankle; 14 mmHg at the mid-calf; and the lowest pressure, 8 mmHg, at the thigh. They are contraindicated with gross oedema (Miller 2011).

Thigh-length GCS distribute the mechanical effect over a higher proportion of the leg which should offer a potential advantage over knee-length GCS, but the evidence is inconclusive as to which are more effective (Caprini 2010, Sajid et al 2012). However, thigh-length GCS are harder to apply and more likely to become blood-stained or rolled down, thereby decreasing compliance. If the GCS are rolled down, there is an increased risk of a pressure ulcer occurring and Sajid et al (2012) caution that rolling down thigh-length GCS may increase the risk of VTE formation. The RCOG (2015) suggest that while properly fitting thigh-length GCS may be advocated for the pregnant woman, knee-length GCS should be considered if the thigh-length GCS are ill fitting or there is poor compliance.

It is important that the GCS are fitted correctly, which involves measuring the woman's legs. Ohayon et al (2013) caution that when GCS are too tight, skin breakdown occurs. If they are too loose, they will not apply the correct pressure and will be ineffective. Ideally the legs should be measured in the morning before the woman has stood up (which is often difficult to achieve). Bowen & Noble (2014) recommend the woman should lay on the bed with her legs extended for at least 15 minutes if she has been sitting down. The leg measurements should also be reviewed on a regular basis as changes may occur (e.g. occurrence or disappearance of oedema). The measurements should be documented in the woman's records, along with the size of stockings issued.

Two measurements are required for knee-length stockings (Fig. 54.3A):

1. from the base of the heel to the popliteal fold (bend of the knee)
2. the widest part of the calf.

For thigh-length stockings, three measurements are necessary (Fig. 54.3B):

1. around the widest part of the thigh
2. the widest part of the calf
3. from the base of the heel to the gluteal fold.

If the legs measure differently, two different size stockings should be used. If the thigh circumference is >91.5 cm (36 inches) or the calf circumference is outside of the specified range recommended for thigh-length GCS, knee-length GCS should be used.

Applying and wearing GCS

GCS should be applied to ensure they are in the correct position so no excess pressure is applied and there are no wrinkles. Knee-length GCS should reach 2–5 cm below the patella and thigh-length GCS should be 2–7 cm below the gluteal fold (Bowen & Noble 2014). When reapplying they should be put on before getting out of bed. They may be

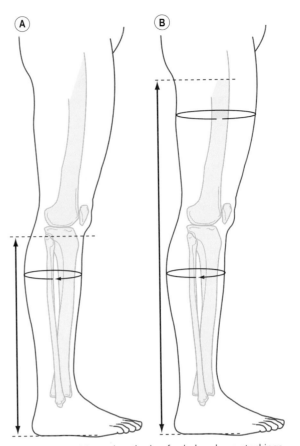

Figure 54.3 A, Measuring the leg for below-knee stockings – the widest part of the calf and the distance from base of heel to just below the knee. **B,** Measuring the leg for full-length stockings – the widest part of the calf, the widest part of the thigh, and the distance from the base of the heel to the gluteal fold.

difficult to put on, moisturizing the legs may assist with this. Alternatively the bag containing the GCS can be placed over the woman's foot and the stocking applied over this. Once the stocking is in place the bag can be removed through the toe opening. Wearing examination or rubber gloves may make it easier to grip the stocking.

The stockings should be removed once a day and the legs examined to ensure there is no deterioration in the skin condition. They can be replaced when dirty to increase compliance and washed according to the manufacturer's instructions.

GCS work when the legs are horizontal as the pressure gradient is interfered with when the legs are not straight. If the woman is sitting out of bed she should be advised to elevate her legs (Miller 2011). The woman should be advised as to how long she should wear GCS, which is often until the woman is fully ambulant to 2 years if a DVT is diagnosed.

PROCEDURE: applying graduated compression stockings

- Discuss the reason for applying GCS and gain consent.
- Wash and dry hands.
- Measure the legs and fetch the correct size of GCS.
- Use handrub and allow to dry.
- Ensure privacy and ask the woman to lie down and remove any clothing around her legs.
- Inspect the condition of the skin on the legs for a baseline and ensure the legs are dry.
- Remove the GCS from their bag.
- Insert one hand inside the stocking and take hold of the seamed heel.
- Holding onto the heel, turn the stocking inside out until the heel pocket is seen.
- Place the stocking over the foot and heel, ensuring the heel is in the centre of the pocket and the toes do not protrude through the toe opening.
- Pull the stocking slowly up the leg, a few centimetres at a time until the stocking is fully in place.
- Smooth out any wrinkles.
- Repeat with the second stocking to the other leg.
- Advise the woman on the use of GCS.
- Dispose of rubbish.
- Wash and dry hands.
- Document leg measurements, condition of skin, size of GCS applied and advice given to the woman.

SEQUENTIAL COMPRESSION DEVICES

Sequential compression devices (SCDs) comprise an extremity sleeve which covers the entire leg or a calf boot extending from the foot to the knee, connecting tubes and an air pump and may be intermittent or sequential. The extremity sleeve contains air chambers that are inflated to a preselected pressure then deflated. Intermittent SCDs alternate inflation and deflation from one leg to the other according to preset times whereas sequential SCDs can inflate legs together or separately but are designed to move the pressure up the leg in increments (Hill 2014). Caprini (2010) recommends inflation pressures of 35–55 mmHg, with a compression cycle of 10–35 seconds and a deflation period of 1 minute to allow the leg/foot veins to refill with blood.

SCDs reduce VTE formation by enhancing blood flow in the lower limbs and stimulating the fibrinolytic system which may help modulate hypercoagulability (Arabi et al 2013, Caprini 2010).

These are often applied in the theatre or in the high dependency/intensive care unit but can also be used for women at high risk of VTE formation who have an epidural during labour. Within the US it is recommended that these are used for all women having a caesarean section, as this is the time when most emboli develop (Clarke 2015). Arabi et al (2013) found a higher reduction in the incidence of VTE when SCDs were used in critically ill patients compared with GCS. Clarke et al (2011) advise only devices marked CE should be used within the UK. It is unclear for how long the SCD should be worn, with recommendations varying from until 'fully ambulant' to 'discharge' (Brady et al 2015).

PROCEDURE: applying a sequential compression device

- Discuss the reason for applying the SCD and gain consent.
- Gather and assemble equipment:
  - SCD insufflator with air hoses attached
  - Adjustable Velcro compression stockings/SCD sleeve.
- Wash and dry hands.
- Ensure privacy and ask the woman to lie down and remove any clothing around her legs.
- Inspect the condition of the skin on the legs for a baseline and ensure the legs are dry.
- Place the SCD sleeve under the woman's leg using the position indicated on the inner lining of the sleeve:
  - the back of the ankle should line up with the ankle position indicated
  - the back of the knee lines up with the popliteal opening.
- Wrap the SCD sleeve around the woman's legs and secure with the Velcro fastening.
- Check the SCD sleeve tightness by placing the pads of two fingertips side-by-side between the woman's leg (by her ankle) and the SCD sleeve.
- Attach the SCD sleeve to the air insufflator and turn on the device.
- Remain with the woman for one full cycle to ensure the sleeves are comfortable and working correctly.
- Assist the woman into a comfortable position.
- Wash and dry hands.
- Document condition of skin, SCD applied and advice given to the woman.

ROLE AND RESPONSIBILITIES OF THE MIDWIFE

These can be summarized as:

- up-to-date knowledge regarding the aetiology of VTE and risk factors pertinent to the pregnant woman
- undertaking a risk assessment at booking, at each hospital admission including labour, following delivery and if the clinical condition changes and referral as necessary
- ensuring the woman does not become dehydrated
- encouraging active exercises for women with reduced mobility
- undertaking competent clinical care, particularly in relation to anticoagulation prophylaxis, application of graduated compression stockings and sequential compression devices
- education of the woman
- contemporaneous documentation.

SUMMARY

- Thromboembolism remains a major cause of maternal mortality; pregnancy alone is a risk factor, other risks include previous VTE, reduced mobility, smoking and obesity.
- Gentle foot and leg exercises, deep breathing, anticoagulation prophylaxis, and the use of graduated compression stockings or sequential compression devices can all contribute to reducing the risk of VTE.
- Immobility and dehydration should be avoided whenever possible.
- Graduated compression stockings must be fitted and worn correctly to be effective.

SELF-ASSESSMENT EXERCISES

The answers to the following questions may be found in the text:

1. Identify the women most at risk of VTE.
2. Why is pregnancy a time of increased risk for VTE formation?
3. What measures can be taken to promote venous circulation?
4. How would the midwife ensure that a knee-length graduated compression stocking is the correct size?
5. How would you fit a sequential compression device?
6. What are the role and responsibilities of the midwife in relation to the prevention of thromboembolism in a woman with restricted mobility?

REFERENCES

Arabi, Y.M., Khedr, M., Dara, S.I., et al., 2013. Use of intermittent pneumatic devices and not graduated compression stockings associated with lower incident of venous thromboembolism in critically ill patients: a multiple propensity scores adjusted analysis. Chest 144 (1), 152–159.

Arya, R., 2011. How I manage venous thromboembolism in pregnancy. Br. J. Haematol. 153, 698–708.

Bennett-Day, S., 2011. Universal risk assessments to guide use of thromboprophylaxis. Br. J. Midwifery 19 (2), 778–785.

Blackburn, S., 2013. Maternal, Fetal and Neonatal Physiology: A Clinical Perspective, fourth ed. Saunders, St. Louis, pp. 228–229.

Bowen, L., Noble, D., 2014. Hygiene. In: Dempsey, J., Hillege, S., Hill, R. (Eds.), Fundamentals of Nursing and Midwifery 2nd Australian and New Zealand Edn. Lippincott Williams & Wilkins, Sydney, pp. 878–880.

Brady, M.A., Carroll, A.W., Cheang, K.I., et al., 2015. Sequential compression device compliance in postoperative obstetrics and gynecology patients. Obst. & Gynecol. 125 (1), 19–25.

Caprini, J.A., 2010. Mechanical methods for thrombosis prophylaxis. Clin. Appl. Thromb. Hemost. 16 (6), 668–673.

Chan, N., Merriman, E., Hyder, S., et al., 2012. How do we manage venous thromboembolism in pregnancy? A retrospective review of the practice of diagnosing and managing pregnancy-related venous thromboembolism at two major hospitals in Australia and New Zealand. Int. Med. J. 42 (10), 1104–1112.

Clarke, R., Grewal, J.K., Sholtes, S., Waller, J., 2011. Perioperative care. In: Dougherty, L., Lister, S. (Eds.), The

Royal Marsden Hospital Manual of Clinical Nursing Procedures, eighth ed. John Wiley & Sons, Chichester, p. 1043 (Chapter 17).

Clarke, S.L., 2015. Peripartum venous thromboprophylaxis. Where do we go from here? Obstet. & Gynecol. 125 (1), 16–18.

Department of Health, 2010. Risk assessment for Venous thromboembolism (VTE). Available online: <http://www.vteprevention-nhsengland.org.uk/images/downloads/National%20Risk%20Assessment%20Tool.pdf> (accessed 22 February 2015).

deWit, S.C., O'Neill, P., 2014. Fundamental Concepts and Skills for Nursing, fourth ed. Elsevier, St. Louis.

Drife, J., 2011. Thrombosis and thromboembolism. In: Centre for Maternal and Child Enquiries (CMACE). Saving Mothers' Lives: reviewing maternal deaths to make motherhood safer: 2006–08. The Eighth Report on Confidential Enquiries into Maternal Deaths in the United Kingdom. Br. J. Obstet. & Gynaecol. 118 (Suppl. 1), 57–65.

Hill, R., 2014. Perioperative care. In: Dempsey, J., Hillege, S., Hill, R. (Eds.), Fundamentals of Nursing and Midwifery 2nd Australian and New Zealand Edn. Lippincott, Williams & Wilkins, Sydney, pp. 878–880 (Chapter 36).

James, A., 2011. Practice bulletin no. 123: thromboembolism in pregnancy. Obstet. & Gynecol. 118 (3), 718–729.

Knight, M., Nair, M., Shah, A., et al., on behalf of the MBRRACE-UK, 2014. Maternal Mortality and Morbidity in the UK 2009–12: Surveillance and Epidemiology. In: Knight, M., Kenyon, S., Brocklehurst, P., et al., on behalf of MBRRACE-UK, (Eds.), Saving Lives, Improving Mothers' Care – Lessons Learned to Inform Future Maternity care from the UK and Ireland Confidential Enquiries into Maternal Deaths and Morbidity 2009–12. National Perinatal Epidemiology Unit, Oxford, pp. 9–26.

Meyer, S., 2010. Leg compression and pharmacologic prophylaxis for venous thromboembolism prevention in high-risk patients. Am. Fam. Physician 81 (3), 284–285.

Miller, J.A., 2011. Use and wear of anti-embolism stockings: a clinical audit of surgical patients. Int. Wound J. 8 (10), 74–83.

Ohayon, R., Rose, R., Ebert, K., et al., 2013. Incidence of incorrectly sized graduated compression stockings and lower leg irregularities in postoperative orthopedic patients. Medsurg. Nurs. 22 (6), 370–374.

Roswell, H., Law, C., 2011. Reducing patients' risk of venous thromboembolism. Am. Fam. Physician 81 (3), 284–285.

RCOG (Royal College of Obstetricians & Gynaecologists), 2015. Reducing the risk of venous thromboembolism during pregnancy and the puerperium. Green-Top Guideline No. 37a. Available online: <https://www.rcog.org.uk/en/guidelines-research-services/guidelines/gtg37a/> (accessed 26 June 2015).

Sajid, M.S., Desai, M., Morris, R.W., Hamilton, G., 2012. Knee length versus thigh length graduated compression stocking for prevention of deep vein thrombosis in postoperative surgical patients. Cochrane Database Syst. Rev. (5), Art. No.: CD007162. doi:10.1002/14651858.CD007162.pub2.

Tritak, A., 2015. Immobility. In: Potter, P.A., Perry, A.G., Stockert, P.A., Hall, A. (Eds.), Essentials for Nursing Practice, eighth ed. Elsevier, St. Louis, pp. 1042–1055 (Chapter 36).

Virkus, R.A., Løkkegaard, E.C.L., Lidegaard, Ø., et al., 2013. Venous thromboembolism in pregnancy and the puerperal period: a study of 1210 events. Acta Obstet. Gynecol. Scand. 92 (10), 1135–1142.

Wik, H.S., Jacobsen, A.F., Sandvik, L., Sandst, P.M., 2012. Prevalence and predictors for post-thrombotic syndrome 3 to 16 years after pregnancy-related venous thrombosis: a population-based, cross-sectional, case-control survey. J. Thromb. Haemost. 10 (5), 840–847.

Chapter 55

Principles of cardiopulmonary resuscitation: maternal resuscitation

LEARNING OUTCOMES

Having read this chapter, the reader should be able to:

- anticipate and recognize maternal collapse
- discuss the modifications necessary for resuscitation of a pregnant woman
- recognize the importance of prompt, effective cardiac compressions
- describe the equipment and how it is used
- demonstrate maternal resuscitation on a manikin.

This chapter focuses on maternal resuscitation and basic life support techniques. While maternal collapse is a rare event, associated with increased morbidity and mortality for the woman and her baby, the frequency of cardiac arrest in pregnancy is increasing (Vanden Hoek et al 2010). McDonnell (2009) suggests that cardiac arrest has an incidence of 1:30,000 during pregnancy. However the Royal College of Obstetricians and Gynaecologists (RCOG) suggest the true rate of maternal collapse lies somewhere between 0.14 and 6 per 1000 births (RCOG 2011). The midwife rarely undertakes cardiopulmonary resuscitation (CPR); thus it is vital the midwife undertakes regular training and practice to ensure she can do this effectively and efficiently when the need arises and can modify the CPR to accommodate the particular needs of the collapsed pregnant woman. There are two 'patients' involved in the resuscitation of a pregnant woman and the best chance for the baby to survive is afforded by maternal survival (Vanden Hoek et al 2010).

Cardiac arrest occurs when the heart stops contracting effectively, e.g. ventricular fibrillation, or at all (asystole). As a result, breathing will stop, although agonal breathing may be seen before cessation of respiration. Travers et al (2010) suggest that there is a substantially better outcome when cardiac arrest is due to ineffective contraction of the heart rather than no contraction.

The Chain of Survival refers to the coordinated set of actions linking the victim of a sudden cardiac arrest with survival. These are specifically:

- early recognition of impending or actual collapse and call for help to initiate the emergency response system
- early CPR – with emphasis on cardiac compression
- early defibrillation

- effective advanced life support
- post-resuscitation care (Travers et al 2010).

When CPR is undertaken immediately, the likelihood of survival for someone with an out-of-hospital cardiac arrest can double or triple (Cha et al 2013, Chalkias et al 2013, Iwami et al 2012). Where cardiac compressions and defibrillation occur within 3–5 minutes of collapse, survival rates are 49–75% (Nolan et al 2010). Each minute that CPR is delayed, the likelihood of survival can decrease by approximately 10% (Yang et al 2014) and for each minute defibrillation is delayed the chances of surviving to discharge from hospital are reduced by 10–12% (Nolan et al 2010). Dellimore & Scheffer (2012) suggest post-CPR survival rates can be extremely low which they partly attribute to the poor quality of compressions – depth, rate and length.

ANTICIPATION OF COLLAPSE

The majority of pregnant women are healthy and at low risk of cardiac arrest but there is the potential for complications from childbearing which may be life threatening. It may be possible to anticipate collapse and be proactive to prevent it occurring. These include:

- massive obstetric haemorrhage
- thromboembolism
- anaphylactoid syndrome (amniotic fluid embolism)
- cardiac disease
- severe sepsis
- drug toxicity or overdose
- eclampsia
- intracranial haemorrhage
- anaphylaxis
- other causes, e.g. airway obstruction (RCOG 2011).

When a woman is unwell it is important she is observed and managed appropriately so that any deterioration in her condition is recognized early and treated promptly. The use of the modified early obstetric scoring chart will assist with this (p. 66) (RCOG 2011).

EQUIPMENT

In the hospital environment, resuscitation equipment should be readily available and is usually kept together in a resuscitation trolley that can be taken to the place where resuscitation is occurring. The trolley will be standardized across the hospital, with equipment always in the same place to make it easier for the resuscitation team to access what they need quickly. It is therefore important that equipment is not added, removed or rearranged. Midwives attending homebirths usually have equipment available for providing oxygen and ventilation breaths; the paramedic crew will bring other equipment as needed, e.g. defibrillator. Equipment and drugs should be checked regularly to ensure they are working effectively and are in date.

The Resuscitation Council (UK) (2013a) have a list of equipment that should be immediately available (within first few minutes of cardiorespiratory arrest) or accessible (available for prompt use when the need is determined by the resuscitation team) within the acute care hospital setting.

Immediate availability

- Oxygen mask with reservoir
- Self-inflating bag with reservoir
- Clear face masks, sizes 3, 4, 5
- Oropharyngeal airways, sizes 2, 3, 4
- Nasopharyngeal airways (and lubrication), sizes 6, 7
- Portable suction with Yankauer sucker and soft suction catheters
- Gloves, aprons, eye protection
- Sharps container and clinical waste bag.

Accessible

- Clock/timer
- Nasogastric tube
- Large scissors
- 70% alcohol/2% chlorhexidine wipes
- Blood sample tubes
- Intravenous (I.V.) extension set and connectors, ports, and caps
- Pressure bags for infusion
- Blood gas syringes
- Blood gas analyzer and testing strips
- Drug labels
- Manual handling equipment
- CPR arrest record forms for patient records, audit forms and do-not-attempt-CPR (DNACPR) forms
- Access to algorithms and emergency drug doses.

There should also be an emergency drug box which may contain drugs required for anaphylaxis management (p. 151):

- Adenosine 6 mg ×5
- Atropine 1 mg ×3
- Adrenaline 1 mg (=10 mL 1 : 10 000) prefilled syringe
- Amiodarone 300 mg ×1 prefilled syringe
- Calcium chloride or calcium chloride 10 mL 10% ×1
- Chlorphenamine 10 mg ×2
- Hydrocortisone 100 mg ×2
- I.V. glucose

- 20% lipid emulsion 500 mL
- Lidocaine 100 mg ×1
- Magnesium sulphate 2G (8 mmol)
- Midazolam 5 mg in 5 mL ×1
- Naloxone 400 mcg ×5
- Potassium chloride
- Sodium bicarbonate 8.4% or 1.26%.

INITIAL ASSESSMENT

Collapse may be witnessed or unwitnessed. With an unwitnessed collapse, resuscitation may be less successful because of the delay in commencing cardiac compressions. The woman may be seen to look unwell, e.g. pale, cyanosed and clammy, and appear to be unmoving. It is important to ensure it is safe to approach the collapsed woman. A quick visual assessment of the area around the woman should be undertaken for hazards such as a wet floor or dangling wires. Personal safety should be considered if there is a lot of body fluids around or the woman is in isolation and personal protective equipment donned as necessary (p. 79).

Assessing responsiveness

The midwife should approach the woman from the side and assess her responsiveness by gently shaking her shoulders (unless a neck or back injury is suspected) and talking loudly to her. Asking her a question such as 'Are you all right?' will usually rouse the woman if she is not unconscious. Bearing in mind that the woman may be hard of hearing in one ear, the midwife should direct her talking to both ears.

Calling for help

If there is no response, help should be sought immediately. In a hospital setting this can be through use of the emergency buzzer or calling for help. It is important to call for the resuscitation team if the hospital has one, using the standard emergency number 2222 (National Patient Safety Agency 2004). The call should include the name of the ward/clinical area and specific location, e.g. first side room. If the ward is locked, a staff member should be positioned at the doors ready to let the team in as they arrive. The Resuscitation Council (UK) (2013b) advise the resuscitation team should be activated within 30 seconds of the call for help. In the community setting a paramedic team should be summoned using the 999 call. If the address is difficult to find, use a family member, if possible, to stand at the driveway to flag down the ambulance. The front door should be left unlocked to enable the paramedic team to enter quickly.

If there is no emergency buzzer or phone available to call for help, the midwife should send someone to call for help or if she is on her own, she will need to leave the woman, make the emergency call or ring the emergency buzzer and then return and continue with the resuscitation. CPR then continues using the ABCD approach – airway, breathing, circulation and defibrillation.

Airway

According to Madams (2008) the tongue is the main airway obstruction in collapsed or unconscious women during the intrapartum period. Opening the airway may be all that is needed to enable the woman to resume breathing. Ideally the woman should be turned onto her back and her airway opened using a head tilt and chin lift so her head is slightly extended and her tongue prevented from falling back and obstructing the airway. This is achieved by placing a hand on the woman's forehead and gently tilting her head back, then using fingertips under her chin to tilt her chin upwards. Occasionally a jaw thrust is required to maintain the open airway during ventilation (Madams 2008) or when a cervical spine injury is suspected (Soar & Davies 2010). The jaw thrust is undertaken with both hands by placing two or three fingers under the mandible and one at the angle of the jaw to push and lift the jaw forwards. Pressure on the soft tissue should be avoided as this can cause oedema which can occlude the airway. Alternatively an oropharyngeal airway can be used if it becomes difficult to maintain an open airway.

An oropharyngeal airway has three parts: flange, body and tip. The flange is the piece that protrudes from the mouth and rests against the lips preventing the airway from moving further into the pharynx once it is inserted. The body is curved and follows the curve of the roof of the mouth, resting on top the tongue. The distal end is the tip that sits at the base of the tongue.

It is important to use the correct size of airway and this is assessed either by holding the flange of the airway against the side of the woman's mouth, with the airway held horizontally so that the curved part of the airway curves around the woman's jaw. It should end at the bottom of her earlobe. Alternatively the flange is placed against the midpoint of the woman's lips (philtrum), with the airway finishing at the angle of the jaw (more difficult in obese people). Large adults generally require a size 5–6, medium adults size 4–5, and small adults size 3–4.

Prior to inserting the airway, tilt the woman's head backwards and hold the airway with the curve up, i.e. the opposite way up to its final position within the oropharynx. This will allow the curved body to depress the tongue, preventing it from being pushed backwards. The airway is inserted following the curve of the woman's airway. As it reaches the junction of the hard and soft palates, the airway should be rotated 180° into the correct position, with the curve down, while continuing to move it further into the mouth. When the airway is lying in the oropharynx, the flange should sit between the woman's teeth. The tilted, neutral head position should be maintained and chin support given as required. It is important to assess the position of the airway intermittently to ensure it has not dislodged.

Any debris seen in the mouth should be removed with a wide-bore suction catheter. It is not advisable to undertake a finger sweep as the woman may bite the fingers and there is a small risk of cross-infection from body fluids. Loose dentures should be replaced in the mouth, as they help to maintain the shape of the jaw and chin tilt/jaw thrust. If the dentures are poorly fitting and keep coming loose, they may need to be removed.

Breathing

No more than 10 seconds should be taken to assess if the woman is breathing. The midwife will do this by bringing her head close to the woman's face and chest and looking for chest rise, listening for breath sounds and feeling for breath on her cheeks. When no breathing is noted, cardiac arrest is assumed as the cause and CPR commenced immediately. Abnormal breathing should be noted as agonal breathing/gasping is present during the first minute after a sudden cardiac arrest in 40% of cases (Koster et al 2010) and so should not prevent initiation of cardiac compressions (Sayre et al 2010). If the woman is not breathing, there is no need to determine whether a pulse is present, as this is often unreliable (Travers et al 2010).

'Rescue breaths' are not given before the commencement of cardiac compressions, as this will delay the initiation of compressions further and it is vitally important that compressions begin as soon as possible. If the cardiac arrest is non-asphyxial in nature, there will be a high oxygen content in the blood initially, rendering ventilation less important than compressions (Handley & Colquhoun 2010).

Circulation

Cardiac compressions increase the chance of survival by maintaining the blood supply to the heart and brain (Travers et al 2010). This is achieved only if there is adequate perfusion of the coronary arteries to oxygenate the myocardium and of the brain for a neurologically intact survival (Cunningham et al 2012). With each compression, coronary perfusion pressure gradually increases, and Cunningham et al (2012) suggest it takes 40–45 seconds of continuous compressions to achieve the optimal perfusion pressure. Each time compressions are interrupted there is a rapid decrease in aortic relaxation (diastolic) pressure which reduces both coronary and cerebral perfusion pressures; thus it is important to minimize interruptions to cardiac compressions (Beesems et al 2013).

Cardiac compressions are undertaken by placing the heel of one hand in the centre of the chest, which positions the hand onto the lower half of the sternum (Sayre et al 2010). The heel of the second hand is placed on top of the first hand with the fingers interlocking to avoid pressure on the ribs (Koster et al 2010) (Fig. 55.1). Cha et al (2013) found cardiac output was increased when using manikins when the compressions were undertaken on the internipple line as opposed to the lower half of the sternum. However, Sayre

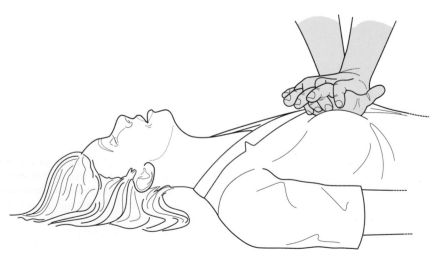

Figure 55.1 Cardiac compression.
(Adapted with kind permission from Peattie & Walker 1995)

et al (2010) suggest the use of the internipple line as a landmark is unreliable and this would be particularly so for women, as the position of their nipples vary according to the size of their breasts.

With arms locked to make full use of upper body weight (Lewinsohn et al 2012), the hands compress the sternum 5 cm (2 inches) or at least one-third of the anteroposterior diameter, although the European Resuscitation Council suggest the depth should be 6 cm (Nolan et al 2012). If undertaking compressions on a soft surface such as a mattress, the effect of mattress compression should be taken into account and the depth of compression increased accordingly. Dellimore & Scheffer (2012) suggest the stiffness of many hospital mattresses is suboptimal for undertaking compressions; however, Sayre et al (2010) warn against the potential for overestimation of compression depth when the person is on a soft surface.

The extended arms should be vertical, at a 90° angle to the chest and Lee et al (2012) caution that resuscitation on the bed makes this difficult unless the height of the bed matches the height of the person undertaking compressions. This reduces rescuer fatigue due to improved posture and produces more effective compressions (Lee et al 2012). Lewinsohn et al (2012) advise the bed height should be at mid-thigh level to generate more effective intrathoracic pressure during compression and reduce fatigue. They found that intrathoracic pressure could be reduced by 22% when the bed was too high for the person undertaking compressions which will adversely affect outcome (Lewinsohn et al 2012). Lee et al (2012) found the use of a step stool for fixed height beds increased the depth, accuracy and quality of compressions, rather than standing on tiptoe. Alternatively, cardiac compressions can be undertaken while kneeling on the bed next to the woman.

The compression rate is 100 per minute, the International Liaison Committee on Resuscitation found there was insufficient evidence to recommend what the upper limit should be and hence do not provide a range for the compression rate. However, the European Resuscitation Council has set an upper limit – 120 (Nolan et al 2012) so that compressions are undertaken at a rate of 100–120 per minute. Idris et al (2012) found the depth of compressions tended to decrease as the rate increased and that a rate of <75 compressions per minute (particularly when there were interruptions for ventilation breaths) was associated with a decreased likelihood of return of spontaneous circulation. Stiell et al (2012) agree, finding a significantly deleterious effect on compression depth as compression rates increased.

Undertaking cardiac compressions is tiring and fatigue affects the both the rate and depth of compression given. Lewinsohn et al (2012) suggest it is common for reduced compression depth to occur after only 1 minute of compressions but that the person undertaking compressions may not be aware of this for 5 minutes. Thus they recommend a switching between persons undertaking compressions every 2 minutes. Lyngeraa et al (2012) found highly motivated and skilled resuscitation participants can maintain the correct depth and rate of compressions for longer, possibly up to 10 minutes, emphasizing the importance of calling the resuscitation team early.

Following each compression, it is important to allow the chest to recoil to its precompression position and failure to release the chest completely during compressions is referred to as leaning. When leaning occurs, the heart does not refill sufficiently, with less blood pumped around the body with the next compression. This will quickly reduce perfusion pressure and reduce the likelihood of a successful outcome (Soar et al 2012).

Defibrillation

An automated external defibrillator (AED) can be used by anyone regardless of the amount, if any, of resuscitation training experienced. When connected, the AED will give voice and visual prompts that are easy to follow. Semi-automatic AEDs may have the facility for the operator to override the commands of the AED and deliver a shock manually, whereas the fully automated AED would not allow this. The AED has two electrode pads that are applied to the woman's chest and which are plugged into the AED. When the machine is operational, it will analyze the heart rhythm and where there is a shockable rhythm (ventricular fibrillation (VF), pulseless ventricular tachycardia (VT)) will advise the delivery of an electric shock. Defibrillation is the only effective therapy for a cardiac arrest resulting from VF or VT (Perkins & Colquhoun 2010). The AED then re-analyzes the heart rhythm after 2 minutes.

The AED should be used early in the resuscitation process (within 3 minutes for an in-hospital collapse), as the delay from collapse to the delivery of the first shock is considered to be the single most important determinant of survival with the chances of successful defibrillation reducing approximately 10% for each minute its use is delayed (Perkins & Colquhoun 2010).

The machine should be turned on as soon as it arrives so that it can go through its self-checking programme. The adhesive electrode pads should be placed on the collapsed woman while compressions are happening – the right pad is placed to the right of her sternum below her clavicle. The left pad is placed laterally in the left mid-axillary line, clear of any breast tissue (Perkins & Colquhoun 2010). Although the pads are labelled right and left and may have a picture on them showing where the pad should be placed, Perkins & Colquhoun (2010) advise that inadvertent placement of the right pad in the left pad's position and vice versa does not matter and time should not be wasted swapping them round. There may be difficulty getting the pads to adhere

to the chest if there is a lot of hair (a quick shave is indicated) or if the skin is wet, e.g. from being in the pool or shower (dry skin quickly).

An analysis of the heart rhythm is undertaken but if there is too much movement this may not be possible; thus the AED may instruct the resuscitators to stand clear when it is analyzing. The person undertaking cardiac compressions can maintain their position with hands poised just above the chest so that when the command is given to recommence CPR, this is undertaken quickly, minimizing the interruption to compressions. If no shock has been given, the AED will continue to analyze until a shockable rhythm is detected or it is turned off.

If a shock is to be administered, a warning noise will sound and all personnel should stand clear of the woman (and bed if she is on one). The person undertaking compressions is the last to stand clear and following a quick check to ensure everyone is clear, the shock button is pressed delivering the electric shock to the woman's heart (Soar & Davies 2010). Immediately, compression should recommence (Koster et al 2010). The risk of someone else receiving an accidental shock if they are touching the woman or the bed she is on is negligible (Nolan et al 2010). If supplemental oxygen is being administered through a facemask, there is a theoretical risk of a spark occurring although there have been no reports of fire when adhesive pads are used (Perkins & Colquhoun 2010). The AED will then wait 2 minutes before undertaking another rhythm analysis.

Pregnancy is not a contraindication to using the AED or receiving a shock. The same amount of charge is used for the shock. Vanden Hoek et al (2010) suggests there is a theoretical risk to the fetus if a cardiotocograph (CTG) monitor is in use when the shock is delivered, as the current may travel through the amniotic fluid and may cause burns to the fetus, or potentially death, and there is a small risk of fetal cardiac arrhythmias occurring. If a CTG monitor was in use prior to the collapse, it would be prudent to remove the two monitors to eliminate these risks and also to avoid the distraction of hearing a severe fetal bradycardia or no heart rate.

Ventilation breaths

Compressions can be combined with ventilation breaths at a rate of 30 compressions to 2 breaths for an adult (15 : 2 for a child). Ventilation breaths for basic life support can be undertaken using a facemask connected to a bag–valve–mask (BVM) system, e.g. Ambu bag, a pocket mask, or mouth-to-mouth. Sayre et al (2010) advise each breath should use a 1-second inspiratory time and a volume of approximately 600 mL. Where higher volumes are used, there is an increased risk of gastric distention (Koster et al 2010). Thus no more than 5 seconds should be used to

administer the two ventilation breaths (Handley & Colquhoun 2010). This is two attempts at ventilation and if one or both are unsuccessful during the 5 seconds, compressions should be recommenced and the breaths re-attempted after 30 compressions; however, Beesems et al (2013) found the median time for 2 ventilation attempts was 7 seconds. The longer the time taken to administer the breaths, the longer the interruption to cardiac compressions and the greater the decrease in perfusion. Chalkias et al (2013) question whether positive-pressure ventilation should be used during the initial stages of CPR, suggesting it may be harmful as it may increase the intrathoracic pressure which will decrease coronary perfusion pressure. Koster et al (2010) agree that hyperventilation is harmful and lessens the chance of survival.

When using a facemask for ventilation breaths, it is important to use the correct size (small, medium or large). Bosson & Gordon (2013) suggest that where the correct size is not available, a seal will be easier to achieve with a mask that is too big than one that is too small. Ideally the mask should not extend over the end of the woman's chin or into her eye sockets. It has a deformable rim that will fit snugly around the woman's nose and mouth when even pressure is applied and an airtight seal formed. It is important the mask is held in place with slight pressure on the firm surface of the mask as pressure on the rim may cause it to deform and lose the seal. The woman's head should be slightly extended. It can be harder to achieve a good seal in the presence of facial hair (use a water-soluble lubricant over the hair to improve contact), lack of teeth, body mass index (BMI) >26, age >55 years, and a history of snoring (Bosson & Gordon 2013). Bosson & Gordon (2013) suggest that the mandible should be lifted to the mask rather than the mask pushed down onto the face.

There are several ways to hold the facemask in place using one or two hands. A common method is the E-C technique where the non-dominant hand is used by creating a C-shape with the thumb and index finger and placing them on the upper and lower part of the mask's firm surface. Gentle downward pressure is applied to create an airtight seal. The remaining three fingers are placed around the mandible in an E-shape to lift the chin up towards the mask. If there is another person available to compress the bag, then two hands can be used to hold the mask in place with a double jaw thrust. Two opposing semi-circles are made using the thumb and index finger of each hand and placed on either side of the facemask. The remaining three fingers of each hand are placed under the mandible and behind the angle of the jaw to pull the chin forwards (Fig. 55.2). A third technique is to place the length of the thumbs along the sides of the facemask to hold it in place using the remaining fingers under the mandible to pull the chin forwards. Care should be taken whichever technique is used to ensure the fingers under the mandible are only

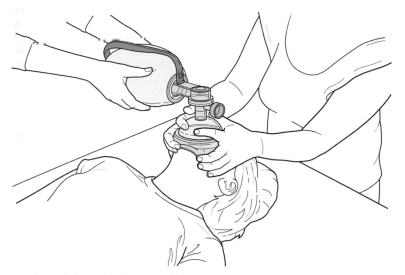

Figure 55.2 Bag–valve–mask ventilation using two resuscitators.

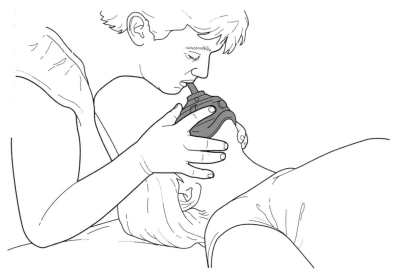

Figure 55.3 Using a Laerdal pocket mask.

applying pressure on bone and not the soft tissue of the neck, as this may result in swelling and airway occlusion.

If a pocket mask is available, it should be placed over the woman's nose and mouth and her airway opened using a chin tilt. The mask should be held on the firm surface to prevent the rim from deforming. The midwife blows through the opening on the pocket mask using a normal expiratory breath as the chest rises (Fig. 55.3). This is repeated once. If there is no chest movement noted, the head and mask position should be checked and corrected

and the two breaths re-attempted after the next set of compressions.

Mouth-to-mouth can be undertaken if the midwife is willing to do so; however, it is acceptable to continue with compressions until suitable equipment arrives for ventilation, as there is a risk of coming into contact with body fluids. Koster et al (2010), however, suggest the risk of disease transmission is extremely low. To undertake mouth-to-mouth, the woman's airway should be opened as described above, the soft part of the woman's nose closed by pinching it between the thumb and forefinger and the heel of the same hand placed on the woman's forehead. The woman's mouth should be opened slightly while maintaining a chin tilt and the midwife then places her mouth over the woman's mouth, ensuring a good seal. Air is blown into the woman's mouth over 1 second using a normal expiratory breath while looking for chest rise (Koster et al 2010). When the breath is finished, the midwife removes her mouth as the woman's chest falls, then this is repeated once more.

In situations where ventilation breaths are not attempted, it is helpful to place an oxygen mask on the woman's face connected to 100% oxygen as this may facilitate the passive exchange of oxygen during compressions.

The facemask can be attached to a self-inflating BVM system and oxygen attached as soon as possible (Madams 2008). Currently the recommendation is for 100% oxygen to be used with cardiac compressions. Nolan et al (2012) agree that the highest possible oxygen concentration should be used initially but suggest this should be altered according to the arterial blood oxygen saturation when they can be obtained reliably by pulse oximeter or arterial blood gas analysis to achieve an arterial blood oxygen saturation of 94–98%.

The bag should be slowly compressed for 1 second for each ventilation then released to refill while chest rise and fall are looked for. It may be difficult to see chest rise with pregnant women, particularly during the third trimester. Lateral chest and/or breast movement may be noted as an indication of lung inflation.

Considerations for the pregnant woman

Although the principles of resuscitation are the same as for any adult, there are physiological changes that occur during pregnancy that can influence resuscitation outcomes. The most important consideration is that of the gravid uterus and the compression effect it has on the inferior vena cava when the woman is lying in the supine position. As a result, venous return is impeded which reduces both the stroke volume and cardiac output by 30–40% (RCOG 2011). Soar et al (2010) suggest that uterine obstruction of venous return may precipitate cardiac arrest in the critically ill woman. The exact gestational age at which aortocaval compression occurs is inconsistent and can vary depending on the size and or number of fetuses (Vanden Hoek et al 2010). The Resuscitation Council (UK) (2015) recommend lateral displacement of the uterus from 20 weeks' gestation or if clinically obvious.

The use of a left lateral tilt under the pelvis and thorax will reduce the effect of uterine weight and increase stroke volume and cardiac output. Vanden Hoek et al (2010) suggest the degree of tilt should be 27–30°; when it is >30° the woman may slide or roll off the inclined plane, whereas Soar et al (2010) advise 15–30° and the RCOG (2011) recommend 15°. Some hospitals have wedges available for the resuscitation of pregnant women – ideally these should be in all areas where resuscitation may be required, e.g. maternity wards, accident and emergency departments. The wedge may be hard (made of wood) or firm (made of foam). Where no wedge is available, improvisation may occur by using a human wedge whereby the woman is tilted against someone who is kneeling back or with pillows (soft wedge). Ip et al (2013) found the use of a hard wedge was better than a firm wedge for stability and maintenance of the tilt but there was no difference in compression depth. The soft wedge, e.g. pillow, had significantly lower stability than the other three types of wedges and did not maintain the tilt well – initially the degree of tilt was 15–30° but this quickly reduced. The human wedge provided a greater degree of tilt but was less stable than the hard and firm wedges and there was a significant reduction in the depth of cardiac compressions – it was also very uncomfortable for the person kneeling, making it more likely that the person would alternate this role with another person, interrupting cardiac compressions. Ip et al (2013) recommend the use of custom made hard wedges when resuscitating pregnant women. Kundra et al (2007) recommend the use of both a wedge and manual displacement of the uterus.

Cardiac compressions may be less forceful when the woman is tilted compared to supine; thus it may be preferable to perform uterine displacement manually. Vanden Hoek et al (2010) recommend the person undertaking the displacement stands on the woman's left and uses both hands to displace the uterus or on the woman's right using one hand. They also suggest that cardiac compressions should be performed slightly higher on the sternum to account for the elevation of the diaphragm and abdominal contents from the gravid uterus.

If the gravid uterus is considered to be interfering with maternal haemodynamics a perimortem caesarean section (CS) should be undertaken within 5 minutes of collapse and is undertaken in the place where the woman has collapsed (RCOG 2011). Castle (2009) cautions that the sterility adhered to within the theatre setting will not be possible. Knight et al (2014) recommend the massive obstetric haemorrhage protocol is triggered once the decision to perform a perimortem CS is made. Delivering the baby gives the woman a greater chance of surviving, depending on the reason for the cardiac arrest. The RCOG (2011) and McDonnell (2009) recommend a perimortem CS pack should be readily available in both the maternity unit and the accident and emergency departments.

Airway management may be more difficult in the pregnant woman due to the changes in airway mucosa, e.g. oedema, increased friability, hypersecretion, hyperaemia, which in conjunction with an airway that may be smaller in the third trimester, makes intubation more difficult (Vanden Hoek et al 2010). McDonnell (2009) advises early tracheal intubation emphasizing the importance of calling for the resuscitation quickly. Cricoid pressure should be used during intubation because of the increased risk of aspiration (due to progesterone relaxing the lower oesophageal sphincter, delayed gastric emptying and raised intra-abdominal pressure secondary to the gravid uterus) (Fig. 55.4).

The pregnant woman can become hypoxic more readily during periods of hypoventilation due to changes in lung function during pregnancy (increased tidal volume and minute ventilation), diaphragmatic splinting (reducing the functional residual capacity) and increased oxygen consumption of the fetoplacental unit which can make ventilation more difficult (RCOG 2011). Thus the RCOG (2011) advise that supplemental oxygen should be administered as soon as possible using high-flow 100% oxygen.

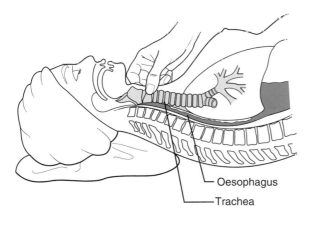

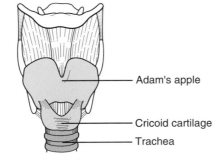

Figure 55.4 Application of cricoid pressure.
(Adapted from Fraser et al 2003)

ADDITIONAL MEASURES

When the resuscitation team arrive, one of them will take overall control of the resuscitation to ensure the resuscitation is progressing as it should. A clear, concise, verbal handover of the history, treatment and response to-date should be given to the team. However, the obstetrician or midwife present will need to guide them on the particular adaptations necessary for the pregnant woman. While compression, ventilation breaths and use of the AED continue, other personnel can site two wide-bore gauge intravenous cannulae and commence fluid boluses or administer drugs as requested and maintain contemporaneous documentation. At this point the midwife also has an important role in supporting the family, setting up the resuscitaire, calling the paediatrician and assisting with resuscitating the baby if it is delivered.

Stopping resuscitation

The resuscitation will stop when there is return of spontaneous circulation, the people undertaking CPR are too exhausted to continue (usually this is an out-of-hospital situation) or a senior team member makes the decision to stop. Because the collapse is usually unexpected, the case will be referred to the Coroner. It is important that any pieces of equipment inserted during the resuscitation remain *in situ*, e.g. airways, endotracheal tubes, cannulae, as these will be reviewed by the pathologist as part of the postmortem examination.

All maternal deaths are notified to MBRRACE-UK (Mothers and Babies: Reducing Risk through Audits and Confidential Enquiries across the UK). MBRRACE-UK is the association appointed by the Healthcare Quality Improvement Partnership to investigate maternal deaths (also stillbirths and infant deaths), collate the information and provide recommendations to support the safe, high-quality, patient-centred delivery of care. They are also continuing the Confidential Enquiry into Maternal Deaths reports. For further information, go to their website https://www.npeu.ox.ac.uk/mbrrace-uk.

When the woman survives, post-resuscitation care will usually be provided in the intensive care unit following time in the operating theatre if a perimortem CS was performed. Debriefing for the woman, her family and staff involved is essential. The Supervisor of Midwives can be a valuable support for midwives involved in any maternal resuscitation but particularly so when it is unsuccessful; this is a devastating event for the family and all involved in the care and resuscitation of the woman.

PROCEDURE: maternal resuscitation

- Recognize the arrest and assess the situation for any potential dangers.
- Assess the level of responsiveness.
- If unresponsive, call for emergency assistance.
- Turn the woman on her back with a wedge under her right side and/or manually displace the uterus and tilt her head so that it is slightly extended.
- Ensure the airway is open, using chin support.
- Assess breathing taking no more than 10 seconds.
- If not breathing, commence cardiac compression at a rate of 100 beats per minute (bpm).
- After every 30 cardiac compressions, undertake 2 ventilation breaths where possible, and maintain the rate at 30:2.
- Apply AED electrodes and follow voice commands.
- Continue with resuscitation until spontaneous respiration or movement seen, or until told to stop by the senior person present (or if too exhausted to continue and there is no one to take over from you).
- If after 4 minutes there is minimal success, preparation should begin for caesarean section (if pregnant) and the baby delivered within the next minute.
- Participate within the multidisciplinary team and undertake other roles as needed, e.g. intravenous cannulation, drug and fluid administration, support of family, assisting with neonatal resuscitation.
- Maintain detailed records of all actions taken.
- Fully debrief following the resuscitation.

ROLE AND RESPONSIBILITIES OF THE MIDWIFE

These can be summarized as:
- keeping up-to-date with changes to the resuscitation guidelines
- attending CPR updates on at least an annual basis
- swift recognition and response in the event of collapse
- undertaking CPR quickly and effectively including cardiac compressions and ventilation breaths
- attaching the AED leads as soon as possible and following the voice prompts
- recognizing the need for and undertaking the adaptations necessary for resuscitating the pregnant woman
- undertaking other aspects of care, e.g. intravenous cannulation, neonatal resuscitation, care of the family
- consultation with others, e.g. risk manager, Supervisor of Midwives, especially if resuscitation is unsuccessful
- detailed contemporaneous records.

SUMMARY

- Maternal resuscitation is a rare occurrence; thus it is important that resuscitation skills are practised at least yearly.
- Calling for help is essential when a non-responsive person is found.
- If the person is not breathing or making gasping noises, cardiac arrest is assumed and compressions commenced.
- Cardiac compressions are the most important component of resuscitation and interruptions should be minimized.
- Cardiac compressions that are delivered at a rate of 100 per minute, a depth of 6 cm, and the chest allowed to recoil between compressions are associated with an increased survival rate.
- A defibrillator should be attached and used early in the resuscitation as this may increase the likelihood of survival.
- Adaptations are required when resuscitating a pregnant woman due to the physiological changes of pregnancy that make resuscitation more difficult: a wedge and/or manual displacement of the uterus and delivery of the baby at 5 minutes.

SELF-ASSESSMENT EXERCISES

The answers to the following questions may be found in the text:
1. What does the Chain of Survival refer to?
2. What conditions may predispose the pregnant or postnatal woman to a cardiac arrest?
3. What actions would you take, in order, when finding a collapsed woman?
4. Describe how to perform effective cardiac compressions.
5. How can effective ventilation be achieved?
6. What adaptations may be needed for a woman being resuscitated at 38 weeks' gestation?
7. Summarize the role and responsibilities of the midwife when resuscitating a pregnant woman.

REFERENCES

Beesems, S.G., Wijmans, L., Tijssen, J.G.P., Koster, R.W., 2013. Duration of ventilations during cardiopulmonary resuscitation by lay rescuers and first responders: relationship between delivering cardiac compressions and outcomes. Circulation 127, 1585–1590.

Bosson, N., Gordon, P.E., 2013. Bag-Valve-Mask Ventilation. Available online: <http://emedicine.medscape.com/article/80184-overview#showall> (accessed 3 March 2015).

Castle, N., 2009. Neonatal and maternal resuscitation. In: Chapman, V., Charles, C. (Eds.), The Midwife's Labour and Birth Handbook, second ed. Blackwell Publishing Ltd, Oxford.

Cha, K.C., Kim, Y.J., Shin, H.J., et al., 2013. Optimal position for external cardiac compressions during cardiopulmonary resuscitation: an analysis based on chest CT in patients resuscitated from cardiac arrest. Emerg. Med. J. 30, 615–619.

Chalkias, A., Vogiatzakis, N., Tampakis, K., et al., 2013. One-hand chest compression and hands-off time in single-lay rescuer CPR – a manikin study. Am. J. Emerg. Med. 31, 1462–1465.

Cunningham, L.M., Mattu, A., O'Connor, R.E., Brady, W.J., 2012. Cardiopulmonary resuscitation for cardiac arrest: the importance of uninterrupted cardiac compressions in cardiac arrest resuscitation. Am. J. Emerg. Med. 30, 1630–1638.

Dellimore, K.H., Scheffer, C., 2012. Optimal cardiac compressions in cardiopulmonary resuscitation depends upon thoracic and back support stiffness. Med. Biol. Eng. Comput. 50, 1269–1278.

Handley, A., Colquhoun, M., 2010. Resuscitation Guidelines 2. Adult Basic Life Support. Available online: <https://www.resus.org.uk/pages/bls.pdf> (accessed 3 March 2015).

Fraser, D.M., Cooper, M.A., Myles, M.F. (Eds.), 2003. Myles Textbook for Midwives, fourteenth ed. Churchill Livingstone, Edinburgh.

Idris, A.H., Guffey, D., Aufderheide, T.P., The Resuscitation Outcomes Consortium (ROC) Investigators, et al., 2012. Relationship between cardiac compression rates and outcomes from cardiac arrest. Circulation 125, 3004–3012.

Ip, J.K., Campbell, J.P., Bushby, D., Yentis, S.M., 2013. Cardiopulmonary resuscitation in the pregnant patient: a manikin-based evaluation of methods for producing lateral tilt. Anaesthesia 65, 694–699.

Iwami, T., Kitamura, T., Kawamura, T., et al., 2012. Chest compression-only cardiopulmonary resuscitation for out-of-hospital cardiac arrest with public-access defibrillation. Circulation 126, 2844–2851.

Knight, M., Kenyon, S., Brocklehurst, P., et al., (Eds.), on behalf of MBRRACE-UK, 2014. Saving Lives, Improving Mothers' Care – lessons learned to inform future maternity care from the UK and Ireland Confidential Enquiries into Maternal Deaths and Morbidity 2009–12. National Perinatal Epidemiology Unit, Oxford.

Koster, R.W., Baubin, M.A., Bassaert, L.L., et al., 2010. European resuscitation council guidelines for resuscitation 2010 Section 2. Adult basic life support and use of automated external defibrillators. Resuscitation 81, 1277–1292.

Kundra, P., Khanna, S., Habeebullah, S., Ravishanka, M., 2007. Manual displacement of the uterus during caesarean section. Anaesthesia 62 (5), 460–465.

Lee, D.H., Kim, C.W., Kim, S.G., Lee, S.J., 2012. Use of step stool during resuscitation improved the quality of chest compressions in simulated resuscitation. Emerg. Med. Australas. 24, 369–373.

Lewinsohn, A., Sherren, P.B., Wijayatilake, D.S., 2012. The effects of bed height and time on the quality of cardiac compressions delivered during cardiopulmonary resuscitation: a randomised crossover simulation study. Emerg. Med. 29, 660–663.

Lyngeraa, T.S., Hjortrup, P.B., Wulff, N.B., et al., 2012. Effect of feedback on delaying deterioration in quality of compressions during 2 minutes of continuous chest compressions: a randomized manikin study investigating performance with and without feedback. Scand. J. Trauma Resusc. Emerg. Med. 20, 16.

Madams, M., 2008. Maternal resuscitation; how to resuscitate mothers who die. Br. J. Midwifery 16 (6), 372–375.

McDonnell, N.J., 2009. Cardiopulmonary arrest in pregnancy: two case reports of successful outcomes in association with perimortem Caesarean delivery. Br. J. Anaesth. 103 (3), 406–409.

National Patient Safety Agency, 2004. Establishing a standard crash call telephone number in hospitals. Patient Safety Alert02. London. Available online: <http://www.google.co.uk/url?sa=t&rct=j&q=&esrc=s&source=web&cd=1&ved=0CCMQFjAA&url=http%3A%2F%2Fwww.nrls.npsa.nhs.uk%2FEasySiteWeb%2Fgetresource.axd%3FAssetID%3D59981%26type%3Dfull%26servicetype%3DAttachment&ei=4zX1VL2eGYTk8AWBlYII&usg=AFQjCNFZhUXL0LrdWiVs8KOc5DkE0JovGg&bvm=bv.87269000,d.dGc> (accessed 3 March 2015).

Nolan, J.P., Perkins, G.D., Soar, J., 2012. Chest compression rate: where is the sweet spot? Circulation 125, 2968–2970.

Nolan, J.P., Soar, J., Zideman, D.A., On behalf of the ERC Guidelines Working Group, et al., 2010. European resuscitation council guidelines for resuscitation 2010 section 1, executive Summary. Resuscitation 81, 1219–1276.

Peattie, P.I., Walker, S., 1995. Understanding Nursing Care, fourteenth ed. Churchill Livingstone, Edinburgh.

Perkins, G.D., Colquhoun, M. 2010 Resuscitation Guidelines 3. The use of Automated External Defibrillation. Available online: <https://www.resus

.org.uk/pages/aed.pdf> (accessed 3 March 2015).

Resuscitation Council (UK), 2015. Prehospital Resuscitation. Available online: <http://www.resus.org.uk/resuscitation-guidelines/prehospital-resuscitation/> (accessed 18 December 2015).

Resuscitation Council (UK), 2013a. Minimum equipment and drug lists for cardiopulmonary resuscitation. Available online: <http://www.resus.org.uk/pages/QSCPR_PrimaryCare_Equip.htm> (accessed 3 March 2015).

Resuscitation Council (UK), 2013b. Quality standards for cardiopulmonary resuscitation practice and training. Acute Care Available online: <https://www.resus.org.uk/pages/QSCPR_Acute.htm> (accessed 3 March 2015).

RCOG (Royal College of Obstetricians and Gynaecologists), 2011. Green Top Guideline 56 Maternal collapse in pregnancy and the puerperium.

Available online: <https://www.rcog.org.uk/globalassets/documents/guidelines/gtg_56.pdf> (accessed 6 December 2014).

Sayre, M.R., Koster, R.W., Botha, M., et al., 2010. Part 5: adult basic life support: 2010 international consensus on cardiopulmonary resuscitation and emergency cardiovascular care science with treatment recommendations. Circulation 122, S298–S324.

Soar, J., Davies, R. 2010 Resuscitation Guidelines 6. In-hospital resuscitation. Available online: <https://www.resus.org.uk/pages/inhresus.pdf> (accessed 3 March 2015).

Soar, J., Perkins, G.D., Gamal Abbas, G., et al., 2012. Cardiac compression quality – push hard, push fast, but how deep and fast? Crit. Care Med. 40 (4), 1363–1364.

Stiell, I.G., Brown, S.P., Christenson, J., The Resuscitation Outcomes Consortium (ROC) Investigators,

et al., 2012. What is the role of chest compression depth during out-of-hospital cardiac arrest resuscitation? Crit. Care Med. 40 (4), 1192–1198.

Travers, A.H., Rea, T.D., Bobrow, B.J., et al., 2010. Part 4: CPR overview: 2010 American heart Association guidelines for cardiopulmonary resuscitation and emergency cardiovascular care. Circulation 122, S676–S684.

Vanden Hoek, T.L., Morrison, L.J., Shuster, M., et al., 2010. Part 12: cardiac arrest in special situations: 2010 American Heart Association guidelines for cardiopulmonary resuscitation and emergency cardiovascular care. Circulation 122, S829–S861.

Yang, Z., Li, H., Yu, T., et al., 2014. Quality of chest compressions during compression-only CPR: a comparative analysis following the 2005 and 2010 American Heart Association guidelines. Am. J. Emerg. Med. 32, 50–54.

Chapter 56

Principles of cardiopulmonary resuscitation: neonatal resuscitation

LEARNING OUTCOMES

Having read this chapter, the reader should be able to:

- recognize a baby who requires resuscitation
- discuss the different ways of maintaining an open airway for the baby during resuscitation
- discuss the rationale for using air to begin the resuscitation and when to increase the percentage of oxygen used
- describe when and how cardiac compressions are given
- describe the equipment and how it is used
- discuss in detail the role and responsibilities of the midwife prior to, during and following a neonatal resuscitation
- demonstrate/simulate a neonatal resuscitation using a manikin, discussing how effective resuscitation is achieved.

Up to 1% of low-risk babies (Rovamo et al 2013) and between 10–20% of all newborns (Schilleman et al 2010, Vento & Saugstad 2011) require ventilatory assistance at birth. Internationally, O'Donnell (2012) advises that between four and seven million babies require resuscitation with 0.06% of babies ≥34 weeks' gestation needing chest compressions; the sequelae of birth asphyxia is estimated to have a mortality of two million a year with 99% of deaths occurring in developing countries (Murilaa et al 2012). The aim of neonatal resuscitation is to restore tissue oxygen delivery before irreversible damage occurs which may affect long-term neurodevelopment and increase the mortality rate (Harach 2013). Prompt initiation of resuscitation is critical (Amin et al 2013) and the quality of care provided during the first few minutes after birth has a significant effect on long-term health (Rovamo et al 2013). Niermeyer & Clarke (2011) suggest that with each minute resuscitation is delayed, the time to the first gasp increases by about 2 minutes and the onset of spontaneous breathing can be delayed beyond 4 minutes. It is therefore vital that the midwife is able to anticipate and recognize the baby that requires resuscitative assistance at birth and provide this efficiently and competently to reduce morbidity and mortality associated with birth asphyxia.

The International Liaison Committee on Resuscitation (ILCOR) is a multinational group with representation from eight international resuscitation councils – American Heart Association (see Kattwinkel et al 2010), European Resuscitation Council (see Richmond & Wyllie 2010), Heart and Stroke Foundation of Canada (see Finan et al 2011), Resuscitation Council of Asia, Resuscitation Council of South Africa, Australian and New Zealand Resuscitation Council (see NZRC), and the Inter-American Heart Foundation. They review and debate the evidence on neonatal resuscitation and their recommendations are produced as guidelines by Resuscitation Councils across the world. There may be subtle differences between the different Resuscitation Councils according to whether or not they adopt the recommendations in their entirety. The midwife who intends to work in a different country is advised to review that country's Resuscitation Council guidelines.

At birth there are a number of adaptations the baby has to make to successfully transition from intrauterine to extrauterine life. The airways of the lungs are fluid filled prior to birth and must quickly change to being air filled for effective ventilation to occur. The alveoli in the lungs expand and maintain this expansion with the assistance of surfactant. A functional residual capacity (FRC) is created following the first few breaths. Pulmonary blood flow dramatically increases which assists in the reversal of blood flow through the ductus arteriosus and the closure of the foramen ovale. Negative pressures as high as -80 cm H_2O can be generated by the baby with the first breaths, with lower pressures required for subsequent breaths. Lung expansion occurs in conjunction with an increase in the alveolar oxygen tension which results in decreased pulmonary vascular resistance and increased pulmonary blood flow. Oxygen saturation levels increase slowly over the first 5–10 minutes. There is a significant difference in pre- and post-ductal oxygen saturation levels during the first 15 minutes of life. At this point, Beşkardeş et al (2012) suggest it is possible the transfer of blood from right to left along the ductus arteriosus has stopped, increasing saturation levels in the extremities.

Babies who cannot produce adequate alveolar expansion develop respiratory failure and the change in pulmonary vascular resistance does not occur, resulting in persistent pulmonary hypertension, decreased pulmonary blood flow, and hypoxaemia.

Very preterm babies can quickly develop surfactant deficiency preventing the alveoli from maintaining their expansion. They also may have weaker lung muscles, underdeveloped airway protective reflexes and a reduced drive to breathe. Post-mature babies may pass meconium into the amniotic fluid which can be inhaled before or during labour causing inflammation of the lungs and airway obstruction.

PATHOPHYSIOLOGY OF ASPHYXIA

Asphyxia refers to inadequate tissue perfusion that does not meet the metabolic demands of the tissues for oxygen and removal of waste (Niermeyer & Clarke 2011) resulting in increasing hypoxia, hypercapnia and acidosis. This will cause a change in metabolism from aerobic to anaerobic creating a metabolic acidosis, initially buffered by bicarbonate. As the bicarbonate is depleted, acidosis worsens. The initial response to asphyxia is an increased heart rate followed by decreased cardiac output and peripheral vasoconstriction in an attempt to maintain the blood pressure so that perfusion of the vital organs occurs. As acidosis worsens, cardiac failure can ensue with a decrease in heart rate and blood pressure.

ANTICIPATION

There may be known maternal, fetal or intrapartum factors that increase the likelihood of the need for neonatal resuscitation. In these cases it is advisable for the woman to birth in a hospital where resuscitative equipment and personnel are at hand. These include:

- maternal disease, e.g. pre-eclampsia
- maternal infection, e.g. chorioamnionitis
- maternal substance abuse
- fetal abnormality, e.g. diaphragmatic hernia
- intrauterine growth restriction
- ante- or intrapartum haemorrhage
- prolonged rupture of membranes
- malposition or malpresentation, e.g. breech
- abnormalities of the fetal heart rate indicative of fetal compromise
- induction and augmentation of labour
- preterm labour
- significant meconium within the amniotic fluid
- heavy maternal sedation
- prolonged labour
- instrumental and operative delivery
- obstetric emergency, e.g. cord prolapse, shoulder dystocia.

However, there will always be the unexpected situation in a low-risk setting that reminds the midwife of the importance of ensuring there is access to resuscitation equipment available for every birth, even the homebirth environment, highlighting the requirement that all midwives are trained in and practice neonatal resuscitation on at least a yearly basis so that there is at least one person at the delivery who is trained in newborn life support (Kattwinkel et al 2010, Richmond & Wyllie 2010). Ideally, two midwives are present at each birth allowing one to attend to the immediate needs of the baby and the other to call for emergency assistance. In the hospital environment this may be through the use of the emergency bell or emergency phone number, while in the community the paramedic service should be accessed through ringing 999 or 112.

Training in neonatal resuscitation should occur in the environment and with the equipment with which the midwife works. Multidisciplinary training is ideal as good teamwork behaviours are correlated with higher quality of care during resuscitation (Sawyer et al 2013). Cusack & Fawke (2012) suggest significant decay in psychomotor skills occurs as soon as 3 months following training in resuscitation and advise refresher training and assessment should occur 6 months after attending a resuscitation course to increase retention of knowledge and psychomotor skills.

EQUIPMENT

The majority of babies require minimal support with resuscitation necessitating only a small amount of equipment. In the hospital environment it is likely that a standard resuscitaire with additional equipment will be available. The advantage of the resuscitaire is that it comes equipped with a flat surface, good heat and light source, and generally a clock, in addition to equipment for ventilation such as a neopuff/self-inflating bag and the ability to blend air and oxygen. The resuscitaire can be switched on in preparation for the birth so that the environment is prewarmed. All of the equipment should be checked to ensure it is working correctly and the clock started when the baby is born. Some hospitals are fortunate to have a resuscitation table that can be placed next to the bed to allow resuscitation to occur at the bedside with an unclamped umbilical cord so the baby has the benefit of delayed cord clamping (see Chapter 32).

In the home environment the equipment should be laid out ready next to a flat surface and away from draughts with a supply of warm towels available when needed. This may be close to the mother so that if resuscitation is required, it can be undertaken with the cord still attached and unclamped.

Ideal requirements for basic resuscitation in hospital include:

- a flat surface
- towels and non-sterile gloves (somewhere to wash and dry hands if time permits)
- a radiant heater
- a clock, with a second hand
- stethoscope
- blended oxygen/air source with flow regulation and adjustable pressure relief valve (these should be

checked prior to the delivery to ensure they are working correctly)
- pulse oximeter and neonatal probe
- T-piece resuscitator, e.g. neopuff or a self-inflating bag–valve–mask (BVM)
- assorted size facemasks, 00, 01
- Guedel airways, sizes 0, 00, 000
- suction apparatus with tubing and catheters
- polyethylene wrap or food-grade plastic wrapping (for preterm babies <28 weeks).

And for more advanced resuscitation:

- laryngoscopes (with spare bulbs and batteries)
- endotracheal tubes, introducers and connectors
- drugs
- needles, syringes, scissors, tape, other extras, e.g. umbilical catheterization pack, intraosseous needle.

PRINCIPLES OF NEONATAL RESUSCITATION

While these follow ABCD – airway, breathing, circulation, and drugs – there are important steps to be taken beforehand which may result in the baby breathing spontaneously without having to resort to these. The baby is born wet and into a cooler environment which means heat loss can occur quickly. It is therefore important to dry the baby as soon as possible, this will also stimulate the baby and encourage him to breathe spontaneously. It allows the midwife to assess the response of the baby, particularly the tone. A quick assessment is made to determine if respiration is being established and whether the heart rate is above 100 bpm. If not, prompt action is taken, the cord is clamped and cut (if the resuscitation area is not by the bedside), and the baby taken to the resuscitation area. Resuscitation takes priority over delayed cord clamping as there is insufficient evidence to recommend a time for clamping in babies who require resuscitation (Finan et al 2011) and positive pressure ventilation should begin within the first minute of life, sometimes referred to as 'the golden minute' (Kattwinkel et al 2010).

It is important to ensure the wet towel is removed and the baby wrapped in a warm, dry towel. Some resuscitaires heat the baby more quickly if the baby is uncovered – it is essential the midwife is aware of how the resuscitaire she is using works to avoid inadvertently preventing the baby from warming up. A cold baby is harder to resuscitate.

There are two exceptions to drying the baby at birth:

1. If the baby is preterm baby <28 weeks' gestation: The baby should be loosely wrapped in a polyethylene bag/sheet from neck to toe without drying the baby – this should ideally be prewarmed by placing under the

radiant heater (not on the radiator as it may melt). The wrapping should take place as close to the time of birth as possible. Once the baby is wrapped, the head should be dried, a hat applied, and the baby stimulated. This will help maintain the baby's temperature by reducing evaporative heat loss but allowing radiant heat to be transmitted to the baby (O'Donnell 2012). It significantly reduces the risk of hypothermia which has an increased risk of morbidity and mortality for the preterm baby (Rohana et al 2011).

2. Where meconium has been passed *in utero* and the baby has not breathed: In this instance the baby's airway should be suctioned under direct vision using a wide-bore suction catheter, removing any visible meconium. After this the baby is dried and stimulated. If the baby has already breathed, any meconium close to the airways will have been inhaled and further suction is usually of no benefit.

The baby should be positioned so that his head is in a neutral position, neither flexed nor extended, to ensure the airway is open to facilitate air entry into the lungs. This is particularly important with the floppy baby as the loss of pharyngeal tone causes the tongue to fall back and occlude the airway. At birth the prominent occiput (often associated with moulding) of some babies can cause the neck to flex, resulting in airway occlusion. Placing a folded towel/blanket, approximately 2 cm in depth, under the baby's shoulders will bring the head and neck in alignment and keep the trachea straight (Fig. 56.1).

ASSESSMENT OF THE BABY

The baby should now be assessed – breathing, heart rate, and tone:

Breathing: Is the baby breathing? If yes, count the rate, depth and symmetry and observe for abnormal respiratory signs and sounds such as gasping and grunting.

Heart rate: The gold standard has been to auscultate the apex beat with a stethoscope. Initially the base of the umbilical cord can be palpated but may be unreliable. If the rate is above 100 bpm, Richmond & Wyllie (2010) consider this to be reliable; however, if it is below 100, the apex should always be auscultated. Katheria et al (2012) found both auscultation and palpation of the cord are unreliable in very low birthweight babies, underestimating the heart rate by 14–21 bpm. They recommend attaching electrocardiograph (ECG) leads at birth for more accurate results. Mizumoto et al (2012) also recommend the use of ECG leads over pulse oximetry for determining heart rate, particularly for bradycardic babies with poor perfusion. van Vonderen et al (2015) suggest that ECG is now the gold standard for assessing the heart rate. They found that the heart rate measured by pulse oximetry was significantly lower than that measured by ECG during the first 7 minutes of life for both term and preterm babies particularly during the first 2 minutes (van Vonderen et al 2015). However, Kamlin et al (2008) acknowledge the difficulty in applying the ECG electrodes to wet skin and that they may damage the skin of an extremely preterm baby. They found pulse oximetry provided an accurate display of the baby's heart rate; pulse oximetry and ECG measure the heart rate differently, particularly in relation to averaging intervals; thus small differences may be seen when both are used (Kamlin et al 2008). When the heart rate changes, the measurement on the pulse oximetry may lag behind the ECG for a few seconds but Kamlin et al (2008) suggest this is not clinically significant. The New Zealand Resuscitation Council (NZRC 2010a) advise that the heart rate should be consistently above 100 bpm within the first minute of life for the uncompromised baby, although Dawson et al (2010) suggest the median heart rate of both the term and preterm babies is

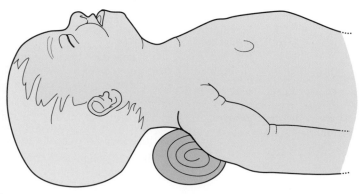

Figure 56.1 Neutral position.

<100 bpm (99 bpm and 96 bpm, respectively). These were babies who did not require any resuscitation even though at 1 minute 17% had a heart rate <100 bpm and 7% had a heart rate <60 bpm and all had good tone and normal respiratory effort (Dawson et al 2010). An increasing heart rate is the most reliable sign that the baby's condition is improving, with a decreasing heart rate associated with a deterioration in the baby's condition. Assisted ventilation should be given if the heart rate is persistently <100 bpm (NZRC 2010a). Tone: Assessment of tone is subjective, a baby with good tone (moving limbs, flexed posture) is unlikely to be compromised enough to require resuscitation. A floppy baby (not moving, extended posture) is usually one that requires resuscitation; however, tone is related to gestation, hence a very preterm baby may have poor tone but not require resuscitation.

1. Breathing: established, crying
   Heart rate: ≥100 bpm
   Tone: good
   No further action required except to ensure the baby is dry, placed skin-to-skin with his mother, and covered with warm towels.
2. Breathing: inadequate or absent and/or
   Heart rate: <100 bpm
   Tone: normal or reduced
   The baby requires ventilatory support with mask inflation which is likely to increase the heart rate and established respiration. Once the baby is breathing regularly and the heart rate is ≥100 bpm the tone will improve.
3. Breathing: inadequate or absent
   Heart rate: low or undetectable
   Tone: reduced
   The baby requires immediate ventilatory support with mask inflation and may require chest compressions.

In the UK, breathing, heart rate and tone should be re-assessed following the first five inflation breaths, then every 30 seconds during resuscitation, as the condition of the baby and the degree of resuscitation required will change. The heart rate should increase in response to adequate ventilation. A pulse oximeter probe should be applied if the baby requires more than a few inflation breaths and then the oxygen saturation reading also becomes part of the 30-second assessment. Note that in some countries, e.g. New Zealand, re-assessment does not occur until 30 seconds of effective ventilation has occurred.

Note that colour is not part of the formal assessment at present, as it can be misleading. It is not unusual for babies to have blue hands and feet and this should not be mistaken for cyanosis. Kattwinkel et al (2010) advise that skin colour is a very poor indicator of oxyhaemoglobin saturation following birth and the lack of cyanosis is also a poor indicator of oxygenation of an uncompromised baby. Additionally, the determination of colour is prone to substantial interobserver variability (O'Donnell 2012). Central cyanosis is noted by observing the mucous membranes inside the lips and gums. If there are concerns regarding the oxygenation of the baby a pulse oximeter should be used to assess the baby's oxygen saturation level.

Airway

If the baby cannot maintain his own airway, assistance must be given to keep the head in the neutral position.

Chin support

This is achieved by placing a finger under the tip of the chin, on the bone to support the chin upwards. Care must be taken to avoid pressure on the soft tissues as this may occlude the airway.

Jaw thrust

This is particularly helpful when the baby has little or no tone. The midwife places a finger at the angle of the jaw to push the lower jaw outwards and forwards. This may be undertaken as a double jaw thrust using a finger on both sides of the jaw. Two fingers can also be placed on the jaw and below the tip of the chin to assist with maintaining the forward, outward thrust of the jaw.

Use of oropharyngeal (Guedel) airway

If there continues to be difficulty maintaining the airway during resuscitation despite the use of chin support/jaw thrust, the baby has a facial or oral abnormality which makes this difficult (e.g. micrognathia) or the midwife is resuscitating the baby with no assistance, an oropharyngeal airway can be used which will maintain airway patency by keeping the tongue forwards.

It important to use the correct size of airway (0, 00, 000); size is assessed by placing the flange of the airway against the baby's philtrum and positioning the airway horizontally so the curved part of the airway curves around the baby's jaw. The correct size will end at the angle of the jaw. Alternatively, measure from the edge of the lips to the bottom of the earlobe. An airway that is too large may cause laryngospasm; one that is too small is ineffective and may worsen the airway obstruction (Johansen et al 2012).

The airway is inserted by opening the baby's mouth by depressing the chin and sliding the airway over the baby's tongue without pushing the tongue backwards. It should slide easily into position. If the tongue is obstructing insertion, use a laryngoscope or tongue depressor to gently press down on the tongue while inserting the airway.

433

Oropharyngeal suction

Occasionally, if the airway is not patent despite the above measures, a direct visual assessment should be undertaken using a laryngoscope. Oropharyngeal suction should only be undertaken by someone experienced with intubation and only when the area is clearly visualized and a blockage seen. It should be undertaken quickly, using a large-bore suction catheter which should not be passed more than 5 cm beyond the lips of a term baby and using a negative pressure not exceeding 100 mmHg (NZRC 2010b). Inadvertent stimulation of the posterior pharynx and larynx with the suction catheter can result in severe vagal bradycardia, quickly exacerbating the situation, as can suctioning of the nasopharynx (Kattwinkel et al 2010). Although meconium can cause tracheal obstruction, routine suctioning is not recommended for babies born through meconium-stained liquor.

Breathing

When the airway is patent, spontaneous breathing may follow. However, if respiratory effort is absent or inadequate, or the heart rate is <100 bpm (Japan Resuscitation Council 2010, NZRC 2010b) it is important to fill the lungs with air as quickly as possible to improve the oxygenation of the blood which will increase the heart rate and prevent further deterioration.

While there is no clear evidence indicating what the initial inflation time should be, the Resuscitation Council (UK) (2010) and Richmond & Wyllie (2010) recommend the first five inflation breaths should be given slowly over 2–3 seconds, suggesting this will help lung expansion. Once the alveoli have been inflated and the lung fluid replaced with air, surfactant will help to maintain the inflation, making subsequent breaths easier. As lung fluid is removed from the airways, chest expansion will be noted which may not be until the fourth or fifth inflation breath. Once there is chest expansion, ventilation breaths should be given at approximately 1 per second until adequate spontaneous breathing occurs.

If there is no chest movement, the most likely cause is either the baby's head is not in the neutral position or the facemask is not correctly positioned and sealed. Reposition the baby's head and/or the facemask and re-attempt chest inflation.

Use of oxygen in resuscitation

Since 2010, 'room air' containing 21% oxygen has been recommended as the gas of choice to initiate ventilation, prior to this 100% oxygen was used. It is now recognized that the administration of high concentrations of oxygen can damage hypoxic cells and tissues due to the production of free radicals and antioxidants (Richmond & Wyllie 2010, Vento et al 2009), contributing to brain injury in perinatal asphyxia (Kapadia et al 2013). These are often neutralized by the antioxidant defence system which develops towards the end of pregnancy; thus preterm babies <30 weeks' gestation are at increased risk from oxidative stress (Dawson et al 2009, Escrig et al 2008). Administration of 100% oxygen will cause a rapid increase in oxygen saturation levels which causes oxidative stress that can last for 4 weeks even in healthy term babies (Bhola et al 2012). Oxidative stress can damage the heart, lungs, brain and kidneys and result in a long-term pro-oxidant status (Vento & Saugstad 2011) and is thought to be an important factor in the pathogenesis of persistent pulmonary hypertension of the newborn (Lapointe & Barrington 2011) and bronchopulmonary dysplasia (Vento et al 2009). Hyperoxia reduces cerebral blood flow in both term and preterm babies even when 100% oxygen is administered for short periods (Davis et al 2004). For hypoxic babies, Bhola et al (2012) suggest that administering a high concentration of oxygen can delay cardiorespiratory recovery and may quadruple the risk of short-term mortality. Thus resuscitation is commenced using air and oxygen levels increased and then decreased according the response of the heart rate and or oxygenation (guided by pulse oximetry) (NZRC 2010b). O'Donnell (2012) suggests that preterm babies initially resuscitated with air frequently need supplemental oxygen to achieve the saturation targets initially but can be weaned off it quickly. Babies <32 weeks' gestation may not achieve the expected level of oxygen saturation in air. Rook et al (2014) recommend that in babies below this gestation, resuscitation should commence with 30% oxygen, while Davis & Dawson (2012) recommend a starting point of 21–30% oxygen. Escrig et al (2008) found that when babies <28 weeks' gestation are resuscitated with low levels of oxygen, they were more likely to be ventilated (if needed) in air rather than oxygen.

Blenders are now fitted to many resuscitaires to enable a blend of air and oxygen to be given. They have a supply of air and oxygen feeding into the blender box and a dial indicating the amount of oxygen that will be administered. The dial should be set at 21% at the beginning of the resuscitation. By turning the dial to the next number (e.g. 30%, increasing by 10% with each turn of the dial), the amount of oxygen can be increased in incremental stages according to the needs of the baby. The baby should be resuscitated with the lowest percentage of oxygen needed to maintain the heart rate above 100 bpm and oxygen saturation levels within the normal range for the age of the baby. When the oxygen percentage has been increased during resuscitation, it should be decreased when the heart rate is above 100 bpm and the oxygen saturation levels are within the normal range.

When the heart rate is above 100, there is no need to increase the amount of oxygen the baby is receiving. Below

60, the oxygen concentration should be increased to 100% for the duration of chest compressions. Saugstad (2012) advises that the ideal oxygen concentration for chest compressions is unknown; this recommendation may change with the future Neonatal Resuscitation guidelines. For babies where the heart rate is 60–100 and effective ventilations have been given for at least 30 seconds, the percentage of oxygen should be increased. The heart rate is re-assessed every 30 seconds and if it is still 60–100, the oxygen percentage is again increased. If it is above 100 bpm, consideration should be given to reducing the oxygen percentage, provided the oxygen saturation levels are normal.

Pulse oximetry

Oxygen saturation levels are assessed using a pulse oximeter and a neonatal probe applied to the right hand or wrist. This assesses the pre-ductal levels which may be 10–15% higher than post-ductal during the first 15 minutes of life (Vento & Saugstad 2011). This is a more accurate indicator of oxygen saturation than colour but may take 1–2 minutes to apply and work and may be unreliable if cardiac output or perfusion is very poor (Kattwinkel et al 2010). During the first 10 minutes of life, the oxygen saturation levels of the baby are lower than that of an adult, a term baby not requiring resuscitation takes a median time of 7.9 minutes to attain an oxygen saturation >90% (Harach 2013). Dawson et al (2012) advise it takes at least 5 minutes for the pre-ductal oxygen saturation to increase from 50–90% in term babies; this is slightly slower in preterm babies. For babies born by caesarean section (CS), Vento & Saugstad (2011) advise they will need approximately 2 minutes longer to achieve an oxygen saturation of 90% than those born vaginally. Zubarioglu et al (2011) suggest this is due to the retention of lung fluid. Reassuringly, Urlesberger et al (2011) found that although the transcutaneous oxygen saturation levels are lower initially for the baby born by CS, there is no difference in the oxygen saturation levels within the brain.

Kattwinkel et al (2010) recommend the use of pulse oximetry if positive pressure is being administered for more than a few breaths, when cyanosis is persistent, or when supplementary oxygen is administered. The machine should be switched on and the probe attached to the baby before the probe is connected to the pulse oximeter, as this facilitates the quickest acquisition of the signal. The probe should be shielded from light (Dawson et al 2012).

The Resuscitation Council (UK) state the acceptable pre-ductal SpO_2 is:

- 2 minutes 60%
- 3 minutes 70%
- 4 minutes 80%
- 5 minutes 85%
- 10 minutes 90%.

If the oxygen saturation is below the normal level for the age of the baby, the percentage of oxygen should be increased to the next amount. If it is above the normal level, and the heart rate is above 100 bpm, the oxygen percentage can usually be decreased.

When using a self-inflating bag-valve-mask (BVM) device that is not attached to a blender, it is still possible to vary the amount of oxygen administered to the baby. The resuscitation should commence with no oxygen or reservoir bag connected to the device – this will result in room air, 21% oxygen, being administered. If a higher percentage of oxygen is needed, the oxygen supply should be turned on – this provides 40–50% oxygen. Should a higher percentage of oxygen be required or chest compressions commenced, the oxygen remains on and the reservoir bag added to the device providing 90–100% oxygen. However, the concentration of oxygen delivered is affected by flow rate and whether the shutter valve is open (Thió et al 2014).

Facemask

The facemask has a deformable rim and should fit snugly around the baby's nose and mouth to form an airtight seal when even pressure is applied. It is important to use the correct size (00, 01) so the facemask does not extend into the eye sockets or over the chin, as it is difficult to achieve a good seal (Fig. 56.2). The facemask is attached either to a T-piece resuscitator or a self-inflating BVM system.

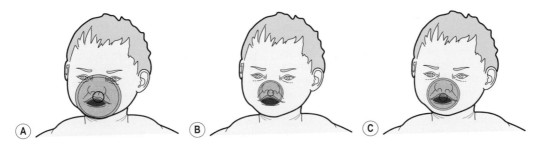

Figure 56.2 Correct positioning of the facemask. **A,** Facemask too large. **B,** Facemask too small. **C,** Facemask correct size.

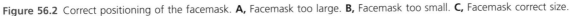

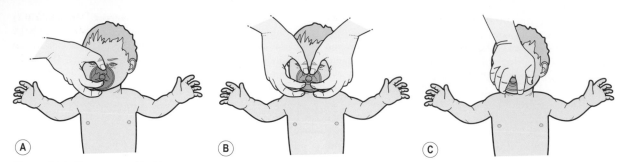

Figure 56.3 Three ways of holding the facemask in position. **A,** Two-point top hold. **B,** Two-handed hold. **C,** Spider hold.

Schilleman et al (2010) suggest the facemask is placed into position by gently rolling the facemask upwards onto the face from the tip of the chin. They caution against holding the stem and the fingers encroaching onto the rim of the facemask. When a good seal is obtained, there is minimal leak and if using a T-piece resuscitator, a high-pitched whistling sound is heard as air escapes through the positive end expiratory pressure (PEEP) valve.

There are thee methods to hold the mask in place (Wilson et al 2014) (Fig. 56.3):

1. Two-point top hold – The thumb and forefinger are placed either side of the mask on the firm surface and the remaining fingers support the jaw either with a chin lift or jaw thrust.
2. Two-handed hold – The same hold as above but using both hands. Tracy et al (2011) suggest this hold will halve mask leak by preventing deformation of the mask rim. A second person is required to occlude the T-piece or squeeze the bag.
3. Spider hold – The stem of the mask is placed between the index and middle fingers and pressure applied with the palm of the hand to hold the mask in place. The fingertips curl around the jaw to apply a chin lift. The fingers cover the face so visual cues from facial movements are not seen but may be felt. There may also be unrecognized compression of the eyes or nose causing airway obstruction and a more palpable leak.

Tracy et al (2011) suggest that a facemask connected to a T-piece resuscitator will have more mask leak on average than a facemask attached to a self-inflating bag due to the positive pressure being maintained throughout inspiration and expiration. Excessive pressure should be avoided, as this may cause facial bruising and may obstruct the airway (Schilleman et al 2010). Mask leak is a common cause of inadequate ventilation, as is excessive pressure, which can lead to variable and inadequate tidal volumes being administered (Schilleman et al 2010). Schmölzer et al (2011) caution that significant airway obstruction and mask leak occurs in about 50% of preterm babies <32 weeks' gestation

during the first couple of minutes of ventilation, which may be associated with putting on hats, placing in the bag, etc.

T-piece resuscitator

This is connected to a supply of compressed gas, ideally air and oxygen that can be blended to provide varying amounts of oxygen to the baby, and two pressure dials. One of the pressure dials is an outlet valve that sets the PEEP which controls the rate at which the gas escapes during expiration; the other is a variable release valve that limits the positive inspiratory pressure (PIP). These should be tested before use to ensure appropriate pressures are used. The gas flows into the T-piece, then into facemask (or endotracheal tube if intubated). The T-piece has an open end through which the gas can escape; this is covered during inspiration.

Positive end expiratory pressure

Providing PEEP is important for the development of the functional residual capacity, especially for the preterm baby (Dawson et al 2011). Morley et al (2010) suggest that failing to provide PEEP can lead to atelectrauma due to repetitive inflation and collapse of the terminal airways and alveoli. PEEP should be set at 5–8 cmH_2O and can be tested by removing the facemask, turning on the gas supply to 10 L, and occluding the open end of the T-piece that connects to the facemask. The dial should be adjusted until the PEEP is correct. High levels of PEEP, e.g. 8–12 cmH_2O, should be avoided, as it may result in reduced pulmonary blood flow and pneumothorax (NZRC 2010b).

Positive inspiratory pressure

PIP should be set at 30 cmH_2O for the term baby and 20–25 cmH_2O for the preterm baby, although at times higher pressures may be needed before chest movement is seen. The T-piece device reaches the target PIP more often than self-inflating bags (Dawson et al 2011). To test the PIP, remove the facemask, turn on the gas supply to 10 L, and occlude both open ends of the T-piece. Adjust the dial until the PIP is correct.

To inflate the lungs using a T-piece, occlude the open end with a thumb or finger for 2–3 seconds, then release if giving inflation breaths or occlude and release at a rate of 40–60 per minute for ventilation breaths allowing 0.3–0.5 seconds for inspiration.

Self-inflating bag–valve–mask (SIB)

The BVM system consists of a 240-mL bag, which is a flexible air chamber (manual resuscitator, Ambu bag) connected to a shutter valve (this allows gases to pass from the air chamber to the facemask but is one-way so expired gases do not pass back into the air chamber), which, in turn, connects to the facemask. A pressure-relief valve, set at 40 cmH$_2$O, prevents excessive pressure being used when the bag is squeezed but the valve can activate at inconsistent and wide-ranging pressures; it can be overridden should a higher pressure be needed (NZRC 2010b). There is a detachable reservoir bag and a connector for air/oxygen tubing to be fed into the air chamber. When the bag is squeezed, air is forced out through the facemask and when the bag is released, it self-inflates either by drawing in ambient air or by drawing from the connected gas supply They are the most frequently used devices for manual ventilation, particularly in resource-poor countries (Hartung et al 2013) and should always be available in case there is failure of the compressed gas supply. Dawson et al (2011) suggest fitting these devices with PEEP valves in these countries and where a reliable gas supply is not available, although Hartung et al (2013) advise that these provide lower pressures than the set PEEP on the T-piece resuscitator. Such PEEP valves are reusable when thermo-sterilized but repeated sterilization can result in insufficient PEEP being generated; hence it is important to test the valves prior to use (Hartung et al 2013). Mask leak can be exacerbated when using a PEEP valve because of the increased pressure within the mask during expiration as well as inspiration (Morley et al 2010).

The pressure-relief valve should be tested prior to use by occluding the outlet and squeezing the bag. As the pressure increases, the valve will make a noise to confirm it is working and safe for use. This valve is often called the 'pop-off' or 'blow-off' valve. If no noise is heard, check the valve to ensure it has not become fixed.

Davis & Dawson (2012) and Kelm et al (2012) caution that SIBs produce highly variable, operator-dependent PIP and tidal volumes, as they usually do not have a pressure-monitoring device. Bassani et al (2012) agree, suggesting these variations are frequently insufficient or excessive for neonatal resuscitation and that both PIP and tidal volume increase when more fingers are used to squeeze the bag. Kelm et al (2012) suggest where these are excessive, they

may contribute to lung disease. Davis & Dawson (2012) recognize that the volume of gas administered is more important than the pressure used for effective ventilation and advise that low volumes result in inadequate ventilation which worsens if there are leaks around the facemask. Tracy et al (2011) warn that twice the tidal volume (10 mL/kg) can be delivered compared to the T-piece 'neopuff' (5 mL/kg), which has the potential to damage the lungs.

Mouth to mouth-and-nose ventilation

Mouth to mouth-and-nose ventilation can be used if there is no equipment available. Keeping the baby's head in the neutral position, the baby's mouth and nose are sealed with the midwife's mouth and air from the midwife's cheeks is gently breathed into the lungs to provide inflation and then ventilation breaths.

Circulation

The heart rate is assessed prior to commencing resuscitation and then every 30 seconds. If during the subsequent assessments the heart rate is <60 bpm (with adequate ventilation), chest compressions should commence at a rate of 120 per minute, approximately 2 per second. A ratio of 3 compressions to 1 ventilation is used which will approximate 90 compressions and 30 breaths per minute. When the heart rate is >60 bpm, chest compressions are stopped. Schilleman et al (2010) advise that chest compressions are rarely needed during resuscitation and suggest it is often secondary to improper ventilation. Binder et al (2014) agree that adequate positive pressure ventilation is the single most important procedure during resuscitation; thus it is important the baby has received 30 seconds of effective ventilation before chest compressions are commenced (Finan et al 2011, Japan Resuscitation Council 2010, Kattwinkel et al 2010, NZRC 2010c). However, the European Resuscitation Council (Richmond & Wyllie 2010) and the Resuscitation Council (UK) (2010) both recommend that the heart rate is re-assessed after the five inflation breaths and if it is <60 bpm, chest compressions should commence if there has been chest movement. It is important for the midwife to be aware of the differences that occur between different countries as to whether to assess the heart rate after the first five inflation breaths or following 30 seconds of ventilation.

The aim of chest compression is to circulate oxygenated blood to the heart and brain. However, Martin et al (2013) suggest that effective closed chest compressions achieve only 50% of cerebral and 15–25% of coronary baseline blood flow levels. It is important to consider the depth and rate of compressions and the chest release force, as one or both of these undertaken ineffectively will reduce the effectiveness of compressions (Martin et al 2013). If the chest is not released completely, higher intrathoracic pressures result; a prolonged compression combined with increased rates results in inadequate chest wall relaxation. Both of these impede venous return to the heart, lowering cardiac output, cerebral blood flow and perfusion pressures (Martin et al 2013).

Two-handed technique

This is the most effective method of chest compression as greater depth is achieved and higher peak systolic and coronary perfusion pressures are generated compared with the two-finger technique (Huynh et al 2012, Kattwinkel et al 2010, Martin et al 2013). Place the pads of both thumbs side by side or on top of each other (depending on the size of the baby and thumbs) on the lower third of the sternum (above the xiphisternum and just below the nipple line) (Fig. 56.4) with the fingers encircling the baby, supporting the back (it is not necessary for the hands to meet behind the baby). The chest is compressed firmly to a depth of one-third of the anteroposterior diameter (1–2 cm) and then released to allow blood to flow into the heart. It is important to keep the thumbs together and ensure only the sternum is compressed to avoid pressure on the soft tissues and ribs, as this will result in ineffective chest compression and has a risk of damage which can exacerbate the situation.

Two-finger technique

This should only be used if the midwife is resuscitating a baby on her own as it is less effective. The fingertips of the index and middle fingers are placed on the lower third of the sternum (above the xiphisternum and just below the nipple line) (Fig. 56.5). Christman et al (2011) found that using the pads of the fingers instead of the tips resulted in less effective compressions. The other hand can support the baby's back if it is not holding the facemask in position. The chest is compressed and released as for the two-handed technique. Kattwinkel et al (2010) suggest this technique may be preferable when access to the umbilicus is needed to insert an umbilical catheter.

If the heart rate does not improve despite adequate ventilation and compression, drug therapy and transfer to a high-dependency unit may be required.

Drug therapy

Fortunately, drugs are rarely required during neonatal resuscitation, Lee et al (2011) suggest the rate is 0.05% and the prescription and administration is the responsibility of the paediatrician. The preferred route of administration is via an umbilical venous catheter. Adrenaline (epinephrine) 1 : 10 000, 10–30 mcg/kg, may be given to increase the heart rate. Fluids may be administered if there is suspected blood loss or the baby appears shocked and has not responded to the resuscitative measures used. Richmond & Wyllie (2010) suggest using a 10 mL/kg bolus of irradiated, leucocyte-depleted group O Rhesus-negative blood or isotonic crystalloids to restore the intravascular volume. Care must be taken to administer volume expanders slowly to

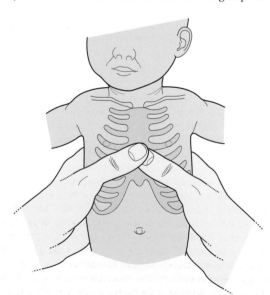

Figure 56.4 Two-handed chest compression.

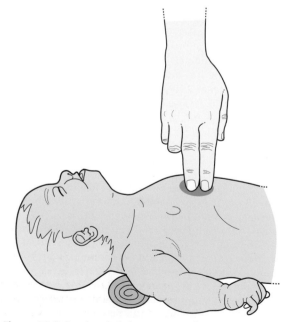

Figure 56.5 One-handed chest compression.

preterm babies, as Kattwinkel et al (2010) caution that rapid infusions of large volume have been associated with intraventricular haemorrhage.

AFTER THE RESUSCITATION

Following a successful resuscitation, the baby will either remain with his parents or, if unwell, be transferred to the neonatal intensive care unit. Both body temperature and blood glucose levels should be monitored as the baby may not be able to maintain these. Early feeding is essential due to the use of glucose during anaerobic respiration. The parents will need support and information to understand what has occurred and to appreciate whether any further concerns exist. The midwife will document the resuscitation details including the time the emergency call was made, when and who arrived, time of onset of respiration, nature of resuscitation, drugs administered and personnel present. For babies who develop moderate to severe hypoxic-ischaemic encephalopathy, there is increasing evidence that therapeutic hypothermia for babies over 36 weeks' gestation reduces the risk of death and neuro-developmental disability at 18 months (Richmond & Wyllie 2010).

Local protocols will vary on when to halt the resuscitation if it is unsuccessful, but the paediatrician will consider making the decision usually when there has been no detectable heart rate for 10 minutes despite full resuscitation support (Finan et al 2011). Considerable care of the parents and the staff involved will be required. A debriefing with staff involved in the delivery and resuscitation can be helpful.

PROCEDURE: neonatal resuscitation (UK)

- Check the resuscitaire prior to delivery; when birth is imminent, switch on the heater and light.
- Dry and stimulate the baby at birth and assess the need for resuscitation.
- Move the baby to the resuscitation area and turn on the clock (if not on), noting the time.
- Dry and stimulate the baby thoroughly, remove the damp towel; wrap in a clean warm towel, with the chest exposed.
- Position the baby's head in the neutral position.
- Assess breathing, tone and heart rate (these are reassessed every 30 seconds):
  - breathing spontaneously, heart rate >100 bpm – keep the baby warm and return him to his parents for skin-to-skin contact

- breathing irregularly with a heart rate >100 bpm – provide tactile stimulation, keep the baby warm and the head in the neutral position. Continue to assess tone, respiratory effort and heart rate, returning the baby to his parents when breathing spontaneously and heart rate >100 bpm
  - no respiratory effort or breathing remains irregular or heart rate <100 bpm – commence resuscitation.
- Send out an emergency call for appropriate personnel (if an anticipated problem the paediatrician should already be present).
- Ensure the baby's head is in the neutral position with an open airway, using chin support, jaw thrust or an oropharyngeal airway as necessary.
- Inflate the lungs using a facemask and T-piece or BVM system with 21% oxygen, providing five effective inflation breaths over 2–3 seconds and looking for chest movement. If no chest movement is seen, check head and mask position and repeat inflation breaths.
- Following the inflation breaths when chest movement seen, assess the heart rate:
  - heart rate >100 bpm – continue with ventilation breaths until spontaneous respiration occurs. Reassess breathing, heart rate and tone every 30 seconds. (Note that in some countries, e.g. New Zealand, the heart rate is not rechecked until 30 seconds of effective ventilation has been provided and will increase oxygen levels if it is <100 bpm)
  - heart rate <60 bpm – commence chest compressions at a rate of 3 : 1 with each cycle lasting two seconds, using 100% oxygen. Re-assess breathing, heart rate and tone every 30 seconds. When the heart rate is ≥60 bpm, stop chest compressions but continue with ventilation breaths until spontaneous respiration occurs with the heart rate >100 bpm.
- Secure a neonatal oxygen saturation probe on the baby's right hand or wrist as soon as possible then include saturation levels in the 30-second assessments:
  - if oxygen saturation levels are below the target level for the age of the baby, increase the amount of oxygen to the next level, e.g. from 21% to 30%
  - once the oxygen saturation level is reached, begin to reduce the amount of oxygen given.
- If the condition of the baby does not improve, the paediatrician will consider venous access and drugs.
- Document the procedure in the baby's notes.
- Discuss the resuscitation with the parents.

ROLE AND RESPONSIBILITIES OF THE MIDWIFE

These can be summarized as:

- ensuring knowledge around resuscitation and resuscitation guidelines is current
- maintaining competent resuscitation skills, including correct use of equipment
- anticipating the need for resuscitation and preparation of the environment and equipment
- undertaking the assessment at birth and recognizing the need for resuscitation
- summoning appropriate medical/newborn life support (NLS) trained assistance if not present
- supporting and assisting others during the resuscitation
- accurate contemporaneous record keeping
- information for, and support of, the parents during and following the event
- appropriate transfer of the care of the woman and baby.

SUMMARY

- The midwife has a responsible role in the recognition and management of neonatal resuscitation.
- Equipment should be accessible and the midwife should be familiar with its use.
- Appropriate help should be sought quickly.
- Management includes drying the baby (>28 weeks' gestation) and assessing tone, respiratory effort and heart rate.
- A baby <28 weeks' gestation should not be dried but wrapped in a polyethylene bag/sheet to maintain his temperature.
- A neonatal oxygen saturation probe should be applied to the baby's right hand or wrist as soon as possible.
- Resuscitation should begin in room air and the oxygen level increased according to the oxygen saturation level and the requirement for chest compressions.
- Cardiac compressions using the two-handed technique is undertaken if the heart rate is below 60 bpm once the lungs have been oxygenated.
- During the first 10 minutes of life, the baby has lower acceptable pre-ductal oxygen saturation levels.
- Colour is not a reliable indicator of oxygenation.
- Manoeuvres to open the airway and ventilate the lungs and chest compression should be undertaken efficiently when required.
- Routine oropharyngeal suctioning is not recommended.
- Drug therapy may be required when the response is poor.

SELF-ASSESSMENT EXERCISES

The answers to the following questions may be found in the text:

1. Identify five situations in which you would anticipate the need for neonatal resuscitation.
2. List the equipment required for neonatal resuscitation, indicating how each piece is used.
3. What would you assess in the baby at birth to determine if resuscitation is required?
4. How can the midwife ensure the baby's airway is patent?
5. What percentage of oxygen would you use to begin resuscitation?
6. When would you increase the amount of oxygen?
7. What would you do differently for a baby <28 weeks' gestation?
8. When would you undertake oropharyngeal suctioning?
9. When are chest compressions required and how are they undertaken?
10. Demonstrate/simulate a neonatal resuscitation, giving verbal explanations for the actions taken.

REFERENCES

Amin, H.J., Aziz, K., Halamer, L.P., Beran, T.N., 2013. Simulation-based learning combined with debriefing: trainers' satisfaction with a new approach to training the trainers to teach neonatal resuscitation. BMC Res. Notes 6, 251.

Bassani, M.A., Filho, F.M., de Carvalho Coppo, M.R., Martins Marba, S.T., 2012. An evaluation of peak inspiratory pressure, tidal volume and ventilator frequency during ventilation with a neonatal self-inflating bag resuscitator. Respir. Care 57 (4), 525–530.

Beşkardeş, A., Salihoğlu, Ö., Can, E., et al, 2012. Oxygen saturation of healthy term neonates during the first 30 minutes of life. Pediatr. Int. 55, 44–48.

Bhola, K., Lui, K., Oei, J.L., 2012. Use of oxygen for delivery room and neonatal resuscitation in non-tertiary Australian and New Zealand hospitals: a survey of current practices, opinions and equipment. J. Paediatr. Child Health 48, 828–832.

Binder, C., Schmölzer, G.M., O'Reilly, M., et al, 2014. Human or monitor feedback to improve mask ventilation during simulated neonatal cardiopulmonary resuscitation. Arch. Dis. Child. Fetal Neonatal Ed. 99, F120–F123.

Christman, C., Hemway, R.J., Wyckoff, M.H., Perlman, J.M., 2011. The two-thumb is superior to the two-finger method for administering chest compressions in a manikin model of neonatal resuscitation. Arch. Dis. Child. Fetal Neonatal Ed. 96, F99–F101.

Cusack, J., Fawke, J., 2012. Neonatal resuscitation: are your trainees performing as you think they are? A retrospective assessment for neonatal medical trainees over an 8-year period. Arch. Dis. Child. Fetal Neonatal Ed. 97, F246–F248.

Davis, P.G., Dawson, J.A., 2012. New concepts in neonatal resuscitation. Curr. Opin. Pediatr. 24, 147–153.

Davis, P.G., Tan, A., O'Donnell, C.P.F., Schulze, A , 2004. Resuscitation of newborn infants with 100% oxygen or air: a systematic review and meta-analysis. The Lancet 364, 1329–1333.

Dawson, J.A., Kamlin, C.O.F., Wong, C., et al, 2009. Oxygen saturation and heart rate during delivery room resuscitation of infants <30 weeks gestation with room air or 100% oxygen. Arch. Dis. Child. Fetal Neonatal Ed. 94, F87–F91.

Dawson, J.A., Kamlin, C.O.F., Wong, C., et al, 2010. Changes in heart rate in the first minutes after birth. Arch. Dis. Child. Fetal Neonatal Ed. 95, F177–F181.

Dawson, J.A., Gerber, A., Kamlin, C.O.F., et al, 2011. Providing PEEP during neonatal resuscitation: which device is best? J. Paediatr. Child Health 47, 698–703.

Dawson, J.A., Vento, M., Finer, N.N., et al, 2012. Managing oxygen therapy during delivery room stabilization of preterm infants. J. Pediatr. 160 (1), 158–161.

Escrig, R., Arruza, L., Izquierdo, I., et al, 2008. Achievement of targeted saturation values in extremely low gestational age neonates resuscitated with low or high oxygen concentrations. a prospective randomized trial. Pediatrics 121 (5), 875–881.

Finan, E., Aylward, D., Aziz, K., 2011. Neonatal resuscitation guidelines update: a case-based review. Paediatr. Child Health 16 (5), 289–291.

Harach, T., 2013. Room air resuscitation and targeted oxygenation for infants at birth in the delivery room. J. Obstet. Gynecol. Neonatal Nurs. 42, 227–232.

Hartung, J.C., Schmölzer, G., Schmalisch, G., Roehr, C.C., 2013. Repeated thermo-sterilisation further affects the reliability of positive end-expiratory pressure valves. J. Paediatr. Child Health 49, 741–745.

Huynh, T.K., Hemway, R.J., Perlman, J.M., 2012. The two-thumb technique using an elevated surface is preferable for teaching infant cardiopulmonary resuscitation. J. Pediatr. 161 (4), 658–661.

Japan Resuscitation Council, 2010. Ch. 4 NCPR; Neonatal Cardiopulmonary Resuscitation. Available online: <http://jrc.umin.ac.jp/pdf/20121011_NCPR.pdf> (accessed 3 March 2015).

Johansen, L.C., Mupanemunda, R.H., Danha, R.F., 2012. Managing the newborn infant with a difficult airway. Infant 8 (4), 116–119.

Kamlin, C.O.F., Dawson, J.A., O'Donnell, C.P.F., et al, 2008. Accuracy of pulse oximetry measurement of heart rate of newborn infants in the delivery room. J. Pediatr. 152, 756–760.

Kapadia, V.S., Chalak, L.K., DuPont, T.L., et al, 2013. Perinatal asphyxia with hyperoxemia within the first hour of life is associated with moderate to severe hypoxic ischemic encephalopathy. J. Pediatr. 163 (4), 949–954.

Katheria, A., Rich, W., Finer, N., 2012. Electrocardiogram provides a continuous heart rate faster than oximetry during neonatal resuscitation. Pediatrics 130, e1177–e1181.

Kattwinkel, J., Perlman, J.M., Aziz, K., et al, 2010. Part 15: neonatal resuscitation: 2010 American Heart Association Guidelines for Cardiopulmonary Resuscitation and Emergency Cardiovascular Care. Circulation 122 (Suppl.), S909–S919.

Kelm, M., Dold, S.K., Hartung, J., et al, 2012. Manual neonatal ventilation training: a respiratory function monitor helps to reduce peak inspiratory pressures and tidal volumes during resuscitation. J. Perinat. Med. 40, 583–586.

Lapointe, A., Barrington, K.J., 2011. Pulmonary hypertension and the asphyxiated newborn. J. Pediatr. 158 (Suppl. 2), e19–e24.

Lee, A.C.C., Cousens, S., Wall, S.N., et al, 2011. Neonatal resuscitation and immediate newborn assessment and simulation for the prevention of neonatal deaths: a systematic review, meta-analysis and Delphi estimation of mortality effect. BMC Public Health 11 (Suppl. 3), S12.

Martin, P.S., Kemp, A.M., Theobald, P.S., et al, 2013. Do chest compressions during simulated infant CPR comply with international recommendations? Arch. Dis. Child. Fetal Neonatal Ed. 98, F576–F581.

Mizumoto, H., Tomotaki, S., Shibata, H., et al, 2012. Electrocardiogram shows reliable heart rates much earlier than pulse oximetry during neonatal resuscitation. Pediatr. Int. 54, 205–207.

Morley, C.J., Dawson, J.A., Stewart, M.J., et al, 2010. The effect of PEEP valve on a Laerdal neonatal self-inflating resuscitation bag. J. Paediatr. Child Health 46, 51–56.

Murilaa, F., Obimbo, M.M., Musoke, R., 2012. Assessment of knowledge on neonatal resuscitation amongst healthcare providers in Kenya. Pan Afr. Med. J. 11, 78. Available online: <www.panafrican-med-journal.com/content/article/11/78/full/> (accessed 3 March 2015).

Niermeyer, S., Clarke, S.B., 2011. Delivery room care. In: Gardner, S.L., Carter, B.S., Enzman-Hines, M., Hernandez, J.A. (Eds.), Merenstein & Gardner's Handbook of Neonatal Intensive Care, seventh ed. St. Louis, Mosby, pp. 52–77 (Chapter 4).

NZRC (New Zealand Resuscitation Council), 2010a. Neonatal Resuscitation Guideline 13.3 – Assessment of the Newborn Infant. Available online: <http://www.nzrc

.org.nz/assets/Uploads/Guidelines/guideline-13-3dec10.pdf> (accessed 3 March 2015).

NZRC (New Zealand Resuscitation Council), 2010b. Neonatal Resuscitation Guideline 13.4 – Airway Management and Mask Ventilation of the Newborn Infant. Available online: <http://www.nzrc.org.nz/assets/Uploads/Guidelines/guideline-13-6dec10.pdf> (accessed 3 March 2015).

NZRC (New Zealand Resuscitation Council), 2010c. Neonatal Resuscitation Guideline 13.6 – Chest Compressions during Resuscitation of the Newborn Infant. Available online: <http://www.nzrc.org.nz/assets/Uploads/Guidelines/guideline-13-4dec10.pdf> (accessed 3 March 2015).

O'Donnell, C.P.F., 2012. Turn and face the strange ..ch..ch..ch..changes to neonatal resuscitation guidelines in the past decade. J. Paediatr. Child Health 48, 735–739.

Resuscitation Council (UK), 2010. Newborn life support. Available online: <https://www.resus.org.uk/pages/nls.pdf> (accessed 3 March 2015).

Richmond, S., Wyllie, J., 2010. European Resuscitation Council Guideline for Resuscitation 2010 Section 7. Resuscitation of babies at birth. Resuscitation 81, 1389–1399.

Rohana, J., Khairina, W., Boo, N.Y., Shareena, I., 2011. Reducing hypothermia in preterm infants with polyethylene wrap. Pediatr. Int. 53, 468–474.

Rook, D., Schierbeek, H., Vento, M., et al, 2014. Resuscitation of preterm infants with different inspired oxygen fractions. J. Pediatr. 164 (6), 1322–1326.

Rovamo, L.M., Mattila, M.-M., Andersson, S., Rosenberg, P.H., 2013. Testing of midwife neonatal resuscitation skills with a simulator manikin in a low-risk delivery unit. Pediatr. Int. 55, 465–471.

Saugstad, O.D., 2012. Hyperoxia in the term newborn: more evidence is still needed for optimal oxygen therapy. Acta Paediatr. 101 (Suppl. 464), 34–38.

Sawyer, T., Laubach, V.A., Hudak, J., et al, 2013. Improvements in teamwork during neonatal resuscitation after interprofessional team STEPPS training. Neonatal Netw. 32 (1), 26–33.

Schilleman, K., Witlox, R.S., Lopriore, E., et al, 2010. Leak and obstruction with mask ventilation during simulated neonatal resuscitation. Arch. Dis. Child. Fetal Neonatal Ed. 95, F398–F402.

Schmölzer, G.M., Dawson, J.A., Kamlin, C.O.F., et al, 2011. Airway obstruction and gas leak during mask ventilation of preterm infants in the delivery room. Arch. Dis. Child. Fetal Neonatal Ed. 96, F254–F257.

Thió, M., Bhatia, R., Dawson, J.A., Davis, P.G., 2010. Oxygen delivery using neonatal self-inflating resuscitation bags without a reservoir. Arch. Dis. Child. Fetal Neonatal Ed. 95, F315–F319.

Tracy, M.B., Klimek, J., Coughtrey, H., et al, 2011. Mask leak in one-person mask ventilation compared to two-person in newborn infant manikin study. Arch. Dis. Child. Fetal Neonatal Ed. 96, F195–F200.

Urlesberger, B., Kratky, E., Rehak, T., et al, 2011. Regional oxygen saturation of the brain during birth transition of term infants: comparison between elective cesarean section and vaginal deliveries. J. Pediatr. 159 (3), 404–408.

van Vonderen, J.J., Hooper, S.B., Kroese, J.K., et al, 2015. Pulse oximetry measures a lower heart rate at birth compared with electrocardiography. J. Pediatr. 166, 49–53.

Vento, M., Moro, M., Escrig, R., et al, 2009. Preterm resuscitation with low oxygen causes less oxidative stress, inflammation and chronic lung disease. Pediatrics 124 (3), e439–e449.

Vento, M., Saugstad, O.D., 2011. Oxygen supplementation in the delivery room: Updated information. J. Pediatr. 158 (Suppl. 2), e5–e7.

Wilson, E.V., O'Shea, J.E., Thio, M., et al, 2014. A comparison of different mask holds for positive pressure ventilation in a neonatal manikin. Arch. Dis. Child. Fetal Neonatal Ed. 99, F169–F171.

Zubarioglu, U., Uslu, S., Can, E., et al, 2011. Oxygen saturation levels during the first minutes of life in healthy term neonates. Tohoku J. Exp. Med. 224, 273–279.

Glossary

Abduction Movement away from the midline of the body.

Adduction Movement towards the midline of the body.

Agglutination Clumping together.

Aortocaval occlusion Occlusion of the inferior vena cava and aorta by the pregnant uterus. Tends to occur if a heavily pregnant woman is asked to lie flat. Avoided by adopting a lateral position or using a wedge under the right hip. Also known as supine hypotension.

Apical The apex of the heart.

Apnoea Absence of respiration for >20 seconds.

Atelectrauma Damage to the alveoli from transient and repeated collapse and inflation during respiration.

Bacteriuria The presence of bacteria in the urine.

Bilirubinuria The presence of bilirubin in the urine.

Biparietal diameter The distance between the parietal eminences, usually 9.5 cm in the term baby. This is the widest transverse diameter of the fetal skull to pass through the pelvic brim (during engagement) and to distend the perineum (during crowning).

Bishop's Score A scoring assessment used to assess the favourability (or ripeness) of the cervix prior to induction of labour. Considers the position, consistency, length and dilatation of the cervix and station of the presenting part within the pelvis. Each factor is awarded a score accordingly; the dose of Prostin may be adjusted according to the total score. A Bishop's Score of 6 or more considers the cervix to be favourable.

BFI Baby Friendly Initiative, the UK Baby Friendly Initiative is based on a global accreditation programme of UNICEF and the World Health Organization. It is designed to support breastfeeding and parent–infant relationships by working with public services to improve standards of care.

Blanching Colour changes in the skin with fingertip pressure, turning the skin white. The colour should quickly return to normal as capillary refill occurs.

Bradycardia A slow heart rate, <60 bpm for an adult, <100 for a baby.

Caput succedaneum An oedematous swelling between the scalp and the periosteum which develops during labour as a result of pressure between the presenting part and the cervix or the perineum. It pits on pressure, crosses suture lines, and will decrease in size following birth.

Commensal An organism that lives on or within another organism, and derives benefit without harming or benefiting the host.

Constipation Infrequent or difficult defaecation resulting from decreased motility of the intestines, which results in faeces remaining in the colon for prolonged periods. This extended time in the colon means that greater than usual amounts of water are absorbed, making the faeces hard and dry. Constipation can be caused by improper bowel habits, spasms of the colon, insufficient bulk in the diet, lack of exercise, and emotions.

Cyanosis Bluish appearance of skin and mucous membranes caused by reduced oxygenation.

Cystocele Bulging of the bladder into the upper part of the anterior vaginal wall.

Denominator The leading part of the fetus, likely to meet the pelvic floor first. For a flexed vertex presentation it is the occiput, for the buttocks it is the sacrum.

Desiccation Extreme dryness or the process of extreme drying.

Diarrhoea Frequent defaecation of liquid faeces caused by increased motility of the intestines. There is not enough time for absorption and it can lead to dehydration and electrolyte imbalance. Diarrhoea has several causes, e.g. infection, stress. Diarrhoea overflow may also occur in the presence of constipation.

Diplopia Double vision.

Diuresis Increased formation and excretion of urine.

Dysuria Difficult or painful micturition.

Erythema Redness.

Erythema toxicum A blotchy red rash, sometimes with yellowish pinhead papules, which occurs usually between days 2 and 8 of age. Cause unknown, no treatment required.

Extravasation Escape of fluid from the vessels into the surrounding tissues.

Extubation Removal of the tube inserted during intubation.

Feeding cues The signs visible in neonates that demonstrate hunger and a readiness to feed (rapid eye movement, turning of head, searching with the mouth, bringing of hand to mouth, sucking hand and fist, moving arms and legs). Late cue: crying.

Fetal lie Relation of the long axis of the fetus to the long axis of the uterus. Where the two are parallel, it is a longitudinal lie. Variations include transverse or oblique.

Fetal pole An extremity or end, e.g. skull or buttocks (when in flexed position).

Fetal position The relation of the denominator on the fetus to a landmark on the fetal pelvis, e.g. occiput facing the left iliopectineal eminence equates to left occipitoanterior (LOA).

Fetal presentation The part of the fetus which is lying in the lower part of the uterus over the cervical os and would therefore 'present' first. Usually head or buttocks but could be face, brow, shoulder, hand, knee or foot.

Fever A cause of hyperthermia, produced in response to the presence of pyrogens in the blood.

Fistula An abnormal connection between two hollow organs or between a hollow organ and the body surface.

Functional residual capacity This is the volume of air remaining in the lungs at the end of passive expiration.

Haematuria The presence of blood in the urine.

Haemorrhoids Varicosities of the rectal vein. Can occur as a result of chronic repetitive straining to defaecate, resulting in enlargement of the venous plexuses.

Helminth Parasitic worm.

Hydronephrosis A collection of urine in the pelvis of the kidney.

Hydroureter Blockage in the ureter causing distension.

Hyperacusia Abnormal acuteness of hearing due to increased irritability

of the sensory neural mechanism; characterized by intolerance for ordinary sound levels.

Hypercapnia An abnormally high level of carbon dioxide in the blood.

Hyperthermia An increase in the core body temperature to >37.5°C. Also referred to as pyrexia: low-grade pyrexia is classified as a temperature up to 38°C, a moderate to high pyrexia is 38–40°C and hyperpyrexia is an excessively high temperature >40°C.

Hyperventilation Increased rate and depth of respiration that results in low carbon dioxide levels in the blood.

Hypoglycaemia A lowered level of glucose in the blood.

Hypothermia A decrease in the core body temperature to 35°C or below.

Hypoventilation Slow or shallow breathing that results in an excess of carbon dioxide and reduced levels of oxygen in the blood.

Hypovolaemia A reduction in the circulating blood volume.

Hypoxaemia Low level of oxygen in the blood.

Induration An area of localized oedema under the skin, often occurring with abnormal reactive hyperaemia.

Intrathecal Within the meninges of the spinal cord.

Intubation The introduction of a tube into part of the body, e.g. for anaesthesia – introduction of an endotracheal tube into the trachea.

IVF In vitro fertilization, fertilization of an egg in an artificial environment, i.e. outside of the body.

Laxative A medicine that helps loosen the contents of the bowel and encourages evacuation. Those with a mild action are referred to as aperients; those with a stronger action are called purgatives.

Meatus Opening or passageway, commonly used when talking about the female urethral opening.

Micrognathia A receding jaw.

Milia Blocked sebaceous glands that appear as small white spots over the nose and cheeks.

Nocturia Excessive urination at night.

Observer bias Can occur when the previous findings are known and the observer subjectively alters their current findings, e.g. looking at a woman's previous blood pressure reading and expecting the current reading to be very similar.

Occiput The back of the head.

Oliguria Diminished capacity to form urine. In the baby, this is a urine output of less than 0.5 mL/kg/hour after 48 hours of age.

Orthopnoea Dyspnoea that is aggravated by lying flat.

Oxytocin A hormone released by the posterior lobe of the pituitary gland, responsible for contraction of the myometrium and epithelial cells within the breast and uterus. Produced synthetically as Syntocinon.

PaCO$_2$ The partial pressure (amount) of carbon dioxide dissolved in arterial blood.

PaO$_2$ The partial pressure (amount) of oxygen dissolved in arterial blood.

Parenterally Administered by any route other than through the mouth.

Paronychia A staphylococcal infection of the nail bed, often associated with hangnails.

Pharmacokinetics The way the body affects the drug, e.g. absorption, distribution, metabolism and excretion.

Philtrum The vertical groove, or medial cleft, in the middle area of the upper lip.

Phimosis A condition in which the foreskin is retracted back from the glans penis and becomes obstructed, causing swelling and pain.

Phlebitis Inflammation of a vein.

Photophobia An abnormal sensitivity to light.

Polydactyly Extra fingers or toes.

Polyuria Voiding large amounts of urine.

Postural hypotension Lowering of blood pressure occurring during a change of position from sitting to standing, or lying to upright. Frequently accompanied by dizziness and light-headedness, and sometimes syncope.

Proteinuria The presence of protein in the urine.

Pruritus Itching caused by localized irritation of the skin, nervous disorders, infection, e.g. fungal infection of the vulva, haemorrhoids, intestinal worms and some forms of jaundice.

Rectocele A prolapse of the lower posterior vaginal wall.

Rigors Uncontrollable, involuntary episodes of intense shivering during which the temperature rises rapidly and then decreases after a short period. Often associated with the presence of bacteria or toxins within the blood, it may occur with severe cases of pyelonephritis in pregnancy.

SaO$_2$ The amount of oxygen bound to haemoglobin in arterial blood.

SpO$_2$ The SaO$_2$ measured using pulse oximetry.

Shoulder dystocia Occurs when the normal mechanism of labour stops as the shoulders attempt to enter the pelvic brim but are unable to do so. Occurs with pelvic abnormalities reducing the pelvic diameters or increased bisacromial diameter (distance between the shoulders). This may be due to one (unilateral dystocia) or both (bilateral dystocia) shoulders becoming impacted.

Sternal recession Occurs when the alveoli fail to remain inflated and the compliant chest wall begins to collapse around the stiff lungs. The sternum is seen to recess in, rather than expand out, with breathing movements.

Stress incontinence As a result of reduced control of the internal and external sphincter, involuntary voiding of small amounts of urine occurs when the intra-abdominal pressure increases, e.g. during bouts of coughing, laughing or sneezing.

Subinvolution The uterus is involuting at a slower rate than expected or remains at the same size for several days. This may be due to the presence of retained products of conception, blood clots within the uterus, uterine fibroids or infection. It predisposes to postpartum haemorrhage and is considered a deviation from normal.

Surfactant A phospholipid present in the lungs of the mature newborn that reduces surface tension in the alveoli permitting the lungs to expand and the alveoli to remain inflated.

Syndactyly Webbing between the fingers or toes.

Tachycardia A fast heart rate, >100 bpm for an adult, >160 bpm for a baby.

Tachypnoea Abnormally rapid rate of breathing, >20 per minute for an adult, >60 for a baby.

Terminal digit preference Occurs when a person recording blood pressure rounds the measurement to a digit of their preference, most commonly zero.

Tetany Intermittent tonic contractions and muscular pain caused by abnormal calcium metabolism.

Threshold avoidance Occurs when the blood pressure is recorded as being lower than the threshold for implementing treatment, when the actual measurement is at or above that level.

Thrombophlebitis Inflammation of a vein with clot formation.

Tinnitus Ringing sound in the ears.

Tonicity The relative concentration of solutions that determine the direction and extent of diffusion.

Torticollis Congenital muscular torticollis occurs when the sternomastoid muscle is shortened or tightened on one side.

Transfusion-related acute lung injury (TRALI) Antibodies in the donor blood react with the host's neutrophils. Inflammatory cells cause leakage of plasma into lung alveoli spaces. The patient has a raised temperature and lowered blood pressure, breathlessness and frothy pink sputum. Care in the intensive care unit is required.

Trisomy 21 A condition where there is an extra chromosome 21 present, resulting in three chromosome 21s in each cell. Also referred to as Down's syndrome.

Urgency The need to micturate immediately.

Urinary frequency Increased need to micturate, often voiding small amounts of urine.

Urinary retention The inability of the bladder to empty resulting in an accumulation of urine in the bladder.

Urticaria A skin rash characterized by the recurrent appearance of an eruption of wheals (raised stripes of skin, similar to whiplash marks) which results in severe skin irritation.

Index

Page numbers followed by "*f*" indicate figures, "*b*" indicate boxes, and "*t*" indicate tables.

Index

Index